D0575745

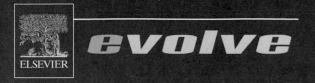

ELSEVIER

evolve

To access your Student Resources, visit the web address below:

http://evolve.elsevier.com/Yoder-Wise/beyond/

- **WebLinks**
  An exciting resource that lets you link to hundreds of web sites carefully chosen to supplement the content of your textbook. The WebLinks are regularly updated with new ones added as they develop.

Beyond Leading
and
Managing

Nursing Administration
for the Future

Beyond Leading
and
Managing
Nursing Administration
for the Future

Patricia S. Yoder-Wise, RN, EdD, CNAA, FAAN
Professor
Texas Tech University Health Sciences Center;
President, The Wise Group
Lubbock, Texas

Karren E. Kowalski, RN, PhD, FAAN
President
Kowalski Associates
Grant Project Director
Colorado Center for Nursing Excellence
Larkspur, Colorado

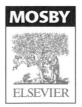

11830 Westline Industrial Drive
St. Louis, Missouri 63146

BEYOND LEADING AND MANAGING: NURSING
ADMINISTRATION FOR THE FUTURE, FIRST EDITION
Copyright © 2006, by Mosby, Inc., an affiliate of Elsevier Inc.

ISBN-13: 978-0-323-02877-6
ISBN-10: 0-323-02877-2

Notices

ISBN-13: 978-0-323-02877-6
ISBN-10: 0-323-02877-2

Senior Editor: Yvonne Alexopoulos
Senior Developmental Editor: Danielle M. Frazier
Publishing Services Manager: John Rogers
Senior Project Manager: Cheryl A. Abbott
Senior Designer: Amy Buxton

Printed in the United States of America

Last digit is the print number: 9 8 7 6 5 4 3 2

This book is dedicated to our husbands, Robert and Walter, and to the families and friends who supported us as we created it; to the faculty who are dedicated to producing the nursing leaders for the ever-changing healthcare services; to the learners who have committed to an exciting career in nursing administration; and to the nurse leaders who face the incredible issues of healthcare every day, who do their best in leading important changes in practice, and who remain committed to the glory of nursing: the care we deliver to patients.

Finally, this book is dedicated to two leaders in nursing who are no longer with us; their mentorship lives on, however, through others.

To Ingeborg Mauksch, a leader in nurse practitioner work and education, and Margretta Madden Styles, a leader in credentialing and the profession.

Lead on ... ¡Adelante!

THE AUTHORS

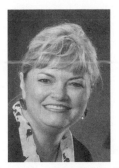

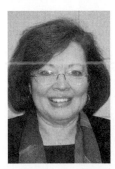

Patricia S. Yoder-Wise, RN, EdD, CNAA, FAAN
Professor
Texas Tech University Health Sciences Center;
President, The Wise Group
Lubbock, Texas

Karren E. Kowalski, RN, PhD, FAAN
President
Kowalski Associates
Grant Project Director
Colorado Center for Nursing Excellence
Larkspur, Colorado

CONTRIBUTORS

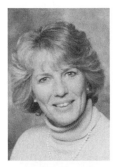

Kathy M. Burke, PhD, RN
Assistant Professor and Assistant Dean of Nursing
School of Nursing Ramapo College
University of Medicine and Dentistry of New Jersey
Mahwah, New Jersey
Chapter 3, Journey to Excellence: The Malcolm Baldrige National Quality Award

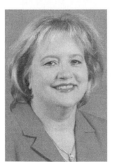

Jacqueline L. Gonzalez, ARNP, MSN, CNAA, BC
Senior Vice President/Chief Nursing Officer
Miami Children's Hospital
Miami, Florida
Chapter 15, Creating a Culture for Promoting Nursing Research and Clinical Scholarship

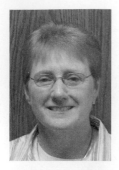

Ginny Wacker Guido, JD, MSN, RN, FAAN
Associate Dean and Director of Graduate Studies
College of Nursing
University of North Dakota
Grand Forks, North Dakota
Chapter 5, *Fostering Legal and Ethical Practices*

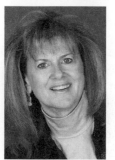

Carol Haun, RN, BS, MA
Director of Human Resources
HCA HealthOne Sky Ridge Medical Center
Lone Tree, Colorado
Chapter 16, *Working with Human Resources to Develop a Strategic Partnership*

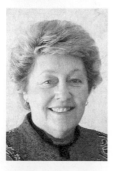

Sharon Hellwig, EdD, RN, CPHQ
Associate Professor of Nursing
Nursing Department
College of Saint Elizabeth
Morristown, New Jersey
Chapter 3, *Journey to Excellence: The Malcolm Baldrige National Quality Award*

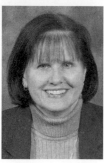

Karen Kelly, EdD, RN, CNAA, BC
Associate Professor and Coordinator of Continuing Education
School of Nursing and Department of Primary Care and Nursing Systems
Southern Illinois University at Edwardsville
Edwardsville, Illinois
Chapter 14, *Financial Leadership and the Chief Nursing Officer*

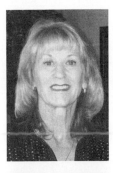

Eleanor T. Lawrence, DBA, MS, BS
President, Human Dynamics
Human Resources and Organizational Behavior Consulting Firm
Colorado Springs, CO
Chapter 16, *Working with Human Resources to Develop a Strategic Partnership*

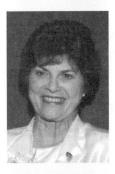

Mary Beth Mancini, RN, PhD, CAN, FAAN
Professor and Associate Dean for Undergraduate Nursing Programs
School of Nursing
University of Texas at Arlington
Chapter 19, *Working with Regulatory and Accrediting Bodies*

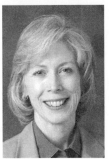

Patricia Messmer, PhD, RN, BC, FAAN
Nurse Researcher
Nursing Department
Miami Children's Hospital
Miami, Florida
Chapter 15, *Creating a Culture for Promoting Nursing Research and Clinical Scholarship*

Sharon Pappas, RN, MSN, CNAA
Chief Nursing Officer and Chief Operating Officer
Administration Department
Porter Adventist Hospital
Denver, Colorado
Chapter 20, *The Chief Nursing Officer as the Chief Operating Officer*

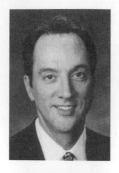

Roy Simpson, RN, C, CMAC, FNAP, FAAN
Vice President Nursing Informatics
Cerner Corporation
Kansas City, Missouri
Chapter 12, Advancing with Technology

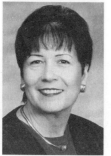

Linda Urden, RN, DNSc, CNA, FAAN
Executive Director of Nursing Quality, Education & Research
Palomar Pomerado Health
Poway, California
Chapter 2, Transforming Professional Practice Environments: The Magnet Recognition Program

THE STORY TELLERS

Virginia Trotter Betts, RN, MSN, JD, FAAN
Commissioner of the Department of Mental Health and Developmental Disabilities
State of Tennessee;
Former President, American Nurses Association
Nashville, Tennessee

Marilyn Bowcutt , RN, MSN
Vice President of Patient Care Services
University Health Care System
Augusta, Georgia

Joyce C. Clifford, RN, PhD, FAAN
President and CEO
The Institute for Nursing Healthcare Leadership

Rheba de Tornyay, RN, EdD, FAAN
Former Dean and Professor Emeritus
University of Washington
Seattle, Washington

Mary Ellen Doyle, RN, BSN, MBA
Chief Nursing Officer
Saint Luke's Hospital of Kansas City
Kansas City, Missouri

Sheila Everly, RN, MS, CNAA, BC, FACHE
Vice President and Chief Nurse Executive
Medical City Dallas Hospital
Dallas, Texas

Georgia Fojtasek, RN, EdD
President and CEO
Foote Health System
Jackson, Michigan

Lillee S. Gelinas, RN, MSN, FAAN
Vice President and Chief Nursing Officer
VHA Inc.
Irving, Texas

Jacqueline L. Gonzalez, ARNP, MSN, CNAA, BC
Senior Vice President/Chief Nursing Officer
Miami Children's Hospital
Miami, Florida

Joyce Johnson, RN, DNSc, FAAN
Senior Vice President Operations and
    Chief Nursing Officer
Georgetown University Hospital
Washington, DC

Maxine Johnson, RN, MBA, CNAA, BC
Administrator, Outpatient Services,
Edwardsville Health Center, Gateway Regional
    Health Services;
Former Chief Nursing Officer for Gateway
Regional Medical Center
Granite City, Illinois

Karlene Kerfoot, RN, PhD, CNAA, FAAN
Senior Vice President, Nursing and Patient
    Care and Chief Nursing Officer
Clarian Health Partners
Indianapolis, Indiana

Phyllis Beck Kritek, RN, PhD, FAAN
courage
Conflict transformation consultation, training,
    coaching, and mediation services
Creating common cause
Richmond, Virginia

Jane Llewelyn, RN, DNSc
VP Nursing Services
Rush Presbyterian St. Lukes Medical Center
Rush University
Chicago, Illinois

Angela Baron McBride, RN, PhD, FAAN
Distinguished Professor and University
    Dean Emerita
Indiana University School of Nursing
Indianapolis, Indiana

**Margaret (Maggie) McClure, RN,
    EdD, FAAN**
Professor, New York University;
Former CNO and Hospital Administrator
New York University Medical Center;
AONE Lifetime Achievement Award Recipient
New York City, New York

Margretta Madden Styles,[†] RN, EdD, FAAN
2005 Christiane Reimann Award Recipient
Past President, International Council of Nurses
Past President, American Nurses Association
Past President, American Nurses Credentialing
    Center
Former Dean, University of Texas Health
    Science Center—San Antonio, Wayne State
    University, University of California at
    San Francisco

Thomas Smith, RN, MS, CNAA
Senior Vice President, Nursing and Patient
    Care Services
The Mount Sinai Hospital
New York City, New York

Lois Sonstegard, RN, MBA, PhD
President
Friends of CHT, Pakistan (a 501 [c] [3]
    organization)
Minneapolis, Minnesota

Pamela Austin Thompson, RN, MS, FAAN
CEO, American Organization of Nurse
    Executives
Washington, DC

Pamela Triolo, RN, PhD, FAAN
Clinical Professor of Nursing
Director, Nursing Leadership and
    Administration in Health Systems
University of Texas Health Science Center at
    Houston, School of Nursing
Houston, Texas

Gail Wolf, RN, DNS, FAAN
Chief Nursing Officer
University of Pittsburgh Health System
Pittsburgh, Pennsylvania

[†]Deceased

REVIEWERS

Martha C. Baker, RN, PhD, CCRN, APRN-BC
Director of BSN Program
Associate Professor of Nursing
St. John's College of Nursing of Southwest Baptist University
Springfield, Missouri

Janice Boundy, RN, PhD
Professor and Associate Dean of Graduate Program
Saint Francis College of Nursing
Peoria, Illinois

Maryanne Garon, RN, DNSc
Assistant Professor
Department of Nursing
California State University Fullerton
Fullerton, California

Patricia E. Kizilay, ARNP-BC, EdD, CS
Associate Professor and Program Director for Adult Nurse Practitioners
Graduate Division
Seton Hall University
South Orange, New Jersey

Carol S. Kleinman, RN, PhD, CNAA
Associate Professor and Director of Health Systems Administration Graduate Programs
College of Nursing
Seton Hall University
South Orange, New Jersey

Kathleen M. Lamaute, BC, APRN, EdD, FNP, CNAA
Assistant Professor and Coordinator FNP Program
Department of Graduate Nursing
Molloy College
Rockville Centre, New York

Ann Marie P. Mauro, RN, PhD
Assistant Professor
College of Nursing
Seton Hall University
South Orange, New Jersey

Joyce Wright, DNSc, RN, CCRN
Director of Accelerated Nursing Program
Georgain Court College off-campus site
College of Nursing
Seton Hall University
South Orange, New Jersey

PREFACE TO INSTRUCTOR

This book is designed to assist future nurse leaders in determining what nursing administrative and leadership positions entail. It takes more, much more, than the basic skills of leading and managing to lead and manage a large group of people who are committed to working toward a mutual goal. Sometimes even getting to the understanding of the mutual goal is itself the challenge. Based on the foundations that appear in the undergraduate text, *Leading and Managing in Nursing*, this book takes selected content that is specifically different for those at the clinical director and higher level positions and provides insight into how nurses at these levels of positions are focused on making key changes in the healthcare system.

Each chapter begins with a well-known quote pertinent to the chapter topic. This strategy is designed to help students think in different ways about the content. After a brief overview, each chapter begins with an introduction and includes key content on the subject. As appropriate, chapters include tables and diagrams to augment the chapter content. Because graduate students should exhibit a level of sophistication in their learning, objectives appear at the end of the chapter as a guide. Each chapter also includes contemplations, the questions and thoughts that create additional thinking about the topic.

In addition to content that is particularly pertinent to leaders at the clinical director and higher levels, we have selected some of nursing's key leaders to provide practical insight into how to apply the content or the relevance of the content in the reality of healthcare today. Their stories in each of the chapters provide practical examples of how the content is applied in healthcare organizations.

Appendix A provides a ready reference about theories and concepts that have been prominent in shaping today's thinking about nursing administration. Content in this appendix is not necessarily included in any of the chapters. Rather it is designed as a ready reference. Appendix B includes additional reading resources for the key topics covered in the text.

Today's key leaders in nursing have access to books, people, and other learning resources about many subjects. Some of these subjects can best be learned from the perspective of specific leadership positions. However, that doesn't mean that new leaders should enter positions without any preparation. So many variances exist in healthcare that are specific to a particular workplace. Hence, it is challenging to transfer learning from one place to another in a directly meaningful way. Additionally, the business and healthcare administration literature is rich with information useful to nurse administrators. Students should be encouraged to secure and use books and articles in areas where they need to focus their personal growth.

Opportunities to engage in the latest thinking about nursing administration and leadership are rich. The challenge is selecting the right learning experiences to augment those gained in a formal academic setting. Students should be encouraged to select continuing education opportunities that help develop them in the breadth and depth of an administrative or leadership position.

Special note: The terms *client* and *patient* are used interchangeably in the text to encompass those we provide care for. *Nurse leader* and *nurse administrator* may also be used interchangeably. *Nurse manager* refers to those leaders with unit level accountability.

ACKNOWLEDGMENTS

As with any publication endeavor, many people other than those whose names appear on the cover, the list of contributors, and the list of interviewees make the actual publication possible. We thank each of the contributors who worked diligently to meet deadlines and content expectations. Without them, this book would be a lot thinner! The nurse leaders who agreed to be interviewed told fabulous stories related to the various chapters. Without them, this book would be much less interesting! What a fabulous group to work with!

We are indebted to our reviewers who provided valuable feedback that helped refine the book. Receiving peer review is critical to any successful publication.

Special thanks go to our editorial team: Yvonne Alexopoulos and Danielle Frazier. They were gently nudging so that this book became a reality. Even more special thanks go to our husbands and best friends, Robert Wise and Walter Kowalski. Bob served as the perfect host while Karren and Pat worked diligently in intense sessions in Lubbock. Walt was very tolerant of Karren's travel to Texas and shared resources and ideas.

Final thanks go to the graduate students with whom Karren and Pat worked over many years and to nurse leaders who expressed ideas about what nurse administrators and leaders need to be successful.

As with the undergraduate text, *Leading and Managing in Nursing,* which serves as the foundation, this book is designed to stimulate thinking and to encourage continued professional development. This book represents current thinking on current complexities of administration. Both the thinking and the complexities will continue to change… and so, hopefully, will you! The passion of nursing and leadership await!

Patricia S. Yoder-Wise
Karren E. Kowalski

CONTENTS

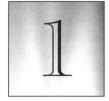

Leading for the Future

A leader is not an administrator who loves to run others, but someone who carries water for his people so they can get on with their jobs. ROBERT TOWNSEND

This chapter provides an overview of nursing administration, the influence of professional expectations, and the differences between leading and managing and reasons both are important. The positions and the expected competencies, education, credentials, and experience of nursing administrators and the administrator's role in patient safety are prescribed.

EVERY GENERATION OF NURSE ADMINISTRATORS believes their challenges are greater than the ones of the previous generation. Whether referring to staffing, financing, accountability, or development of the organization, each generation is right. As the intensity of these elements has increased, so have the challenges and opportunities, whether technological, regulatory, or professional. Therefore the role of the nurse administrator has evolved into a dramatic new influence in quality care. Because of nursing's prominence in patient safety, quality standards, and excellence, this administrative role will be even more influential in the future.

Despite the size or type of the organization, the chief nursing officer (CNO) is accountable for ensuring the quality of comprehensive services performed in the name of nursing. The CNO is frequently the "face" and "voice" of nursing. Through the CNO, many community members interact with the organization and gain perspective about the kind of care to expect. This perspective must be reflected at the point of service; otherwise the discrepancy between expectations and reality threatens the organization's credibility. The CNO's means of interaction with staff members to ensure quality, timeliness, and positiveness is critical. The clinical and service directors (e.g., nurse managers, clinical leaders, or directors) within the nursing service organization and the CNO interact cooperatively to enhance each leader's influence. In addition, this group of leaders must have synergistic interactions with staff nurses to exchange their influence for quality patient care. This synergism creates enthusiasm and opportunities.

LEADING THE OPPORTUNITIES THAT EXIST FOR NURSING

In a March 1, 2004, *Wall Street Journal* advertisement (p. A18), the Morgan Stanley Investment Corporation advertised for CEOs. The position required applicants to be stellar risk managers with strong personnel skills; understand new technologies; have the abilities to separate fantasy and hope from reality; and most importantly, have integrity. The advertisement concluded with this statement: "Who runs the show matters." That can be said for nursing, too!

All the job requirements detailed in the advertisement for CEOs are applicable directly to CNOs. Although an organization may have many leaders, the CNO must be a positional leader; that is, by position alone the CNO is designated a leader. Sadly, "clinicians do not value management" (Bolton, 2004, p. 33). A lack of trust and respect for each other has created a "we/they" phenomenon and has the potential to undermine the effectiveness of the nursing organization. The devaluing of management creates problems in the clinical arena and the profession. The negative view of leadership is a deterrent to recruiting capable nurses into leadership positions, interferes with effective succession planning, isolates leaders from those they are trying to lead, perpetuates a culture of blame and conflict, spurs leader burnout, creates unsafe environments for staff and patients, and prevents individuals and organizations from achieving their full potential (Bolton, 2004, p. 34).

However, according to Kimball (2004), "Nurse managers can make a significant difference in how nurses perceive and embrace their jobs." Therefore eliminating or minimizing the "we/they" struggle is critical to the success of staff nurses, managers, CNOs, and ultimately the patient.

CNOs must be able to lead people toward positive patient outcomes and create positive work environments. The leader often is accountable for the challenge of "raising the bar" (Kerfoot, 2001). Helping people achieve expectations they thought impossible is challenging and exciting. Leadership is about the challenge of improving the practice of nursing, the focus on creating the vision for the future, and the expenditure of energy to convert the vision into reality. Leadership requires consistent hard work to achieve success.

Leadership differs from management. The former focuses on facilitating; the latter focuses on controlling. Leadership is future oriented; management is engrossed in the present. Leadership focuses on developing people so that they will break the rules (and therefore make improvements); management focuses on ensuring that others abide by the rules. Both elements are necessary for an effective operation. Achieving change without absolute chaos requires a delicate balance between these two key roles of nurse administrators. When either element becomes the sole focus of a nurse administrator, stagnation or chaos results.

Management is critical to the success of an organization's smooth operation on a daily basis. However, the ongoing attention to leadership and management produces new ways of solving today's problems so that new challenges can be met tomorrow. Being proactive in relation to an issue allows those individuals involved to shape its direction. This kind of leadership creates opportunities for the future. Current issues may undergo minor redirections, or dramatically new insights into emerging issues may arise. Leadership is about creating the influence that relationships and networks provide (Gladwell, 2000).

Maxwell (1999) suggested that three types of competent people exist: those who see what needs to happen (good assessors); those who can bring about change (good implementers); and those who "can make things happen when it really counts" (p. 35) (transformational leaders). Although the current literature tends to focus on the latter, all three elements are critical to effect exceptional leadership.

Leadership has many facets. It is not positional, although people in key positions are expected to lead. Leadership requires seeing the big picture, translating the picture to action, sharing data, and telling the story. This means that CNOs must envision potential and translate that view into practical and essential steps to move the organization forward. Achieving this requires sharing data about current performance and progress made toward the vision. Telling stories about successes and failures is an effective tool to help staff focus on progress. "For most leaders, the great challenge is not understanding the practice of leadership: It is practicing their understanding of leadership" (Goldsmith & Morgan, 2004, p. 6). Furthermore, shared stories of success and progress promote understanding.

> *Managers are people who do things right, while leaders are people who do the right thing.*
> WARREN BENNIS

Influence of Professional Expectations

Several professional expectations exist for the execution of the nurse administrator role. Some derive from basic documents within the profession, such as *Nursing's Social Policy Statement* (ANA, 2003) and the *Code of Ethics for Nurses* (ANA, 2001). Specific expectations derive from the profession in the form of the *Scope and Standards for Nurse Administrators* (ANA, 2004), the AONE *Nurse Executive Competencies* (2005), the Joint Position Statement on Nursing Administration Education (AACN & AONE, 1997), or the Council on Graduate Education for Administration in Nursing (1995). Others derive from a broader healthcare perspective, such as the Core Competencies in Healthcare (Ross, Wenzel, & Mitlyng, 2002) or the competency model from the National Center for Healthcare Leadership (2004). Additionally, rules and regulations from state boards of nursing and health departments, in addition to standards related to accreditation and recognition of healthcare organizations, influence nurse administrators.

Nursing's Social Policy Statement

Nursing's Social Policy Statement (ANA, 2003) defines six qualities essential to professional nursing:

1. Caring relationships that facilitate health and healing
2. Consideration of the range of human experiences and responses
3. Integration of objective data with the knowledge gleaned from the client's subjective experience

4. Use of judgment and critical thinking in diagnosis and treatment
5. Scholarly inquiry that advances professional nursing knowledge
6. "Influence on social and public policy to promote social justice" (p. 5)

Each of these six qualities contributes to professional nursing; however, in some situations it is difficult to see the full impact of professional nursing within the organization. When CNOs create an environment in which nurses can flourish, nursing moves beyond patient care and focuses on the way in which nurses make exquisite decisions based on substantive judgment that advances nursing's scholarship and evidence-based practices. This kind of nurse leadership contributes to social justice and a healthcare organization's efforts to make a difference in a community. This phenomenon can happen regardless of size, locale, or type of organization. As society entrusted a legal relationship with nurses through licensure, nurses committed to fulfill their contract with society by executing the six qualities of nursing for the public good.

Code of Ethics for Nurses

The *Code of Ethics for Nurses* (ANA, 2001) shapes the ethical performance of the nurse executive, just as it shapes that of nurses in direct patient care and those in education. The *Code* identifies such elements as being committed primarily to the patient. This is an important factor in administrative roles. The professional nurse's first obligation is to the patient, not to the institution. Therefore in matters of conflict between what is right for the institution and what is right for the patient, the nurse administrator is guided by the *Code* to support the patient first. Another example can be found when the *Code* calls for nurses to work to improve healthcare environments and conditions of employment. Although all nurses carry this responsibility, the nurse administrator has a greater obligation as head of the service of nursing.

Curtin (2000) defined an additional set of ethical principles distinct to the role of the CNO (Table 1-1). These principles use basic ethical

Table 1-1 ETHICAL ADMINISTRATION

Principle	Example
Frugality and therapeutic elegance	The right amount of economy and resources to ensure competent care
Clinical credibility through organizational competence	Applying practice guidelines, peer evaluations, consistent policies
Presence	Mutual trusting and collaboration
Responsible representation	Carrying the message forward for decision making
Loyal service	Focuses on organization not personal career
Deliberate delegation	Delegation of sufficient authority
Responsible innovation	Examination of the impact of potential change on patient care
Fiduciary accountability	Value for the dollar (safety, quality, relevance)
Self-discipline	Careful deliberation creates the decision
Continuous learning	Investment of time and resources to promote competence and excellence

From Curtin, L. L. (2000). The first ten principles for the ethical administration of nursing services. *Nursing Administration Quarterly*, *25*(1), 7-13.

standards and combine the accountability of an ethical nurse with that of an ethical administrator. For example, the principle of frugality and therapeutic elegance suggests that CNOs would seek high-quality staffing levels and equipment and simultaneously not create expectations for rarely used staffing levels or equipment because either might be needed. Responsible representation is critical for a CNO to perform in an ethical manner. The CNO presents the "voice" of nursing at high-level administrative meetings and in governance situations. Carrying the message accurately and confidently is important to ensure trust between staff and the CNO.

Scope and Standards for Nurse Administrators

The *Scope and Standards for Nurse Administrators* (ANA, 2004) also explicate the role of the CNO. These are the translation of leadership actions within the nursing organization and convey the accountability of the CNO within an organization.

Box 1-1 illustrates examples of the 14 standards applicable to nurse administrators.

Nurse administrators are accountable for operating on data, creating systems that produce data, and devising approaches about the provision of nursing care within a given service. To achieve these standards, nurse administrators must be able to do more than just manage effectively. They must be able to lead a group of healthcare workers, composed primarily of nurses, toward the best possible outcomes for patients and for the healthcare team.

Nurse Executive Competencies

The American Organization of Nurse Executives (AONE) created a set of competencies that it believes are integral to executive leadership. This set is built on the model from the Health Care Leadership Alliance, which includes AONE, physician executives, healthcare financial managers and information and management systems, medical group managers, and the American College of Healthcare Executives. Five major competency areas are defined: communication and relationship building, healthcare environment, professionalism, business skills, and leadership.

Box 1-1   Examples of the Standards for Nurse Administrators

STANDARDS OF PRACTICE

Standard 3. Identification of Outcomes

The nurse administrator develops, maintains, and evaluates information systems and processes that promote desired, patient/client/resident-defined, professional and organizational outcomes.

Standard 5. Implementation

The nurse administrator develops, maintains, and evaluates organizational systems that support implementation of plans and delivery of care across the continuum.

STANDARDS OF PROFESSIONAL PERFORMANCE

Standard 9. Professional Knowledge

The nurse administrator maintains and demonstrates current knowledge in the administration of healthcare organizations to advance nursing practice and the provision of quality healthcare services.

Standard 10. Professional Environment

The nurse administrator is accountable for providing a professional environment.

Standard 12. Collaboration

The nurse administrator collaborates with nursing staff at all levels, interdisciplinary teams, executive leaders, and other stakeholders.

Standard 13. Research

The nurse administrator supports research and its integration into nursing and the delivery of healthcare services.

From American Nurses Association. (2001). *Code of ethics for nurses with interpretive statement.* Washington, DC: Nursebooks. Reprinted with permission from American Nurses Association. (2004). *Scope and standards for nursing administrators.* Silver Spring, MD: nursebooks.org.

Table 1-2 provides examples of the elements within each of the five major competency areas. This model is designed to include all administrative positions with the expectation that the competencies would vary by position needs.*

Each of the five areas is important, but the interaction of the areas and the synergy of each

influencing all others create quality performance of the role.

AACN/AONE Joint Position Statement

This statement provides for the educational context of nurse administrators. A core of curriculum expectations is augmented with courses from business, psychology, economics, sociology, and/or health services administration. Specific content expectations include such aspects as strategic planning, leadership, policy development, information systems, marketing, and negotiation strategies. Additionally, the future direction of

*This document is also available at the *Nurse Leader* web site, http://www.nurseleader.com, so all nursing leaders could study this set of competencies and consider how they apply in various situations.

Table 1-2 AONE Nurse Competencies: Examples of the Five Competency Areas

Competency Area	Examples of Specific Competencies
Communications and relationship building	Effective communication
	Relationship management
	Shared decision making
	Medical staff relationships
Healthcare environment	Healthcare economics knowledge
	Understanding of governance
	Knowledge and dedication to patient safety
	Outcome measurement
Professionalism	Career planning
	Ethics
	Active membership in professional organizations
Business skills	Understanding of healthcare financing
	Marketing
	Information management and technology
Leadership	Personal journey disciplines
	Ability to use systems thinking
	Succession planning

From American Organization of Nurse Executives. (2005). AONE nurse executive competencies. *Nurse Leader, 3*(1), 15-21.

educational programs identified the intent to focus on interdisciplinary work. Although this position statement is fairly old (1997), the core abilities are reflective of the demands on the role today.

Council on Graduate Education for Administration in Nursing's Essentials for Master's Education

Nursing administration is defined as an advanced practice that is "based on a synthesis of research and knowledge in nursing science, business administration and other related disciplines" (CGEAN, 1995, p. 6). Four key areas make up the suggested curriculum basis: nursing science and social science, nursing administration/ management, business administration/public administration/healthcare administration, and methodology. Nursing science and social science cognates include various theories and policy development. Nursing administration/manage- ment includes ethical and legal issues, patient and staff education, nursing care delivery system,

and system career paths and development. Business administration/public administration/ healthcare administration includes strategic planning, public policy, environmental health, and mentoring. Finally, methodology includes research, standards, and consultation. Further, the Council on Graduate Education for Adminis- tration in Nursing (CGEAN) acknowledges various issues surrounding production of a competent graduate. These issues range from time constraints to faculty preparation and from textbooks to dual-degree programs.

Core Competencies in Healthcare

Because the CNO is a member of the senior exec- utive team, the standards for non-nurse executives in healthcare organizations also should be con- sidered. Ross et al. (2002) divided competencies into two broad categories: system and personal leadership competencies. System competencies encompass such elements as governance, strategic development, ethics and values, and health policy and law. Personal leadership competencies include decision making, risk taking, team building, and mentoring. Ross et al. suggest that 10 knowledge areas underlie what leaders in healthcare need to know. For example, some of the areas are governance and organizational dynamics, human resources, communications and public relations, and organizational and healthcare policy. Each of these competencies and the requisite knowledge contribute to the more effective functioning of an organization when leaders understand and can execute the competencies. Many of these competencies overlap those within nursing's expectations.

In addition, the National Center for Healthcare Leadership developed a competency model to describe "technical and behavioral characteristics that leaders must possess to be successful in positions of leadership across the health professions—administrative, medical and nursing" (NCHL, 2004, p. 1). This model consists of three interlocking circles, or domains, that make up health leadership. One circle represents people and such skills as self-confidence, team leadership, professionalism, and relationship building. A second circle represents execution and such skills as communication, organizational awareness, performance measurement, and project management. The third circle represents transformation and such aspects as analytical thinking, finance skills, information seeking, and strategic orientation. Of the total 26 competencies, only 7 are technical.

Relevance for the Profession

Regardless of which reference set is used, they all share a focus on several key elements. The core focus is on patients and their safety. The manner in which that happens from a CNO's perspective relates to the organizational environment/culture that supports the best performance of the people in the organization. To achieve the culture, exquisite communication is critical. Part of that communication is about securing necessary resources and maximizing the business skills of the organization. To achieve all of this, the nurse administrator must be highly professional and committed to his or her own leadership development.

The Value of Nurse Leaders

Exceptional leaders put people first; they are the first thought about any strategy (Collins, 2001). "Successful organizations do one thing: they quickly adapt to the necessary changes in the environment to achieve eternal success" (Kerfoot, 2001, p. 301). These ideas suggest that the real value of leaders is how people are treated so that they can respond to the ongoing changes in the environment. Committing to people and their development so that the whole is improved, leaders redirect their focus from the traditional tasks of management such as controlling and supervising to the futuristic tasks of communicating, coaching, and developing.

NURSE ADMINISTRATORS AND NURSE MANAGERS

The persons who head nursing organizations are known by different names. They may be called CNO, chief nurse executive, nurse administrator, director of nursing, chief nurse, department head, vice president (for nursing or patient care services), or executive vice president. Sometimes the title for the official nurse leader is linked with another title, such as chief operations officer, vice president for patient services, or director of clinical operations. Regardless of the title, nurses who head nursing organizations have responsibility for the largest number of employees in the typical healthcare organization and also the largest financial and other resources. Therefore the success of healthcare in an organization depends on many factors, one of which is the nurse administrator's method for leading the nursing service. How that nurse leader supports the work environment, the professional autonomy, and the resources for the nurses providing direct care to the public determines the effectiveness of nurses.

Effective nurse leaders are bicultural. They have to be able to relate as well to nursing and its culture of patient care as to business and its culture of fiscal accountability. They have to be able to relate as well to the daily work and its culture of accountability as to the future and its culture of possibilities. Marrying those elements creates new opportunities and multiple challenges that CNOs face regularly. These elements are inherent in the *Scope and Standards for Nurse Administrators* (ANA, 2004) and the AONE Nurse Executive Competencies (2005). The positions of CGEAN (1995) and AACN/AONE (1997) also support these elements.

Scope and Level of Practice

According to the American Nurses Association (2004), the scope of practice for nurses in administration can be seen in one of two key aspects: executive or manager. Table 1-3 outlines key differences between executives and managers. The nurse executive is defined as the person with the ultimate accountability for the services known as nursing. These services in a nursing setting include practice, education and professional development, research, administration, and services (ANA, 2004). The nurse manager, on the other hand, is someone who manages defined areas of nursing services, such as population or disease-based services. Managers report to the executive level and have the designated authority and accountability for the management of those elements that occur within the defined areas of service. Nurse managers tend to be much more clinically focused and are the direct bridge between administration and other departments with the nursing staff. Therefore nurse managers must hold comparable values and goals with the nurse executive if the nursing organization is to progress.

Obviously, not every nurse wishes to be an administrator or manager and not every nurse is considered prepared to assume such roles. Historically, the best clinical nurse was promoted to the role of nurse manager (typically known as head nurse) because he or she had excelled in clinical nursing. Now, however, many organizations make appointments to administrator or manager based on a combination of clinical, leadership, and managerial abilities.

EXPECTATIONS FOR PREPARATION AND QUALIFICATIONS OF ADMINISTRATORS AND MANAGERS

Three factors seem to be among the requisites for the position of administrator: education, credentials, and experience. Each is important; together they form expectations for quality leadership.

Education

In the 2000 National Sample Survey of Registered Nurses (BHP, 2002), only 10% of registered nurses held a master's or doctoral degree. Although this percentage remains small, it has doubled since the 1980 National Sample Survey. Approximately 14.1% of the nursing population represents administrative roles (head nurse, supervisor, or administrator). According to the survey, only 26.5% of administrators held a master's or doctoral degree; supervisors 6.6%; and head nurses 10.8%. The greatest educational preparation for the various administrative positions was administrators, 30.7% with an associate degree; supervisors, 38.3% with an associate degree; and head nurses, 37% with a bachelor's degree. On the other hand, an American Nurses Credentialing Center (ANCC) presentation at the 2003 Magnet conference indicated that 100% of the CNOs in Magnet facilities held a graduate degree, although not necessarily in nursing (Allison & Monarch, 2003).

These data are important. In the 1995 ANA *Scope and Standards for Nurse Administrators*, the desired educational level for nurse executives was a baccalaureate degree in nursing and a graduate degree in nursing, *or a related field*; and for

Table 1-3 COMPARISON OF EXECUTIVE AND MANAGER LEVELS OF ADMINISTRATION*

Level	Definition	Focus	Educational Expectation	Certification	Certification Examination Focus (% of Questions in Each Area in 2004)
Executive	The person with the ultimate accountability for the services known as nursing	Practice, education and professional development, research, administration and services[†]	Goal: Baccalaureate and master's degrees in nursing; doctorate recommended Reality: 26.5% hold master's or doctorate; 30.7% hold associate degree[‡]	CNAA: Certified in Nursing Administration, Advanced	Organization and structure (27.3%); Economics (24.7%); Human resources (16.6%); Ethics (12.0%); Legal and regulatory (19.3%)
Manager	Someone who manages defined areas of nursing services, reports to the executive level and has designated authority and accountability for the management of those elements in a defined area of service	More clinically focused; direct bridge of administration and nursing	Goal: Baccalaureate in nursing; master's in nursing recommended Reality: Supervisors: 6.6% hold graduate degree; 38.3% hold associate degree Head nurses: 10.8% hold graduate degree; 37% hold baccalaureate[‡]	CNA: Certified in Nursing Administration	Organization and structure (19.3%) Economics (20.7%) Human resources (24.0%) Ethics (15.3%) Legal and regulatory (20.7%)

*ANCC, 2004.
[†] ANA, 2004.
[‡] BHP, 2002.

nurse managers, a baccalaureate degree in nursing, *or a related field* (ANA, 1995). The new standards, however, articulate the need for a baccalaureate and master's degree in nursing with a doctorate recommended (nurse executive) and a baccalaureate degree in nursing with a master's degree in nursing recommended (nurse manager) (ANA, 2004). CGEAN (1995) and AACN/ AONE (1997) support the placement of nursing administration preparation at the graduate level.

Although these tend to reflect the expectation of society for more education than previously held, nursing clearly has a huge gap to fill if nurse administrators are to be prepared at the recommended levels. Furthermore, if Aiken, Clarke, Cheung, Sloane, and Silber's research (2003) is carried beyond the study of surgical patients, the presence of nurses educated with a minimum of a baccalaureate degree in nursing can have positive outcomes related to mortality and failure-to-rescue rates. If this is true for direct interactions with patients, nurse administrators must hold at least a baccalaureate degree. Furthermore, the Magnet Commission of the ANCC in March 2004 established the following standard: The CNO must possess a baccalaureate degree and a master's degree. Either the baccalaureate or master's degree must be in nursing.

Many graduate programs preparing administrators offer dual degrees in either public administration or business administration. Additionally, many of the programs no longer carry the title nursing administration. Frequently, the programs use titles such as healthcare management or administration or health systems administration because of the need to administer services beyond nursing. Matisoff-Li (2004) suggested that the advancement of nursing's position is a result of nurses obtaining advanced business degrees. Yet, this degree may not meet future needs.

Credentials

In addition to education, which produces an academic credential, two other major credentials are associated with nurse leaders. One is licensure, a requirement for all positions in nursing, and the other is certification. Achieving certification (CNAA is recommended for executives and CNA is recommended for managers) is an option. Because the certification examinations use the scope and standards for a given practice area, the assumption is that an individual who passes the certification examination at either the executive or manager level is able to reflect the standards in actual practice.

Licensure

Nurses who serve in an administrative role must be licensed in their respective states to practice professional nursing. All nurses are held to the same standards of legal practice within a specific state, with some variations related to role or specialty preparation. Many laws, such as those governing hospitals, cite the expectation for ensuring licensure of the staff.

Certification

The Scope and Standards for Nurse Administrators (ANA, 2004) forms the basis for certification in nursing administration. *Standards for Nurse Administrators* are divided into two sets of standards: practice and professional practice. The first set, practice, follows the nursing process. Therefore assessment, problems/diagnosis, identification of outcomes, planning, implementation, and evaluation are elements applied to the way in which nurse administrators influence the system to enhance patient care. The second set, professional performance, focuses on elements associated with administrative practices. These elements are quality of care and administrative practice, performance appraisal, professional knowledge, professional environment, ethics, collaboration, research, and resource utilization.

According to the ANCC website, the 2005 nursing administration, advanced examination (designed for CNOs) and the nursing administration certification examination (basic for the management level of administration) use five areas of questions: organization and structure, economics, human resources, ethics, and legal and regulatory. Differing emphases are evident in the two examinations and can be explained by understanding the level of the organizational interaction that prevails for most individuals in the two types of positions. These types of tests are developed based on role delineation studies to reflect the predominant practices. Their focus on the major elements of the nurse administrator role reflects the reality of the work that most in those roles perform on a regular basis.*

An additional certification that some CNOs pursue is in a broader context. The healthcare credential relates to a certified healthcare executive. The competencies described by Ross et al. (2002) form the basis of the content related to this examination. As stated earlier, these competencies focus on two broad categories: system and personal leadership.†

Experience

As is true in almost every other kind of position in nursing, no standard or specific expectation exists for a CNO regarding prior experience. However, in general, an individual should have had increasingly accountable positions in terms of management and leadership to attain the background for dealing with many of the issues facing the executive. For example, one career trajectory consists of moving from a position of charge nurse, to nurse manager, and to clinical director before moving to an executive role. Therefore a given number of years' experience in a specific type of position or a specific type of setting commonly is expected. Clearly, however, the person needs to have all of what Covey (1989) calls the levels of leadership (Figure 1-1). Moving from the inner circle of personal leadership outward,

*Detailed information is available at http://www.nurse credentialing.org.
†More information can be found at http://www.ache.org/policy/Bdcert.cfm.

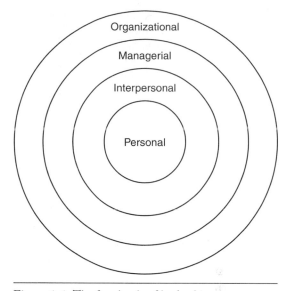

Figure 1-1 The four levels of leadership. Modified from Covey, S. R. (1989). *The 7 habits of highly effective people: Powerful lessons in personal change.* New York: Simon and Schuster.

the nurse leaders are expected to have broad influence. First, these leaders need to be secure individuals and to have positive interpersonal leadership abilities. Second, they must be able to influence nursing management and the entire organization. Each level of leadership, however, enhances the other and produces the overall experience leaders have to lead effectively. As evidenced by numerous Gallup poll results about the most trusted professionals, the power of professional nurses has influence beyond organizations to the community.

NURSE ADMINISTRATORS AND PATIENT SAFETY

Everyone's job in healthcare revolves around patient safety. However, nurses frequently are the final source of protection from having an untoward event occur. As the head of the nursing organization, the CNO therefore has a major influence on how safety issues are addressed and how patients and their families are protected from harm.

Nurse leadership is a valued commodity. The evolution of the role of the CNO to an executive one is reflective of such recognition. The Institute of Medicine (IOM), as an example, focused one of its major reports in 2004 on nursing and the leadership that nurse professionals can bring to the issue of patient safety.

The IOM calls for five specific actions:

1. Balance the tension between production efficiency and reliability (safety)
2. Create and sustain trust throughout the organization
3. Actively manage the process of change
4. Involve workers in decision making pertaining to work design and work flow
5. Use knowledge management practice to establish the organization as a "learning organization" (IOM, 2004, p. 8)

Although the IOM focused this work on patient safety, the key focus is found in the subtitle of this report, Transforming the Work Environment of Nurses. Dr. Lucian Leape gives one example about transforming the environment: "I can talk to any three nurses in a unit for an hour about what bothers them, and come out with a safety agenda that will keep me busy for a year." (HealthGrades Quality Study, 2004, p. 8). That same strategy holds true for the CNO. Listening to the messages from the bedside and acting on them can transform the work environment in many more ways than patient safety, although patient safety is the core of healthcare.

BALANCING THE TASKS OF LEADING AND MANAGING

Leadership is about making things better for the future. It has to do with creating visions and then finding ways to bring those visions to reality. Management, however, is about the daily, short-term changes and the problems of reality. If all of the usual daily work is not accomplished, the future may not be as planned. Therefore the key is to balance the elements of leadership and management so that the work is accomplished to ensure that the organization's goals are met. As Bossidy and Charan (2002) suggest, the work must be completed to implement the next dream.

Even in terms of interaction, both concepts, leading and managing, have to be used to promote a successful environment. Although most administrators would love to work with inspiring others and helping to develop knowledge, skills, and abilities, sometimes compassionate confrontation is necessary to hold someone accountable for basic performances. Even at the administrative level, management skill sets are critical to an administrator's success. Thinking and, even worse, acting as if only leadership skills are important is erroneous.

LEADING TO THE FUTURE

The Arista 3 report (Sigma Theta Tau, 2004) defined the top three areas in which nurses could make the strongest contributions for healthy communities: (1) the delivery of evidence-based care, (2) policy development, and (3) professional advocacy. Although numerous roles in nursing have these three elements as part of the role expectations, they clearly are expectations for those in nursing administrative roles. These aspects of leadership must be inherent in the nurse administrator role for nursing to survive and thrive.

As healthcare has moved from less formal approaches in care to an evidence-based approach, numerous practices have changed. However, the *2000 Yearbook of Medical Informatics* indicated that it takes 17 years for a new approach to move from clinical trial to practice. With that kind of time frame, the lag of translating knowledge into practice must be reduced. The opportunity to make a dramatic impact on healthcare could reside in nursing's ability to decrease that lag time so that patient care is improved in a more timely manner.

Although much of the policy work that CNOs engage in is internally focused, addressing external policies is equally important, especially in terms of healthcare and employee public policy issues. The action of the U.S. Congress in 2004 to limit overtime payment for a wide group of U.S. workers, including nurses, is an example of the need for CNOs to be engaged in policy development. Often the CNO is the nurse selected to represent the "voice of nursing" on a relevant policy issue. Therefore that individual must be acutely aware of the numerous issues affecting nurses and their patients.

Leaders provide for their people what the people cannot provide for themselves.
JOHN C. MAXWELL

This focus on policy also translates into professional advocacy. In addition, a supportive and informed CNO allows numerous opportunities for nurses to be supported in their roles and viewpoints. Professional advocacy promotes nurses being "at the table" and having well-represented positions related to the issue under consideration. It also ensures that in the efforts toward an interdisciplinary approach to healthcare that nurses are included and assured of input into decisions.

The Healthcare Context for Nursing Administration

Healthcare is at a place that Gladwell (2000) would call the tipping point, the point at which numerous factors come together to effect change. Gladwell defined three characteristics of a tipping point: (1) several little things in an environment that can make a big difference, (2) contagiousness, and (3) potential for sudden change. Many events and elements in any healthcare organization can make a difference. The impetus for change, as one example, can be seen as contagious (i.e., once one person is committed to an idea for action, others join in); and when sufficient movement occurs, change can seem to happen in one dramatic moment. Although all nurses in an organization have accountability to move nursing care to a new level, the CNO has the organizational accountability to ensure this movement occurs.

Everything in life relates to a context. In nursing administration, that context relates to healthcare. The current system, or as many would observe, nonsystem, is based heavily on illness care. Even in situations in which preventive services exist, the majority of the nation's expenses are focused on illness care. However, as individuals assume more accountability for direct costs and decisions, as healthcare costs continue to escalate, and as awareness of the impending costs of current lifestyle behaviors grows, a shift is occurring for services needed. The range of organizational constructs includes major systems that include preventive, wellness, long-term, residential, acute, chronic, home, and telephonic services in addition to free-standing services in each of those areas of expertise. These changes suggest that the CNO is prepared to move resources and to develop new approaches to remain ready for the changes in what the public expects of healthcare.

Impact of the Complexity of Today's Healthcare System Issues

Today's healthcare is complex in service and in operation. With an increasing emphasis on basic patient safety, healthcare organizations are under greater scrutiny. The list of "never events" (those events that should never occur) is expanding, and sentinel events (those events that result from inadequate system activities and that result in a major patient problem) are required to be reported. The Centers for Medicare and Medicaid Services has increasing expectations for quality measures being met; the public also expects no less. The culmination of continuing increased costs, losses of health benefits (or increased costs to the worker), the pressure for movement to quality, and the public's expectations of access has resulted in a challenging situation for nurse administrators.

In addition to managing these issues at the macro level, and sometimes at the micro level, today's administrator in nursing is faced with numerous challenges within the discipline in addition to the focus on administrative practice improvement tasks. The new skills sets that administrators need include those that are designed for success in the emerging world of work. According to Porter-O'Grady (2003), one of the key skills involves accelerating disruptive change. He identifies six elements to achieve this acceleration:

1. Sufficient dissonance to make workers sufficiently uncomfortable—thus it is untenable to maintain the status quo
2. Clear definition of activities to be sacrificed to make way for new critical functions
3. Continual assessment of patient expectations
4. Reconfiguration of work based on education and preparation of other providers and patients
5. Focus on the potential for the future, not the loss of the known work
6. Movement from patterns of dependence on past practice as the filter for new endeavors

Some could argue that healthcare workers are sufficiently uncomfortable and have, in fact, led the movement for dissatisfaction with the status quo. An ongoing conflict, for example, occurs between decisions concerning what to give up and what to carry forward as new tasks and skills are assumed. Perhaps one of the greatest

challenges in nursing relates to the reconfiguration of work based on education. When Aiken et al. (2003) suggested that surgical patient outcomes related to educational level, various groups quickly responded to support or refute this study. Similarly, considerable discussion, some not evident publicly, surrounds the American Association of Colleges of Nursing's proposal for the clinical nurse leader, a role designed to change clinical practice (AACN, 2004). Clearly, multiple changes are occurring that affect nursing administrative philosophy and goals; such changes will continue.

SUMMARY

To lead and manage effectively, the CNO has to connect to numerous groups of people and various standards and strategies for the future. Adequate educational preparation, prominent position in the organization, and ability to balance leadership skills and management skills allow the CNO to advance the organization and lead it to a successful future.

KEY POINTS TO LEAD

1. Analyze essential qualities and abilities of CNOs.
2. Analyze the balance of and differences between leading and managing.
3. Evaluate how CNO interaction with staff nurses advances the organization's goals.

Literature Box

The story of Bill Bratton, former New York City police commissioner, is an example that conveys the concept of the tipping point. Bratton's story is the basis for this article because of his successful leadership in turning around organizations.

One of the skills emphasized in helping an organization move toward and beyond the tipping point is to focus on solutions as opposed to focusing on the problem. Often administrators become consumed with the nuances of the problem and potential scapegoats rather than thinking creatively about solutions. However, the latter demonstrates the full strengths of leadership.

The use of a four-step process is what can effect change within the context of limited resources.

Literature Box

The four steps are viewed as hurdles to overcome: cognitive, resource, motivational, and political. Cognitive and resource hurdles are those that organizations face in strategy development. Motivational and political hurdles are those that, if met, ensure a rapid execution. So, when all four processes are "tipped" (think of the "breaking point"), change occurs quickly.

The use of communication within the department and with the external community is highlighted to illustrate how perceptions often are misaligned. For example, what a member of the community considers important may not coincide with the view of the provider of services. The use of budget is equally important. When a budget is limited, some administrators determine that a problem cannot be addressed at this time. However, Bratton did what experts would advocate: concentrate resources where the greatest change is needed and where the greatest potential for payoff exists. Concomitantly, creating streamlined paperwork increases the productivity of people working to solve a problem.

To ready the whole team for the need for change, the leader has to explain how limited resources will not prevent success. In addition, key influencers (the people with the power to influence others or secure resources) have to support the change. These people, once engaged, dramatically influence others and so all employees within an organization have joined the effort.

Another strategy represented in this article is to make results and responsibilities clear so that a culture focused on performance is created. The art of framing the specific goals also was addressed. Bratton framed each challenge as a series of specific goals relevant to officers at various levels. This made the overall change seem possible, because it started small and grew.

Finally, an equal amount of preparation should be devoted to those who would influence negatively. As change progresses, those who are opposed to it increase their attempts to damage or destroy the change. Therefore being ready for such attacks and neutralizing the prospective arguments when possible can limit the influence or the damage any naysayers may have.

More information about Bill Bratton's leadership may be accessed online at www.heritage.org/Research/Crime/HL573.cfm.

Kim, W. C., & Mauborgne, R. (2003, April). Tipping point leadership. *Harvard Business Review*, 60-69.

Contemplations

- In times of limited staff availability, what is the best approach to working with staff to ensure adequate staffing levels to guarantee quality care?
- Does one set of standards or competencies fit particular work settings better than others?
- Does the *Code of Ethics for Nurses* pose potential conflicts between nurses in direct care and nurse administrators, or is any difference explainable by a direct versus nondirect care perspective?

- Should the minimum level of educational preparation for a CNO be a graduate degree in nursing?
- Should nurse administrators be certified in their clinical area of expertise (e.g., cardiac, gerontology), should they be certified in their functional area of expertise (i.e., nursing administration), or should they be certified in both?
- How can a nurse administrator push a patient safety agenda?

LEADER STORY

Lillee S. Gelinas
Vice President and Chief Nursing Officer
VHA, Inc.
Irving, Texas

When we talk about the future, we sometimes think it is foggy and complicated but not concrete. However, the future is concrete in terms of where we need to go. We know that we have a healthcare system that is unsafe and unsatisfying to patients, their families, and healthcare workers. We know so through the data from patient satisfaction surveys, from the sentinel event data reported to JCAHO, and from the employee satisfaction data for nurses. Certain hospitals exhibit outstanding performance: the Baldrige winners in healthcare, and the designated employers of choice and Magnet hospitals. However, out of 6000 hospitals in America, approximately a maximum of 500 hospitals have performance excellence designations. How do we close the gap?

Today's consumer expects safe, cost-effective, reliable, timely, efficient healthcare. CNOs have a tremendous role in helping to close that gap. Their educational experience allows them to see the healthcare system as a whole. Holistic and global education is found in few professions. That description of global education, knowledge, and ability to execute strategy has an upside and a downside. The upside is that broad sense of knowing the entire healthcare system as it plays out within the entire patient. The downside is knowing where to focus. When we look at the role of CNOs today, they have one of the broadest roles within the organization. It is really difficult to focus.

CNOs need to consider seriously where they will have the most influence and where they will have the best ability to be an advocate for patients. Superfluous duties should be eliminated.

One of the most informative and useful exercises a CNO can do is to create the stop-doing list. The stop-doing list is all of the activities and tasks you do that do not add value, are just soaking up a whole lot of time, and are not really areas that you can influence.

Let me give you a great example. I heard a CNO speak. He was talking about the fact that he was on three blood pressure medications and his physical health was suffering because he was working 12 to 16 hours every day, going home feeling that his inbox was still full, that the e-mail wasn't done, and neither was the voice mail. He felt that he never went home with a sense of satisfaction. He realized how much time he was spending on medical staff issues. However, in his role as CNO, he does not credential physicians, he does not have a role of coaching or mentoring them clinically or operationally, he does not have the authority to fire them, and he has no role in performance management with them. So he asked, "Why am I spending so much time with medical staff issues that the chief medical officer should handle?" He shared that question with his CEO. He indicated the need for those issues to be removed from his plate so that he had time to make rounds on nursing units and deal with nursing issues and patient issues. He pointed out that he could not do those things if he spent so much time with medical staff issues.

Another example of a stop-doing item related to workforce is doing exit interviews with nurses and others. Why perform an exit interview? It is too late. These employees are leaving; you can do nothing to change that, yet you are investing all of these hours to find out what you did wrong.

We need to spend time talking with staff, asking how long they intend to stay. Do we as CNOs really understand retention intent? Retention intent is how long nurses plan to stay in an organization. Far more productive would be conversations regarding why they would intend to leave or where they would plan to go and whether decisions might be personal or professional. Those are two examples of how we continue to practice without changing our behavior or our use of our time. A good way to begin to change is to critically evaluate how you spend your time.

Imagine that your boss asked for a report of where you spent your time over the past year, the past month, and the past week and requested that you divide that time up into the critical areas of what your role is. What does your job description say you are responsible for doing? Does the amount of time you are spending match what the role indicates you should be doing? If you in your role are serving as a patient advocate in your organization and yet you can determine the amount of time devoted to that area is limited, are you really achieving your role expectations? This type of analysis shows you if your actual time spent is misaligned with your job responsibilities. To lead in the future, your role has to be consistent with the job.

One of the greatest challenges is understanding how to get the organization to support the role matching the job. We really tolerate insanity in healthcare today. We establish a job description and hire people with credentials and skills. Then we put those very talented people in roles in which they cannot effectively implement their skills, and then we wonder why CNO turnover is so high. Reading into the future requires close attention to the role matching the job and what we do daily, monthly, and yearly.

In April of 2004 at a VHA Leadership Conference, we asked a group of several hundred CNOs to think about how their role needs to change for the future. CNOs looked at themselves in four major categories of influence and judged how effective they were in each. The four categories were CNO as leader, CNO leadership in the care delivery organization, CNO in the care delivery support organization, and CNO leadership in the community and in a patient-focused industry.

The first category, CNOs as leaders, is the most important role. The CNO is best positioned to champion the patient because he or she is responsible for the care delivery organization. As a patient advocate, the CNO leads the organization, affects the support organization of the healthcare facility, and then influences areas outside the hospital in the community and the industry. The model of the CNO role in the ideal healthcare system of the future reflects the communication and influence as a two-way process. The CNO has to be in a position to interact with other components of the healthcare organization. Being able to hold crucial conversations is one of the most essential skills of the CNO as leader. Think about how we are educated: are we really educated around exquisite communication skills, negotiation skills?

The second category, the role of the CNO within the care delivery organization, really shows the CNO has responsibility for the areas that touch and affect the patient. So, does the CNO have a really good sense of how the care delivery organization is built? So many hospitals have expanded the CNO's scope and role into areas that traditionally have not reported to the CNO, such as dietary and pharmacy. Nutrition and pharmaceuticals are two essential components of what happens to the patient in the hospital and are part of the care delivery organization.

A couple of key elements in this role illustrate what is needed for the future. For example, implementing a measurement system is critical. I have had the privilege of working with the National Quality Forum (NQF) on their project, nursing care performance measures, the first set of which produced endorsed nursing-sensitive performance measures. When you ask CNOs if they know their failure-to-rescue rate, they usually say no. However, the NQF has found failure-to-rescue rate is one of the single most important components that hospitals can measure to look at nursing care performance.

CNOs' unique leadership roles specific to the hospital and care delivery organization are a measurement system of nursing care performance, patient care unit design for safe and efficient care, healthy relationships with the medical and nursing staff, and designing nursing roles for best patient outcomes. CNOs who are leading within the healthcare system need to make sure an accurate measurement system is in place and that the correct measurements are being taken. An important part of that measurement effort is making sure that patient care units are designed for safe, effective care. How we design hospitals is not based on evidence. The Robert Wood Johnson Foundation publication, *Designing the Twenty First Century Hospital*, reveals that we are building hospitals based on what we can pay the architects and what we can build. It has nothing to do with evidence-based physical plants.

Quality measurement is impossible without healthy relationships with the medical staff, which relates to how we work with our physician colleagues. Nursing staff roles, too, must be designed for best patient outcomes and high nurse and patient satisfaction.

CNOs must also be leaders in the care delivery support organization. This makes up the third category. Examples of CNO leadership in this area include influencing the organizational culture, having a healthy culture, having a culture with an intense focus on performance excellence, making leadership development a priority for the entire organization, and making sure the performance measurement system (the review "annual" process) is tied to our culture and our strategy. One of the most important roles in this category is making sure nursing is entwined throughout the whole organization. In the past, nursing was too often described as functioning in

a silo. A patient care delivery organization needs to be totally entwined in its services. Contributing to organizational culture results in organizational excellence and making leadership development a priority.

The fourth area is related to the external focus of community and industry. That focus is on managing outward. Without presence in the community, we do not have a reputation and credibility. The role of the CNO includes work in this area too.

The CNOs' descriptions of their roles in relation to these four discrete and concrete areas were enlightening. These four areas encompass the foci that CNOs need to have for the future and they are a way to look at strengths and needs for growth. For the majority of CNOs, the role in the support organization needs the most attention. Usually CNOs excel in the first two areas or they would not be in a leadership position. CNOs need the greatest development in understanding all the various parts of the organization and how they fit together and the expense/revenue and important business aspects. CNO leadership in the community has improved over the years, especially with joint appointments in schools of nursing and the hospital and becoming involved in Kiwanis and Rotary.

Only when CNOs have skills balanced across these four categories can they help lead their organizations into the future. When skills are not present in important areas, the organization actually is held back from achieving its potential. An analogy is a sea anchor when you are trying to move a ship forward in the white water (of change) and yet the anchor is down in the silt. The ship cannot move effectively. The anchor represents skills and competencies that are not there; you do not know what you do not know. Therefore you cannot be a good navigator; you are held back by the skill set deficit. The public and politicians will demand the healthcare organization of the future to be a high-performing organization. For the organization to be high performing, the CNO also must be high performing.

The required skills and competencies are having the ability to look honestly at skill sets and competencies, honing the ability to take a hard look at where they are spending their time, using exquisite communication skills (because conversations are how we build relationships and our leadership skills), and being able to ask why.

Jim Collins mentions in his book, *Good to Great*, the notion of strategic humility. We are educated as nurses to know what we have to do when. When we participate in a code on a patient, we have to know the algorithms of performance. It is a linear scientific process. One of the hardest transitions we make is going from scientist and linear thinking around evidence to being nonlinear thinkers and having to deal with the abstract rather than the concrete. That transition from the concrete thinking of scientist to the abstract thinking of leader can be difficult. It can be enlightening, uplifting, and revealing to understand that the best skill you need as a leader is to be able to ask why and to be able to say, "I don't know." We are taught in nursing school to ask why; that is part of differential diagnosis. However, we are not taught as much around the idea of uncertainty and how to deal with that abstraction.

I am concerned about the turnover of CNOs, which is a threat to clinical quality. We have the public and politics that are ramping up the public performance of hospitals, public disclosure of data, pay for clinical performance, and payers not paying for poor performance. The pressure to achieve clinical excellence has never been greater. A CNO in a hospital/health system is critical to the pursuit of clinical excellence. Instability in that role results in instability in achieving clinical excellence. Therefore understanding the dynamics of the high turnover of CNOs in the United States will be an important component to a hospital and health system's quest for clinical excellence.

We are in the most perfect storm of pressure now. I wonder if the turnover of CNOs is not like the canary in the analogy. Canaries were used to determine when the gases in mines were at dangerous levels. If the canary died, the miners knew not to go in. Perhaps the turnover of CNOs and other nursing leaders is the warning of dangers in the healthcare organization. Wouldn't it be interesting if the CNOs were the equivalent of the canaries in the mines? Once again, the analogy speaks volumes about the instability of the system and poor care. CNOs understand and the nursing staff knows it too. It speaks volumes about the instability in leadership overall. As we looked at the NQF nursing care performance measures project, we know strength of evidence surrounds 15 key indicators that describe nursing care. In the ideal healthcare system the goal is that all 15 are measured and that nurses clearly play an instrumental role in the patient outcome.

How can hospitals function to achieve clinical excellence around those 15 elements if no CNO is present or the job keeps turning over? I have asked CNOs how long it was before they felt really comfortable in their job and role. Most CNOs say this takes 3 years. Year one is figuring out about who is who and what is what. Year two is about developing relationships with other leaders, and year three is deciding where those four categories of the CNO role can be played out. We are looking at improvement work at VHA and how long it takes for change to stick and be sustainable. In our transformation in the ICU work VHA has been doing, we know it is in the third year. Therefore a skill imperative to future success will be tenacity because change takes time.

The ideal healthcare system of the future is one in which care is safe, evidence-based, and provided by competent physicians, nurses, and staff. It is scary to think about the future. We know we will not have sufficient nurses. Physicians are exhausted from the hassles of care, and pharmacists feel so overcontrolled. The economic pressure erodes the clinical role and it deserves a lot of attention for the future. The erosion of the clinical role prevents us from achieving what we can do.

The core of the healthcare system focused on excellence requires a strong CNO at the center.

The data all make that clear. We have seen the role expand over the years and we have studied the role here for years. Broadening the skill set is critical to include financial outcomes, data management and analysis, marketing initiatives, human resource management, and strategic visioning and planning.

Lillee Gelinas was also co-chair of the NQF Committee which produced the NQF Voluntary Consensus Standards for Nursing Sensitive Care: An Initial Performance Measure Set (2004) to Endorse National Voluntary Consensus Standards for Nursing Sensitive Care.

Chapter References

Aiken, L. H., Clarke, S. P., Cheung, R. B., Sloane, D. M., & Silber, J. H. (2003). Educational levels of hospital nurses and surgical patient mortality. *Journal of the American Medical Association, 290,* 1617-1623.

Allison, M. M., & Monarch, K. (2003, October). Magnet recognition program: an update. Paper presented at the Magent Conference, Houston, TX.

American Association of Colleges of Nursing. *The clinical nurse leader: developing a new nursing role.* Retrieved from http://www.aacn.nche.edu/NewNurse/index.htm August 21, 2004.

American Association of Colleges of Nursing and American Organization of Nurse Executives. (1997). *Joint position statement on nursing administration education.* Washington, DC: AACN.

American Nurses Association. (1995). *Scope and standards for nurse administrators.* Washington, DC: The Association.

American Nurses Association. (2001). *Code of ethics for nurses with interpretive statement.* Washington, DC: The Association.

American Nurses Association. (2003). *Nursing's social policy statement.* (2nd ed.). Washington, DC: The Association.

American Nurses Association. (2004). *Scope and standards for nurse administrators.* (2nd ed.). Washington, DC: The Association.

American Nurses Credentialing Center. (2004). Retrieved February 20, 2004, from http://www.nursingworld.org/ancc/cert.html.

American Organization of Nurse Executives. (2005). AONE nurse executive competencies. *Nurse Leader, 3*(1), 15-21.

Bolton, J. G. (2004). Valuing leadership: Transforming the "we/they" dichotomy in nursing organizations. *Nurse Leader, 2*(4), 33-35.

Bossidy, L., & Charan, R. (2002). *Execution.* New York: Random House.

Bureau of Health Professions. (2002). *The Registered Nurse Population. National Sample Survey of Registered Nurses.* Washington, DC: Health Resources and Service Administration, US Department of Health and Human Services.

Collins, J. (2001). Level 5 leadership. *Harvard Business Review, 79*(1), 67-76.

Council on Graduate Education for Administration in Nursing. (1995). *Essentials of baccalaureate nursing education for nursing leadership and management and master's nursing education for nursing administration advanced practice.* CGEAN.

Covey, S. R. (1989). *The 7 habits of highly effective people: Powerful lessons in personal change.* New York: Simon and Schuster.

Curtin, L. L. (2000). The first ten principles for the ethical administration of nursing services. *Nursing Administration Quarterly, 25*(1), 7-13.

Gladwell, M. (2000). *The tipping point: How little things can make a big difference.* Boston: Little, Brown and Company.

Goldsmith, M., & Morgan, H. (2004). Leadership is a contact sport: The "follow-up factor" in management development, *Strategy+Business,* 36.

HealthGrades Quality Study. (2004). *Patient safety in American hospitals.* Lakewood, CO: HealthGrades.

Institute of Medicine. (2004). *Keeping patients safe: Transforming the work environment of nurses.* Washington, DC: The National Academies Press.

Kerfoot, K. (2001). The art of raising the bar. *Dermatology Nursing, 13,* 301-302.

Kim, W. C., & Mauborgne, R. (2003, April). Tipping point leadership. *Harvard Business Review*, 60-69.

Kimball, B. (2004, May). Health care's human crisis—Rx for an evolving profession. *Online Journal of Issues in Nursing*. Retrieved from http://www.nursingworld.org, June 17, 2004.

Matisoff-Li, A. (2004, April). Chief nursing officers: A seat at the table. *Healthleaders*, 35-44.

Maxwell, J. C. (1999). *The 21 indispensable qualities of a leader: Becoming the person others will want to follow.* Nashville, TN: Thomas Nelson Publishers.

National Center for Healthcare Leadership. (2004). *Health leadership competency model.* Chicago: The Center.

Porter-O'Grady, T. (2003). A different age for leadership, part 2: New rules, new roles. *Journal of Nursing Administration, 33,* 173-178.

Ross, A., Wenzel, F. J., & Mitlyng, J. W. (2002). *Leadership for the future: Core competencies in healthcare.* Chicago: Health Administration Press.

Sigma Theta Tau. (2004). *Arista 3: Nurses and health: A global future.* Indianapolis, IN: The Society.

Yearbook of Medical Informatics. (2000). Heidelberg, Germany: University of Heidelberg.

Transforming Professional Practice Environments

THE MAGNET RECOGNITION PROGRAM

Linda Urden

Every system is perfectly designed to achieve exactly the results it gets. New levels of performance can only be achieved through dynamic system-level redesign. ROBERT PORTER LYNCH

This chapter describes a program to transform the professional practice environment into one that attracts and retains nurses, empowers staff, promotes interdisciplinary collaboration, fosters lifelong learning, supports evidence-based practice, and results in excellent outcomes for persons to whom nursing care and services are provided. Specifically, the Magnet Recognition Program™ is described from a historical perspective. The program framework is delineated, along with suggestions for implementation of the program tenets. Finally, clinical and organizational outcomes related to Magnet-designated work environments are summarized.

TURBULENT SOCIETAL AND ECONOMIC challenges are having a direct impact on healthcare institutions and providers. Current and predicted

shortages of healthcare providers in all categories are imminent and threaten the health and services of our communities nationally and globally. The nursing workforce is aging, and nurses are changing careers or retiring early because of physical and emotional constraints. The number of applications for nursing education programs appears to be increasing, although history has shown that this is cyclic. Regardless of the actual applications, enrollment may not be consistent because of lack of sufficient numbers of available faculty, who are also retiring with insufficient numbers to replace them.

The healthcare work environment is demanding and stressful in all settings and specialties. Each particular setting carries its own specific challenges that can directly affect relationships, clinical care, safety, and clinical and organizational outcomes. The good news, however, is that research has demonstrated factors that positively influence the practice environment, which leads to retention of nursing staff, excellence in clinical outcomes, and organizational effectiveness. The Magnet Recognition Program was created by the American Nurses Credentialing Center (ANCC) to celebrate the demonstration of excellence.

HISTORICAL OVERVIEW

The genesis for the current Magnet Recognition Program was the work of a Task Force on Nursing Practice in Hospitals of the American Academy of Nursing in 1981. At this time, the supply of nurses was inadequate and a large number of vacancies existed in hospital nursing positions. This group was charged "to examine characteristics of systems impeding and/or facilitating professional nursing practice in hospitals" (McClure, Poulin, Sovie, & Wandelt, 2002, p. 1). The task force recognized the serious nursing shortage and at the same time acknowledged that facilities across the country were able to attract and retain nurses and provide excellent care. Because these institutions were successful in attracting and retaining nurses, the term "magnet" was used to identify them (Figure 2-1). Subsequently, the Academy commissioned a study to examine the characteristics of these facilities.

A national sample of organizations was identified, with 155 respondents, 46 of which were selected as Magnets for the purposes of the study. Group interviews were held in each of the eight regional locations with directors and staff of the organizations. Post-interview comments were solicited from the participants regarding activities, programs, and policies believed to enhance professional and personal satisfaction of nurses. All data were reviewed with the emergence of three broad categories of characteristics: administration, professional practice, and professional development. The congruence regarding the existence of the characteristics among hospitals, regardless of bed size, geographic location,

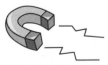

Figure 2-1 Like magnets, Magnet facilities attract. In the case of Magnet facilities, in addition to attracting nurses, they attract physicians, other employees, and patients.

or role of the study participants was impressive. The research team discussed the difficulty in operationalizing a professional practice environment and the challenge that the Magnet organizations had in maintaining such an environment. However, a consistent theme was the existence of continual efforts toward improvement in all aspects of the environment (McClure & Hinshaw, 2002).

CREDENTIALING AND RECOGNITION

The ANCC was formed in 1991 and is a subsidiary of the American Nurses Association (ANA). ANCC provides formal, systematic mechanisms by which individuals and organizations voluntarily may seek credentials that recognize quality in professional practice and continuing education. Credentialing services offered by ANCC include (1) accreditation for organizations or approval bodies that meet continuing education standards; (2) certification of individuals by validating that the requisite knowledge, skills, and abilities to practice in a given specialty are present; and (3) recognition by evaluating an organization's adherence to excellence-focused standards. The recognition service of ANCC is operationalized through the Magnet Recognition Program.

Upon completion of a pilot project in 1994 that included five facilities, the first facility designated as a Magnet by ANCC was the University of Washington Medical Center in Seattle, Washington. Programmatic and operational details were revised and streamlined before the launch of the national program that was then known as the Magnet Nursing Services Recognition Program. In 1998 the program expanded to include long-term care facilities, including subacute, chronic, and rehabilitation services. After another pilot project, the program expanded again in 2000 to include international healthcare organizations and any setting in which nursing is practiced, regardless of geographic location. Clearly, the issues and challenges facing healthcare delivery and nurses worldwide are similar and the standards and conceptual basis for the program apply and can be integrated wherever nursing is practiced.

The volunteer governing body that oversees the Magnet Recognition Program is the ANCC Commission on Magnet Recognition (Commission). Commission members are appointed by the ANCC Board of Directors and represent a variety of roles and related nursing organizations. This Commission is accountable for (1) approving all aspects of the program criteria, policies, and guidelines; (2) establishing standards and qualifications for program appraisers, along with selection and training; (3) making final decisions regarding Magnet status; (4) providing a mechanism for the systematic review and evaluation of the Program; and (5) establishing advisory groups, expert panels, and work groups deemed necessary to carry out the program functions and evolution. Program integrity is the overarching and key focus of the Commission.

MAGNET RECOGNITION PROGRAM FRAMEWORK

The purpose of the Magnet Nursing Services Recognition Program (now Magnet Recognition Program) is to recognize excellence. Excellence is recognized in four major areas:

1. The management, philosophy, and practice of nursing services
2. Adherence to national standards for improving the quality of patient care services
3. Leadership of the nurse administrator in supporting professional practice and continued competence of nurses
4. Understanding and respecting the cultural and ethnic diversity of patients, their significant others, and healthcare providers

The program framework incorporates the characteristics found to be present in Magnet organizations described by McClure and colleagues and

standards of practice and professional performance defined by the ANA. The Forces of Magnetism™ illustrate an organization's overall culture in 14 areas. Organizations must demonstrate that the Forces of Magnetism are present and that a level of excellence has been achieved on all measurement criteria to receive the ANCC Magnet designation.

Forces of Magnetism

The 14 Forces of Magnetism, summarized in Box 2-1, are based on the original research and are described in more detail below.

Quality of Nursing Leadership

Nursing leaders were perceived as knowledgeable, strong risk-takers who followed an articulated philosophy in the daily operations of the nursing department. Nursing leaders also conveyed a strong sense of advocacy and support on behalf of the staff.

Organizational Structure

Organizational structures were characterized as flat, rather than tall, and by unit-based decision making. Nursing departments were decentralized;

Box 2-1 FORCES OF MAGNETISM

Quality of nursing leadership
Organizational structure
Management style
Personnel policies and programs
Professional models of care
Quality of care
Quality improvement
Consultation and resources
Autonomy
Community and the hospital
Nurses as teachers
Image of nursing
Collegial nurse/physician relationships
Professional development

strong nursing representation was evident in the organizational committee structure. The nursing leader served at the executive level of the organization, and the chief nursing executive reported to the CEO.

Management Style

Hospital and nursing administrators were found to use a participative management style, which incorporated feedback from staff members at all levels of the organization. Feedback was characterized as encouraged and valued. Nurses serving in leadership positions were visible, accessible, and committed to communicating effectively with staff members.

Personnel Policies and Programs

Salaries and benefits were characterized as competitive. Rotating shifts were minimized, and creative and flexible staffing models were used. Personnel policies were created with staff involvement, and significant administrative and clinical promotional opportunities existed.

Professional Models of Care

Models of care were used that gave nurses the responsibility and authority for the provision of patient care. Nurses were accountable for their own practice and were the coordinators of care.

Quality of Care

Nurses perceived that they were providing high-quality care to their patients. Providing quality care also was seen as an organizational priority, and nurses serving in leadership positions were viewed as responsible for developing an environment in which high-quality care could be provided.

Quality Improvement

Quality improvement activities were viewed as educational. Staff nurses participated in the quality improvement process and perceived the process as one that improved the quality of care delivered within the organization.

Consultation and Resources

Adequate consultation and other human resources were available. Knowledgeable experts, particularly advanced practice nurses, were available and consulted. In addition, peer support was given within and outside the nursing division.

Autonomy

Nurses were permitted and expected to practice autonomously, consistent with professional standards. Independent judgment was expected within the context of a multidisciplinary approach to patient care.

Community and the Hospital

Hospitals that were best able to recruit and retain nurses also maintained a strong community presence. A community presence was seen in a variety of ongoing, long-term outreach programs. These outreach programs resulted in the hospital being perceived as a strong, positive, and productive corporate citizen.

Nurses as Teachers

Nurses were permitted and expected to incorporate teaching in all aspects of their practice. Teaching was one activity that reportedly gave nurses a great deal of professional satisfaction.

Image of Nursing

Nurses were viewed as integral to the hospital's ability to provide patient care services. Other members of the healthcare team regarded the services provided by nurses as essential.

Collegial Nurse/Physician Relationships

Interdisciplinary relationships were characterized as positive. A sense of mutual respect was exhibited among all disciplines.

Professional Development

Significant emphasis was placed on orientation, inservice education, continuing education, formal education, and career development. Personal and professional growth and development were valued.

In addition, opportunities for competency-based clinical advancement existed, along with the resources to maintain competency (Urden & Monarch, 2002) (Figure 2-2).

Standards of Practice and Professional Performance

The *Scope and Standards for Nurse Administrators* (ANA, 2004) is a foundational document upon which the Magnet Recognition Program is based. The standards apply to nurse administrators in any specialty, setting, and geographic location. Standards reflect values and priorities of the profession and are authoritative statements that delineate responsibilities for which its practitioners are held accountable. This document also can be used as a framework to create the infrastructure for a professional practice environment for nursing practice. The 14 program standards with related criteria delineate expectations associated with measurable program standards. These criteria are referred to as measurement criteria. Standards are divided into Standards of Practice and Standards of Professional Performance (Box 2-2). Reading the full document reveals specific details and measurement criteria. The following is a brief explanation of the standards.

Standards of Practice

Assessment. This standard is met by having methods to assess nurse-sensitive indicators, resources to support data collection, systems for efficient data collection and data retrieval, and processes to modify information systems to meet changing data requirements and needs. Use of research findings and guidelines and standards to modify data collection elements is important. Analysis of the workflow related to effectiveness and efficiency of assessment processes in the target environment is essential. Evaluation of the assessment processes sensitive to the unique and diverse needs of individuals and populations served is required. Confidentiality of data must be ensured. Another essential component of this standard is the facilitation of a unified assessment process developed in collaboration with other healthcare disciplines across the continuum of care.

Problems/Diagnosis. The nurse administrator must advocate for resources for decision analysis in collaboration with other departments. Staff must be developed and maintain competency in the diagnostic process, and the organizational climate must support validation of diagnoses. Interdisciplinary collaboration in data analysis and decision-making processes is essential as is a format for documentation of diagnoses that facilitates a client-centered plan of care and determination of outcomes.

Identification of outcomes. The nurse administrator must participate in the design and implementation of multidisciplinary processes to maintain standards consistent with the identified outcomes of clients and facilitate staff participation in interdisciplinary processes. Databases that include nurse-sensitive outcomes must be identified

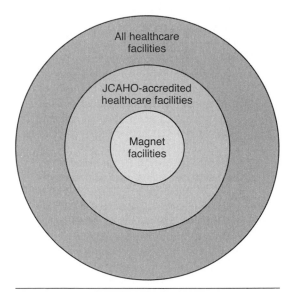

Figure 2-2 Magnet in the context of healthcare. Only a small percentage of healthcare organizations have achieved Magnet status.

Box 2-2   ANA SCOPE AND STANDARDS FOR NURSE ADMINISTRATORS

STANDARDS OF PRACTICE

Standard 1: Assessment

The nurse administrator develops, maintains, and evaluates patient/client/resident and staff data collection systems and processes to support the practice of nursing and delivery of patient/client/resident care.

Standard 2: Problems/Diagnosis

The nurse administrator develops, maintains, and evaluates an environment that empowers and supports the professional nurse in analysis of assessment data and in decisions to determine relevant problems and diagnoses.

Standard 3: Identification of Outcomes

The nurse administrator develops, maintains, and evaluates information systems and processes that promote desired patient/client/resident-defined, professional, and organizational outcomes.

Standard 4: Planning

The nurse administrator develops, maintains, and evaluates organizational systems to facilitate planning for the delivery of care.

Standard 5: Implementation

The nurse administrator develops, maintains, and evaluates organizational systems that support implementation plans and delivery of care across the continuum.

Standard 6: Evaluation

The nurse administrator evaluates the plan and its progress in relation to the attainment of outcomes.

STANDARDS OF PROFESSIONAL PERFORMANCE

Standard 7: Quality of Care and Administrative Practice

The nurse administrator systematically evaluates the quality and effectiveness of nursing practice and nursing services administration.

Standard 8: Performance Appraisal

The nurse administrator evaluates personal performance based on professional practice standards, relevant statutes, rules and regulations, and organizational criteria.

Standard 9: Professional Knowledge

The nurse administrator maintains and demonstrates current knowledge in the administration of healthcare organizations to advance nursing practice and the provision of quality healthcare services.

Box 2-2   ANA SCOPE AND STANDARDS FOR NURSE ADMINISTRATORS—CONT'D

Standard 10: Professional Environment

The nurse administrator is accountable for providing a professional environment.

Standard 11: Ethics

The nurse administrator's decisions and actions are based on ethical principles.

Standard 12: Collaboration

The nurse administrator collaborates with nursing staff at all levels, interdisciplinary teams, executive leaders, and other stakeholders.

Standard 13: Research

The nurse administrator supports research and its integration into nursing and the delivery of healthcare services.

Standard 14: Resource Utilization

The nurse administrator evaluates and administers the resources of nursing services.

Reprinted with permission from American Nurses Association. (2004). *Scope and standards for nursing administrators.* Silver Spring, MD: nursebooks.org.

and used. Nurse participation in monitoring and evaluating nursing care in accordance with professional, regulatory, and organizational standards must be ensured. Clinical, human resource, and financial data must be integrated and used to make decisions. Continuous quality improvement of clinical guidelines linked to outcomes that provide direction for care processes are important.

Planning. Emphasis is heavy on the nurse administrator's contribution to the development and continuous improvement of organizational systems related to the delivery of nursing services. Interdisciplinary planning and collaboration that focus on specific populations are required. Applicable contemporary management and organizational theories, nursing, and related research findings must be integrated into the planning process. Systems for preventing and reporting abuse of clients' rights, and incompetent, unethical, or illegal practices by healthcare providers must be evidenced. Appropriate use of staff at all levels of practice in accordance with the state's

nurse practice act and professional standards of practice must be demonstrated.

Implementation. Organizational systems must integrate policies and procedures with regulations, practice standards, and clinical guidelines and resources that support interventions that are consistent with the established plans of care. Systems and resources must ensure safe, effective, efficient, and culturally competent interventions. Interventions must be implemented by the most appropriate personnel, and a mechanism must be in place to ensure appropriate and efficient documentation of interventions.

Evaluation. Processes and resources that deliver data and information to empower staff to make decisions must be evidenced. Nurse administrators must advocate for educational opportunities for staff members specific to current interventions, technologies, and other skills to enhance their skills and abilities for their roles. Appropriate research methods in place and use of research findings are required to improve care processes, systems, and outcomes. Policies, procedures, and guidelines must be based on research findings, and data generated from outcomes research are used to develop innovative changes in care delivery. Participation and recognition of staff members in formal and informal organizational committees and work groups are required. Resources sufficient to provide time for critical assessment and evaluation of outcomes must be ensured. A process of governance that includes participation of all nurses must be in place. The nurse administrator must participate in the peer review and privileging process for advanced practice nurses.

Standards of Professional Performance

Quality of care and administrative practice. The nurse administrator must identify key quality indicators for monitoring and evaluation and analyze data and information to identify improvement opportunities. Systems and processes must be developed, implemented, and evaluated that enhance the overall organizational plan for process improvement. Participation in interdisciplinary evaluation teams is crucial.

Performance appraisal. The nurse administrator engages in self-performance appraisal on a regular basis and identifies areas for strength and areas for professional and practice development. Constructive feedback regarding practice is sought, and action is taken to achieve goals.

Professional knowledge. The nurse administrator seeks additional knowledge and skills by development of and participation in educational programs and activities, conferences, workshops, interdisciplinary professional meetings, and self-directed learning. Experiences are sought to expand and maintain skills and knowledge bases; appropriate formal education and certification are accomplished. Networks with peers in the state/region/nation are evidenced to share ideas and conduct mutual problem solving.

Professional environment. The nurse administrator promotes understanding and effective use of organization, management, and nursing theories and research and contributes to nursing management education and professional development of others. Knowledge and skills are shared with colleagues, and acting as a role model and mentor is valued as is the creation of a climate of effective communication.

Ethics. The nurse administrator advocates on behalf of services and personnel and fosters a nondiscriminatory climate in which care is delivered in a manner sensitive to sociocultural diversity. Privacy, confidentiality, and security of patient, client, staff, and organization data are maintained. The *Code of Ethics for Nurses* (ANA, 2001) is followed, and a system is in place to address ethical issues within nursing and the organization.

Collaboration. The nurse administrator collaborates with nursing staff and other disciplines at all levels in the development, implementation, and evaluation of programs and services and facilitates collaboration of others within the organization. Evidence exists of nursing collaboration with administrative peers in determination of acquisition, allocation, and use of organizational fiscal and human resources. Collaboration with the human resources staff regarding recruitment and retention programs is important. Ongoing communication with nursing staff and other providers within the healthcare system is essential.

Research. The identification of priority areas for nursing research is fostered, the conduct and use of research and other scholarly activities is supported, and resources to facilitate research are provided. Procedures for review of proposed research studies are provided, and knowledge-driven nursing practice is promoted.

Resource utilization. The nurse administrator must evaluate factors related to safety, outcomes, effectiveness, cost, and social impact when developing practice changes and innovations. Responsibilities appropriate to the licensure, education, and experience of staff are delegated, with negotiation for appropriate role expansion and delimitations. Appropriate utilization of staff is monitored and evaluated, and organizational acceptance of appropriate roles or role changes are designed and negotiated. Evidence of advocacy is important to secure appropriate fiscal and human resources to meet the goals of the services and programs.

MAGNET APPRAISAL AND DESIGNATION PROCESS

The appraisal process consists of four phases: (1) application; (2) submission of written documentation and evaluation process; (3) site visit; and (4) the decision.

Application

Phase one usually begins when an individual or representative of the nursing department obtains an application manual and reviews the eligibility criteria and standards to assess an approximate level of readiness to apply for Magnet status. Information is shared with others and a decision is made whether to embark on the process. A person within the organization is designated as the project coordinator, an application timeline is prepared, and the application is submitted by the applicant organization to the ANCC Magnet Program office.

Submission of Written Documentation and Evaluation Process

Phase two starts when the applicant compiles and submits to ANCC written documentation that comprehensively reflects how the organization meets program standards. Appraisers are appointed to review the written documentation to determine whether criteria have been met. If a range of excellence score has been obtained, phase three commences.

Site Visit

Phase three is that phase of the application process in which the site visit occurs. The number of appraisers and the number of days dedicated to a site visit depend on the size of the applicant organization. The site visit is used to amplify, verify, and clarify the information contained in the applicant's written documentation. After the site visit, appraisers prepare a report for the ANCC Commission on Magnet Recognition. Phase three ends when the appraisers issue their final report to the Commission.

The Decision

The ANCC Commission on Magnet Recognition reviews the report, confers with appraisers for clarification or elucidation, and determines whether to confer Magnet status. This portion of the application process is referred to as phase four, or "Making the Decision" phase.

Magnet status is awarded when the organization has been deemed to exhibit the Forces of Magnetism and to demonstrate adherence to standards at a level of excellence. Magnet status is awarded for 4 years. To ensure that organizations continue to uphold program standards and requirements, annual reports are submitted that address continued observance of standards and maintenance of the Forces of Magnetism. In addition, a redesignation procedure is available for organizations that wish to extend their Magnet status beyond the initial 4-year period. The annual reports are analyzed carefully, and if questions remain after requests for further documentation, should such be needed, a site visit is scheduled. Although this is not an unannounced visit, it is conducted with short notice to validate actual current practices.

BENEFITS AND OUTCOMES RELATED TO MAGNET ORGANIZATIONS

Magnet designation denotes validation of excellence and has taken years of commitment on the part of a nursing leader's vision and well-developed strategies to create a professional practice environment for nurses. Many nurse executives use the program tenets as the framework by which to create the infrastructure to support professional nursing practice. It is during these years that the transformation really takes place through shared leadership for decision making, evidence-based practice, enhanced interdisciplinary relationships, quality focus, career advancement, peer review, support for educational endeavors, professional care delivery models, and assurance that appropriate resources and consultation are in place. This process is often referred to by all who go through the process as "The Journey." The actual designation as a Magnet is the "crowning touch," or "icing on the cake," acknowledging the processes that have been put into place by the organization. It is also the impetus to continue to enhance the current structure and processes and to look to the future, "beyond" levels of performance and innovations.

The spirit, the will to win, and the will to excel are the things that endure. These qualities are so much more important than the events that occur.
VINCE LOMBARDI

Magnet designation is an important recognition of nurses' worth, quality of the nursing enterprise, and the importance of nurses to the success of the entire organization. Recognition of excellence through the ANCC Magnet designation may be publicized by the recipient and used in its marketing strategies directed toward consumers and potential nursing staff.

Magnet designation is a major factor in nursing recruitment and retention. ANCC Magnet-designated healthcare organizations consistently outperform their peers in recruiting and retaining nurses, resulting in increased stability in patient care systems across the organization. These "nurse friendly" organizations benefit from reduced costs as a result of low turnover, which results in greater institutional stability (Magnet, 2004).

A competitive advantage is created through Magnet designation. A recent survey found that 93% of the public would have more confidence in the overall quality of a hospital if the hospital had passed the rigorous standards required to be a Magnet. The same survey found that 85% of the public would have more confidence in long-term care facilities that had passed similar nursing standards. Through recognition of an organization as being among the best in the nation for nursing care, consumers can be sure they have chosen the best provider, and health plans can be assured of the organization's commitment to high-quality patient care (Magnet, 2004).

Research documents that high-quality nurses are one of the most important attributes in attracting high-quality physicians. Therefore achieving this status creates a positive "halo" effect beyond the nursing services department that permeates the entire healthcare team. In fact, experience demonstrates that an organization with Magnet status for the nursing department also demonstrates the Forces of Magnetism throughout the entire organization, across departments and disciplines.

Because this recognition award indicates excellence in nursing services, the recipient is a model for other nursing and healthcare organizations. The many innovations and new scientific knowledge promulgated by Magnet-designated organizations are shared through presentations and publications, thus expanding new knowledge to the entire nursing community worldwide. In this aspect, excellent nursing service variables may be emulated by others, which contributes to upgrading the quality of nursing services in the nation's healthcare delivery systems. Additionally, staff nurses within the recognized Magnet nursing service system also may be contacted by other nurses for consultation. Nurses in Magnet facilities are leaders and active participants in nursing, healthcare, and related professional organizations, thereby influencing standards and policy.

Empirical evidence related to Magnet facilities and organizational outcomes has been documented in the literature. Attributes important to the professional practice environment, such as collaborative relationships, professional practice models, autonomy, and effective leadership, have been explicated over the years. The positive impact of these variables on nurse retention and job satisfaction is consistent among studies (Scott, Sochalski, & Aiken, 1999). Apparent differences exist in nursing infrastructure and outcomes between the ANCC Magnet–designated facilities and those without the designation. Those with Magnet designation had a distinct nursing department, a nurse researcher with a doctoral degree, and the chief nurse executive's perception of control over nursing practice. In addition, Magnet hospitals reported higher levels of support for autonomy, control over practice, and stronger nurse-physician relationships (Havens, 2001).

Magnet-designated facilities had higher levels of job satisfaction linked with greater visibility and responsiveness of nurse leaders and better support of autonomous decision making by clinical nursing staff. In addition, greater support for a professional nursing practice setting in Magnet organizations seemed to exist (Upenieks, 2003). (See the Literature box at the end of the chapter.) Structural empowerment (i.e., the social structure within the work environment that provides staff with essential elements so that they can accomplish their work in ways meaningful to them) has been linked to Magnet characteristics. Specifically, relationships were present between empowerment and autonomy, control over practice environment, and positive nurse-physician relationships. Additionally, access to empowering work environment conditions and Magnet characteristics were significantly predictive of nurses' satisfaction with their jobs (Laschinger, Almost, & Tuer-Hodes, 2003).

ORGANIZATIONAL COMMITMENT TO THE JOURNEY TO EXCELLENCE

The decision to use the Forces of Magnetism and ANA standards as an organizing framework for the nursing enterprise is one that necessitates careful deliberation and commitment from the nursing leadership team and the executive members of the organization. Although embarking on the Magnet process is a substantial undertaking, it creates a great opportunity to highlight excellence that already exists and take other programs to higher levels than currently exist. Because the journey takes time to build the infrastructure to support a professional nursing practice environment, the chief nurse executive's strategic plan is essential in reaching the vision and achieving the goal of recognition through Magnet status. Internal and external consultants and experts in multiple areas may be brought into the organization to inject new knowledge or energize the team. Often an outside facilitator can be used as an impartial person to move groups along and reach higher levels of planning more quickly. The decision to use any consultant or facilitator will rest on the CNO's assessment of the organization, talent, and "starting point" of the department in the process. Questions and considerations in determining the decision to move forward or not with the Magnet journey can be found in the Contemplations section at the end of the chapter.

A starting point is usually a gap analysis to assess readiness of the organization and the ability to meet the standards and exhibit the Forces of Magnetism. Because of organizational uniqueness, titles and roles may vary, but a coordinator or project manager usually is appointed to organize and facilitate all of the Magnet-related activities. Other important early discussions and decisions include timeframes. The timeline for planning and implementing or revising systems and structures varies, depending on the level of maturity (if already in existence) or a need to create and implement. A balance must exist between establishing an aggressive timeline and the reality of the ability to fully meet all of the standards, with Forces of Magnetism present. Experience suggests more positive outcomes are related to more fully developed and implemented changes. Having a more mature system that all nurses can speak to allows validation of outcomes. Each organization, nursing department, and system is unique and will arrive at decision points in different ways, using various mentors and resources.

SUMMARY

Magnet is an outcome and a process. It designates the best about nursing care delivery. It allows for staff recognition and unification around processes designed to continue improvements in healthcare. Primarily, it assures the public of the best in care.

The challenges in creating and maintaining a professional practice environment for nursing continue to confront nurse leaders now and into the future. During the various cycles of nursing shortages over the years of experience, many interventions have been put into place to address issues important to nursing. Many of these "solutions" have been short-lived and have not delved into the real underlying issue: the practice environment and the personal and professional needs of the nurses. The Magnet Recognition Program is a program built on evidence, with

demonstrated positive organizational and professional outcomes. It reaches into the real root of the problem and can have long-lasting effects. The fact that the program "works" in all settings and specialties, nationally and globally, speaks to the universality of the issue and the solution. The program standards and tenets impact nursing and other disciplines, departments, and ultimately the community served. It is truly a transformational model for nursing and healthcare.

KEY POINTS TO LEAD

1. Critique the history of credentialing and recognition of nursing excellence.
2. Explore important organizational elements that form the basis for a professional nursing practice environment.
3. Analyze in detail the ANA Scope and Standards for Nurse Administrators and how they can be used to create an infrastructure to support professional practice.
4. Assess the organization and nursing mission and vision for congruence with the Forces of Magnetism.
5. Conduct a gap analysis for ability to meet standards and tenets of the Magnet Recognition Program.
6. Assess factors to determine the decision to move forward with the Magnet journey to excellence.
7. Analyze research findings related to Magnet for incorporation into practice.

Literature Box

PROBLEM/PURPOSE

Research published regarding Magnet has examined primarily nurse job satisfaction and retention of nurses in the organization. The effectiveness of the nurse leaders in Magnet organizations has not been studied. The purpose of this study was to identify leadership qualities considered to be essential in today's healthcare settings. Specifically, the opinions of Magnet and non-Magnet nurse leaders were examined in the areas

of leadership traits, organizational structures, and methods for creation of a successful organization.

METHODOLOGY

An exploratory descriptive design was used that incorporated inductive and deductive content analysis techniques. Sixteen nurse leaders were selected from Magnet (M) and non-Magnet (NM) facilities. Tape-recorded interviews ranged from 60 to 90 minutes. A core set of questions,

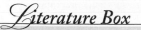
based on Magnet hospital literature and recommendations from expert nurse leaders, was formulated by the researcher. The interviews included one nurse leader per interview session and were informal with additional questions as needed for clarification. Content analysis was done with categories emerging from the data.

RESULTS

Magnet nurse leaders described their most consistent attributes as being honest, supportive, visible, accessible, positive, collaborative, and empowering; as possessing business acumen; and as being a good listener and a strong advocate for nursing. NM leaders delineated attributes as being credible, direct, self-assured, flexible, fair, passionate about nursing, accessible, knowledgeable, and having business sense. The two groups differed regarding their perception of the presence of elements that support professional nursing practice: supportive organizational climate (M = 86; NM = 67); collaborative nurse-physician relationships (M = 72; NM = 56); autonomous climate (M = 86; NM = 67); career ladders/

continuing education (M = 100; NM = 45); participatory management (M = 72; NM = 55); flexible schedules (M = 43; NM = 33).

CONCLUSIONS AND IMPLICATIONS

The researcher concluded that many of the traits identified by Magnet leaders reflect on their empowering and people-oriented skills and may indicate that Magnet facilities attract leaders with strong people skills. It also may be a reflection on the Magnet program standards and focus on the environment conducive to professional nursing practice. Differences existed in the presence of all elements identified as important for the success of an organization in supporting professional nursing practice by nurse leaders in Magnet and non-Magnet organizations. Challenges and organizational vision and priorities affect the ability to implement the elements considered important for a professional practice environment.

From Upenieks, V. V. (2003). What constitutes effective leadership? Perceptions of Magnet and nonmagnet nurse leaders. *Journal of Nursing Administration, 33,* 456-467.

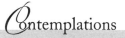
Contemplations

- What is the vision for the organization, nursing, and patient care services?
- What is the culture of the organization and nursing?
- Does the organization have an overarching focus on quality?
- Does an expectation exist for evidence-based practice and the conduct of research?
- Are there data collection systems in place with evaluation of data and action plans and follow-up on practice changes?
- Does the organization have a commitment to education and career development for both clinical and leadership positions? Is academic advancement encouraged?
- Are nurses encouraged and expected to practice autonomously?

- Does a cohesive, collaborative environment exist among departments and disciplines?
- Are policies and programs in place to address diversity of staff and patients?
- Do staff members have respect for each other's area of expertise, values, and experience?
- Do nurses deliver care through professional models?
- Are rewards and/or acknowledgements in place for excellence in care, outcomes, teamwork, and achievements?
- What stakeholders in the organization and external environment need to be brought into the discussion and implementation of systems and processes?

LEADER STORY

PAMELA KLAUER TRIOLO
CLINICAL PROFESSOR OF NURSING
DIRECTOR, NURSING LEADERSHIP AND
ADMINISTRATION IN HEALTH SYSTEMS
UNIVERSITY OF TEXAS HEALTH SCIENCE CENTER
AT HOUSTON, SCHOOL OF NURSING
HOUSTON, TEXAS

One of the main reasons I chose to come to the Methodist Hospital, Houston, Texas, in April of 1998 was because I was in search of a hospital that had the potential to be a Magnet hospital. It had been my dream for many years to take a hospital to Magnet status because I believed that this process was the path to a great nursing organization.

Early in the process while Methodist was recruiting me, when I talked with the physicians, directors, and staff, it was evident that people really valued the critical role of nursing in high-quality patient care. Nursing must be viewed as a key ingredient for success by the team. The medical staff is especially important. In my experience, two general cultures of medical staff exist: the culture in which physicians want to keep nurses in their place and the culture in which the medical staff seeks talented team members. The Methodist medical staff wanted the best nurses. Therefore a key ingredient in assessing a potential work culture are administrative and physician support for strong nursing services. Strong support from the managers and staff is critical for nursing to be the best. Methodist possessed those strengths.

Methodist was also in an environment that had a huge number of resources, a strong financial base, and academic connections to many schools of nursing. The Texas Medical Center is such a large and vibrant place and is the largest employer of nurses in the world. All of the key elements to achieve Magnet status were there.

When I went to Methodist, I began talking about what it might be like to be a Magnet facility,

"painting the picture" of what it would look and feel like and what nurses would be doing. I believe in the "planting seeds" leadership gardening metaphor, where you start with the seeds and develop the ground. It has to be a multifocal strategic path. To achieve Magnet status, we had to do a great deal of the development of the environment. When I arrived in 1998, we had no nursing governance and no leadership development. Few directors were prepared at the graduate level, the clinical ladder was outdated, performance management systems were based strictly on tenure, and the culture suffered from layoff survivor sickness.

While we conducted a gap analysis of the existing systems and infrastructure against the Magnet Standards, we did a lot of development of the environment. We found that although the values of "being the best" were there, the systems and programs to make Methodist a Magnet facility were not. So, we sent people to school. We developed a cohort of master's-prepared directors in 2 years (through the University of Texas Health Science Center–School of Nursing, Houston). We held educational programs for staff, and we encouraged them to go back to school. We obtained foundation funding for scholarships and innovative student programs. We dismantled the classic nursing education center and built what we called the "Center for Professional Excellence," which served as the hub for professional nursing practice. We were getting the environment ready for a more educated and skilled group of nurses. The foundation of our belief was that if you have the best nurses, you create the best patient care.

As the Chief Nurse Executive and Senior Vice President, my role was to lead by example, clearly articulate the vision, and communicate, communicate, communicate. So I did that through regular open forums with staff, rounds, letters to staff at home, talking to new orientees about expectations at Methodist, teaching CE programs and graduate courses, and reaching staff through the Nursing Intranet web site. We guided and pushed staff in terms of presentations and posters, joining and becoming active in professional organizations, applying evidence-based practice, getting them involved with research, and applying research at the unit level.

Medical staff members will say to you that nursing really began to change in April of 2001 when we launched our "pay for performance" strategy. I had been planting the seeds for this for some time, so when it happened, it was no surprise. It was time for a market correction in salaries, and the Texas Medical Center is a highly competitive place for nurses. So we conducted an analysis of every nurse on every unit, assessing to determine if a correlation existed between pay and performance. We looked at years of experience, performance rating, and salary and found to our dismay that no correlation existed. High-performing nurses were compensated poorly and some low-performing nurses were compensated highly. So instead of doing an across-the-board salary increase for all staff members as was done in the past, we did a staff-by-staff correction based on performance and compensation ratio. The bottom line was that high-performing staff got the increases and the lower performers got, in some cases, nothing. We believed in a consequence model to shape performance.

We continued the drive toward Magnet status, building programs and systems, even when Tropical Storm Allison crippled us in June of 2001. The flooding brought 40 vertical feet of water into our basements, knocking out power, food services, pharmacy, computers, elevators, water systems, and more. Once we evacuated 90% of our patients, although we lived without air conditioning for 6 weeks in the heat and humidity of a Houston summer, our nursing directors continued to collect and develop the documentation to submit our Magnet application in October of 2001. They rented a room and a computer at the Marriott, pulled up the soggy carpet, and kept at it.

Methodist became the fifty-fourth and second largest Magnet Hospital in July of 2002, the summer I was diagnosed with and began treatment for breast cancer. Although we celebrated our Magnet status with banners, parties, and a candlelight pinning ceremony in the chapel, the momentum built over the past 4 years continued to swell, and we increased the standards for nursing performance. We launched what we called a "visibility campaign" to encourage nurses to submit abstracts to key professional meetings and worked hard to nominate outstanding nurses for appropriate local and national awards. For 5 years in a row, District 5 of the Texas Nurses Association named a Methodist nurse in the ranks of the 20 Outstanding Nurses of the Year.

We believed that students were our future and we developed scholarship programs with five schools of nursing. We accepted students as juniors, assigned them to a specific unit, and groomed them for work as a graduate. The number of students in clinical experiences at Methodist rose to 660 and our summer student program, which started with 7 students, bloomed to 25 seniors from colleges all over the United States.

The crown jewel of our performance management, reward, and recognition model was finalized after we achieved Magnet status, the summer of 2003. This copyrighted model was called the Nursing Clinical Career Progression Model. The model is based on the philosophy that nursing is leadership, art, and science, and nursing progresses from novice to expert. So the model has five levels, is a differential practice model, and was designed to be a stretch model, which means that it was designed to take the staff into the future. In July of 2003, we also made the decision to hire only baccalaureate-prepared new graduates to increase the percentage of nurses with college degrees and improve the quality of our care.

The Nursing Clinical Career Progression Model starts with the Clinical Apprentice. This is for the new graduate or nurse new to the hospital. It is designed so that they are "cocooned" in support. The focus is on entrée in the complexity of urban, tertiary care. The plan for this level was to dovetail the model into the University Health System Consortium/American Association of Colleges of Nursing (UHC/AACN) residency that had been developed. From clinical apprentice, a nurse moves to clinical colleague, a full partner in care. When we transitioned all of our nurses to the model in 2003, many of our seasoned nurses chose to stay a clinical colleague versus moving up to clinical mentor, which required increasing work in the science of nursing, professional practice and certification, and development of others.

The fourth level of the model, clinical leader, requires a baccalaureate degree. When we launched the model in 2003, we believed that our nurses did not know how to practice at the clinical leader level, so we opened up only three levels. We realized that we would have to teach them how to do this new work. The fifth level of the model was the unit-based advanced practice nurse, clinical expert. This role was designed to support clinical teaching by nurses working clinically with students, conducting research, and serving as a master teacher and researcher. We saw clinical experts serving as nurse practitioners, nurse researchers, and adjunct clinical faculty.

Because we believed that the role of clinical nurse leader would transform care at the bedside

(we were simultaneously building our new patient care delivery model based on the philosophy of relationship centered care), we worked with the University of Texas Health Science Center, School of Nursing–Houston to design a 3-hour course that we would offer for graduate credit or CEUs to prepare this role. The clinical nurse leader was designed as the nurse at the bedside who would serve as the link between management and staff, sharing the global perspective of management issues (e.g., team builder, healthcare finance, organizational dynamics) and applying this knowledge in daily patient care at the bedside.

We launched the new course "Transforming Health Care through Clinical Nursing Leadership" in the spring of 2004 with 33 nurses from the Texas Medical Center. We used experts in the fields of finance, spiritual integrity at work, organizational performance improvement, and regulatory issues as guest teachers. As the primary faculty for this course, teaching them about leadership, team building, and global issues in nursing, I watched the lights come on in their eyes as they began to understand the "why" behind the "what" we needed from them in terms of patient care. We assessed their Myers-Briggs styles and oriented them to systems thinking through such simulations as "Friday Night in the ER," a learning game. Through application papers, they applied their learnings on the units, everything from improving physician relationships to analyzing supply costs. The transformation process was amazing and immensely rewarding.

Because renewal is a vital part of being a successful leader, in March of 2004, I left the Methodist Hospital for what one of my dear friends called my "sabbatical." I was healthy and at the peak of my career, but it was time to rest, reflect on what I wanted to do for the remainder of my career, and do many of the things that I had put off for 30 years: leisurely lunches with friends, improving my golf game, polishing my piano, and writing my mystery novel. As I look back on this chapter in my career life, I smile because we created all of these wonderful things for nurses through the talents of a great team and our love for nursing and each other. Now, my new career is devoted to creating future Magnet leaders, a new way to support talents, and love of the profession.

Chapter References

American Nurses Association. (2001). *Code of ethics for nurses with interpretive statements*. Washington, DC: The Association.

American Nurses Association. (2004). *Scope and standards for nurse administrators*. (2nd ed.). Washington, DC: The Association.

Havens, D. S. (2001). Comparing nursing infrastructure and outcomes: ANCC Magnet and nonMagnet CNEs report. *Nursing Economics, 19*(6), 258-266.

Laschinger, H. K. S., Almost, J., & Tuer-Hodes, D. (2003). Workplace empowerment and Magnet hospitals characteristics. *Journal of Nursing Administration, 33,* 410-422.

Magnet. (n.d.). Retrieved February 17, 2004, from http://nursecredentialing.org/ingworld.org/ancc/magnet/benes.html.

McClure M. L., & Hinshaw, A. S. (Eds.). (2002). *Magnet hospitals revisited*. Washington, DC: American Nurses Publishing.

McClure, M. L., Poulin, M. A., Sovie, M. D., & Wandelt, M. A. (2002). Magnet hospitals: Attraction and retention of professional nurses (the original study). In McClure, M. L., & Hinshaw, A. S. (Eds.), *Magnet hospitals revisited*. Washington, DC: American Nurses Publishing.

Scott, J. G., Sochalski, J., & Aiken, L. (1999). Review of Magnet hospital research. Findings and implications for professional nursing practice. *Journal of Nursing Administration, 29,* 9-19.

Upenieks, V. V. (2003). What constitutes effective leadership? Perceptions of Magnet and nonMagnet nurse leaders. *Journal of Nursing Administration, 33,* 456-467.

Urden, L. D., & Monarch, K. (2002). The ANCC Magnet recognition program: Converting research findings into action. In McClure, M. L., & Hinshaw, A. S. (Eds.), *Magnet hospitals revisited*. Washington, DC: American Nurses Publishing.

Journey to Excellence

THE MALCOLM BALDRIGE NATIONAL QUALITY AWARD

Sharon Donahue Hellwig

Kathleen Burke

It is not the strongest of the species that survive, or the most intelligent, but the one most responsive to change. CHARLES DARWIN

This chapter describes a comprehensive self-assessment process designed to drive change and continuous improvement in all sectors of a healthcare organization. The process, known as the Malcolm Baldrige National Quality Award assessment criteria, is a framework of core values and concepts that encourage organizations to use an integrated approach to improve organizational performance practices, capabilities, and results. The Baldrige philosophy and assessment criteria framework are described, along with examples from healthcare organizations that have earned the award.

HEALTHCARE ADMINISTRATORS, PRACTITIONERS, and payer organizations are faced with considerable challenges in the current environment. All are in search of strategies to ensure the provision of effective healthcare services in a time of increased customer expectations, diminishing resources, and intense competition. This search has led many in healthcare to look to the business community for new approaches that might be applied to healthcare. One such approach is the Malcolm Baldrige National Quality Award (MBQA) Program, which recognizes organizations for achievements in quality and performance. It is a national award managed by the National Institute of Standards and Technology (NIST), a part of the U.S. Department of Commerce. NIST participates in government/private sector relationships with a goal of assisting U.S. businesses to access the information and expertise necessary to improve their competitiveness in the national and global marketplace.

Healthcare organizations have found the MBQA criteria to be a useful tool in strengthening their performance by creating a performance improvement process driven by customers and data. The criteria offer a planned and integrated approach to quality improvement and a framework to assess and measure performance (Kaye & Anderson, 1999). It is based on the management philosophy of total quality management (TQM), a philosophy that has been adopted by the Joint Commission on Accreditation of Healthcare Organizations (JCAHO) and many successful healthcare organizations throughout the country (Perrott, 2002). TQM establishes a set of practices to ensure ongoing improvement. Proponents of this management philosophy claim that the principles of TQM applied through an organized, integrated system of continuous quality improvement (CQI) can be applied to any type of business or organization and will generate improved quality of products and services, reduce costs, create more satisfied customers and employees, and improve financial performance (Perrott, 2002). Activities necessary to ensure CQI, or performance improvement as it is more commonly known, are seen to include meeting customer needs, reducing rework, thinking long-range, increasing employee involvement and teamwork, valuing redesign and competitive benchmarking, solving problems, measuring results, and building closer relationships with suppliers (Powell, 1995).

The MBQA criteria, based on the TQM philosophy that drives continuous improvements, contrast dramatically with the quality assurance (QA) approach historically used in healthcare. The Baldrige criteria are a comprehensive self-evaluation tool designed to drive change and continuous improvement in all sectors of the organization, whereas QA is intended to meet mandatory and often minimum standards set by outside auditors. QA uses the audit method to collect large amounts of data and provide a snapshot of how things happened in the past. The concern, however, was that it lacked a mechanism for finding the root cause of problems. QA represented a circular approach of monitoring, evaluating, and remonitoring. In traditional QA, an arbitrary threshold for compliance set the bar at average and maintained business as usual. "A compliance audit that revealed no significant non conformances was considered a success, while a Baldrige assessment that reveals no opportunities for improvement is considered a failure" (Hutton, 2000, p. 603).

The traditional QA approach provided only part of the solution to quality improvement because it did not complete the improvement loop by providing a mechanism for finding the root cause of a problem or for the creation of improvement strategies. TQM, by contrast, is a management structure that creates the organizational culture of individual empowerment. When TQM is combined with CQI, a process that uses the tools and techniques of data collection to analyze a process and develop an improvement plan, a systematic process for achieving sustained organizational improvement emerges.

HISTORY OF BALDRIGE

In the mid-1980s, CQI was introduced to healthcare through the work of three physicians: Paul Batalden, Donald Berwick, and Brent James. All followed the quality philosophy of W. Edward Deming, which was designed to transform organizations. An approach designed by Deming is known as **FOCUS-PDCA:**

Find a process to improve
Organize a team that knows the process
Clarify current knowledge of the process
Understand causes of process variation
Select the process improvement
Plan-**D**o-**C**heck-**A**ct cycle

This approach is used today by many healthcare organizations to provide a common language and an orderly sequence for implementation of the cycle of continuous improvement (McLaughlin & Kaluzny, 1999).

In the early 1990s, groups, particularly from large employers in the business community who were besieged with increasing costs of annual healthcare premiums, were interested in supporting healthcare organizations in their efforts to become more efficient and effective. The principles embodied in the MBQA were seen as aligning with the dual challenges of performance improvement and cost containment in healthcare (Hertz, Reimann, & Bostwick, 1994).

The MBQA is the highest level of national recognition for quality that a U.S. company can receive. The award was created by an act of Congress in 1987 and named for Malcolm Baldrige, the twenty-sixth U.S. Secretary of Commerce. Initially awards were given in three categories: manufacturing, service, and small business.

The early service organization winners, such as the Ritz Carlton Hotel Company, L.L.C. (in 1992 and 1999), created customer-focused best practices in many areas related to service. For example, many healthcare organizations have benchmarked the hotel room food preparation and delivery processes to assist them in the improvement of patient satisfaction with hospital food. In 1995 a successful Baldrige Health Care Pilot Study resulted in establishing a healthcare award category in 1999. The first Baldrige Health Care Award was granted in 2003.

THE AWARD

The award criteria known as the "criteria for performance excellence" create a common language for quality measurement and a framework for performance management and improvement. The seven basic criteria are designed to help organizations enhance their competitiveness by focusing on two goals: delivering ever-improving value to customers and improving overall organizational performance. The Baldrige measurement system is simple and complex, because it asks the organization to define itself and to demonstrate that it does what it says it is doing. The beauty of the criteria is that they offer organizations a cost-effective, system-wide self-assessment and education process encompassed within an award.

The underlying philosophy of the MBQA is much more than an award competition. It is intended to give American businesses a roadmap that can lead the way to achieving performance excellence (Berglund, 2001). Using data from 220 hospitals, Mayer and Collier (2001) tested the causal relationships in the Health Care

Pilot criteria. The findings supported that many of the hypothesized causal relationships in the Baldrige model were statistically significant. Four healthcare organizations earning a national MBQA were SSM Health Care (SSMHC, 2002), based in St. Louis, Missouri (see Literature Box at the end of the chapter); Baptist Hospital, Inc. (BHI, 2003), a subsidiary of Baptist Health Care that includes two hospitals in Florida; Saint Luke's Hospital (SLH) of Kansas City, Missouri (2003); and Robert Wood Johnson University Hospital Hamilton of New Jersey (2004).*

BALDRIGE INDEX

Considerable evidence exists to show that adopting the Baldrige criteria as a way of doing business leads to business success. The Department of Commerce completed periodic studies to determine if Baldrige-winning companies achieved greater financial success. The "Baldrige Index," a hypothetical stock fund comprising U.S. companies that received the MBQA, has historically outperformed the Standard & Poor's 500 by approximately four to one (Fisher, Dauterive, & Barfield, 2001). These studies demonstrate that the Baldrige approach to quality management and performance improvement increases the chances of achieving high performance (Hutton, 2000).

The MBQA is based on an organizational assessment reflective of established criteria. The healthcare criteria have three vital roles in strengthening healthcare competitiveness (Baldrige National Quality Program, 2005, p. 1):

1. To help improve organizational performance practices, capabilities, and results
2. To facilitate communication and sharing of best practice information among

---

*Baldrige award winners are listed at http://www.baldrige.nist.gov/Award_Recipients.htm.

healthcare organizations and among U.S. organizations of all types
3. To serve as a working tool for understanding and managing performance and for guiding organizational planning and opportunities for learning

BALDRIGE CRITERIA

The Baldrige criteria comprise a framework of core values and concepts that encourage organizations to use an integrated approach to improve organizational performance management. The Health Care criteria specifically are designed to assist organizations in the following:

- Delivery of ever-improving value to patients and other customers, contributing to overall healthcare quality
- Improvement of overall organizational effectiveness and capabilities as a healthcare provider
- Organizational and personal learning

Health Care criteria are built on the interrelated core values and concepts found in Table 3-1 (Baldrige National Quality Program, 2005, p. 1).

The systems perspective is listed in Table 3-2. The driver is senior leadership's focus on strategic directions and on patients and other customers and markets. It means that the senior leaders monitor, respond to, and manage performance based on organizational results. Systems alignment includes using measures/indicators to link the organization's key strategies with their key processes and to align resources for the improvement of overall performance. A systems perspective means managing the whole organization and its components to achieve excellence.

Organizations that earn an MBQA complete a three-part application process beginning with a 50-page application. The company submits a five-page profile of the organization. This profile is critically important because it sets the stage for the whole assessment process. It gives a snapshot of the organization and provides information about elements important to the organization, the competitive environment, strategic challenges, and performance improvement system. The examiners and judges use it in all stages of the application review.*

The MBQA criteria are divided into seven interrelated categories. Figure 3-1 illustrates how the categories contribute to each other.

The Health Care criteria are a set of 19 performance-related requirements divided into seven categories:

1. Leadership (120 points)
2. Strategic planning (85 points)
3. Focus on patients, other customers, and markets (85 points)
4. Measurement, analysis, and knowledge management (90 points)
5. Staff focus (85 points)
6. Process management (85 points)
7. Organizational performance results (450 points)

Points are assigned for scoring MBQA applicants, and the point values reflect the importance of the item in the overall view of the organization. The fact that category 7, organizational results, has such a high point value clearly indicates the significance of the JCAHO (1999) question, "What did the organization actually achieve?"

Category 7 is concerned with *results*. The factors used to evaluate results include the current performance, the performance relative to appropriate benchmarks, rate and breadth of the performance improvements, and the linkage of the results to the important patient care, healthcare market, and process and action plan requirements identified as important to the organization.

An Updated Plan-Do-Check-Act Cycle

The Baldrige criteria are not prescriptive and are adaptable to the particular culture of the individual

---

*For further information about the application process, refer to the following web site: http://www.baldrige.nist.gov.

Table 3-1 BALDRIGE HEALTH CARE CRITERIA

Baldrige Core Values	Examples
Visionary leadership	Senior leaders set direction, values, and high expectations; serve as role models; communicate; plan; and demonstrate ethical behavior.
Patient-focused care	The quality and performance of the care delivered to patients are key determinants of patient satisfaction; patient-focused excellence demands an awareness of emerging patient populations and needs.
Organizational and personal learning	Learning includes a proactive approach, continuous improvement, and adaptation of change leading to new goals and approaches.
Valuing staff and partners	An organization commits to the growth, satisfaction, well-being, skill development, and flexible high-performance work practices of staff. Internal (e.g., unions) and external partnerships (e.g., preferred relationship with supplier of OR instrumentation) are needed to allow the organization to better accomplish strategic goals.
Agility	The organization has the ability to rapidly respond to the changing healthcare environment with the timely design/redesign of healthcare delivery systems.
Focus on future	The assessment system is focused on healthcare outcomes resulting in evidence-based practice and the proactive development of all stakeholders. Continuous movement forward is implied.
Managing for innovation	Innovation and adaptation to continuous growth is a part of the daily culture of this healthcare organization.
Management by fact	The actual performance of the organization in areas of healthcare outcomes, community health, epidemiologic data, clinical pathways, practice guidelines, staff competencies, cost, and financial performance provide the information for the strategic plan.
Social responsibility and community health	Organizations must meet all local, state, and federal laws and regulatory requirements and must demonstrate ethical behavior and responsibility to the community.
Focus on results and creating value	The key question for the organization becomes, "How well did the organization actually do and of what value was the performance?"
Systems perspective	An integrated systematic perspective is in place for the entire healthcare organization.

Modified from Baldrige National Quality Program, 2005, pp. 2-4.

organization. The first six categories are considered *process* items, in which the organization is asked, "What is the overall *approach* that you use to meet the criteria requirements?" The factors used to evaluate *approach* items include (1) the appropriateness of the methods to the requirements; (2) the effectiveness of use of the methods and the degree to which the *approach* is repeatable and consistently applied, the embodiment of

evaluation/improvement/learning cycles, and the basis of reliable information and data; (3) alignment with the organizational needs; and (4) evidence of beneficial innovation and change.

Deployment refers to the extent that the *approach* is applied throughout the organization. Beyond determining how an organization establishes an *approach* and actually *deploys* it, the Baldrige philosophy focuses on process and

Table 3-2 The Baldrige Health Care Criteria as a System

Input	Identification of customers and their needs
Driver	Mission, vision, values, and leadership
Data measures	Define desired outcomes and collect data
	Develop strategic planning process
Processes/ systems	Ensure customer satisfaction
	Create systems that promote staff
	Manage processes for improvement
Results	Achieve organizational performance results

organizational improvement *(learning)* and *integration* with other organizational initiatives. These four factors, Approach, Deployment, Learning, and Integration (ADLI), may be viewed as an updated Plan-Do-Check-Act (PDCA) cycle (Baldrige National Quality Program, 2004, p. 59).

Category 1: Leadership

In the leadership category senior leadership's central role in setting the direction of the organization is examined. Senior leadership is composed of the head of the organization and the leadership team. These leaders are viewed as the drivers of the entire quality process. The chief nursing officer, as a member of the senior leadership team, plays an important role in achieving the goals of this category.

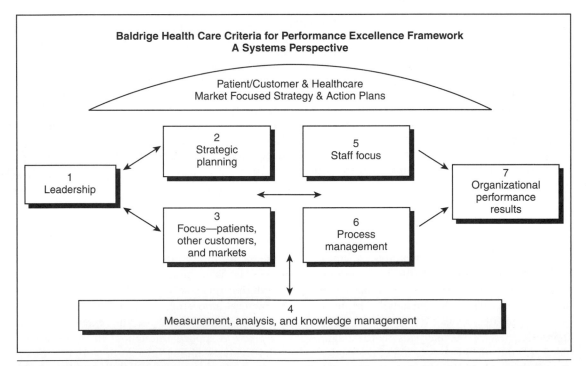

Figure 3-1 Baldrige Health Care Criteria for Performance Excellence Framework. (Reprinted with permission of Malcolm Baldrige Award.)

This category examines the role of senior leadership in guiding the organization to define organizational values and set direction and performance expectations. It addresses how senior leadership creates an environment of empowerment, employee learning, innovation, and organizational agility. Increasingly this requires creation of a means for rapid and effective application of knowledge. The organization's governance and how the organization addresses its public and community responsibilities also are examined. For example, at BHI, an MBQA recipient, community responsibility was demonstrated in revenue allocation to indigent patients. In one fiscal year, 6.7% of its total revenue was dedicated to the care of indigent patients compared with 5.2% and 4% for its competitors (Baldrige Award Recipients, 2003).

Attention is given to how senior leaders communicate with employees, review organizational performance, and create an environment that encourages high performance. The criteria address such questions as the following:

- How do the senior leaders become actively involved in communicating the vision, mission, and values of the organization to employees?
- How do senior leaders support employee participation in performance improvement at all levels of the organization?
- Do leaders "walk the talk"?
- What percent of leaders' time is spent in performance improvement activities?
- Do the leaders demonstrate that they are the champions of the quality process?

An example of how senior leaders support employee involvement can be seen at SSMHC, another MBQA winner. Nearly 3000 employees and physicians participated in focus groups across the system to define a more concise and memorable mission statement, "*Through our exceptional health care services, we reveal the healing presence of God.*" A "Meeting in a Box" tool kit was designed, to include a video, brochures, and pocket cards used to facilitate consistent deployment and

reinforcement of the mission and core values (Dunn & Santamour, 2003).

Similarities exist between the Magnet Recognition Program™ (ANCC, 2004) (see Chapter 2) and the MBQA Program particularly in the area of leadership. The Baldrige leadership criterion focuses in part on examining how senior leaders create an environment of empowerment, innovation, and employee learning. The shared governance practice model used by many Magnet healthcare organizations aligns with the Baldrige philosophy in building a management structure that creates ownership and accountability for patient care at the bedside.

Category 2: Strategic Planning

Category 2, strategic planning, assesses the organization's method of preparing for the future. It has a dual focus: strategy development and strategy deployment. It examines how the organization sets strategic direction and how it develops key strategies, plans, and goals needed to succeed in the increasingly complex environment of healthcare. The vision, mission, and values of the organization are the framework for the strategic planning process. The vision is the starting point, a step into the future to capture what a leader wants to have happen. It is the root of long-term and short-term goals and objectives from which success can be measured. The values are the foundation of the business strategy, they determine how actions are prioritized, and they influence all the business decisions. In addition, this criterion focuses on how the organization converts its strategic objectives into action plans and deploys the plans throughout the organization to achieve the key strategic objectives. Key here is evidence of a proactive approach in aligning the organization's capabilities with external opportunities. At BHI, for example, the core strategies are people, service, quality, finances, and growth. Specific strategies for each of these core strategies have been identified along with specific action goals for each of the strategies. Their strategic plan identifies system goals that cascade into leader goals, 90-day action plans, senior management priorities, and budgets.* BHI's senior management priorities and budgets are then cascaded throughout all levels of the organization.

Leggitt and Anderson (2001) noted, by contrast, that most healthcare organizations undertake a strategic planning process on an annual basis. A typical plan might assign ownership of a specific strategic goal to an individual or small group. Yet rarely do individual department goals or employee goals align with each other's or the strategic goals of the organization. This alignment of goals throughout the organization is an important component of the Baldrige philosophy. An example of goal deployment to the level of each employee is SSMHC's "Passport to Exceptional Health Care Services," a program designed to deploy strategic goals and action plans to all employees and align network, entity, department, and individual plans with overall organizational strategy. Each employee carries a "passport card" that spells out the system's mission and values and the individual employee's goals that link to the system's goals.

Accomplishment of action plans requires resources and performance measures, in addition to the alignment of department, supplier, and partner plans. Each department must identify the priorities and ongoing improvement activities needed to support the strategic objectives. In addition, human resource plans to support the new strategic objectives must be identified clearly. These could be, for example, the initiatives that have been developed to foster knowledge sharing and organizational learning, the changes in the compensation and recognition systems to acknowledge the work of teams, or the educational and training designed to support new initiatives.

The strategic planning process also must evidence a proactive approach in aligning organizational capabilities with external opportunities (Baldrige National Quality Program, 2004).

*http://www.nist.gov/public_affairs/releases/bhitrauma.htm

This requires that the organization have a capacity for rapid change and flexibility to manage the ever-shorter cycles for introductions of new healthcare services. The essence of the strategic planning process is *choosing the right things to do.*

Category 3: Focus on Patients, Other Customers, and Markets

This category focuses on how the organization seeks to understand the expectations and requirements of patients, other customers (e.g., physicians, healthcare insurers, suppliers, families, and community members), and the marketplace. Patients are identified separately from other customers in this criterion. The organization identifies what is important to the customer. The focus is also on features that affect healthcare-related loyalty and customer perception of clinical and service quality. For example, the perception of clinical excellence is important for patients willing to travel a distance for hospitalization at one of "America's Best Hospitals." Patient rooms with Internet access may be of importance to the high-powered executive and family who choose a particular hospital for elective surgery. Other patient-centered features may include assistance with billing paperwork and extended visiting hours. Rapid bill payment for suppliers and rapid turnaround on billing for insurance payers may be examples of service quality important to other customers.

This criterion also looks at the ways that the organization remains current and future oriented in the marketplace. A hospital that supplies limited maternal-child services may note an anticipated increase in the number of young families in the area upon review of the current and projected census data for its market locale. Such information might then lead to a change in the maternal-child services to meet the projected need of the changing community. Conversely, as a population ages, demographic data may suggest that an organization needs to expand services focused on an aging population.

Nationwide, nurses have become familiar with the focus on patient satisfaction and the measures used to collect such information. The most recognized surveys used in the determination of patient satisfaction are the surveys designed by the Press Ganey organization (Press Ganey, 2004). High patient satisfaction levels are of particular importance in areas characterized by competition for patients. When patients have a choice of hospitals, they most often will choose the institution where they have had a good experience or one that has been positively referenced by a friend or colleague. This relationship building results in patient loyalty, an important component in a competitive environment.

This part of the criteria reviews the methods used to determine the patient satisfaction of the various segments of patients in the institution (e.g., outpatient, inpatient, elective, or the emergency department) and the selection of the tools used to collect the data. As with the other criteria, the focus needs to be current and future oriented.

Category 4: Measurement and Analysis of Organizational Performance

As shown in Figure 3-1, category 4 is the underlying support for all criteria. This category evaluates the selection, use, and improvement of all performance and organizational data, information, and knowledge assets. Central to the Baldrige core value is management by fact. Such fact-based decision making requires thoughtful selection, collection, and integration of data. Organizations claim the existence of an overload of information collected and available on a daily basis. As Wilson and Porter-O'Grady (1999) have said, it is not the "quantity of information but the prevalence of misinformation that is the problem. If you are getting the right information, you can never get enough of it" (p. 5).

The organization leaders are asked to describe how they measure, analyze, and improve performance data as a healthcare provider at all levels and in all parts of the organization (Baldrige National Quality Program, 2005, p. 23). Nurses are familiar with the collection of the nursing sensitive indicators (Gallagher & Rowell, 2003). Indicators about skill mix, nursing hours per patient day, pressure ulcers, falls, patient satisfaction with overall care, patient satisfaction with nursing care, patient satisfaction with pain management, patient satisfaction with education, nosocomial infection rate, and staff satisfaction offer the nursing administrator the opportunity to evaluate the nursing care within and across the organization. Reporting unit-specific and organization-specific results on nursing sensitive indicators offers nursing administrators a way to assess department and unit progress toward strategic goals (Gallagher & Rowell, 2003).

Goal performance also requires the use of comparative data. These data are obtained by benchmarking and also by seeking competitive comparisons. The patient satisfaction data are ranked in terms of similar institutions in the region and nation. Such comparative information is also available for other areas of performance. Financial market share is compared with the local competitors. Pay rates and employee satisfaction are compared with the local and regional competition. Length of stay data and clinical performance outcomes also are benchmarked in this competitive environment. Measures of performance in other healthcare processes, such as time in the admission process, waiting time for clinic appointments, and lag time for billing, also can be related to the comparative data. In this highly competitive market, healthcare institutions are concerned with how their performance relates to local competition and to those organizations identified as "Best in Class."

Although the proper information and analyses for organizational decision making are imperative, the timing of the availability of the data also is vital. Patient satisfaction data that are 3 months old are of little value in analysis of a current situation. Equally important to having accurate, reliable, and secure data is having those data meet all confidentiality requirements of the regulators.

The timeliness of all data sets is of utmost importance in a rapid improvement cycle. Proper individuals or groups of individuals must have the information necessary for them to work and improve. For example, patient satisfaction data for the operating room is probably of little value to the oncology unit.

In this time of information overload, another part of this criterion evaluates how the organization maintains the currency of the data and information collected and analyzed. This includes the evaluation of the data and information collected for alignment with organizational plans. If information is no longer necessary, it does not need to be collected. Conversely, if a new organizational goal requires different comparative information, it needs to be selected, collected, and analyzed. The continuous evaluation of the appropriateness of data/information available to the organization needs to be part of the continuous improvement process.

Category 5: Staff Focus

The staff focus is directed toward those practices that create and maintain a high-performance workplace. A high-performance workplace reflects the core Baldrige value of agility. An agile workplace requires a staff empowered to adapt to change. An agile staff is the result of an organization that gives staff the necessary information to improve their outcomes in relation to those of the organization.

High-performance work is characterized by flexibility, innovation, knowledge, and skill sharing. Skill sharing is especially important in an environment of continuous improvement. One unit may have found that a change in new RN orientation resulted in a more satisfactory experience for the new RN and that the new employee turnover rate on that unit decreased. If this "lesson learned" is not shared with the other patient care units, the improvement will not be seen across the institution.

High-performance work systems in healthcare also are characterized by shifting more decisions down the organization's hierarchy to the level of ownership of the decision: for example, staff nurses in an ICU making changes in the visiting hours for their unit. Nurses working in organizations with decentralized decision making reported higher commitment to the organization and a significantly lower intent to leave (Gifford, Zammuto, & Goodman, 2002). Rousseau and Tijoriwala found preconditions for the implementation of such decision making include a relationship of trust between senior leadership and staff (as cited in Page, 2004), thus emphasizing the interconnectedness of the leadership category and the staff focus category.

The criterion also looks at staff learning and motivation. The manner in which the organization meets the ongoing needs for staff licensure, education, and credentialing and the manner in which they encourage career development lead to the success of the organization in its creation of a high-performing workplace. This is alignment of the organization goals, the unit/department goals, and individual employee goals.

Staff well-being and satisfaction activities are included in this category. Healthcare organizations are different than many of the other business organizations in that their operations continue all day every day with a diverse workforce spread across many shifts. This segmentation of staff is important in review of staff well-being and satisfaction issues and approaches. The employees working the night shift may have very different satisfaction issues than the day shift. Staff parking may be an issue of great concern to the day and evening shift workers, whereas the night shift may identify the lack of employee food service as a satisfaction issue. A strong staff focus assists the organization in alignment of organization, department-specific, and individual goals.

Category 6: Process Management

This criterion examines the major aspects of the organization's process management in all departments and work units. The concept of process management is one of the most difficult areas to understand for individuals who do not work in manufacturing areas. In manufacturing, the process of producing a "widget" usually follows a well-defined sequence of activities, whereby a "widget" eventually is produced. In healthcare the term *process* refers to linked activities with the purpose of producing a service for patients (Baldrige National Quality Program, 2005, p. 38).

Process management in healthcare is concerned with two major issues: (1) the way in which the organization identifies and manages its key processes for the delivery of patient healthcare services and (2) the manner in which the organization identifies and manages the key business and other processes that support the overall healthcare processes. In some instances processes may require a specific sequence of activities with documentation of procedures and requirements, some of which may have defined measurement and control steps. An example of such a process would be the steps involved in the interpretation of a laboratory specimen. In healthcare, processes include a preferred sequence of events such as a clinical pathway, or the "process" of admitting a patient.

The overall process of patient care is affected by the actual operation of key processes. Length of stay is a major issue for healthcare institutions across the country. The length of stay outcome has direct correlation with the financial results of most institutions. This issue is affected by a wide variety of delivery of healthcare and support processes. Examples of delivery of healthcare processes are physician ordering, the process of progressing a patient from pre-admission to discharge, the process of transferring a patient from unit to unit, and the delivery of meals. Examples of support processes that affect the length of stay variable are the acquisition of the newest technology, medical record-keeping processes, the processes of billing and submission to payers, and the process of hiring and orienting qualified personnel.

This criterion examines how the organization identifies and shares best practices. Magnet hospitals routinely share the best practices that make the nursing practice of their organization "best in class." On an internal level, the organization must share best practice or lessons learned with all areas of the institution. An example would be with an employee satisfaction survey that listed "lack of supplies" as a major concern. Individual departments were encouraged to develop their own processes for ordering supplies. Upon a repeat survey, the satisfaction rates increased, but the results were not segmented to reflect individual departments. Such an implementation did not allow for a determination of which action plans succeeded and for a sharing of the successes.

As with all areas of the Baldrige evaluation, the manner in which the organization defines, manages, improves, and keeps all processes current is of the utmost importance in evaluation of the continued growth of the organization.

Category 7: Organizational Performance Results

As the point value of this criterion (450 points out of a total of 1000) suggests, this is the most important of all categories. It is no longer enough to see what the organization is doing or planning on doing; what they actually have done and how well it was done are what is important. The measure of quality of performance requires a comparative analysis or benchmarking. The Baldrige Award requires a maturity of both *approach* and *results,* so a number of cycles of improvement are required. Being able to ascertain that the improvements can be replicated on a continuous basis is important. Seeing a single improvement is not enough. Rather a pattern of improvement and continual growth must emerge. The Baldrige criteria form the framework for a continual culture of data-driven, future-oriented growth.

The results reported here include healthcare results; patient- and other customer–focused results; financial and market results; staff and work system results; and organizational effectiveness results.

Healthcare Results

Healthcare results, as reported by SLH of Kansas City, Missouri, are one example. Because SLH is a tertiary care, level one trauma center, it provides care to the sickest types of patients. The high severity of illness affects all healthcare outcomes, such as mortality, length of stay, and infections. Sicker patients tend to stay longer and require more resources to be expended in their care. These factors come into play in comparison of SLH performance against that of other organizations. Table 3-3 shows that SLH patients are considerably sicker than patients of any other area hospital, with a severity index of 257 compared with the metro average of 100. At the same time, SLH's mortality and length of stay results show that it is among the best performers, despite the high severity index.

Patient- and Other Customer–Focused Results

Patient- and other customer–focused results are reflected in this material reported by SLH. They reported that Consumer's Checkbook, a consumer education organization, ranked their hospital thirty-fifth in the nation, out of 4500 evaluated. SLH received an overall score of 7669 compared with the national average of 5418. The similar rating for SLH physicians was 86% compared with a national average of 33%.

An example of patient satisfaction results, reported by SSMHC in their award-winning application, indicates a strong degree of satisfaction (Figure 3-2). The systemwide patient satisfaction and loyalty survey process provides in-depth insight into the needs and requirements of SSMHC's patients. Loyalty is a key measure for SSMHC, because it indicates a patient's willingness to recommend services. Inpatient loyalty is a system-level indicator of exceptional patient satisfaction. A word-of-mouth referral from a friend or neighbor is a key factor in a person's selection of a healthcare provider. Loyalty is calculated monthly from patient satisfaction survey responses for inpatients, emergency department patients, outpatient surgery patients, and home care patients. Long-term care (nursing home) satisfaction is assessed annually. The loyalty indices are calculated from key summary questions in the surveys addressing the respondents' overall satisfaction, willingness to recommend to others, and overall performance relative to their expectations.

Respondents are placed into one of three categories: "loyal," "in-play," and "at risk." SSMHC uses impact analysis to engage in process improvements

Table 3-3 Medicare Marketplace Comparison: Top Competitors

Hospital	RDRG Severity Index			ALOS Index			Mortality Index		
	1999	2000	2001	1999	2000	2001	1999	2000	2001
SLH	293	290	257	99	98	96	88	91	82
HOSP B	175	173	180	107	87	80	105	84	76
HOSP C	186	197	201	127	98	99	126	101	102
HOSP D	242	228	214	97	98	102	119	113	122
HOSP E	113	116	120	109	109	117	90	83	78
HOSP F	124	113	109	115	99	112	106	88	135
HOSP G	141	142	127	137	109	115	117	101	118

Source: Solucient Sachs.
Used with permission from http://www.baldrige.nist.gov/PDF_files/Saint_Lukes_Application_Summary.pdf.
RDRG, Refined diagnosis related groups; *ALOS,* average length of stay.

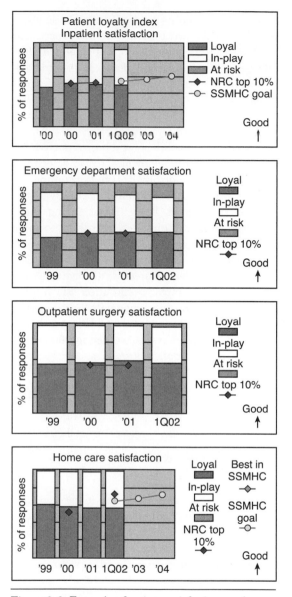

Figure 3-2 Example of patient satisfaction results. (Used with permission from SSM Health Care, St. Louis, MO.)

to increase "loyal" and decrease "at risk" and "in-play" respondents. *Loyal* refers to those respondents who are very highly satisfied, very willing to recommend, and found the service to be more than they expected. *In-play* refers to those respondents who give inconsistent ratings, neither high nor low, to the summary questions. *At-risk* refers to respondents who were dissatisfied, not willing to recommend, and found the service to be less than expected. National benchmarks for patient loyalty are taken from the NRC *Health Care Market Guide*. SSMHC uses the scores of hospitals performing in NRC's top 10% (best in class). SSMHC inpatient loyalty increased from 47.5% in 1999 to 50.0% in 2001, nearing NRC's top 10% national benchmark of 51.6%. In 2000 and 2001, SSMHC ranked above the national benchmarks for patient loyalty in emergency department services, outpatient surgery, and home care.

Financial and Market Results

Financial and market results reported by SSMHC indicated the following "cash on hand" results (Figure 3-3). SSMHC maintained an average of 211 days' cash on hand while increasing capital spending throughout the system. The reliance on government payers greatly reduces SSMHC's ability to manage the timing of payments effectively. The reduction of 9 days in accounts receivable in 2001 represents $36 million in additional cash on hand. Not-for-profit healthcare providers are dependent upon their own financial

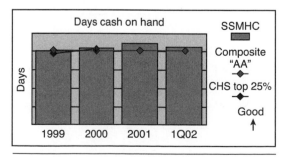

Figure 3-3 "Cash on hand" results. (Used with permission from SSM Health Care, St. Louis, MO.)

outcomes to fund their capital needs, because the stock markets are unavailable to them. SSMHC is the industry benchmark for AA-rated health systems.

Staff and Work System Results

Staff and work system results serve as an evaluation of the organization's work system performance, staff learning and development, and staff well-being and satisfaction. BHI reported: The employee turnover rate has improved at BHI from 27% in 1997 to 13.9% in 2003 and Gulf Breeze Hospital (GBH) has improved from 31% in 1997 to 14% in 2003. These levels for both hospitals are more favorable than the northwest Florida average and the national average and are at the best-in-class level (Baldrige Award Recipient Profile, 2003).

Organizational Effectiveness Results

Organizational effectiveness results encourage the organization to develop unique, innovative, and organization-specific measures and results. SSMHC shows a result in this area in Figure 3-4. Despite significant growth in volume, SSMHC has engaged in a disciplined approach to staffing and, as a result, has been able to manage successfully paid hours per adjusted patient day at a slower rate of increase than the increase in patient volume. This has resulted in efficiencies in staffing while accommodating volume growth

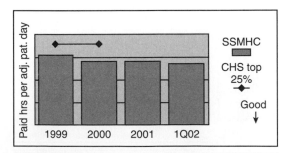

Figure 3-4 Paid hours per adjusted patient day. (Used with permission from SSM Health Care, St. Louis, MO.)

without compromising patient care. Productivity is managed daily at SSMHC at the department level to better predict and anticipate volume changes that affect staffing needs. Improved daily management resulting from more stringent monitoring has contributed to SSMHC's ability to manage this critical component of expense management.

Social responsibility results, reported by BHI, illustrate this element. Health screenings and physicals provided by BHI to the community are increasing. For example, through the HeartFirst program, heart risk screenings have increased from 1100 in fiscal year 2000 to more than 2400 in fiscal year 2003. BHI's new Women's Heart Advantage program was established to improve awareness of heart disease among women, provide education on healthy lifestyles, and provide women with easy access to cardiac testing and treatment. BHI's goal was to provide 2500 screenings to women in 2003.

All of these sample reported results areas cross all aspects of the organization. All of these results have a part in the other six categories. This is the systematic integrated approach of the Baldrige criteria.

ROLE OF NURSING LEADERSHIP

The achievement of CQI is not an easy process. The essential ingredient is leadership commitment. Successful leaders must have a vision that has its origins in a commitment to quality. Leadership's responsibility is to ensure that this quality vision is firmly embedded in the culture of the organization (Scarnati & Scarnati, 2002). Employees will embrace the quality process if they know how their department and their personal work contribute to the direction set by the leaders of the organization (Leggitt & Anderson, 2001).

Future leaders of healthcare need the skill sets to manage and lead in an increasingly competitive environment, an environment in which change happens at an accelerated pace and the competition is located not only down the street but also in other states and nations. Vokurka (2001, p. 364) described the skill transitions required of individuals in the future as moving from "functional expertise to cross-functional expertise; decision making based on experience and knowledge to data-based decision making and analytical skills; and supervisory skills to team development skills." Future leaders must relinquish (or not acquire) the autocratic leadership practices of the past and work through others to achieve the goals of the organization. Leaders must empower employees at every level to take ownership in the outcome of their work and have a vested interest in the organization's success (Scarnati & Scarnati, 2002).

SUMMARY

Organizations interested in using the Baldrige framework to improve performance practices, capabilities, and results can begin the journey by becoming involved in their regional or state quality award process. Many states have Baldrige-based state quality awards, sometimes called "baby Baldriges." States that offer the awards generally provide education and training programs to assist organizations in completion of the self-assessment and evaluation. State and regional awards provide an excellent introduction to the Baldrige criteria and self-assessment process. The MBQA offers a free self-assessment tool, *Are We Making Progress,* on its web site.* Beginning any journey to quality helps organizations remain relevant to changing needs. Achieving the Baldrige award conveys high success in this venture.

KEY POINTS TO LEAD

1. Critique the development of the MBQA.
2. Analyze the criteria for the award and how they can be used to create an infrastructure to support professional practice.
3. Assess the organization and nursing mission and vision to see where the strengths and limitations are so that these areas can be addressed for congruence with the award itself.

*http://www.baldrige.nist.gov/Progress.htm

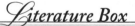

Literature Box

This interview with the CEO, Sister Mary Jean Ryan, who is also a registered nurse, highlights how SSMHC began applying for the Baldrige award in 1999 and was unsuccessful. One of the comments related to the fact that the system had not defined exceptional healthcare services, which is in the mission statement. According to Sister Mary Jean, this was a wake-up call.

To redirect the energy in the organization, everyone focused on improvement. The work ahead was viewed as an opportunity to do a self-examination and create goals for improvement. Even in the year SSMHC was successful, they received 100 pages of recommendations for improvement. Achieving the Baldrige award was a journey toward excellence.

One example of exceptional work is the Passport Program, which carries the strategic plan for the system all the way to the individual employee. This activity ensures alignment of individual goals with the overall system goals.

The focus on quality has allowed the organization to create stretch goals and to create a blame-free environment. Finally, the Career Development Program is a system that supports succession planning.

Each of these activities leads to improvement in the organization with the goal of ensuring excellence.

Smith, A. P. (2003). Magnet and Baldrige: SSM Health Care's journey for excellence (Part I of II). *Nursing Economics, 21*(2), 71-74, 93.

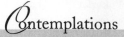

Contemplations

- How does the nurse executive ensure that employees represent diverse ideas, cultures, and thinking?
- How does the nurse executive provide for effective succession planning for leadership and management positions?
- How does the nurse executive translate organizational performance review findings into breakthrough improvement and opportunities for innovation?
- In an increasingly competitive healthcare marketplace, how does the nurse executive determine which customer groups and market segments to pursue for future services?
- Agility, cost, and cycle time reduction are increasingly important in the management of key patient care processes. How does the nurse executive develop key measures for tracking these aspects of key processes?
- Increasingly organizations interact with customers through a variety of "real time" listening and learning methods. What methods do nurse executives employ to determine key customer requirements and changing expectations for services and products?
- What is the nurse executive's role relating to current trends of work system performance to issues such as staff retention, internal promotion, and staff satisfaction?
- How does the MBQA enhance healthcare? What is its contribution to nursing? Is there a relationship between Magnet and the Baldrige? How can CNOs build on the best of both recognitions to improve resources for nursing?

LEADER STORY ✍

MARY ELLEN DOYLE
CHIEF NURSING OFFICER
SAINT LUKE'S HOSPITAL OF KANSAS CITY
KANSAS CITY, MISSOURI

Saint Luke's Hospital, a Baldrige award recipient, actually started on this journey in 1995 when the organization made a decision to adopt the Baldrige framework as its management model. The award was not our main focus; rather we recognized Baldrige would meet our needs from a management philosophy perspective. At the same time we applied and received the Missouri Quality Award (MQA), which is modeled after the Baldrige criteria. When Baldrige created a category for healthcare in 1999, we made the commitment to pursue recognition at a national level.

One of the greatest benefits in completing the Baldrige application and undergoing a Baldrige site visit is the feedback report that is generated. This report details the observed strengths within your organization and opportunities for improvement (OFI). We have used this report to drive performance improvement within Saint Luke's Hospital.

A collegial and collaborative relationship always has existed among the CNO, nursing leadership, and our clinical staff. Saint Luke's Hospital has had a shared governance model since 1988 and our nurses are actively involved in decisions about practice and how care is delivered. Through Baldrige and our Magnet journey we have examined and improved our care delivery processes.

We use a Transformational Model of Professional Nursing Practice. We believe this model is congruent with our Baldrige management philosophy. Key to this model is transformational leadership.

During our Magnet site visit the Magnet appraiser discussed authority for decision making, and she commented, "Authority really doesn't seem to be the right word to use in this organization." I agree. So much collegiality and sharing occur within our organization that you do not feel the walls of authority. It was gratifying for me to have one of our Magnet appraisers recognize how well the staff members at Saint Luke's Hospital work together in an empowered environment.

One of the challenges always has been bringing aboard the medical staff. Interestingly we listed physicians in our Baldrige application as partners, not as customers; that is an important distinction for us. We have worked hard over the past 12 to 15 years to partner with our physicians. The medical staff officers and medical staff are involved in decisions made in this organization. The medical staff officers partner with executives to co-lead the balanced scorecard perspectives. We are open in sharing information and information is power. As a result of our performance, Saint Luke's Hospital was recognized by AARP as one of the top 50 hospitals in the United States. Many examples of partnering within nursing exist. For example, the medical staff and nursing staff are working together to ensure evidence-based medicine is practiced at Saint Luke's Hospital.

In the clinical arena, nursing and medical staff partner to improve patient care. For example, we have a formal patient safety plan. One of the pieces of the plan is medication delivery. We measure medication errors and the severity of medication errors. The data appear within our patient safety index on our balanced scorecard. We have a group that meets once a week to review every single incident report related to medication near misses or medication errors, and we have a physician that is part of that group. This physician has a particular interest in medication safety, so he is a co-leader of the team. As a result of the analysis of data by this group, we elected to form a performance improvement team led by a physician and a nurse to study medication errors related to insulin administration. The team revised the medication administration record and is now in the process of completing a total revision of insulin order administration.

The Baldrige philosophy has served us well. If you are truly living the philosophy, you understand your environment and the significant issues facing your organization. You develop strategies to address the significant key issues. You are forced to look at the significant issues that will affect the organization over time. In nursing we have become focused and disciplined about what we work on; we work on those things that we know will have a significant impact.

Our goal is to establish a culture of cooperation and learning, we want an empowered work force, we know we need to be fully aligned, we want to manage by fact, and we have to be flexible and able to respond quickly to our ever-changing environment.

Structure helps set the culture for our performance management process. We pay for performance. Our four core values are the heart and soul of this organization. We have a formal coaching process. We listen for and get feedback from individual practitioners and from their peers about that individual's performance. We look at an individual's performance against our core values and work with him or her to identify opportunities for improvement. We are clear regarding expectations; if an individual does not meet expectations, we ask them to leave the organization.

Kansas City faces many challenges, like many areas of the country. Workforce shortages and skyrocketing malpractice fees have affected the medical staff. Revenues have declined as a result of a highly managed market. We have a nursing shortage, but nurses who work here are expected to live our core values of quality and excellence, teamwork, customer focus, and resource management.

Saint Luke's Hospital has had an RN clinical ladder since 1988. It was revised 3 years ago and is now behavior based and outcome focused. Our career advancement program now requires a professional nurse to demonstrate consistent behaviors and contributions to positive outcomes over time. We reward consistency and sustained performance. It has not been easy, but I think we are going in the right direction.

We provide nursing leaders opportunities to develop their leadership skills. If you are not performing at the expected leadership level, you are asked to change positions. We are diligent about placing the right people in leadership roles. We use behavior-based interviewing and we also believe in promoting our own. We know what our people are like before they go into leadership roles, and we hold them accountable.

Saint Luke's Hospital has measured its clinical outcomes for quite some time. We have not always been process focused. With use of the Baldrige model, we now design and monitor the effectiveness of our healthcare and business processes more efficiently with use of process scorecards.

Our core values drive us; our goals are clear. Our vision statement is simple; we want Saint Luke's Hospital to be "The best place to get care, the best place to give care." And does that not say it all?

Chapter References

American Nurses Credentialing Center. (2004). *Magnet Recognition Award*. Retrieved May 4, 2004, from http://www.nursingworld.org/ancc.

Baldrige Award Recipient Profile. (2003). Retrieved October 20, 2005 from www.nist.gov/public_affairs/releases/bhitrauma.htm.

Baldrige National Quality Program. (2004). *Health care criteria for performance excellence*. Gaithersburg, MD: National Institute of Standards and Technology.

Baldrige National Quality Program. (2005). *Health care criteria for performance excellence*. Gaithersburg, MD: National Institute of Standards and Technology.

Berglund, R. (2001). Using a Baldrige based tool to get results from your quality process. *Quality Congress. ASQ's Annual Quality Congress Proceedings*. Milwaukee, WI: American Society for Quality, 353-369.

Dunn, P., & Santamour, B. (2003). How health care won its first Baldrige. *Hospitals and Health Networks, 77*(9), 67.

Fisher, C., Dauterive, J., & Barfield, J. (2001). Economic impacts of quality awards: Does offering an award bring returns to the state? *Total Quality Management, 12*(7, 8), 981.

Gallagher, R. M., & Rowell, P. (2003). Claiming the future of nursing through nursing sensitive quality indicators. *Nursing Administration Quarterly, 27*(4), 273-284.

Gifford, B., Zammuto, R., & Goodman, E. (2002). The relationship between hospital unit culture and nurses' quality of work life. *Journal of Healthcare Management 47*(1), 13-25.

Hertz, H. S., Reimann, C. W., & Bostwick, M. C. (1994). The Malcolm Baldrige national quality award concept: could it help stimulate or accelerate health care quality improvement? *Quality Management in Health Care, 2*(4), 63-72.

Hutton, D. (2000). Beyond compliance: A Baldrige-based approach. *Quality Congress. ASQ's, Annual Quality Congress Proceedings*. Milwaukee, WI: American Society for Quality, 599-606.

Joint Commission on Accreditation of Healthcare Organizations. (1999). *Assess for success: achieving excellence with Joint Commission Standards and Baldrige Criteria*. Chicago: JCAHO.

Kaye, M., & Anderson, R. (1999). Continuous improvement: The ten essential criteria. *International Journal of Quality and Reliability Management, 16*(5), 49-52.

Leggitt, M., & Anderson, R. (2001). Quality Congress. *ASQ Annual Quality Congress Proceedings*. Milwaukee, WI: American Society for Quality, 462-469.

Mayer, S., & Collier, D. (2001). An empirical test of the causal relationships in the Baldrige health care pilot criteria. *Journal of Operations Management, 19*, 4.

McLaughlin, C., & Kaluzny, A. (1999). *Continuous quality improvement in healthcare*. Gaithersburg, MD: Aspen.

Page, A. (Ed.). (2004). *Keeping patients safe*. (p. 121). Washington, DC: The National Academies Press.

Perrott, B. (2002). Strategic implications of quality management in health care. *Journal of Change Management, 3*(2), 159.

Powell, T. C. (1995). Total quality management as competitive advantage: A review and empirical study. *Strategic Management Journal, 16*, 15-37.

Press Ganey. (2004). *Press Ganey the leader in health care satisfaction measurement and improvement*. Retrieved May 4, 2004, from http://www.pressganey.com.

Scarnati, T., & Scarnati, B. (2002). Empowerment: The key to quality. *The TQM Magazine, 14*(2), 110-120.

Vokura, R. J. (2001). Using the Baldrige criteria for personal quality improvement. *Industrial Management & Data Systems, 101*, 363-370.

Wilson, C., & Porter-O'Grady, T. (1999). *Leading the revolution in health care*. Gaithersburg, MD: Aspen.

CHAPTER

4 Theories That Guide Administrators

The person who knows "how" will always have a job. The person who knows "why" will always be his boss. DIANE RAVITCH WRITER

This chapter provides a brief overview of leadership and management theories that administrators use to guide their work. The purpose of this chapter is to help readers become familiar with a wide array of leadership and management theories.

ADMINISTRATION IS DESIGNED TO ENCOURAGE others to achieve greater goals. Administrative activities are evident every day. Two people may approach the same situation and respond in two different ways. Each may be right, and each may be theory driven.

Numerous ways exist for looking at the theories and realities of administration. The literature is full of management and leadership theory. Sometimes what is called leadership is in fact management, and vice versa. Sometimes only classic views of theory are considered, and sometimes only those clearly rooted in business are referenced. All of these different theories may contribute to the theory and practice of nursing administration. As the Literature box illustrates, theory is important to effective leadership and management.

ETHICAL THEORIES

Theories that derive from a predominant view of ethics tend to focus on the motives and attitudes behind a person's actions and the effect of those actions on individuals. Ethics frequently is used in popular media to suggest the basic concept of "doing right." The problem with that simplistic view is that many opinions exist regarding what is "right." Although not one specific theory exists regarding leadership and management ethics, the recent scrutiny with which top positions in organizations of all kinds, and especially business, have been examined would indicate this would be a good place to start a discussion about theories affecting administrative roles. Therefore, if the goal is to develop staff members and help them improve their performance, leaders may be forgiven if they stumble. But, if leaders are focused on how they advance or how they can look better in a situation, it will not matter if they execute a brilliant strategy. They have lost the critical element of the situation: the trust and valuing of those they represent.

Ethical Principles

The universal ethical principles that relate to all disciplines' respective codes of ethics are those undergirding nursing and administrative practices.

Therefore nursing and administrative practices share a common set of principles that influence practice. Table 4-1 identifies the principles and their key meaning. These eight principles interact with one another in any given situation. One principle may dominate in certain situations, or one principle may overtake another as a situation changes. Many nurses believe, however, that the most important one, especially in administration, is respect for others. Maintaining respect for others encourages acceptance of differing viewpoints. This also helps to maintain a viewpoint of value of others and to accept bad news as well as good.

The Theories

The primary ethical theories are utilitarian, altruistic, and egoist. They derive from ancient times, and the words derive from ancient Greek.

Table 4-1 ETHICAL PRINCIPLES AND THEIR MEANING

Principle	Meaning
Autonomy	Having personal freedom; the right to choose
Beneficence	Promoting good
Fidelity	Keeping promises; loyalty
Justice	Treating people equally/fairly
Nonmaleficence	Doing no harm
Paternalism	Making decisions for another (especially when that person is limited in his or her ability to make decisions)
Respect for others	Acknowledging the rights of others to make decisions that may differ from one's own
Veracity	Telling the truth

The utilitarian theory focuses on the consequences of any decision. The outcome of this theory can be summarized in the following phrase: the greatest good for the masses. Therefore, when a nurse administrator recommends a new approach to creating reports that streamlines that paperwork, the administrator may be operating from a utilitarian perspective that all will benefit.

Altruistic theory involves placing others before self and historically has been a framework for the way in which nurses function. At the staff nurse level, not taking a scheduled break because "my patients need me" is an example of placing others before self. At the administrative level, taking the criticism for the actions that occurred on a given patient unit without having the involved nurses receive the criticism directly also could be an altruistic approach.

Egoist theory relates to being concerned with the best solution for self. Sometimes a person may choose an egoist perspective. However, when a healthcare administrator chooses this path, other members of the group may become concerned that the administrator has placed personal interests above those for whom the administrator is accountable, the patients and the staff. A common example is when the CEO or members of the executive team accept a bonus for performance at a time when other employees are experiencing flat wages or when layoffs have taken place.

Servant Leadership

The seven habits that Stephen Covey (1989) defined magnified the original work of Robert Greenleaf who coined the term *servant leadership*. These seven habits (Box 4-1) may be considered common sense. Despite some criticism, the seven habits remain a solid part of modern-day thinking about leadership.

Being proactive means people take action rather than waiting for something to happen to them (i.e., being reactive). Covey said that what matters is not so much what happens but rather a

Box 4-1   COVEY'S 7 HABITS OF HIGHLY
          EFFECTIVE PEOPLE

Be proactive
Begin with the end in mind
Put first things first
Think win/win
Seek first to understand, then to be
    understood
Synergize
Sharpen the saw

Covey, S. R. (1989). *The 7 habits of highly effective people: Powerful lessons in personal change.* New York: Simon & Schuster.

person's response. Therefore the more proactive a person can be, the less likely it is that things will just happen and that a hurtful outcome will result.

Being goal directed is beginning with the end in mind. For example, a CNO knows that he wants to have shared governance well established by June of the following year. Because he is proactive, he has had to create a vision of shared governance in his organization and the steps to achieve this goal to ensure the vision for June of the following year becomes a reality.

Put first things first derives from a two-by-two model with the x axis and y axis representing importance and urgency. The first cell is urgent and important: those are activities and work that always get done. The second cell is the nonurgent and important: those are the activities and work that, if done, could revolutionize productivity. However, this cell often is not addressed. The third cell is urgent and not important. Although it seems logical, at first glance, that activities and work in this category could be ignored, the reality is that the urgency often overtakes the importance, and so time is wasted dealing with something that does not contribute to the overall goal. Examples of work in this cell could range from phone calls (because it is urgent for the person on the other end of the line) to drop-in visitors to a request to change plans for later in the day to

accommodate a new activity. Cell four represents not urgent and not important. Although nothing in this cell suggests that a person needs to deal with any of the work represented here, often the sheer volume of input in this area creates a time-consuming activity. Whatever an individual describes as trivial could be an example of work in this cell.

The fourth habit, *think win/win,* is built on the concept of mutual benefit. Framing a situation from a dichotomous or polar one to one of mutual satisfaction requires energy and leads to new solutions to ongoing problems. Thinking win/win suggests that the ethical perspective of egoist would not fit well here.

Seek first to understand, then to be understood means that communication must focus mainly on listening, not talking, and asking, not telling. In many difficult conversations, the person hearing negative news begins to formulate a "defense" before the speaker is even finished speaking. Important information may be missed while the responder prepares to respond. Therefore Covey suggests careful listening, or being "present" (not thinking of other things or preparing the response) in the conversation. Only after the message is fully understood should the listener be ready to form a response.

Synergy refers to how all of the various parts work together to create more than the sum of its parts would suggest was possible. Synergy requires that the individual think about how each element of the seven habits contributes to and gains from each of the others.

The seventh habit, sharpen the saw, refers to personal rejuvenation. Changing physical activity and securing adequate rest is one example. Taking time to read publications not normally read may provide a new perspective and is an example of mental rejuvenation. Social and spiritual rejuvenation require time to interact with others and also to meditate. These are examples of ways to increase personal energy and motivation to continue high-level performance.

To be a great leader, a person first must serve others. This is a value-driven concept, not just a set of techniques or activities an administrator can perform. An example of this theory can be seen in staff development activities. Some organizations provide the minimum requirements and focus heavily on checking off basic requirements. Other organizations provide those requirements and others focus on whether employees have what they need to function at higher levels. If an administrator talks about the growth of staff and is truly proud of what they can do, servant leadership is alive.

Habit is defined by Covey (1989) as the intersection of knowledge, skill, and desire. All three of these elements are essential to transform a behavior into a habit. Forming habits is not a concept to be learned and applied in specific situations. However, increasing the skills that enhance the potential for forming habits is possible. Larry Spears (2004), the CEO of the Greenleaf Center, identified the following 10 characteristics of servant leadership:

Listening. Today's focus on "active listening" reflects this skill. Hearing what the message says is more important than crafting a brilliant response to a statement. Therefore the leader must be focused on what is being said and how it is being said.

Empathy. Listeners put themselves in the speaker's place, which helps listeners feel accepted and that their messages have been heard.

Healing. This concept focuses on making one's self and others whole.

Awareness. Although being aware of others' needs is important, the real focus of this characteristic is on self. When the administrator knows his or her role in a situation, movement toward higher goals is likely.

Persuasion. Convincing or manipulating people, in the positive sense, is the way to influence others rather than to create punishments.

Conceptualization. Servant leaders are great at creating visions and because of their commitment to people can apply themselves to moving people toward that vision.

Foresight. This, according to Spears, relates the past, present, and future.

Stewardship. The key message is that organizations are held in trust for the greater good of society. So, servant leaders make decisions based on "what is right."

Commitment to the growth of people. The focus of this characteristic is to work with others to make them as dynamic and contributing as possible in all aspects of their lives.

Building community. This characteristic might be viewed as thinking of the workplace as a microcosm of the larger community and that within this smaller community various people have distinctive contributions to the benefit of the whole.

Servant leaders are evident by their focus on others and their specific strategies, such as coaching to develop others. They believe in the best of people and are devoted to making people the best. They have great hopes and act on the hopes that tomorrow will be better.

In 2004 Covey produced the eighth habit. This final habit is *finding your voice and inspiring others to find their voice.* Deciding what an individual wants and needs and giving voice to those wants and needs is a choice. Moving beyond the task of finding a person's own voice relates to expanding influence to others to help them use their voice too. As a result, leadership evolves into a choice and not a position. "The 8th Habit gives you a mindset and a skill-set to constantly look for the potential in people" (Covey, 2004, p. 271). Furthermore, like Bossidy and Charan (2002), Covey believes that any of these habits are worthless if they are not executed consistently and well.

Code of Ethics for Nurses

Although the profession's guide to ethical practice is not a theory, it does influence heavily the way in which all nurses practice. The *Code of Ethics for Nurses with Interpretive Statements* (ANA, 2001) provides the basic ethical framework for all nurses to adhere to, regardless of their roles. The Code is built on ethical principles and theories and is designed to state what is distinctive about the profession of nursing in practicing ethically in society. Each of the provisions is stated broadly, such as practicing with compassion or the primary commitment to the patient. Each broad statement is followed with clarification of the elements within the statement and then includes an interpretative statement about the relevance of the elements to current practice.

The nurse administrator is just as accountable to advocate for the patient as the staff nurse providing care. Those provisions are enacted in a different manner at the administrative level, but they are inherent in administration just as they are at the practice level. One common example of advocation for patients is staff nurses who document inadequate staffing levels. When the nurse administrator presents data that indicate insufficient salaries or positions within nursing to provide safe care, the nurse administrator too is advocating for the patient. Staff and administrative nurses must be in concert in their view of ethical action. For example, if a staff nurse reports a medication error (a part of advocating for patients) and then is not supported by nursing administration for doing so, the actions are not in concert at both levels.

Based on differing information that may be available to various positions within the organization, two nurses may reach different conclusions and be using the same provisions to "explain" those decisions. In other words, all people see the world from where they are in it.

LEADERSHIP AND MANAGEMENT THEORIES

Most leadership and management theories originated in business settings or colleges. Appendix A contains a brief description of many of these theories for quick reference, and the framework of the various theories is included in this chapter. These theories are presented in alphabetical order rather than chronologic development or complexity order.

Contingency

The focus of this theory is on fitting the response or action to the situation. In other words, successful action is dependent on the fit of the leader's style with the situation. This would suggest, for example, that clinical directors are not necessarily interchangeable. If one director's style is always to allow for full and open discussion and the typical situations on a clinical unit relate to crisis management, the director might not be seen as valuable to the leadership of that unit. Therefore failure of a clinical director could be as much about the setting as it is about the leader because to be successful, the leader's style must be matched with the appropriate setting.

The original attribution probably belongs to Fiedler (1964). Considerable research has focused on this theory, so it tends to be well accepted, predictive, and useful. This theory is criticized because it contains many unexplainable elements. In the leaders studied, styles were found to be either more task oriented or more relationship oriented. Task-oriented styles relate to being goal oriented. Leaders who are highly task oriented talk about attaining the goal, they talk about the various steps in the plan, and they are deadline focused. Relationship-oriented styles relate to knowing each other, hearing what others have to say, and maintaining close ties with each other. Leaders who are highly relationship oriented talk about how others are feeling about their progress toward goals, they talk about what would facilitate next steps, and they are focused on preserving the relationship as movement toward the goal is made. The instrument that determines preferences for relationships or tasks is known as the least preferred co-worker measure.

Situation variables make up relationships, task structure, and positional power. The relationship component takes into account such factors as loyalty and trust. When staff members trust in the leader, they tend to describe the situation as positive. When positional power is used to enhance trust, for example "sticking up for staff," further loyalty occurs. The task structure refers to the details involved in a task and the amount of personal control an individual has to accomplish a task. Collecting quantitative data in a clinical setting usually is well structured with little flexibility about which data to include or not. Assessing staff performance, on the other hand, requires a great deal of individual control in terms of which data to include and what value to place on the performance behaviors. Power related to a position relates to the leader's authority. In some settings, managers at the unit level have authority to hire and fire (high positional power); in others, managers do not have this independent authority (low positional power).

Exchange Theory

Exchange theory (or leader-member theory) is focused on the process of the interaction. It is based on a dyadic relationship between the leader and the follower. This distinctive theory thus places as much weight on the follower as it does on the leader. The name most commonly associated with this theory is Graen (1976). One of the major features about this theory, as the nature of the relationship suggests, is that the leader works differently with each of the people with whom interactions occur. This theory often is used to explain the "in group"/"out group" phenomenon. The "in group" comprises those followers with whom interactions generally are viewed as positive. The "out group" comprises those followers with whom interactions generally are viewed as negative. A key concept of this theory is the willingness of the followers to expand their respective role responsibilities.

The "in group" seems to receive more information than does the "out group." The "ins" also are more dependable, and, as might be anticipated, experience less turnover and better career development than exist in the "out" group. The "out group" might even feel ostracized from the leader. Because, in this theory, the leader creates relationships on a dyadic basis, a person can move from one group to the other. Because of the fact that the leader builds relationships with each of the followers on an individual basis, this is a time-intensive leadership approach. Further, the movement from a new employee or an "out group" member to an "in group" member is fairly systematic. Initial interactions with new employees and with established "out group" members start as fairly formal exchanges. Movement begins with indication by either the leader or the follower of the potential for additional responsibility and career development. The leader may offer to help the follower develop his or her career. Or, the follower may indicate a desire to assume more responsibility. When full movement to the "in group" occurs, a more equal exchange of benefits occurs. Typically, greater trust is evident and a true partnership emerges.

Path Goal

Based on expectancy theory, this theory relates to how leaders motivate followers toward designated goals. This theory interrelates the leader's style with the follower and the work setting. Most of the early research was done by House (1971) and colleagues. Rather than matching the situation (as with contingency theory), this theory suggests the leader matches style with the follower's motivation. The leader's task is to fill the void in the work setting that limits the follower's movement toward goals. Of all leadership theories, this one is based most closely on motivational theory and methods for working with the follower's motivation to move toward goals. This theory also seems to be fairly pragmatic because it suggests that leaders should do what seems almost intuitive: get the obstacles out of the way for people to do their jobs. Some of these obstacles may be intangible: for example, creating the atmosphere of personal success in achieving a goal. Other obstacles are tangible: for example, securing different equipment so that no physical lifting is required of the person providing direct care.

Leader behaviors consist of direction, support, participation, and achievement-orientation. Direction involves clearly stated outcomes, timelines, and sometimes specific details about how to accomplish a task. Support involves viewing staff as equals and creating a pleasant and facilitative work environment. Participation is consulting with staff and setting mutually agreed upon decisions. Achievement-orientation consists of establishing high expectations and a focus on continuous improvement. Each of these behaviors, according to this theory, is at the disposal of the leader who decides which approach to use based on the situation or the need of the individual staff member.

Follower needs frequently focus on affiliation and control. Those followers who have need for affiliation respond well in supportive leadership situations. Those followers who have need for control seem to respond well to a participative approach by the leader.

In general, the influence of tasks on this leader-follower relationship is based on the structure and clarity of a task. For example, vague tasks have minimal structure; therefore involvement of leaders is needed and valued. When tasks are clear, involvement of the leader can be interpreted as interfering.

Although a connection exists between what the leader does and the follower's motivation, the actual connection is not well explained through research on this theory. In fact, the research has produced mixed results.

Situational Leadership®

This model, developed by Hersey (Hersey and Blanchard, 1969), is among the most popular because people can see how it applies in daily work. When asked what they would do in a particular situation, leaders have said, "It depends." That is because action often is modulated by the specifics of a situation. Therefore delegating in one situation might be the right leader behavior, and telling might be the right leader behavior in another situation. According to Hersey, leader behavior should be based primarily on an assessment of a person's ability to perform in a given situation.

Situational Leadership® is a registered trademark of the Center for Leadership Studies.

Therefore as a person grows in relation to specific tasks, the leader would change behaviors for working with that person even though the situation specifics might not have changed.

The underlying responsibility of the leader is to assess the individual's performance needs in relation to a specific situation and task. Thus the leader's focus is to match his or her style to the assessment outcome. The Situational Leadership model is based on relationship behaviors and task behaviors (Figure 4-1). Each of those elements ranges from high to low. The intersection of these elements suggests how the leader interacts with the follower. Follower readiness is determined by the leader's assessment of how able and willing a

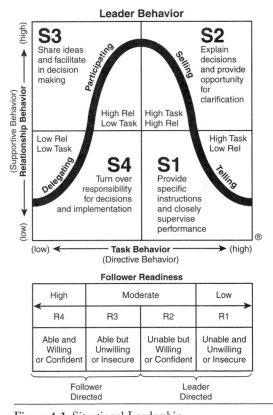

Figure 4-1 Situational Leadership.
From Hersey, P., Blanchard, K.H., & Johnson, D.E. (2001). *Management of organizational behaviors: Leading human resources.* (8th ed.). Upper Saddle River, NJ: Prentice Hall, p. 182.

follower is in relation to a task. So, for example, when a leader assesses an individual's willingness and ability as being *high* (both able and willing), the style of interaction a leader chooses to "fit" the situation would be delegating. If, on the other hand, the leader assesses an individual's willingness and ability as being *low* (unable and unwilling), the style of interaction a leader chooses would be *telling*. The four basic styles of leadership, based on the high to low range of readiness of the followers, are the following:

- Telling/directing
- Selling/coaching
- Participating/supporting
- Delegating/monitoring

Telling is based on an assessment of being unable and unwilling. An example of this style of interaction can be found in emergent situations when a member of the team isn't familiar with the protocols and is insecure in functioning in such situations. Telling the person what to do can provide support for quick and appropriate actions.

Selling is best when the follower is unable yet willing in relation to a specific task and situation. As Chapter 11 suggests, this is an intense process because the leader is vested in the relationship and the person and has very specific task expectations. Selling works best in such situations as when a nurse is working with a terminally ill client and wants to do her best but is unable to decide how best to interact with the client. The focus is on helping the person to perform.

Participating suggests that the follower is able but unwilling to perform a task. Therefore the leader relies on the follower to know and execute the details with full administrative support. This type of situation may be found when the nurse previously described is able to work with the dying client but the motivation to work through one more death is challenging.

Delegating involves working with followers who are fairly sophisticated in relation to the task; they are both willing and able. They don't need much support, and they need little task orientation. They are quick and effective. After the leader assesses the follower as both willing and able, the leader needs to make clear that the follower is "in charge" of the situation and create the climate in which all support the leadership of that individual.

Because any team consists of a mix of all types of followers, the leader must commit to a constant assessment of the members and their willingness and abilities in relation to specific tasks and situations. Without attention to the staff and the situation, only the tasks become better. Despite the lack of a robust research backing, this approach remains common in many organizations.

Style

The predominant view of this theory is Blake and Mouton's Managerial Grid (1978). This grid was used to explain how managers move people toward goals based on concerns for work and concerns for people. The former relates to the tasks and the

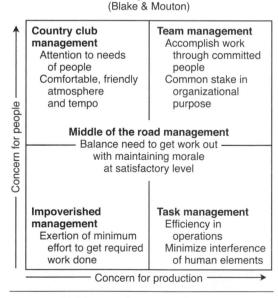

Managerial Grid
(Blake & Mouton)

Figure 4-2 Blake and Mouton's managerial grid. From Blake, R. R., & Mouton, J. S. (1978). *The new managerial grid*. Houston: Gulf.

latter refers to interactions that promote commitment to the goals of the organization. Blake and Mouton defined five styles (Figure 4-2):

1. *Task management* refers to a major focus on the tasks and requirements. This is the historical view of the people at the top: demanding, goal oriented, unconcerned with people.
2. *Country club management* refers to the person who is very much concerned with people and much less so with tasks. People using this style have the goal to create a "good place to work."
3. *Impoverishment* refers to the detached person. This person seems unconcerned with people and with tasks. This management style generates no enthusiasm for others or for the work to be done.
4. *Team management* focuses on both tasks and people. Managers using this style are highly involved with both and generate enthusiasm for people and the work to be done.
5. *"Middle-of-the road"* managers are those who balance people and tasks. They are not the drivers; but they are not disconnected. These people are usually good maintainers of the status quo.

This theory focuses on behaviors that can be observed. Perhaps the biggest concern with this theory is that it is difficult to fit the theory into various situations to explain why certain behaviors are evident.

Trait

Perhaps the oldest theory about management is trait, or characteristics. This theory, sometimes referred to as "great man" theory, was used to explain the world's key leaders. In essence, researchers observed that someone in a key position demonstrated a certain personal quality, such as communication ability. They then observed it in another person in a key position. Soon lists were generated of traits that were attributed to "great men." Zaleznik (1977) is one of the early authors on this theoretic approach to leadership. In U.S. society, for example, sociability is one of the traits that has been found to differ between people who are seen as leaders and others. Most of the traits of leaders are attributed to personality factors, such as better education, sharper thinking, superior contacts, and greater communication skills. This theory is clearly about the leader, not the followers or the situation or the work to be done, although the traits that leaders have must relate to the situation in which leadership is expected. No definitive list of leadership traits has emerged from the various studies that have focused on this aspect of leadership.

Transactional

Transactional leadership refers to a complex exchange theory. First documented by Burns (1978), this theory is based on promises administrators make for people who perform in specific ways. The theory is focused heavily on performance achievements. Transactional leadership focuses on the work at hand and how the leader and followers work together through "trading" (whether tangible, such as a bonus, days off, or recognition, or intangible, such as feeling more a part of a winning team). The more common or conventional approach is basic reward and punishment. When a follower performs as the leader desires, a positive reward occurs. If the follower does not perform as desired, punishment occurs. Although punishment may not be articulated openly, it usually is understood in a culture in which this approach to leadership is evident. This theoretic approach works well in situations in which followers are focused on money and rewards. Transactional leaders tend to be successful in maintaining the status quo because they accept the "givens" in a situation: the structure, the culture, the vision, and the reward and punishment system. These leaders tend to support the current structure and how it operates. The culture of rewards and punishment is potentiated by all levels of administration. Furthermore, positional power is the source of the reward and punishment.

This style of leadership is successful in situations in which absolute adherence to policies, procedures, and standards is expected. It is found in organizations in which chain of command is critical to the culture or functioning of the organization.

Transactional leaders attempt to motivate followers based on their own self-interests whether those relate to rewards to be gained or punishment to be avoided. When transaction is the dominant approach a leader uses, it works for the short term, but it usually does not work for the long term. Transaction helps deal with current crisis but seldom contributes to the creation of a work environment seen as empowering. Transactional leadership relies heavily on control. Providing feedback (and the reward or punishment) makes a major contribution to the effective implementation of this theory.

Transformational

This is the current popular theory of explaining how interactions occur for the best within health-care situations. Transformational leadership refers to the synergistic effect of the leaders and followers. Each encourages the other to perform at new levels. The actions of leaders influence followers and the actions of followers influence leaders. This theory, which emerged into some prominence because of the work of Burns (1978), focuses on all members of the team understanding the vision and each individual fitting within the whole to meet the vision. In this intense interaction, everyone is committed to everyone else, and the group moves forward.

Transformational leadership works from the perspective of inspiration rather than reward and punishment. A heavy focus is on self-management. In other words, the "manager" manages the nature of the inspiration provided rather than managing the followers as they execute their work. Bass and Avolio (1990) defined four transformational factors.

1. *Charisma/idealized influence* refers to serving as highly influential role models. Others want to follow these individuals.
2. *Inspirational motivation* involves conveying high expectations of performance. As a result, followers feel compelled to do their best.
3. *Intellectual stimulation* refers to the fact that people, in general, wish to try new approaches and test new ideas. This factor promotes critical thinking.
4. *Individualized consideration* incorporates the concept of intense listening. As a result of this listening activity on the part of leaders, they are able to coach each follower to perform to his or her personal best.

Persons who are seen as transformational often are described as charismatic. They often are seen as strong role models, and they develop trust in their followers. Leaders also convey high expectations for the whole group's performance. Communication plays an important role in this theoretic approach, because communication is about inspiring others to do their best rather than providing details about policies and performances that could be cited in organizational documents.

Transformational leadership is thought of as a value-driven model. The commitment within a team to each other means that no team member wants any other team member to fail. The team works to enrich those who need new skills, and those who have skills within the team share those talents with others. The notion of transformational leadership includes the potential to revise the workplace completely because everyone is contributing ideas in a professional exchange. Transformational leadership is seen as a way for everyone to perform at his or her best on a fairly consistent basis. In doing so, new levels of performance behaviors are established, and thus the quality within an organization improves on an ongoing basis. Additionally, feedback about less-than-desired performance is done so by exception. In other words, performance is noted and when it is less than it should be, the performer is made aware of the discrepant performance.

MOTIVATIONAL THEORIES

Motivational theories are really about human needs, not just leadership. However, leaders use them to explain their interaction with followers. Motivational theories range from Maslow's Hierarchy of Needs to theories specific to management, such as Theory X and Theory Y and later, Theory Z.

Maslow's Hierarchy of Needs

The most common motivational theory is, of course, Maslow's Hierarchy of Needs (1954). Figure 4-3 presents the basic concepts of the hierarchy. The needs are presented in ascending order with the expectation that those needs at lower levels must be met before needs at higher levels can be addressed.

Although Maslow's hierarchy normally is applied to patients and their human needs, it is equally applicable in understanding some of the basic relationships experienced in administering nursing services. For example, if a director is

worried about a dying relative, he or she is not interested in learning new development strategies. If a nurse manager has teenagers who are sports enthusiasts, he or she wants to be available to attend those events. Managers cannot give much attention to higher-level activities if they are concerned with safety for the staff members as they arrive at work.

McGregor's Theory X and Theory Y and Ouchi's Theory Z

McGregor (1960) is seen as the developer of Theory X and Theory Y. Basically Theory X suggests that workers do not want to work, they have to be watched and given incentives. Further, the theory suggests, workers are not eager to create new solutions and actually are limited in their ability to create such outcomes. X is based on the view that people actually are not very smart, and a goal of the manager is to catch people doing something wrong. Using this perspective, money and security are the primary motivators for people. So, in situations in which these two factors are well addressed, the primary motivators no longer influence followers.

Theory Y suggests that workers actually like to work, work is what their life is about, they

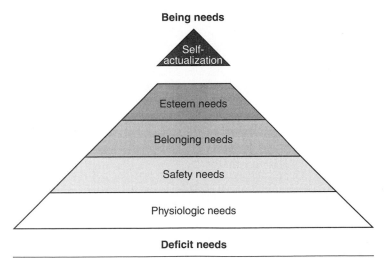

Figure 4-3 Maslow's Hierarchy of Needs.

motivate themselves, and they see value in what they do. In Theory Y, workers are focused on quality and productivity and want to improve work through their creative problem solving. This theory supports workers to do what they believe they need to do to further the work of the organization. Theory X operates primarily on punishment; Theory Y operates primarily on reward.

Theory Z (Ouchi, 1981) was developed in response to a period when the Japanese culture was viewed as far more productive than the U.S. culture. Theory Z combines Theory Y with Japanese best practices. Theory Z focuses decision making at the level of the work. The "local group" (whether a plant division or a hospital unit) is viewed as loyal and vested in its team. Theory Z focuses heavily on concern for the employees and their benefit. Quality circles, in which the people most directly involved with an issue are the ones charged with solving it and making the situation more positive and productive, are a part of Theory Z. The manager who uses this theoretic approach has a goal to help followers feel they are part of a productive endeavor.

SUMMARY

Regardless of how someone performs in a key role in the organization, a theoretic perspective exists to explain it. Theory drives how managers relate with followers and whether they are consistent or variable in their approaches. Theoretic perspectives provide greater insight into ways to work with others and to develop greater abilities in working with others. Knowing that not all people operate from the same theoretic perspective is an added value to understanding the dynamics of the organization.

KEY POINTS TO LEAD

1. Critique the types of theories in terms of the work setting.
2. Contemplate the application of at least three theories to personal performance.
3. Analyze recent personal performance, using one or two theories.

Literature Box

"Theory often gets a bum rap among managers, because it's associated with the word 'theoretical,' which connotes 'impractical.' But it shouldn't. A theory is a statement predicting which actions will lead to what results and why" (p. 68). Christensen and Raynor suggest that managers tend to read management theory and either reject it because it is theory or adopt it without carefully analyzing if the theory is applicable to the user's situation. In addition to approaches to predictions, theories also should be applicable to the current situation and explain why something is happening. Furthermore, theories should help focus on important future changes.

Christensen and Raynor advocate for an emphasis on studying failures in addition to explaining outcomes and making predictions. Further, they advocate for highly detailed field research to observe causal processes firsthand. One of their concerns is that many managers discover a new theoretic approach to an issue that applies to their situation. Unfortunately, the researchers have *not* always identified the circumstances in which the theory does not result in success. "Circumstance-contingent theories enable managers to understand what it is about their present situation that has enabled their strategies and tactics to succeed" (p. 71). Focusing on when or why something does not work is critical to aid managers in making decisions about using a particular theory. In other words, managers must know as much about what their work situation is *not* like as they know about

Literature Box

what their situation *is* like. Knowing how a theory varies as a company's situation changes is extremely important to the manager who is consuming the research.

Five cautions are proposed to managers as they consider research they read:

1. Early work that describes a phenomenon is useful, but it typically does not explain the circumstances under which the theory can be applied.
2. Work that urges revolutionary change should be viewed with caution.
3. If the work is about classifying a phenomenon based on its attributes, this is a useful, preliminary study and is not ready for application in practice.

4. "Correlations that masquerade as causation often take the form of adjectives" (p. 73).
5. Progress occurs when theories explain situations in which they previously failed.

Theory is critical to the approach of administration. An administrator faces the challenge of knowing what is useful and reliable.

Christensen, C. M., & Raynor, M. E. (2003, September). Why hard-nosed executives should care about management theory. *Harvard Business Review*, 66-74.

Contemplations

- Based on your own practice, which theory best explains your approach to working with others?
- How can nurse leaders work more effectively with staff from a theoretic perspective?
- After analyzing your own manager's apparent theoretic perspective, how does your perspective

fit with or conflict with your manager's perspective?
- In developing staff for leadership positions, how would you guide their thinking from a theoretic perspective?

LEADER STORY

Margaret (Maggie) McClure
Professor, New York University
Former CNO and Hospital Administrator,
New York University Medical Center
Recipient AONE Lifetime Achievement Award

One of the advantages of advanced education is that it helps me think analytically and conceptually about everyday problems. In nursing, we do not, in fact, use enough theory in our practice. We also therefore cannot really say that we are doing evidence-based practice. We often don't read the research that has been published and, when we do, we aren't necessarily persuaded by it to change our practice. But the truth of the matter is that if we are trying to move our programs or our processes forward rather than just grinding away in the same old fashion, we are handicapped without current information. The bottom line is that we simply don't apply the evidence that could be useful to making positive change.

My doctoral work caused me to be much more focused on evidence-based administrative practice and to try to be conceptual about the way that our efforts fit into changes occurring in the larger environment. Early on in my tenure at NYU, I was asked to teach a graduate course entitled "Theories Underlying the Delivery of Nursing Services" in the nursing administration program. Clearly everyone who took it had some interest in being prepared as a nurse administrator. You do not know anything so well as when you teach it, and therefore teaching continually kept me abreast of what theories existed and how scholars had looked at administrative practice. So I was lucky enough to spend the better part of my career examining theories and trying to show students, and therefore myself, how they might apply to practice. Of course, examples are critical to students' understanding. Application then became the really interesting part of the classes.

That experience led me to develop my own conceptual model of what nursing is and what it does. This, in turn, shaped my own ability to identify the resources needed for nursing practice, which play a large role in administration. If you aren't able to conceptualize your contribution to the larger organization and you can't conceptualize the work and what it means, you really handicap yourself. What I have observed over time is that some people think that the best way they can administer is by making sure everyone knows why nursing is different and "whining" about what they need to make nursing practice safe and adequate.

My own point of view is that you have to present the nature of nursing care in a clear manner; otherwise, you hardly can defend what you need and the value of what you are trying to achieve. Of course, in this regard, we are not really different from other fields. Even presidents of major corporations generally do not practice based on theory. They may be conceptual thinkers, but their thinking is not necessarily theory based. One of the best examples is the work I have been doing in recent years, which has undergirded my approach to explaining nursing to others.

I am convinced that without the assistance of scholarly works, we are just doing a job. Without theory a person could not really make a case for anyone pursuing an advanced degree in nursing administration. They might just as well get an MBA. The reason, of course, is that nursing has unique and interesting problems that will never be addressed by other disciplines. Even the application of theories from other fields often requires somewhat different interpretation when applied to our discipline. Furthermore, we certainly need to develop more of our own administrative scholars so that they, in turn, will produce the evidence on which we can base our practice.

Two theorists who helped me to figure out nursing practice and make it explicit are the organizational theorists Lawrence and Lorsch. Although their research is old, it is very useful and has formed the basis for the writing I am currently doing, including a book (*Understanding Nursing*). I am using the differentiation-integration theory (Lawrence & Lorsch, 1967) to explain how nursing runs the institution. They have a very interesting way of looking at complex organizations. By definition, complex organizations comprise large numbers of highly specialized ("differentiated") departments. Their framework describes the way in which an "integrator" naturally arises in these organizations. This role essentially is responsible for pulling together the output of all the differentiated departments and thereby creating the actual product. Lawrence and Lorsch believe that if such a role did not exist, the work would just sit there, department by department. In the past, we may have called this work "coordination" in nursing, but I really like the idea of integration better because it conveys such a sense of wholeness. I think this portion of our responsibility often has been a puzzle to nurses, and it certainly was to me. For example, as a head nurse, I might arrive at work and be greeted by a physician irate with me because an X-ray wasn't done the evening before. I could look at him and say in my own mind, "I wasn't here last night and I don't run the X-ray department, why are you talking to me about this?" Somehow, though, I always knew, deep down, that this was our responsibility. However, if you cannot explain it well, then you can't improve it. The exquisite definition of integration and the understanding that this concept brings to our work is invaluable. The nurse is and always has been the integrator, a powerful role requiring a very high level of performance.

The interesting thing is that there really aren't any theories that I haven't found useful. They have led to my own understanding of what is evolving in my own organization and my ability to do my job as an administrator.

Consideration of any of these ideas influences practice. I look back on the time when I was part of the team that did the Magnet Hospital study. To a large extent, some of us would say that the findings supported what we always had thought and believed. On the other hand, I know that some of what I learned changed what I did, especially regarding the ways that I interacted with the staff and how I arranged to do that.

One concrete example comes to mind. Before the Magnet study, I was the CNO at a 700-bed hospital. I routinely held scheduled meetings with the staff. I had a conference room next to my office, and I would arrange to have quarterly open meetings with the staff. We would serve refreshments and have a kind of open house/meeting during the course of all three shifts. People would come from the units to talk with me, and they were free to discuss whatever they wanted. I really thought I was reaching a lot of staff and that it was effective.

After the Magnet study, I changed what I did. Instead of opening up a conference room to meet with the staff, I went to them. I made an appointment to meet with every unit on each shift on a regular basis. I sat down with the staff in the "back room," and we basically addressed their agenda. Over time they developed formal agenda. When we were finished with their topics, I would then fill them in on what was going on in the larger organization. What I realized was that under the old approach, the same people came all the time; more important, the same people *didn't* come. With the new approach, no one had to plan to leave the unit. The service directors would arrange for coverage from other units. This made the sessions much more inclusive.

The meetings changed over time. In the beginning, people were a little quiet; they weren't sure what they were supposed to say. I would remind them that I represented them to the top administration, including the board, and that it was important that I be fully informed on any issues that mattered to them. I also tried to make sure that at some point we talked about clinical care so that I could understand their perspective and also so that I could translate that information to others. When people shared problems, I tried to deal with them. I wanted them to know that meeting with me brought results.

One example comes to mind: Our hospital was a single tower with central elevators. We had no real escort service; rather, there was an "escort" elevator, specifically staffed to move patients. Nursing was responsible for phoning for that car and then delivering the patient to the pick-up point. Problems often occurred when the escort elevator did not arrive. The choices were for the staff member to leave the patient unattended and

return to the unit to place another call or to move the patient back to the unit, which wasn't good either. The staff suggested that telephones be placed next to the elevators, and we were able to do that. I also was direct and honest when suggestions were made that weren't feasible, so they knew that too, and in general, they accepted the information well. The staff always seemed to value this open dialogue and opportunity for input.

You learn from everything; if you are not learning from everything, you aren't really practicing. Administration, because it is practice, is eclectic in its use of theory. I don't think you can choose just one. The use of theory drives my practice.

Chapter References

American Nurses Association. (2001). *The Code of Ethics for Nurses with Interpretive Statements*. Washington, DC: American Nurses Association.

Bass, B. M., & Avolio, B. J. (1990). The implications of transactional and transformational leadership for individual, team, and organizational development. *Research in Organizational Change and Development, 4*, 231-272.

Blake, R. R., & Mouton, J. S. (1978). *The new managerial grid.* Houston: Gulf.

Bossidy, L., & Charan, R. (2002). *Execution.* New York: Random House.

Burns, J. M. (1978). *Leadership.* New York: Harper and Row.

Christensen, C. M., & Raynor, M. E. (2003, September). Why hard-nosed executives should care about management theory. *Harvard Business Review*, 66-74.

Covey, S. R. (1989). *The 7 habits of highly effective people: Powerful lessons in personal change.* New York: Simon & Schuster.

Covey, S. R. (2004). *The 8ᵗʰ habit: From effectiveness to greatness.* New York: Free Press.

Fiedler, F. E. (1964). A contingency model of leadership effectiveness. In L. Berkowitz (Ed.). *Advances in Experimental Social Psychology, 1*, 149-190.

Graen, G. B. (1976). Role-making processes within complex organizations. In M. D. Dunnette (Ed.). *Handbook of industrial and organizational psychology.* Chicago: Rand McNally.

Hersey, P., & Blanchard, K. H. (1969). Life-cycle theory of leadership. *Training and Development Journal, 23*, 26-34.

House, R. J. (1971). A path-goal theory of leader effectiveness. *Administrative Science Quarterly, 16*, 321-328.

Lawrence, P., & Lorsch, J. (1967). *Organization and environment.* Cambridge, MA: Harvard University Press.

Maslow, A. H. (1954). *Motivation and personality.* Upper Saddle River, NJ: Prentice-Hall.

McGregor, D. (1960). *The human side of enterprise.* New York: McGraw-Hill.

Ouchi, W. G. (1981). *Theory Z: How American management can meet the Japanese challenge.* Reading, MA: Addison-Wesley.

Spears, L. (2004). 10 Principles of servant-leadership. Retrieved on August 27, 2004, from http://www.butler.edu/studentlife/hampton/principles.htm.

Zaleznik, A. (1977, May-June). Managers and leaders: Are they different? *Harvard Business Review, 55*, 67-78.

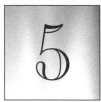

Fostering Legal and Ethical Practices

Ginny Wacker Guido

Law is a magic mirror, wherein we see reflected not only our own lives but also the lives of those who went before us. OLIVER WENDELL HOLMES

This chapter focuses on legal and ethical issues from the perspective of nurse leaders in healthcare organizations. It explores these legal and ethical issues from the perspective of therapeutic jurisprudence, a concept that seeks to incorporate the positive effects that law and ethics play in enhancing the health and lives of individuals, families, groups, and communities.

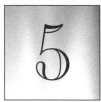

NURSE LEADERS CONTINUOUSLY STRUGGLE to provide competent, quality nursing care delivered in a humanistic and holistic manner. To meet these expectations, nurse leaders must be cognizant of the multiple legal and ethical concepts that occur in all levels of nursing care delivery and in all clinical settings. Therapeutic jurisprudence identifies either the positive or negative effects of legal and ethical decisions and outcomes, which allows individuals to respond by alteration or enhancement of the healthcare delivery system to ensure quality, ethical care of all patients and clients.

THE FIRST NURSING ADMINISTRATOR

Florence Nightingale's service in caring for the sick and injured set the standard for the organization of nursing service evident today. On her arrival, the military hospital in the Crimea had no laundry and no serviceable kitchen; beds were made of straw; and the sick and injured were lying on canvas sheets in the midst of filth and vermin. Within 10 days of her arrival, the newly established kitchens were feeding more than 1000 soldiers a day; within 3 months, 10,000 were receiving clothing, food, and medicine. The ultimate result of her leadership was that the death rate was reduced from 40% to 2% (Isler, 1970). In her writings, Florence Nightingale observed the following:

A good nursing staff will perform their duties more or less satisfactorily under every disadvantage. But while doing so, their head will always try to improve their surroundings, in such a way as to liberate them from subsidiary work, and enable them to devote their time more exclusively to the care of the sick. (Byrnes, 1982, p. 1089)

Given the enormity and effectiveness of her organizational and administrative style, it is no wonder that Florence Nightingale is considered to be the first nursing administrator. Although nursing today is significantly different than it was in the time of Nightingale, the tasks are no less enormous or important. As nursing becomes more complex, the element of risk to the patient increases, in addition to increased potential for nurses to be exposed to malpractice lawsuits and ethical dilemmas. The challenge for the nurse executive is how to promote quality care in today's ever-changing environment.

THERAPEUTIC JURISPRUDENCE

Therapeutic jurisprudence developed over the past several years to begin to describe the extent to which law and ethics affect the way in which healthcare is delivered. Co-founded by Wexler and Winick in the late 1980s (Wexler & Winick, 1991), therapeutic jurisprudence seeks to assess the therapeutic and counter-therapeutic consequences of the law and its application. Therapeutic jurisprudence is a mental health approach to law and ethics that uses the tools from the behavioral sciences to assess therapeutic effects of the application of legal and ethical principles and improve the psychologic functioning and emotional well-being of those affected. As Wexler (2002) noted:

Therapeutic jurisprudence concentrates on the law's impact on emotional life and psychological well-being. It is a perspective that regards the law (rules of law, legal procedures, and roles of legal actors) itself as a social force that often produces therapeutic or anti-therapeutic consequences. It does not suggest that therapeutic concerns are more important than other consequences or factors, but it does suggest that the law's role as a potential therapeutic agent should be recognized and systematically studied. (p. 1)

Nursing's covenant with the public encompasses a commitment to improve the healthcare of individuals, families, groups, and communities. Evidence-based nursing practice has resulted as

a means of testing and evaluating the effectiveness of this nursing care. Parameters of nursing care are developed through the guidance of legal and ethical theories and principles, including deontological theories and the ethic of caring (Beauchamp & Childress, 2001). Beneficence, the duty to do good, coupled with legal principles, begins to provide this framework for nursing care.

ETHICAL ISSUES

Ethical Principles

Ethical principles are the foundation that the nurse executive should employ in decision making. These principles, used in conjunction with legal concepts, set the basis for therapeutic jurisprudence. Although each of these principles can stand alone, in clinical practice settings it is much more common to see more than one ethical principle used when decisions are made. Table 5-1 gives an overview of the ethical principles used by the nurse executive.

Autonomy

The principle of autonomy addresses personal freedom and the right to choose. This principle underlies the daily decisions of chief nursing officers (CNOs) as they consider the impact of decisions and directions on those who must abide by these decisions and directions and the impact for the patients whom these individuals serve.

Perhaps the most difficult aspects of preserving autonomy occurs when nurse executives are employed initially in an institution, because the expectation typically is that they will follow blindly the board of governor's directions. When nurse executives disagree and refuse to allow policy and procedure to occur that will be detrimental to staff members and patients, they often are omitted from the major decision-making process. This leaves the nurse executive essentially "voiceless" and unable to lead. Over time, this type of ethical dilemma has the potential to undermine the quality of nursing care, the institution's ability to

Table **5-1** ETHICAL PRINCIPLES AND
SELECTED APPLICATIONS

Principle	Application
Autonomy	The right to select a course of action.
Beneficence	The actions that promote "good" or appropriate outcomes.
Nonmaleficence	The duty to avoid harm when enforcing new policies.
Veracity	Telling the truth about decisions to the persons these decisions will affect.
Justice	Treating all staff members fairly and equally.
Paternalism	Assisting persons in making difficult decisions.
Fidelity	Keeping promises; not promising what can't be enacted.
Respect for others	Treating all individuals, regardless of their heritage, color, or gender, with equal respect and concern.

attract and retain excellent nursing staff, and the type of nursing leader needed to develop quality nursing services.

Beneficence

The principle of beneficence states that actions should promote good. In healthcare settings, good can be defined in a variety of ways. Boards of governors often define as good those policies that solely support the institution's legal needs without regard to how the implementation of these policies may affect patients and nurses. Similarly, the nurse executive may be requested to make decisions that serve the needs of the organization but have negative effects on the nursing staff. An example of such a policy could be the implementation of a policy to reduce the funding for staff development and in-service programs. Although such a policy meets the current budget crisis, the long-term effect on quality nursing care may be compromised.

Nonmaleficence

The corollary of beneficence, the principle of nonmaleficence, states that a person should do no harm. Although not often referenced in nursing, this principle would be employed if the board of governors issued a policy that involves unfair hiring or firing practices or one that mandated that all medication errors, regardless of severity, reason, or circumstances, would be automatically reported to the state board of nursing.

Veracity

Veracity concerns truth telling and incorporates the concept that individuals always should tell the truth. The principle also compels that the truth be told completely. Nurse executives uphold this principle when they ensure that nurse managers are informed about decisions in a prompt and truthful manner. New policies are described fully, including the positive and negative aspects of the policy. If the nurse executive must maintain confidentiality, this fact is stated to nurse managers.

Justice

Justice concerns the issue that persons should be treated equally and fairly. This principle usually arises in times of short supplies or when competition for resources or benefits occurs. With the current nursing shortage, justice often comes to the forefront in ethical decision making. Nurse executives uphold this principle when they work to ensure adequate numbers and classifications of personnel are maintained on nursing units despite the need to "trim" the budget or when they ensure all units have competent nursing staff in relation to the acuity of patient care.

Paternalism

The principle of paternalism involves making decisions for another and often is seen as a negative or undesirable principle. Paternalism assists persons to make decisions when they do not have sufficient data or expertise to make an informed decision. Nurse executives may use this principle when they help nurse managers and nursing staff members to understand the impact of a newly developed policy, especially if the policy is complex and involves aspects of state and federal laws.

Fidelity

Fidelity is keeping promises or commitments. Nurse executives employ this principle when they are careful not to promise what they cannot deliver, such as additional full-time nursing positions or additional supplies when such positions or supplies are not forthcoming. This principle also is employed when the nurse executive works to improve the quality of nursing care as promised in the institution's stated values.

Respect for Others

The principle of respect for others often is thought to be the highest principle; it incorporates all other principles. Respect for others acknowledges the right of individuals to make decisions and to live by these decisions. Respect for others also transcends cultural differences, gender issues, and racial concerns. The nurse executive positively reinforces this principle daily in actions and communications with employees, patients, and peers. This principle also is reinforced when promotions for which the nurse executive is responsible are made based on excellence and merit rather than on personal preference.

Ethical Issues and Nursing Research

Recent research articles have acknowledged the multiple ethical issues encountered by chief nursing executives in clinical settings. Cooper, Frank, Gouty, and Hansen (2002) studied the key ethical issues encountered in healthcare institutions today.

They found that 4 of the top-rated issues and 7 of the 12 top-rated issues related to perceived failure of healthcare organizations. This widespread disappointment with the quality of care delivery entailed the following:

- Failure to provide service of the highest quality in the eyes of the consumer, regardless of social and economic status, personal attributes, or the nature of the health problems
- Failure to provide service of the highest quality consistent with the standards of the nursing profession
- Failure to provide service of the highest quality because of economic restraints determined by the organization
- Failure to provide honest information regarding resources, employee competence, or service
- Showing partiality toward clients perceived as influential
- Showing partiality toward providers perceived as influential (Cooper et al., 2002, p. 335)

Although economic factors were seen as issues in this failure to provide quality of service, an alternative factor was the failure of healthcare executives to manage effectively the conflict that arises between organizational and professional philosophy and standards.

Cooper et al. (2002, p. 334), quoting Silva, recommended that a holistic systems approach be used when this type of conflict exists, requiring that all levels of individuals involved ascribe to "common, sound, and shared ethical values." Such an approach could be initiated at the nurse executive level and incorporate the concepts of improving quality healthcare while maintaining costs.

The study underlines the following fact:

Despite the promulgation of a Joint Commission on Accreditation of Healthcare Organizations accreditation standard requiring each healthcare organization to develop and operate under a code of organizational ethics and despite considerable discussion in recent years of the need to deal holistically with business and professional ethics in healthcare organizations, the conflict between clinical and organizational ethics is still seen as a key barrier to the delivery of service of the highest quality by healthcare organizations. (Cooper et al., 2002, p. 336)

Perhaps such a reality will exist only when an institution truly can develop an organizational structure based on shared ethical values.

A study by Redman and Fry (2003) explored the ethics and human rights issues experienced by nurses in leadership roles, with particular emphasis on how disturbed the nurse leaders were by the issues and how the issues were handled. These authors identified six top ethical and human rights issues:

1. Protecting patients' rights and dignity
2. Respecting/not respecting informed consent to treatment
3. Use/nonuse of physical/chemical restraints
4. Providing care with possible risks to registered nurses' health
5. Following/not following advanced directives
6. Staffing patterns that limit patient access to nursing care (Redman & Fry, 2003, p. 152)

When the respondents were asked to identify the most disturbing ethical and human rights issues, the top six items were as follows:

1. Staffing patterns that limit patient access to nursing care
2. Prolonging the dying process with inappropriate measures
3. Working with unethical/incompetent/impaired colleagues
4. Implementing managed care policies that threaten the quality of care
5. Not considering the quality of the patient's life
6. Caring for patients/families who are uninformed/misinformed about treatment, prognosis, or medical alternatives (Redman & Fry, 2003, p. 153)

Based on the findings of this study, the implications for the nurse executive are immense.

Nurses must be supported in their roles as patient advocates. The nurse executive is in a position to be a role model for this behavior and ensure (1) the nurses are supported fully and (2) they understand how to advocate effectively for patients and their families. Nurses must understand and support patient rights issues, whether it is the patient's right to informed consent, decision making about acceptable treatments and procedures, or the right to be free from restraint. The nurse executive should ensure that staff members and nurse managers fully understand legal and ethical rights. Again, being a role model and mentoring may be two of the most effective means to ensure that nurses in the clinical setting incorporate these issues in their care of patients.

Providing care with possible risks to the nurses' health and safety also has great implications for the CNO. Concerns about these types of issues could manifest as discrimination for selected patients. The nurse executive must enforce institutional policy that prevents any type of neglect in patient care and policy that prevents risk of harm to the nursing staff members. Such issues may place the nurse executive in the middle of three competing concerns: quality of patient care; protection of staff members; and enforcing institutional policy. Although this is a difficult role for nurse executives, they must conclude how to implement this role effectively. A beginning understanding of how to implement this complex role can be found in the Literature box at the end of the chapter, which describes a study that explored the CNOs' congruence with personal and perceived organizational values and their individual leadership behaviors.

Perhaps the sixth issue, staffing patterns that limit patient access to nursing care, may be the most difficult to affect today. The issue is affected greatly by the current nursing shortage, which is a documented national issue (Siegel, 2004). Implications for the CNO include attention to staffing patterns, continued quality of patient care, collaboration with other administrators to restrict admission to nonurgent patients as appropriate, and reallocation of staff to areas of increased patient acuity as possible. Redman and Fry (2003) note this particular issue was raised by all respondents in multiple clinical settings, which further indicates this is an issue that deserves added attention and study.

Ethics education and resources may be necessary for nurse executives to accomplish their role as they supervise and serve as role models for nursing personnel in the institution. Although ethics education will not necessarily eliminate the personal disturbance levels that nurse executives experience in their roles, it may provide the tools needed for more clearly defining the issues and effectively addressing them in clinical settings. Hopefully, this clarification of ethics will enable the nurse executive to encourage the nursing staff to become more aware of ethics and its implications in patient care settings.

Ultimately, nurse executives are accountable for different outcomes and to different stakeholders than are nurses who staff the nursing units and provide direct patient care. For nurse executives, this outcome is the fiscal viability of the institution coupled with the delivery of competent, ethical nursing care. For the staff member at the bedside, the outcome is related more directly to serving as the patient advocate during delivery of competent, ethical nursing care. The principle of therapeutic jurisprudence mandates that both levels of nurses, executives and staff members, find the most effective means of merging these two diverse outcomes so that patients and their families receive the highest quality of healthcare in the most fiscally responsible manner.

LEGAL ISSUES

The nurse executive is responsible for the supervision of individuals who assist in the daily operations of the organization. Authority for the role of the nurse executive is derived directly, in most institutions, from the board of governors of the institution, and the nurse executive is directly responsible to the board of governors.

Roles and Responsibilities

Roles and responsibilities for the nurse executive include implementation of the policies of the governing board to staff members and interpretation of the policies as needed. Appropriate action must be taken if issues of noncompliance with the policies exist. Periodic reports to the board of governors regarding policy implementation are also an expectation.

Occasionally the nurse executive may believe that following the directions of a governing board may create an unsafe environment for staff members and/or patients. If the nurse executive knows or should have known that a danger or unreasonable risk of harm to staff members or patients would be created by enacting these policies or procedures, the nurse executive must take action to prevent such an outcome. Communication is the first step in prevention of potential harm, and it involves all levels of management and staff.

Communications are often the most effective strategy that the nurse executive can employ when working with subordinates, whether they are nurses or members of other professions. Communications may involve the need for confrontation to ensure the efficient and continued operation of the institution. Although confrontation should not be the first approach in solving issues, it may become necessary to resolve underlying issues. Used correctly, confrontation can be a powerful and effective communication skill in resolution of major issues and prevention of potential legal issues. Strategies for effective confrontation are found in Box 5-1.

Nursing executives also are charged with ensuring that (1) nurse managers and staff members adhere to policies and procedures of the institution and (2) ancillary departments/personnel perform in a manner that allows nursing personnel to provide competent, safe care to patients. In these aspects, effective communication styles and content are again vital for nurse executives. Appropriate, frequent communications with nursing staff members begin to ensure that each

Box 5-1   STRATEGIES FOR EFFECTIVE CONFRONTATION

Use confrontation selectively and only when corrective action can be taken.

Communicate personal respect for the person you are confronting.

Avoid an attitude of anger.

Facilitate taking personal responsibility rather than blaming.

Use personal communication, rather than written communiqués.

Incorporate humor, as appropriate.

Time the confrontation strategically, remembering that both the timing and the setting of the confrontation are critical.

Davidhizar, R., & Cathon, D. (2002). Strategies for effective confrontation. *Radiological Technology, 73*(5), 476-478.

person is performing appropriately. Also such communications allow the nurse executive to work with other individuals, such as ancillary department managers and the medical director, who are involved in the delivery of patient care.

Vicarious Liability

One of the most important legal doctrines that affects nurse executives is the doctrine of respondent superior or vicarious liability. This doctrine, sometimes referred to as substituted liability, allows the legal system to hold employers accountable for the negligence of their employees. The rationale underlying the doctrine is that the employee would not have been in a position to have caused the wrongdoing unless hired by the employer and that the injured party will be allowed to suffer a double wrong merely because most employees are unable to pay damages for their wrongdoings. Nurse executives can best avoid these issues by ensuring that the nursing staff they supervise know and follow hospital policy and procedure, deliver competent nursing care, and serve as advocates for patients and their families.

Perhaps this is one of the largest areas concerning therapeutic jurisprudence as it relates to legal issues. Studies such as the report by the Institute of Medicine (1999) first alerted the public and the healthcare delivery system to monumental issues surrounding medication errors in healthcare facilities across the United States. Subsequent studies on the correlation between nurse staffing and patient mortality (e.g., Aiken, Clarke, Sloane, Sochalski, & Silber, 2002) continue to note the effect of corporate policies and practices on patient outcomes and adverse effects. Potential liability from such errors rests on the individual practitioners and on the entire corporate structure, in particular the nurse executive, under the doctrine of respondent superior. Nurse executives must begin to make an impact on these issues through forceful implementation of existing polices and through the creation and adoption of additional policies. Through therapeutic jurisprudence, the well-being of individuals should be enhanced. Policies must address the economic issues and their physical and psychologic effects on staff members and patients. Some of the underlying principles of therapeutic jurisprudence are to bring "well-being" into focus as a goal of the law and the legal system and begin to demonstrate connections more clearly.

Medicare Fraud in Healthcare Settings

One of the most significant issues that nurse executives may need to address concerns issues of fraud in the institution. Perhaps the most significant area of fraud in healthcare systems today is in the area of Medicare fraud. Since its inception in 1965, Medicare fraud has been estimated at greater than 1 trillion dollars (Rehnquist, 2001). Established in 1976, the Office of the Inspector General (OIG) identifies and eliminates fraud, waste, and abuse in programs sponsored by the Department of Health and Human Services.

Medicare fraud can be committed in a variety of ways:

- False Medicare claims submitted for services that were never rendered to a patient or patients

- Charges for medications that were not dispensed to patients or charged for at a brand name level when generic equivalents were actually dispensed
- Referral fees for services not rendered or rendered solely on paper documentation without the patient ever being fully examined by the referral primary healthcare provider
- Laboratory, services, or supplies kickback fees to third parties
- Nursing home fraud in which residents' charges for services and treatments never encountered were forwarded to Medicare
- Falsification of nursing care

Perhaps the greatest source of fraud is in the area of home healthcare, because this is also the area hardest to track. As an ever-escalating number of elderly receive healthcare at home, the number of scams involving claims for services not received, claims for beneficiaries not homebound, claims for visits not made, and claims for visits not authorized by primary healthcare providers has increased greatly. To combat these abuses in home healthcare, the OIG has established Operation Restore Trust, which targets such scams by home care agencies, nursing homes, and durable medical equipment suppliers.

Corporations, through their boards of governors and executive staffs, have a fiduciary responsibility that includes a duty of care principle. This duty of care principle requires a director or executive to act in good faith with the care that an ordinarily prudent person would exercise under similar conditions. Reasonable inquiry is embedded within this concept. Directors and executives should make inquiries to obtain information necessary to satisfy the duty of care. As outlined in *In Re Caremark International, Inc. Derivative Litigation* (1996):

A director's obligation includes a duty to attempt in good faith to assure that a corporate information and reporting system, which the Board concludes is adequate, exists, and that failure to do so . . . may render a director liable for losses caused by non-compliance with applicable legal standards. (at 964)

Directors and managers, though, have separate obligations. Members of the board of governors of a corporation have the duty of oversight; they do not manage the daily operations of the corporation. Executives at the administrative level have the duty to manage on a daily basis, which includes the responsibility to ensure that none of these fraudulent practices exist within an institution.

A compliance program is the first step to ensure such abuses are not occurring. Benefits of a compliance program include the following:

- Formation of effective internal controls to ensure compliance with statutes, regulations, and rules
- Concrete demonstration to employees and the community at large of the institution's commitment to responsible corporate conduct
- Ability to obtain an accurate assessment of employee behavior
- Increased likelihood of identification and prevention of unlawful and unethical behavior
- Ability to react quickly to employees' operational compliance concerns and effectively target resources to address these concerns
- Improvement in the quality, efficiency, and consistency of providing services
- Mechanism to encourage employees to report potential problems and allow for appropriate internal inquiry and corrective action
- Centralized source for distributing information on healthcare statutes, regulations, and other program directives
- Mechanism to improve internal communication
- Procedures that allow prompt and thorough investigation of alleged misconduct
- Thorough, early detection and reporting, minimizing loss to false claims, and thereby

reducing the institution's exposure to civil damages and penalties, criminal sanctions, and administrative remedies (Compliance Program Guidelines, 2000, p. 14290)

The institution should take the following steps to enact such a compliance program:

- Implement written policies, procedures, and standards of conduct
- Designate a compliance officer and compliance committee
- Conduct effective training and education
- Develop effective lines of communication
- Enforce standards through well-published disciplinary guidelines
- Conduct internal monitoring and auditing
- Respond promptly to detected offenses and develop corrective action (Compliance Program Guidelines, 2000, p. 14289)

Responsibilities for the nurse executive in this area of the law include ensuring that (1) such a program is part of the institution's policy, (2) nursing staff know why it is important and when to report suspicious actions or circumstances, and (3) mid-management level nurses comply with the program. If the nursing managers or staff members have concerns, the nurse executive must follow the institution's policies to report these concerns.

FEDERAL AND STATE LAWS

Laws that nurse leaders must understand and enforce include state and federal enactments. To be effective and legally correct, the nurse executive must be familiar with these laws and how individual laws affect the institution and labor relations. This is true even if the nurse managers have hiring and firing authority. Although some degree of fear of the legal system may exist because of personal experience or the experiences of colleagues, this fear usually is directly attributable to uncertainty with the law or partial knowledge of the law. By understanding and correctly following federal employment laws, nursing administrators at all levels actually may lessen potential liability

because they have complied appropriately with either federal or state laws. Table 5-2 gives an overview of key federal employment laws that the CNO should know.

Equal Employment Opportunity Laws

Several federal laws have been enacted to expand equal employment opportunities by prohibiting discrimination based on gender, age, race, religion, handicap, pregnancy, and national origin. These laws are enforced by the Equal Employment Opportunity Commission (EEOC). Additionally, states have enacted statutes that address employment opportunities, and the nurse executive should consider both when hiring and assigning nursing employees. If the nurse managers are responsible for hiring and assigning new personnel, then the responsibility of the nurse executive is to ensure that these individuals are following proper procedures.

The most significant legislation affecting equal employment opportunities today is the amended 1964 Civil Rights Act (43 Fed. Reg.1978). Section 703 (a) of Title VII makes it illegal for an employer "to refuse to hire, discharge an individual, or otherwise to discriminate against an individual, with respect to his compensation, terms, conditions, or privileges of employment because of the individual's race, color, religion, sex, or national origin." Title VII also was amended by the Equal Employment Opportunity Act of 1972 so that it applies to private institutions with 15 or more employees, state and local governments, labor unions, and employment agencies.

A number of exceptions exist to Title VII. For example, it is lawful to make employment decisions on the basis of national origin, religion, and gender (never race or color) if such decisions are necessary for the normal operation of the business, although the courts have viewed this exception very narrowly. Promotions and layoffs based on bona fide seniority or merit systems are permissible (*Herrero v. St. Louis University Hospital*, 1997), as are exceptions based on

Table 5-2 SELECTED FEDERAL LABOR LEGISLATION

Year	Legislation	Legislation's Purpose
1935	Wagner Act (National Labor Relations Act)	Unions, National Labor Relations Board established
1947	Taft-Hartley Act (Labor-Management Relations Act)	Equal balance of power between unions and management
1962	Executive Order 10988	Allowed public employees to join unions
1963	Equal Pay Act	Became illegal to pay lower wages based on gender
1964	Civil Rights Act	Protected against discrimination as a result of race, color, creed, national origin, etc.
1967	Age Discrimination in Employment Act	Protected against discrimination because of age
1970	Occupational Safety and Health Act	Ensured healthy and safe working conditions
1974	Wagner Amendments	Allowed nonprofit organizations to unionize
1990	Americans with Disabilities Act	Barred discrimination against disabled workers
1991	Civil Rights Act	Amended the Civil Rights Act of 1964 to address sexual harassment in the workplace
1993	Family and Medical Leave Act	Allowed work leaves based on family and medical needs
1996	Health Insurance Portability and Accountability Act of 1996	Addressed portability of health coverage, fraud and abuse issues, and confidentiality of protected health information

From selected Federal Registers.

business necessity. The CNO is the person responsible for requesting these exceptions, as applicable in the institution.

In 1991 the amended Civil Rights Act was signed into law. This act broadened the issue of sexual harassment in the workplace and supersedes many of the sections of Title VII. Sections of the new legislation define sexual harassment, its elements, and the employer's responsibilities regarding harassment in the workplace, especially prevention and corrective action. The Civil Rights Act is enforced by the EEOC as created in the 1964 act; the EEOC's powers were broadened in the 1972 Equal Employment Opportunity Act. The primary activity of the EEOC is processing complaints of employment discrimination in three phases: investigation, conciliation, and litigation. Investigation focuses on determining whether the employer has violated provisions of Title VII. If the EEOC finds "probable cause," an attempt is made to reach an agreement or conciliation between the EEOC, the complainant, and the employer. If conciliation fails, the EEOC may file suit against the employer in federal court or issue to the complainant the right to sue for discrimination under its auspices, including those relating to staffing practices and sexual harassment in the workplace. The EEOC defines sexual harassment broadly, and this generally has been upheld in the courts.

Nurse managers, through guidance and direction from the nurse executive, must realize that it is the duty of employers (management) to prevent sexual harassment in the workplace. The EEOC issues policies and practices for employers to implement to sensitize employees to this problem and to prevent its occurrence. Nurse managers should be aware of these policies and practices and seek guidance in implementing them if sexual harassment occurs on their units.

Age Discrimination in Employment Act of 1967

The Age Discrimination in Employment act of 1967 made it illegal for employers, unions, and employment agencies to discriminate against older men and women. The law, in a 1986 amendment, prohibits discrimination against persons over the age of 40. The practical outcome of this act has been that mandatory retirement is no longer seen in the American workplace.

As with Title VII, this act has some exceptions. Reasonable factors, other than age, may be used when terminations become necessary. Appropriate reasonable factors to plead include a performance evaluation system and some limited occupational qualifications, for example, the tedious physical demands of a specific job.

Americans with Disabilities Act of 1990

The Americans with Disabilities Act (ADA) of 1990 provides protection to persons with disabilities and is the most significant civil rights legislation since the Civil Rights Act of 1964. The purpose of the ADA is to provide a clear and comprehensive national mandate for the elimination of discrimination against disabled individuals and to provide clear, strong, consistent, enforceable standards addressing discrimination in the workplace. The ADA is related closely to the Civil Rights Act and incorporates the antidiscrimination principles established in Section 504 of the Rehabilitation Act of 1973.

The act has five titles, and Table 5-3 shows the pertinent issues covered by each title. The ADA has jurisdiction over employers, private and public; employment agencies; labor organizations; and joint labor-management committees. It defines disability broadly. With respect to an individual, a disability is (1) a physical or mental impairment that substantially limits one or more of the major life activities of such individual, (2) a record of such impairment, or (3) a condition regarded as having such an impairment (42 U.S.C. § 12102[2]). The overall effect of the legislation is

Table 5-3 AMERICANS WITH DISABILITIES ACT OF 1990

Title	Provisions
I	Employment: defines purpose of the act and who is qualified under the act as disabled
II	Public services: concerns services, programs, and activities of public entities and public transportation
III	Public accommodations and services operated by private entities: prohibits discrimination against disabled in areas of public accommodations, commercial facilities, and public transportation services
IV	Telecommunications: intended to make telephone services accessible to individuals with hearing or speech impairments
V	Miscellaneous provisions: certain insurance matters; incorporation of this act with other federal and state laws

Americans with Disabilities Act of 1990, 42 U.S.C. 5 12101 *et seq.* (1990).

that persons with disabilities will not be excluded from job opportunities or adversely affected in any aspect of employment unless they are not qualified or are otherwise unable to perform the job. The ADA thus protects qualified and disabled individuals in regard to job application procedures, hiring, compensation, advancement, and all other employment matters.

Since its enactment, the number of lawsuits filed under the ADA continues to be extensive. Recent cases have assisted in defining disability eligibility. Conditions that do not constitute a disability include (1) the finding that a nurse with a lifting disability is not qualified under the ADA (*Thompson v. Holy Family Hospital*, 1997); (2) erratic behavior does not give notice to the employer that the individual is suffering from mental impairment (*Webb v. Mercy Hospital*, 1996); (3) depression and anxiety are not disabling conditions (*Cody v. Cigna Healthcare of St. Louis, Inc.,* 1998); (4) a nurse taking medications for depression is not disabled (*Wilking v. County of Ramsey,* 1997); (5) migraine headaches and latex allergies are not disabilities (*Howard v. North Mississippi Medical Center*, 1996); and (6) pregnancy is not a disability (*Jessie v. Carter Health Care Center, Inc.*, 1996).

The act requires the employer or potential employer to make reasonable accommodations to employ the disabled. The law does not mandate that disabled individuals be hired before fully qualified, nondisabled persons. It does mandate that the disabled not be disqualified merely because of an easily accommodated disability.

This last point was well illustrated by the court in *Zamudio v. Patia* (1997). The court stated that the employer would be required to inform Ms. Zamudio when a position that she required as reasonable accommodation became available. She would be allowed to apply, but "as a disabled employee seeking reasonable accommodation, she did not have to be given preference over other employees without disabilities who might have better qualifications or more seniority" (*Zamudio v. Patia*, 1997 at 808).

The court also will not impose job restructuring on an employer if the person needing accommodation qualifies for other jobs not requiring such accommodation. In *Mauro v. Borgess Medical Center* (1995) the court refused to impose accommodation on the employer hospital merely because the affected employee desired to stay within a certain unit of the institution. In that case, an operating surgical technician who was HIV positive was offered an equivalent position by the hospital in an area in which no patient contact would occur. He refused the transfer, desiring accommodation within the operating arena and was denied such accommodation by the Michigan court.

The act also provides for essential job functions. These are defined by the ADA as those functions that the person must be able to perform to be qualified for employment positions. Courts have assisted in determining these essential job functions. For example, in *Jones v. Kerrville State Hospital* (1998), the court found that an essential job function for a psychiatric nurse is the ability to restrain patients. In *Laurin v. Providence Hospital and Massachusetts Nurses Association* (1998), the ability to work rotating shifts was held to be an essential job function.

Finally, the act specifically excludes from the definition homosexuality and bisexuality, sexual behavioral disorders, gambling, kleptomania, pyromania, and current use of illegal drugs (42 U.S.C. § 12211 [a] and [b][1]). Moreover, employers may hold alcoholics to the same job qualifications and job performance standards as other employees even if the unsatisfactory behavior or performance is related to the alcoholism (42 U.S.C. § 12114 [c][4]). As with other federal employment laws, nurse managers should have a thorough understanding of the law as it applies to the institution and their specific job descriptions and should know whom to contact within the institution structure for clarification as needed.

Affirmative Action

The policy of affirmative action (AA) differs from the policy of equal employment opportunity (EEO). AA enhances employment opportunities of protected groups of people, whereas EEO is concerned with the use of employment practices that do not discriminate against or impair the employment opportunities of protected groups. Therefore AA can be seen in conjunction with several federal employment laws; for example, in conjunction with the Vietnam Era Veterans' Readjustment Assistance Act of 1974, the AA requires that employers with government contracts take steps to enhance the employment opportunities of disabled veterans and other veterans of the Vietnam era.

Equal Pay Act of 1963

The Equal Pay Act makes it illegal to pay lower wages to employees of one gender when the jobs (1) require equal skill in experience, training, education, and ability; (2) require equal effort in mental or physical exertion; (3) are of equal responsibility and accountability; and (4) are performed under similar working conditions. Courts have held that unequal pay may be legal if it is based on seniority, merit, incentive systems, and a factor other than gender. The main cases filed under this law in the area of nursing have been by nonprofessionals.

Occupational Safety and Health Act

The Occupational Safety and Health Act of 1970 was enacted to ensure that healthful and safe working conditions would exist in the workplace. Among other provisions, the law requires isolation procedures, placarding areas containing ionizing radiation, proper grounding of electrical equipment, protective storage of flammable and combustible liquids, and the gloving of all personnel when handling bodily fluids. The statute provides that if no federal standard has been established, state statutes prevail. CNOs must ensure that nurse managers know the relevant Occupational Safety and Health Administration (OSHA) laws for the institution and their specific work areas. Frequent review of new additions to the law also must be undertaken, especially in this era of AIDS and infectious diseases, and care must be taken to ensure that necessary gloves and equipment as specified are available on each unit.

Family and Medical Leave Act of 1993

The Family and Medical Leave Act of 1993 was passed because of the large number of single-parent and two-parent households, in which the single parent or both parents are employed full time, which places job security and parenting at odds.

The law also supports the growing demands that aging parents are placing on their working children. The act attempts to balance the demands of the workplace with the demands of the family and allows employed individuals to take leaves for medical reasons, including the birth or adoption of children and the care of a spouse, child, or parent who has serious health problems. Essentially, the act provides job security for unpaid leave while the employee is caring for a new infant or other family healthcare needs. The act is gender-neutral and allows men and women the same leave provisions. To be eligible under the act, the employee must have worked for at least 12 months and worked at least 1250 hours during the preceding 12-month period. The employee may take up to 12 weeks of unpaid leave. The act allows the employer to require the employee to use all or part of any paid vacation, personal leave, or sick leave as part of the 12-week family leave. Employees must give the employer 30 days notice before using the medical leave or such notice as is practical in emergency cases.

Employment-at-Will and Wrongful Discharge

Historically, the employment relationship has been considered as a "free will" relationship. Employees were free to take or not take a job at will, and employers were free to hire, retain, or discharge employees for any reason. Many laws, some federal but predominantly state, have been slowly eroding this at-will employment relationship. Evolving case law provides at least three exceptions to the broad doctrine of employment-at-will.

The first exception is a public policy exception. This exception involves cases in which an employee is discharged in direct conflict with established public policy (Pozgar, 1999). Some examples would be discharging an employee for serving on a jury, for reporting employers' illegal actions (better known as "whistleblowing"), and for filing a workers' compensation claim.

Several recent court cases attest to the number of terminations in healthcare settings as retaliation causes of action. More commonly known as "whistleblowing" cases, the healthcare provider is terminated for one of three distinct reasons: (1) for speaking out against unsafe practices; (2) for violations of federal laws; or (3) for filing lawsuits against employers. In *Roulston v. Tendercare (Michigan), Inc.* (2000), a social services director was dismissed after she confronted the director of nursing for what the social services director termed patient abuse. The social services director had reported instances of patient abuse to the state Department of Consumer and Industry Services and the Health Care Fraud Unit of the state attorney general's office. The nursing director first attempted to debate the definition of patient abuse, then told the social services director that she had better start thinking like everyone else who worked at the nursing home. The court was satisfied that the social services director's lawsuit for retaliation against the nursing home was appropriate.

In *Fleming v. Correctional Healthcare Solutions, Inc.* (2000), a nurse in a correctional facility was dismissed for reporting financial mismanagement. The nurse was terminated for insubordination, and she sued her former employer for retaliation under the New Jersey whistleblower act. The court upheld her right to sue for wrongful dismissal. Similarly, the court in *UTMB v. Hohman* (1999) allowed a nurse to bring suit for wrongful dismissal when she was discharged for reporting a physician's alleged abuses.

The court in *Taylor v. Memorial Health Systems, Inc.* (2000) enumerated the conditions that must be present to file a valid employer retaliation lawsuit. (1) The whistleblower must disclose or threaten to disclose an allegation in writing and under oath to the state department of professional regulation. (2) The allegation must have been about an activity, policy, or practice of the employer that is or was a violation of a state or federal law, rule, or regulation. (3) The employee must have given the employer written notification

and a reasonable time to correct the problem. (4) The employee must have suffered retaliation in the form of some actual harm (*Taylor v. Memorial Health Systems, Inc.*, 2000, at 755). Although states may vary slightly on these elements, this court essentially outlines for nurses the elements to consider in contemplation of a whistleblower lawsuit.

The second exception to wrongful discharge is situations involving an implied contract. The courts generally have treated employee handbooks, company policies, and oral statements made at the time of employment as "framing the employment relationship" (*Watkins v. Unemployment Compensation Board of Review*, 1997). For example, in *Trombley v. Southwestern Vermont Medical Center* (1999), the court found that the employee handbook outlined the procedure for progressive discipline, mandating that such procedure must be followed before a nurse could be terminated for incompetent nursing care.

The third exception to wrongful discharge is a "good faith and fair dealing" exception. The purpose of this exception is to prevent unfair or malicious terminations, and the exception is used sparingly by the courts. An older case illustrates its use by the court. In *Fortune v. National Cash Register Company* (1977), an employee was discharged just before a final contract was signed between his employer and another company for which the employee would have received a large commission. The court held that he was discharged in bad faith, solely to prevent payment of his commission by National Cash Register.

Nurse executives must ensure that those who have hiring and firing privileges within the institution know and enforce the respective state law concerning this growing area of the law. Nurse executives and nurse managers should review institution documents, especially employee handbooks and recruiting brochures, for unwanted statements that imply job security or other unintentional promises. Managers also need to know that they should not say anything during the preemployment negotiations and interviews that might be construed as implying job security or other unintentional promises to the potential employee. To prevent successful suits for retaliation by whistleblowers, nurse executives should monitor carefully the treatment of an employee after a complaint is filed and ensure that performance evaluations are performed and placed in the appropriate files. The nurse executive also should take steps to address immediately the whistleblower's complaint or ensure that other, more appropriate, personnel address the issue in a prompt and efficient manner.

Health Insurance Portability and Accountability Act of 1996

One of the means to prevent fraud and abuse in the healthcare system is found in the Health Insurance Portability and Accountability Act (HIPAA) of 1996. This law mandates the development of a centralized electronic database containing all health records for every patient in the United States as a means of administrative simplification. It also mandates that standards for the electronic exchange of individually identifiable health information be developed and implemented. A final enactment date for the provisions of the act was April 2003.

Among the many provisions of HIPAA, the following are found:

- The portability of healthcare coverage
- An antifraud and abuse program
- Streamlining transfer of patient information between insurers and providers
- Tax incentives toward the acquisition of health insurance and accelerated benefits
- Establishing the federal government as a national healthcare regulator

Challenges for the nurse executives in this area of the law are multiple and varied. First, nurse executives must understand the provisions that concern patient privacy, including when confidential information may be shared and how to best protect the information while sharing with others entitled to the information. Second, they must ensure that those they oversee also understand the law and are complying with the confidentiality provisions of the rules. Third, the nurse executives must follow up on areas in which noncompliance with the rules is occurring, whether this noncompliance is observed by nurse executives directly or is reported by concerned staff members. Finally, as additional rules are written and enforced, nurse executives must be aware of these additional regulations and ensure that all nursing personnel also are alerted to their existence.

Mandatory Overtime

Although few states have enacted legislation regarding this issue, mandatory overtime has become a major issue in nursing today. A direct product of the current nursing shortage, mandatory overtime may become one of the most potentially liable means of addressing short staffing issues. Nurses are placed in a unique position when confronted by the demand for overtime. In a time characterized by an aggressive national movement to reduce adverse patient outcomes, fatigued nurses and other healthcare providers routinely are requested to work extra hours. Often this demand for additional work coverage is heralded with the institution's threat of patient abandonment or institution of actions to remove the nurse's license. Numerous attempts have been made to legislate that no registered nurse would be required to work more than 8 hours in a given day or 80 hours in a 14-day period.

Ethical nursing practice mandates that nurses not engage in practice that can compromise patient outcomes. The American Nurses Association's (ANA) *Code of Ethics for Nurses* (2001) addresses these ethical issues in the following sections:

Provision 3: "The nurse promotes, advocates for, and strives to protect the health, safety, and rights of the patient."

Provision 4: "The nurse is responsible and accountable for individual nursing practice and determines the appropriate delegation of tasks consistent with the nurse's obligation to provide optimal patient care." (ANA, 2001, p. 4)

Patient abandonment is the unilateral termination of care and treatment by a healthcare provider without the patient's consent. Although generally made against physicians, such a claim could be brought against a nurse. Mitigating factors that may be pled by the nurse in such legal actions include the fact that the nurse had worked the scheduled hours and that the nurse was physically and mentally unable to continue to care competently for patients.

Nurse executives must work to ensure that competent care remains the standard of the institution and work to ensure that mandatory overtime is not a concept used within their institutions if they work in states that have no restrictions on mandatory overtime. Nurse executives in states where statutes preventing mandatory overtime have been enacted should ensure that these statutes are followed. Finally, nurse executives should begin to work for passage of federal legislation that addresses this issue.

Regulatory Agencies

Legal responsibilities of the nurse executive include the correction of any nursing-related deficiencies found during accreditation surveys by governmental agencies, such as the Centers for Medicare and Medicaid (CMS) and nongovernmental agencies, such as the Joint Commission on Accreditation of Healthcare Organizations (JCAHO). These corrective actions commonly are delegated to the appropriate nurse manager by the nurse executive. During the on-site visit by team members of the surveying agency, team members may provide the organization with either written citation or consultative remarks. Consultative remarks usually highlight areas of concern that the institution should address. These consultative remarks should be given the same attention for correction as written reports.

Finally, the nurse executive must have a thorough understanding of legal principles as they pertain to clinical settings. Such underlying legal principles include the purpose of nurse practice acts; tort law, including intentional, quasi-intentional, and nonintentional torts; staffing issues and potential liability for nursing shortage related issues; delegation and supervision; and informed consent doctrines. Although these individual issues are more the accountability and responsibility of nurse managers, nurse executives are ultimately responsible and accountable for ensuring the actions of those whom they oversee.

SUMMARY

Therapeutic jurisprudence is a positive approach to ethical and legal issues for nurse executives. The concept of therapeutic jurisprudence addresses the quality improvement section of all of healthcare today, by focusing on the human impact of legal and ethical issues rather than on the more common aspect of merely attempting to apply these concepts. By using therapeutic jurisprudence as the base, patient advocacy and human rights are the center of nursing care delivery in healthcare settings.

KEY POINTS TO LEAD

1. Analyze the concept of therapeutic jurisprudence as applied from a legal and an ethical perspective in healthcare.
2. Analyze ethical principles and their application from the perspective of the nurse executive.
3. Evaluate the results of selected research studies involving ethical issues encountered by nurse executives.
4. Critique the roles and responsibilities of the nurse executive.
5. Analyze the role of the nurse executive in the area of Medicare abuse.
6. Analyze key aspects of employment laws from the perspective of a nurse executive.
7. Apply ethical and legal principles in analyzing one nurse executive's perception of her current job.

Literature Box

Currently, healthcare organizations struggle with balancing service delivery with the need to remain fiscally solvent in an ever-changing marketplace; nurse leaders struggle with these same concepts. How can a nurse provide humanistic and holistic care consistent with nursing values while maintaining economic solvency? The purpose of this study was to examine the relationship between nurse executives' perceived congruence with personal and organizational values and their leadership styles: transformational, transactional, and laissez-faire. Value similarity between leaders and the organization were thought of to affect organizational performance positively because of shared interpretation of environmental events, a common system of communication, and clearer role expectations.

Three leadership styles were included in the study. Transformational leaders create and share a vision, defining where the group is headed and giving meaning and clarity to the organization's identity. Transactional leaders approach followers with the intent of determining what can be exchanged as rewards for services rendered, which makes the enticement of potential rewards the guiding direction. Laissez-faire leadership is a nontransaction or the absence of leadership. This leadership style involves no long-range plan and little impetus to work with others in management positions (Perkel, 2002).

A survey was mailed to 900 nurse executives, and the resulting sample consisted of 411 nurse executives employed by American Hospital Association institutions located east of the Mississippi River. Three instruments (Values Analysis Worksheet, Multifactor Leadership Questionnaire, and a researcher-designed socio-demographic questionnaire) were mailed to the identified sample population. Participants in the study were primarily female (92.4%), ranged in age from 31 to 67 years of age with a mean age of 49.96, 64.9% had master's degrees, and the mean length of time in their current position was 4.99 years. Participants in the study were employed primarily by not-for-profit hospitals (85.1%).

Descriptive statistics were used to evaluate the relationship between the personal and organizational values; the sample ranked their personal values higher that the organizational values, with a mean self score of 82.56 versus a mean organizational values score of 68.84. Personal values that ranked highest were integrity, honesty, respect, and loyalty; organizational values ranked highest by the sample were commitment to quality, integrity, belief in high performance, and loyalty. The study also found four areas of greatest incongruity between personal and organizational values to be honesty, sense of humor, feedback systems, and willingness to help others.

The second research question, which examined the relationship between perceived value congruence, level of education, years of administrative experience, and for-profit versus not-for-profit status of the employing agency to leadership behaviors, used descriptive statistics to find that the transformational leadership style was the most commonly used leadership style by these respondents (M = 3.44), followed by transactional as second (M = 2.01), and laissez-faire (M = 0.52) the least utilized leadership style. Multiple regression analysis was then performed, which indicated that no part of the variance in the leadership behavior scores could be accounted for by the four independent variables: values congruence; education; years of administrative experience; or for-profit versus not-for-profit status of the employing agency.

The highest-ranked values of the organization that were not the highest ranked by the nurse executives, the author concluded, were those not in conflict with the values that the nurse executives held the highest and thus did not seem to impede effective leadership style. The nurse executives' personal and organizational values were incongruent, which prompted the author to question how important these areas of incongruence were for the nurse executives. The author concluded that such incongruence could be problematic in the area of decision making, especially in the areas of allocation of resources and handling personnel issues (Perkel, 2002).

Literature Box

Several possible explanations exist for the correlation seen in this study between perceived personal and organizational values. Perhaps the nurse executive's perception upon being employed in this position is that personal values and the actual values held by the organization are incongruent. A second possible explanation is that nurse executives adapt to the organizational values as a means of survival in the corporate world. Third, the results may indicate that when nurse executives experience an intolerable degree of value incongruence, they merely leave the organization. Day (1990) found that executives develop "threshold criteria" that consist of a combination of individual experiences and organizational perceptions. When an individual was pushed too far beyond his or her threshold limit, he or she tried to change the threshold by redefining personal values, redefining perception, or simply by leaving the situation. Thus those nurse executives who experienced significant values incongruence possibly were not participants in this study because they had already resigned their nurse executive positions. This latter fact may be supported by the fact that the mean years of experience in the nurse executive's current position was 4.99 years.

One explanation for the findings of the present study could be that decision making is affected more directly by values conflict than is leadership style. Nurse executives may use flexible leadership styles rather than a single leadership style, and the particular leadership style employed depends upon the situation or people involved at a given time.

Perkel (2002) concluded that nurses who strive to be exceptional transformational leaders must find a means to continue to lead effectively in organizations in which their personal values conflict with the overall organizational values. To accomplish this, nurse executives must first clearly identify their own values and then assess the values of the organization in which they are employed. They must then determine the importance of congruence in these values and begin to assess where areas of value conflict will be a barrier to their ability to provide the leadership necessary to support nursing and the organization for which they work.

The need for exceptional nursing leadership is critical in the rapidly changing and complex world in which healthcare environments exist today. Equally important for nursing leadership is that one's values must be preserved and reflected in behaviors. This study remains one of the first nursing research studies identifying the interplay of personal values and leadership style. Further studies need to be undertaken to understand more fully the relationship of the perception of the congruence of personal and organizational values on effective leadership styles.

Perkel, L. K. (2002). Nurse executives' values and leadership behaviors. *Nursing Leadership Forum, 6*(4), 100-107.

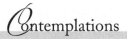

Contemplations

- Which of the ethical principles are most important for the nurse executive to portray?
- If you were the nurse executive, which legal issues would be the most problematic for you and how would you begin to address them?
- What legal issues did the nurse executive in the Leader Story encounter?
- How might you begin to mitigate (lessen) your potential legal liability?

- Do nurse executives have different values than those of staff nurses or nurse managers?
- Do nurse executives reflect the values of the board of governors in their actions?
- What would you recommend to nurses in the scenario about lessening their potential legal liability?

I have been the CNO at my institution for 3½ years. The institution is a 400-bed acute care facility with an active hospice outpatient program, home healthcare program, and a durable medical equipment distributorship. The majority of the registered nurse staff members are prepared at the associate degree level, with approximately 16% prepared at the baccalaureate level. Although the institution policy is to have nurse managers prepared at the master's level, currently only three master's prepared nurses are in these positions.

I joined the institution because I was impressed with its reputation in the community and the positive comments that nurses employed by the institution made regarding patient care and their working environment, and because I was recruited specifically by a member of the board of governors. Since I joined the institution's administrative staff, several of the members of the board of governors are new and the chief operating officer (COO) is now beginning his second year with the facility. Additionally, as in other institutions in this region, we have been affected negatively by the nursing shortage.

Since the arrival of the new COO and the change in the membership of the board of governors, a lack of understanding is apparent regarding the role of nursing, excellence in care delivery, the need for a strong and reliable nursing float pool, and permanent versus agency staff. Indeed, even the COO seems not to comprehend much of what makes up the role of nursing within the institution and its various clinical sites. Compounding this lack of general knowledge about the role of nursing in this institution is the fact that, at least to me, there is no desire for the COO, CEO, or board to understand these critical issues. The bottom line always appears to be financial concerns.

As the nurse executive, I continue to remind them that this is a healthcare business, not a plant or a production center, but a business dedicated to assisting sick individuals. For my part, I believe that they think I am merely someone to be tolerated and ignored, and I feel powerless to make any kind of impact at this point. The worst part is that the board of governors is now excluding me from much of the decision-making process because they know I will not support their decisions. Perhaps it is time for me to think about relocating and seeking alternative employment.

Having read about therapeutic jurisprudence, I tried to begin to introduce the application of this issue at the board meetings to which I was invited. The response was extremely slow at first, with individual members of the administration of the institution giving at least some verbal acknowledgement of the issues involved and the benefits of reexamining these issues from the perspective of the impact at the human level as opposed to merely the fiscal impact. When the executor of a deceased patient's estate sued the institution, the administrative board finally began to look in earnest at why therapeutic jurisprudence was so important a concept. In that lawsuit, it was obvious to all the administrative board that staffing patterns did count and that we could no longer continue to staff high-acuity units with more medical technicians and licensed practical nurses than registered nurses. We also were forced to reconsider our policy on mandatory overtime, especially in light of the fact that the principal nurse at the center of this specific lawsuit had worked 78 hours in a given 7-day work period.

Although the case settled out of court for a fraction of what the executor had requested, it was the "wake-up call" that began a change in corporate policy making.

For myself, I still struggle with helping the administrative staff with the long-range effects of policies. They still create some policies that I feel are unsafe for staff members and patients, and I continue to fight against those policies. But I am now part of all board meetings, even though I still am outvoted on a variety of issues. I have learned, though, to save my comments for the issues that are truly unsafe and potentially disastrous for the institution. I also have incorporated more involvement at the unit level so that I can use realistic examples from those settings in my descriptions of the potential outcomes of less-than-desirable policies. Finally, we did reexamine the staffing ratios and mandatory overtime policies and have made major changes in those policies, although I still work for more improvements in those policies.

For now, I have decided not to seek alternative employment. I know that the values I hold most dear still are not recognized fully by the administrative staff, but I am making inroads slowly and, because of my greater involvement with individual nurses, I want to stay and see this institution succeed.

Chapter References

Aiken, L. H., Clarke, S. P., Sloane, D. M., Sochalski, J., & Silber, J. H. (2002). Hospital nurse staffing and patient mortality, nurse burnout, and job dissatisfaction. *Journal of the American Medical Association, 288,* 1987-1993.

Americans with Disabilities Act of 1990, 42 U.S.C. § 12101 *et seq.* (1990).

American Nurses Association. (2001). *Code of ethics for nurses.* Washington, DC: Author.

Beauchamp, T. L., & Childress, J. F. (2001). *Principles of biomedical ethics.* (5th ed.). New York: Oxford University.

Byrnes, B. (1982). Non-nursing functions: The nurses state their case. *American Journal of Nursing, 82,* 1089.

Cody v. Cigna Healthcare of St. Louis, Inc., 139 F. 3d 595 (8th Cir. 1998).

Compliance Program Guidelines. (2000). *Federal Register, 65*(52), 14289-14306.

Cooper, R. W., Frank, G. L., Gouty, C. A., & Hansen, M. C. (2002). Key ethical issues encountered in healthcare organizations. *Journal of Nursing Administration, 32*(6), 331-337.

Davidhizar, R., & Cathon, D. (2002). Strategies for effective confrontation. *Radiological Technology, 73*(5), 476-478.

Day, J. R. (1990). The interaction of executive and organizational values in healthcare: An exploratory study. Unpublished doctoral dissertation, The Fielding Institute, Santa Barbara, CA.

Fleming v. Correctional Healthcare Solutions, Inc., 751 A. 2d 1035 (New Jersey, 2000).

Fortune v. National Cash Register Company, 272 Mass. 96, 264 N. E. 2d 1251 (1997).

Herrero v. St. Louis University Hospital, 109 F. 3d 481 (8th Cir. 1997).

Howard v. North Mississippi Medical Center, 939 F. Supp. 505 (N. D. Miss., 1996).

In Re Caremark International, Inc. Derivative Litigation, 698 A. 2d 959 (Del. Ch, 1996).

Institute of Medicine of the National Academies. (1999). To err is human: Building a safer health system. [Report] Washington, DC: Author.

Isler, C. (1970). *Florence Nightingale: Rebel with a cause.* Oradell, NJ: Medical Economics.

Jessie v. Carter Health Care Center, Inc., 926 F. Supp. 613 (E. D. Ken., 1996).

Jones v. Kerrville State Hospital, 142 F. 3d 263 (5th Cir., 1998).

Laurin v. Providence Hospital and Massachusetts Nurses Association, 150 F. 3d 52 (1st Cir., 1998).

Mauro v. Borgess Medical Center, 494 CV 05 (Michigan, 1995).

Perkel, L. K. (2002). Nurse executives' values and leadership behaviors. *Nursing Leadership Forum, 6*(4), 100-107.

Pozgar, G. D. (1999). *Legal aspects of health care administration.* (7th ed.). Gaithersburg, MD: Aspen.

Redman, B. A., & Fry, S. T. (2003). Ethics and human rights issues experienced by nurses in leadership roles. *Nursing Leadership Forum, 7*(4), 150-156.

Rehnquist, J. (2001). *Beneficiary awareness of Medicare fraud: A follow-up.* Washington, DC: Department of Health and Human Services.

Roulston v. Tendercare (Michigan), Inc., 608 N. W. 2d 525 (Mich. Ct. App., 2000).

Siegel, S. (2004). The nursing shortage, patient care, and facility liability. *Health Care Law Monthly, 3*(3), 3-10.

Taylor v. Memorial Health Systems, Inc., 770 So. 2d 752 (Fla. Ct. App., 2000).

Thompson v. Holy Family Hospital, 122 F. 3d 357 (9th Cir., 1997).

Title VII of the Civil Rights Act of 1964, Pub. L. 88-352. 43 *Federal Register,* 1978, section 703(a).

Trombley v. Southwestern Vermont Medical Center, 738 A. 2d 103 (Vermont, 1999).

UTMB v. Hohman, 6 S. W. 3d 767 (Tex. App., 1999).

Watkins v. Unemployment Compensation Board of Review, 689 A. 2d 1019 (Pennsylvania Commonwealth, 1997).

Webb v. Mercy Hospital, 102 F. 3d 958 (8th Cir., 1996).

Wexler, D. (2002). Therapeutic jurisprudence: An overview. Retrieved April 22, 2004, from http://www.law.arizona.edu/depts/upr-intj/intj-o.html.

Wexler, D. B., & Winick, B. J. (1991). *Essays in therapeutic jurisprudence.* Durham, NC: Carolina Academic Press.

Wilking v. County of Ramsey, 983 F. Supp. 848 (D. Kan., 1997).

Zamudio v. Patia, 956 F. Supp. 803 (N.D. Ill., 1997).

 Forecasting: Providing Direction to Success

One cannot manage change. One can only be ahead of it. PETER DRUCKER

This chapter focuses on the need for the nurse leaders in any healthcare organization to be able to predict future trends in society and how they influence healthcare organizations and services. Some predictions and trends illustrate the diversity of forecasts to consider. The chapter emphasizes the importance of careful consideration of all of the predictions and trends before a course of action is selected.

BEING ABLE TO ADDRESS CURRENT NEEDS IS an overwhelming challenge. However, a successful organization must go beyond this challenge. Being ahead of change is crucial. An organization that deals only with today's issues soon will be behind and ultimately out of business. Preparing for the future is frequently a process engaged in at the executive level. Although nurse leaders are seldom solely responsible for such planning, they must be well versed in the process, sources, and predictions to be at the front of the wave of new demands from healthcare consumers and workers. If only one future existed (i.e., the future was unaffected by what choices are made now), this process

might be accomplished readily. The reality is, however, that multiple futures exist, and they depend on current actions and interpretations of predictions for the future. Therefore the future is the product of current efforts, which depend on the ability of nurse leaders to engage successfully in forecasting activities.

FORECASTING

Forecasting is a thoughtful statement about the future. It is a decision or judgment about the insight into probable events in advance of their actual occurrence. Forecasting is a sophisticated process of probabilities and insight into society in terms of productivity and future wants and needs. It is based on current developments and decisions, because these form the basis for future advancement.

When added to all of the other demands of the role of chief nursing officer (CNO), the time required to engage in forecasting activities may add stress. However, forecasting keeps the whole organization in tune with society and creates new and exciting strategies that benefit nurses and clients. This creative process allows for thinking in new ways so that new solutions and strategies are seen as possibilities. Conducted on an ongoing basis, forecasting allows for those engaged in the process to know what emerging products, trends, ideas, and services will or could affect what nursing services do. The key, however, is to be engaged actively. The goal is to be an intelligent, involved, creative thinker about potential future trends so that nurse leaders remain in control of their careers and envision small changes that will lead to big outcomes. The CNO must be a forward thinker and proactive in making decisions. In addition to creating a clear vision about the future direction of nursing, the CNO instills the vision and the enthusiasm for it in his or her colleagues.

Forecasting, a deliberate process, forces nurse leaders out of the present to think in the future. Thinking expands from changes in current activities and strategies to what the new activities and strategies—the possibilities—of the future could be. In short, forecasting is a process designed to consider how current changes might evolve; how new events, products, techniques, and technologies will shape current actions; and how the value of society will shape what healthcare provides. It is not mere observation of current activity projected forward. Rather, it is a deliberate deconstruction of observations and ideas to determine future durability and overall themes. "Innovations that could turn the world of an established hospital, health plan or pharmaceutical company upside down tomorrow don't have to be invented; they are already here, in use or in development" (Ellis, 2004, p. 39).

CHAOS THEORY, COMPLEXITY THEORY, AND NONLINEAR THEORY

Chaos theory, complexity theory, or nonlinear theory or science is a theoretical construct for considering the complexity of what appears to be randomness of events and developments but actually is a related process. In a sense, it means that the outcomes of current events do not necessarily correspond with what logically would be anticipated.

As scientists study the influence of various events, they see the complexity of the world and the universality of change. Historically, change has been viewed as linear (Figure 6-1). Most commonly, people talked about cause and effect. However, current thinking suggests that linear change is a narrow way of viewing a complex process. Thus current thinking is that one small change is likely to have numerous direct and indirect outcomes. Rather than a straight line effect, a "starburst" or web effect occurs (Figure 6-2). For example, although not all changes are driven by technology, it certainly has a major impact on the rate and intensity of the changes. Therefore a change in one part of the world has the potential to affect individuals, regardless of where they live and work.

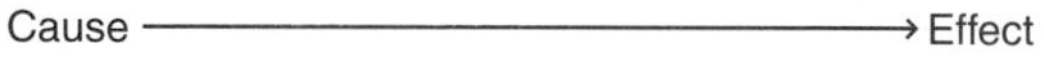

Cause ————————————————→ Effect

Figure 6-1 Linear change.

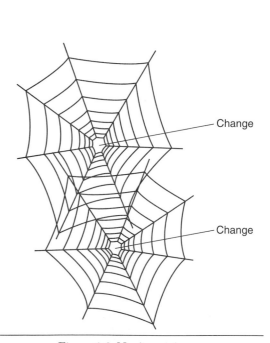

Figure 6-2 Nonlinear change.

If you can dream it, you can do it. Never lose sight of the fact that this whole thing was started by a mouse.
WALT DISNEY

RULES OF FORECASTING

In forecasting, the word *rules* seems almost contradictory. However, thinking about some rules or requirements for engaging in forecasting activities is important.

- **Think productively.** Productive thinking is the most important element in any forecasting session. In other words, being proactive about what leaders can derive from a discussion is an effort that can produce positive results.
- **Think novelty.** Rather than thinking, "I've heard this before," think about how else to view the content or in what new way something could be used.
- **Think in dichotomies.** Because so many aspects of the world today seem dichotomous, to think this way is important. Consider the polar opposite of some factor and then identify a corresponding response. This could help develop skills to deal with the numerous stresses of work involved in forecasting.
- **Think in context.** Ask what else is going on in the world that relates to or influences a specific event or how something else is affected by the focus of your attention.

KEY CONCEPTS

Several key concepts drive the considerations for forecasts and the resultant meaningful products: patterns, proximity, numbers, key data, and context. *Patterns* relate to conceptual structures about behaviors or operations. In a sense, identifying patterns means finding common themes or threads. *Proximity,* in relation to forecasting, refers to the timeframe of consideration; how close or how remote an event or approach is to the time in which it is being considered. *Numbers* suggest that the more people who agree on a particular

thought, the more powerful that thought is. *Key data* refer to those elements that most forecasters track on a regular basis, because they influence so many considerations. *Context* refers to what else is evolving as decisions about the future are made. Each of these elements is important singularly; their interrelationships are even more important.

Patterns

Weather analysis is a common analogy, and it is relevant to healthcare forecasting. Meteorologists have found two distinct patterns to weather: simple and tangled spaghetti. Simple spaghetti appears in a rather tight line, and this kind of weather pattern can be readily predictable. Tangled spaghetti appears as loose connections, and weather in this analysis cannot be predicted accurately. That idea also makes sense in terms of healthcare. When too many "loose ends" (tangled spaghetti) exist, managing the situation is difficult. So, when loose relationships exist, making accurate predictions is difficult. The tighter (simple spaghetti) the various data and information, the more likely a prediction can be made more easily and accurately. An example in healthcare is how the need for tracking payments, the need for access to patient information, the development of better security, and the relatively low cost of computers converged to form a pattern of creating electronic medical records.

Proximity

Predictions that affect behavior are more accurate based on how far in the future the predicted event is. Therefore, continuing to use the weather as an analogy, weather predictions for tomorrow are much more accurate than those for next week. Similarly, forecasts about what might happen in terms of healthcare are much more accurate if the prediction is for the next year versus 5 years in the future. For example, requirements that are activated in the next fiscal year are considered when shaping next year's budget. Those that are anticipated for enactment in several years often are not addressed in part because too many intervening variables are anticipated. Yet, they must be considered.

Numbers

The more weather forecasters who say to expect rain tomorrow, the more likely we are to carry umbrellas. Therefore finding trend in forecasts is important. In other words, the more forecasters who provide comparable predictions, the more likely that idea is to be a solid one for the future. For example, in healthcare, this idea may mean that the more insurers say that they expect their subscribers to access their information via the Internet, the more likely it is that healthcare organizations should provide access to help their clients know how to find the information they need. Just like being prepared for rain by carrying an umbrella, numbers help nurse leaders be prepared to weather the future.

Key Data

Forecasters track several key data sources. These data sources appear in Box 6-1. *Demographics* refers to such factors as gender, age, causes of mortality, and population shifts. These data inform healthcare providers about where to locate services, what services to offer, what preventive

Box 6-1   KEY DATA SOURCES

Key data sources forecasters track the following:
   Demographics
   Environment
   Technology
   Economics
   Culture
   Healthcare
   Government

strategies must be employed, what languages need to be used in developing educational materials, and what marketing approaches to consider.

Environment refers to various factors such as pollution and climatic changes. These data can be used to predict healthcare problems such as an increase in respiratory diseases where air pollution is intense.

Technology usually incorporates inventions and the adoption of technology. Although technology predictions often drive people to purchase the latest developments, they also can influence people to wait for the next iteration of a technologic development.

Economics is focused on earnings, cost of living increases, rates of exchange, and gross national productivity. In addition to indicating proposed tax bases for those healthcare organizations that are public institutions, economic factors also can suggest the amount of disposable income a population might have to engage in healthcare services not normally covered by any insurance plan.

Culture specifically considers differences among groups and the advancement of society in general. One example might relate to the expectations a community has for the betterment of its citizens' overall health and education and result in healthcare services being available in conjunction with grocery stores or other businesses.

Healthcare includes the way in which services are provided and the approaches to morbidity and mortality causes. When data correlate living in certain places with a higher incidence of cancer, for example, the consideration for services and financial coverage would emerge as an issue for discussion.

Government includes all levels of government from federal to local levels and the changes occurring in each. If changes in Medicare or Medicaid altered coverage eligibility, changes in healthcare services or financing of those services would be necessary.

Although other data elements may be included, the majority of forecasters track these seven areas.

Each may be considered individually; however, the real value is in integrating as many of these categories as possible. For example, healthcare happens in the context of governmental policies (federal, state, county, city, and hospital districts) and economics (funding is seldom increased when the economy is not solid), and it clearly is affected by demographics (e.g., the baby boomer generation uses more healthcare services in general, so healthcare has created various programs to address these potential consumers). These interrelationships affect each category directly and all other categories simultaneously. Deciding what to track is a critical decision. How one organization considers these data sources may produce distinctive results from that of another organization.

Context

Despite a growing emphasis on looking to the future, the future must be considered in context of the past and the present. Each person has been influenced by personal and societal experiences. Everyone functions in context of a society that may span from a neighborhood to the world. In addition, the "second translation block" is a concern. It refers to the transfer from clinical trial to practice. In 2000 that time gap was 17 years (Alternative Futures, 2004)! Although understanding the history of some current trend would certainly be valuable, that historical perspective should be focused in terms of future considerations. In some cases, thinking about the past can limit thinking about the possibilities of the future. For example, some groups focus on what did not work in the past and eliminate that from further consideration. In reality, what did not work in the past may readily work in the future.

With all of these changes, Ellis (2004, p. 42) said that the future will be the death of science fiction and "the end of disease, doctor, nurse, hospital and health insurance as we know them today."

Integration of Concepts

One important example related to integration of these various concepts derives from changing demographics. The two most dramatic changes are the number of persons 65 years of age and older and the number of ethnic minorities, especially those who are Hispanic. For example, the Kaiser Family Foundation found that less than one third of persons 65 and older had ever used the Internet for information. However, more than two thirds of persons 50 to 64 years old, the emerging generation of persons 65 and older, had used the Internet (Kaiser Family Foundation, 2005). Therefore knowing about technology and aging and healthcare produces a direction for providing services and information to Medicare-eligible citizens. Further, this knowledge suggests that healthcare providers must be cognizant of Internet sources and the accuracy of information on various sites.

The number of ethnic minorities, especially Hispanics, influences healthcare services that are culturally sensitive and that meet the federal expectations for decreasing healthcare disparities. In addition, the nature of educational materials and marketing campaigns are influenced by an increased population of clients with a Hispanic background.

FORECASTING SOURCES

Several publications exist that relate strictly to the future and forecasts. Discounting popular "sci-fi" literature, several authors and a few journals are consistent, reliable sources. In nursing, *Quantum Leadership* by Porter-O'Grady and Malloch (2002) is an example of futuristic thinking. Sam Hill's *60 Trends in 60 Minutes* (2002) uses the organizing framework of economic and geopolitical trends, technology trends, societal trends, consumer trends, business trends, and workplace trends. Although his focus is not healthcare, the ideas he provides are thought provoking for those in healthcare. *Next Trends for the Near Future,* by Matathia and Salzman (1999), for example, cites several trends that are useful to service executives. Furthermore, for additional clarification, Faith Popcorn and Adam Hanft's *Dictionary of the Future* (2001) contains numerous terms that are related directly to healthcare. Recent editions of such publications can form a context for considering the future.

Laermer (2002) suggested 10 ways to spot trends. Even if a trend is not desirable for a particular healthcare organization, determining trends is important because competitors will be looking at the same information and may choose to act on data in a different manner. Key among those ways to spot trends are the following:

- *Trend tracking* requires establishing a deliberate process (or using a specific resource) to think about specific changes that affect the nursing profession.
- *Book browsing* can be an easy introduction into trending information. Other types of publications such as newsletters or journals may be used. Nurses can trend information by selecting recent editions of various nursing and healthcare journals. Reading the editorials can create a sense of key issues that need to be addressed.
- *Experts* exist, and their readily available resources should be used.
- *Trivia tracking* involves having wide interests and remembering small facts and ideas that might seem irrelevant to forecasting or the nursing profession. Alan Greenspan, as chairman of the Federal Reserve, used this strategy to reach conclusions about what action the Federal Reserve would take.

The following activity is one example of book browsing. Choose as many nursing journals as possible from the past 6 months. Read the nursing editorials. Designate a two- to three-phrase statement to describe an issue each editorial evokes. From those phrases, create three to six broad themes. Create a brief statement about what these themes mean for your organization and your professional future. These themes might, for example, create the trend to track. Experts might be evident, and in the process some trivia may emerge that could provide direction for the future.

Five common sources are related to forecasting. Table 6-1 shows classifications and examples.

1. Newsstand documents are frequently timely and, depending on the focus of the publication, may include specific forecasts and trends. Books by authors focusing on trending are obviously valuable, but they do require "translation" into healthcare.

2. Special publications are usually timely and can be valuable to nurse leaders. Most of these publications, however, require that nurse leaders contemplate the implications in terms of healthcare.

3. Discipline-specific sources are among the least timely and most valuable to nurse leaders. These works are the result of volunteers coming together and thinking through various scenarios. This process is much more drawn out than that used by full-time futurists. However, the results are related directly to healthcare and do not require reconsiderations of abstract ideas.

4. Reliable Internet sources, such as those listed in Table 6-1, typically are useful, if for no other reason than their status within the scientific community. Data presented on the related web sites are usually the result of extensive, well-controlled studies.

5. The least common and often unanticipated source, informed conversations, can provide insight into future trends or validate the nurse leader's existing forecasts. Informed conversations are seldom planned, because scheduling interactions with experts in the field is challenging. However, taking advantage of such opportunities can produce positive results to reinforce earlier thinking.

Table **6-1** FORECASTING SOURCES

Classification	Examples
Newsstand	Magazines: *Time, Newsweek* Newspapers: *Wall Street Journal, New York Times* Books: John Naisbitt, Faith Popcorn, Gary Hamel
Special publications	*World Watch Institute* *World Future Society (Futurist, Outlook)* *Kiplinger Letter* *Futurescan*
Discipline-specific	Arista reports (Sigma Theta Tau) Institute of Medicine reports Foundation reports related to nursing and healthcare Healthy People (2010)
Internet	The Center for the Health Professions (http://www.futurehealth.ucsf.edu) Health Resources and Services Administration (http://www.hrsa.gov) Institute of Medicine of the National Academies (http://www.iom.edu) (Some of the society and federal government publications are also available on-line.) http://morris.wharton.upenn.edu/forecast
Informed conversations	World Future Society Convention Other formal and informal dialogues

Each of these sources is valuable. However, the integration of the various elements provides the richness of information for thinking about the future.

KEY TRENDS AND PREDICTIONS

Many trends and predictions exist. Although many revolve around the changes in technology, other areas are important to explore. For example, the Literature box includes Bell's (2004) ideas regarding the common values in humanity, which are worth consideration in an ever-evolving world.

Table 6-2 presents some key trends that affect healthcare. The list is not comprehensive. Rather, it is designed to provide a sense of how complex change is in today's world.

Other examples of information related to healthcare include the following. Kiplinger (November 26, 2003) predicted (1) a 77% increase in hospital spending by 2013, with an anticipated increase of 200,000 hospital beds and

(2) that employers who provide drug coverage to retirees, generic-drug manufacturers, physicians, rural hospitals, and pharmacy benefit managers all would benefit from the Medicare changes in 2003. The legislation to alter overtime pay was predicted to have mixed results because of who is or is not affected by this change (Kiplinger, November 26, 2003). For example, people who rely on additional income from overtime pay will have less disposable income, or they will seek employment external to their current employers. Many hospitals, however, decided to maintain overtime pay for nurses due to the shortage.

According to Bell (2003), the growth of technology is exponential, and what was thought to be never ending (infinity) actually has a finite timeline. Modis (2003) suggested that that finite date is around 2028.

Each of these predictions suggests that considerable change will occur for healthcare organizations; taken together, these changes will have a profound impact on the near future. Mironov (2003), a tissue engineer, proposed that in the near

Table 6-2 TRENDS AND EXAMPLES

Trend/Prediction	Descriptors/Implication Examples
CDHP: consumer driven health plan	The consumers are in charge of selecting their own healthcare. This concept operates like personal retirement plans: employers make a contribution, and the employee manages it.
Transparency	Information about quality is public information, so consumers know which hospitals and practitioners are the best.
Conflict resolution	New ways to resolve conflict will allow more options for reaching conclusions that help all people adopt a new approach to work and issues associated with work.
Continuing cultural diversification	Finding culturally appropriate strategies to work with others will be a key concern for managers and leaders. Thinking globally will broaden opportunities for interactions and the potential for more diversity.
Free agency	This term appeared in the late twentieth century as a term to reflect how workers of the future would view employment. Rather than being loyal to one position/organization, free agents, as in baseball, make themselves available and seek the best options. This approach places individuals in charge of their careers, and relationships are more about exchanges of needs and fulfillments. (See Manion, 2002.)
Intensity and rapidity of change	Although this is nothing new, the key is to be in relationship with people to help them deal with the people issues surrounding transitions.
High value for emotional intelligence	Leaders will need to be highly skilled in this ability to work effectively with others.
Instant gratification promoted by broadband influence	Waiting to receive healthcare will become unacceptable. People will have the expectation of immediate knowledge.
Basic, repetitive tasks performed by robots	Personal assistance with healthcare needs will be available in a new form: the robot. Some robots could be designed for specific tasks; others could provide a range of repetitive tasks.
Grassroots movements as a result of lack of interest in politics	Part of the local political activity involves healthcare reforms. Knowing the informal community leaders and being connected to them will provide good insight into changes.
Increased isolation resulting from use of Internet experiences	Psychologic disturbances can occur because of this isolation. Knowing how to relate to the people who experience this phenomenon will be an example of creating a service for an emerging market.
Seeking improved health becoming urgent need for Americans	New and increasing demands will be placed on healthcare.

Table **6-2** TRENDS AND EXAMPLES—CONT'D

Trend/Prediction	Descriptors/Implication Examples
People becoming more concerned with the greater good	As a result, people will expect to have greater involvement in social issues.
People required to be connected to their work at all times as a result of increasing business pace	The potential for increased stress because of limited personal time will become more dramatic.
Foundations formed by companies and employees encouraged to be part of charitable works	As a result, individuals will be supported in service activities and will have greater involvement with social issues.
Human resources department becoming central focus for change	Creation of new policies to acknowledge work and personal life could result in a true "cafeteria" plan of benefits from hiring through retirement.
Definition of family evolves into new meanings	Knowing what "the family" is becomes more challenging in making healthcare decisions, especially with genetic information more readily available to link us to others.
Individual cures provided by microchips	Demand for this simple solution will escalate.
Storing human embryos possible	This prediction would result in a new meaning for "planned childbirth."
Uniting of Western and Eastern medicine	People will have multiple healthcare treatment options.
Shortage of obstetric practitioners	The potential for midwives to increase practice options will exist.
Shortage of registered nurses	New models of care with RN as care coordinator, rather than primarily direct care provider, could emerge.
Employer costs for healthcare continue to escalate	Employer insurance plans will rank hospitals based on price and quality.
Talking lids for medication containers	This technology will help remind people when medications are due.
Increased number of high-risk pregnancies	Dichotomous ages of pregnant women, teenagers and over 40, will result from lifestyle considerations.
Portable, wearable technology	One unit will serve multiple functions and be small enough to be portable; this will transfer to imbedded chip technology. Think handheld PDAs to wrist to imbedded transitions.
Increased reliance on higher being	Whether the belief is in God, Mohammed, or some other higher being, people are connecting more with powers beyond the human perspective. This will influence how they approach healthcare decisions and treatments.
Second languages	Although English is the basis for many global businesses, in healthcare, a second language related to the population served will be critical.

Continued

Table **6-2** TRENDS AND EXAMPLES—CONT'D

Trend/Prediction	Descriptors/Implication Examples
Equally important quality and finances	The bottom line will now refer to quality and cost. Therefore the CNO will need to be a member of the executive team and to have full access to the board.
Focus on the experience versus the service	Although services must be safe and quality oriented, the key is that patients determine their view of a hospitalization on the full experience, not just one aspect. Care will focus on meeting the patient's expectation.
Boutique services	Whether this refers to a major healthcare organization or a specialized hospital, the key is to deliver the service in a manner focused on the patient.
On-the-job learning	This is not related to preparing new workers as it has been in the past. It now refers to how to access information about the latest technology and procedures in the workplace when they are needed.
Movement from management to leadership	The management functions remain important but alone are insufficient to meet the needs to create and sustain the quality organization of the future. Although this is true now, it is a trend that will intensify.
Interactive television	This strategy would allow viewers to stop a television program and learn more about a set of symptoms or a disease process.
Noninvasive tests	The "pill" technology will make typically invasive procedures more acceptable to more people.
Shift from healthcare providers as experts to healthcare providers as resources	The role of the patient has shifted over the past few decades, but the trend will increase in rapidity.
Universal healthcare	The belief is that this will be an outgrowth of genetic research so that our genetic backgrounds work against us.
Virtual patients	Healthcare students and practitioners will learn complex procedures in a risk-free environment.
Retail pharmacies	These will change to a Home (Health) Depot offering various technologies to assist in health. (Ellis, 2004)
Microtechnology	New networks could provide us with greater insight into our behavior.

Modified from Laermer, R. (2004, March). The Center for the Health Professions, *Kiplinger Letter* and Hall.

future new tissue will be manufactured easily and simply by using a few cells to meet specific needs. The predicted labor shortage suggests that new ways to conduct business must be devised, in healthcare and other businesses, so that fewer people can accomplish positive effects. Challenger (2003) suggested that enhancement of public image is critical, that mentoring programs should be started or expanded, and that ways to retain older (and typically more experienced) employees must be creative.

Even this textbook will be different in the future based on available technology. The smart-paper book will be read as an e-book, in printed form with the potential to display animated visual data (Stavely, 2003).

Broad Categories

Another way of looking at predictions is to think in broad categories, such as general, generational, and healthcare. Box 6-2 presents a sample of information from these three categories.

Coile (2003) provided an analysis of details related directly to healthcare and used "broad" categories that relate directly and currently to healthcare. Box 6-3 identifies those key categories. Coile's approach is a further modification of broad categories, in this case relating only to healthcare. However, those same categories could be used in other societal endeavors to address forecasts in a broad perspective.

Box 6-2   BROAD CATEGORY PREDICTIONS FOR THE FUTURE

GENERAL

- Dichotomies will be the norm. We have the opportunity to work globally or at home.
- Loyalties are to teams, projects, and professions, not to an institution.
- We are approaching a 24-hour society with a resultant expectation of services being available during evening hours.
- On-line surveys and voting will become available.
- By 2025, the United States will have a national, universal healthcare system.
- Many "jobs" in the future will be that of "knowledge entrepreneur." Knowledge will be the world's most precious resource.

GENERATIONAL

- Generation M (those born around 1982) are civic minded, determined to achieve positive social change, place high value on teamwork and group achievement, and are more bottom-line oriented.
- Advanced nations will have an advancing age population...average age? 41.
- Another Baby Boom will occur in the United States during the first 12 years of the twenty-first century.

HEALTHCARE

- Medical histories will belong to a person, not to an institution or practitioner.
- Smart cards will contain multiple information, including health histories.
- Drugs will be custom designed for specific needs.
- By 2025, more than 4000 genetic conditions will be controlled as the result of diagnostic and treatment procedures.

From Nursing 5371 syllabus, Professional Issues in Nursing, Texas Tech University Health Sciences Center, Lubbock Texas. Based on predictions of the World Future Society and other groups.

Box 6-3   Coile's Categories for Forecasting Healthcare Trends

Demand: The demand for inpatient services is now on the increase except in the rural areas. And baby boomers expect high-tech care.

Consumerism: As more costs of healthcare are derived from individuals, more consumers are driving the changes.

Competition: Factors such as the IOM suggestion to create a national report card are making competition more intense.

Reform: The passage of the Medicare pharmacy benefit and the passage of malpractice reform may open the door for further changes in the way in which healthcare is delivered.

Technology: Dramatic changes such as genomics and high-tech equipment can dramatically alter the future.

Costs: Inflation rates are again increasing in health insurance and health-related products.

Digital hospitals: Movement to a paperless organization has increasing pressure.

Safety: The IOM recent work has focused on issues of safety, and that has helped escalate this issue to new levels.

Workforce: Labor shortages exist in several disciplines, not just nursing.

Trust: The basic trust in the healthcare system is eroding.

Modified from Coile, Jr., R. C. (2003). *Futurescan 2003: A forecast of healthcare trends 2003-2007.* Chicago: Society for Healthcare Strategy and Market Development, American Hospital Association.

Interrelationships of Trends: An Application to the Workforce

Chaotic times are the only times of effective change.
LEE FORD

Interlacing various themes are evident in the graying of the world (a growing population of persons more than 65 years old is not a phenomenon unique to the United States), the diminished number of new potential workers (because of the diminished birthrate of two decades ago), changes in retirement age (working beyond 65 years of age), and the demands of the economy for workers who have various commitments to the "work ethic." Those "employment" type factors may be combined with what is happening in healthcare, where less invasive procedures are being used, people are more in tune with their healthcare needs, and people are most concerned with health insurance. Those elements working together dictate many job redesigns to keep the older worker engaged in the workforce. How will the profession of nursing use its talents without

the physical demands of various positions and settings? How will ongoing professional development be provided that will be needed to help nurses keep current with the numerous changes? What human resource changes will be made to accommodate different interests of different workers? Nurse leaders have the challenge to make these changes happen in timely and effective ways to enable the transition to the next phase of the profession without concerns for an increased shortage.

SUMMARY

In the present rapidly changing society, to think about the future is as important as it is to think about the present. CNOs are responsible for helping the organization bridge from the present to the potential future. To be effective, CNOs must understand and value the concepts inherent in forecasting. They need to apply rules of forecasting to their approaches to current issues and value the meaning of complexity theory. Using various forecasting sources to consider key trends and predictions better prepares the CNO to be a leader in the organization. Without making considerable efforts in this activity, CNOs will be less able to influence the direction the healthcare organization takes.

KEY POINTS TO LEAD

1. Evaluate various sources of forecasting data.
2. Value the complexity of forecast work.
3. Critique the role of the CNO in forecasting.

Literature Box

Cultural differences that create divisions within geographic areas are more important to consider than between-country differences. In general people tend to accommodate and cooperate to ensure a positive living experience. The development of a worldwide economy is not about the increasing influence of the Western culture; actually, a global culture is emerging. This global culture can be threatening because it implies change. Elements of various cultures enrich other cultures. The linkage of people with common interests irrespective of geographic locale creates this new global perspective.

Headlines seldom focus on positive values in the world. Therefore differences and strife often are more evident. However, many positive shared values exist among people in various cultures. For example, many similar concepts exist within the major religions. Similarly, common elements may be found in concerns for the environment. Bell believes that shared human values exist, which include "truthfulness, responsibility, respect for life, granting dignity to all people, empathy for others, kindliness and generosity, compassion and forgiveness" (p. 33). He concludes this article with the following thought, which could drive behavior in healthcare: "We can include all people in our circle of concern, behave ethically toward everyone we deal with, recognize that every human being deserves to be treated with respect, and work to raise minimum standards of living for the least well-off people in the world" (p. 35).

Bell, W. (2004, September-October). Humanity's common values: Seeking a positive future. *The Futurist*, 30-36.

Contemplations

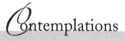

The following are taken from *Transformational Change: A Ten-Point Strategy to Achieve Better Health Care for All* (Davis, 2005):

1. Agree on shared values and goals.
2. Organize care and information around the patient.
3. Expand the use of information technology.
4. Enhance the quality and value of care.
5. Reward performance.
6. Simplify and standardize.
7 Expand health insurance and make coverage automatic.
8. Guarantee affordability.
9. Share responsibility for healthcare financing.
10. Encourage collaboration.

Use the previous 10 points as the basis for determining the following:
- What needs to change in the current societal context to achieve one or more of the points?
- How could the CNO instigate movement toward achieving the strategies within the organization?
- How can you contribute toward such movement?
- How does each of the predictions in Box 6-2 influence a healthcare organization with which you are affiliated?
- Which ones have direct meaning?
- Which ones need to be eliminated because they are not related to the organization or the direction it is taking for the future?
- Which ones need to be modified to be most relevant for further consideration?

LEADER STORY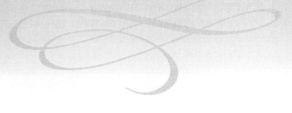

VIRGINIA TROTTER BETTS
COMMISSIONER OF THE DEPARTMENT OF MENTAL
HEALTH AND DEVELOPMENTAL DISABILITIES
STATE OF TENNESSEE
FORMER PRESIDENT, AMERICAN NURSES
ASSOCIATION
NASHVILLE, TENNESSEE

Forecasting? Sometimes I don't think I can see beyond 5 minutes ahead! I say this because so many changes are occurring so quickly that it is almost impossible to stay current. If you really want to think about forecasting, you need to have the manpower to run the data and to scan the environment. It is important anymore to be able to turn on a dime. Fast is critical.

One successful tactic is to stay on top of the likely, recurring problems. We all can identify current problems so dominant they evidently will be problems in the future. If you do nothing else, keep track of those problems and how they are evolving. Although the details of the problem may change, if it is prominent and nothing is happening to eliminate it, the problem will be a part of the future.

I always am focused on mental health workforce shortages. We do have some solid data about acuity of people with these diagnoses, and we know that more dual diagnoses exist. However, we didn't predict the 26% increase in pharmaceutical costs that we experienced this past year. Such dramatic changes in a short period devastate any existing plans.

I wouldn't have taken this job if I thought it would become worse during my tenure. Because we are in the process of disenrolling people in the state plan, I have had to focus on potential improvements in our situation by creating a safety net.

Think about the events of September 11, 2001. President Bush most likely expected some continued terrorism activities. But who would have predicted the magnitude of the events of that day? So, sometimes, even when you have thought about how things might be in the future, you can't predict the magnitude or length of an event or change.

With the budget restrictions that have hit the states, I decided that I needed to have some group to rely on to develop strategy. We needed to think about the expected and the unexpected. An important rule is to view this from an energizing perspective, rather than to think about how overwhelming all of the information can be.

I went home one weekend and seriously thought about whether I was in the right place. I went to work on Monday and called a special meeting. I said to everyone, "If you're staying on, let's plan to mitigate the effects of what we are facing." We are dealing with a whole set of negativity. "If anyone can solve this problem, we can. We're the ones with the experience and know how. We need to know what is needed. We need to know what the costs are and we need to know what the options are. Once we know all of that, we can make an effective plan."

You have to see what you are doing and how it ties in with others' values. When I took on this job, we approached the future with hope. Then as budget changes hit, we were faced with greater fear about the limitations of what we could do. I had to change my context as I worked with the city and county officials. I still want to convey hope to them. But now, I am using a different strategy. Every city and county has a jail or prison (or both), and officials don't like to see those facilities full. So, I approach them with the fact that many people with mental health problems get into trouble because they don't have access to basic services.

My experience at ANA was invaluable. We had to deal with federal, state, and local government on multiple issues.

When events disrupt your view of the future, you still need to know where you are headed. Therefore visioning is really important. That way, when multiple things bombard you all at once and you get turned around, you still have the hope of coming out and heading in the right direction.

We always should study the context. We should look inside ourselves, too, to identify our real values. In a group we have some who are focused on the present, some who are focused on the distant future, and some who are thinking about the near future. Alone, any one of those individuals could be completely wrong about what to do next. Together, great synergy exists and many concerns are addressed. Everyone, however, has to focus on the context. Then you can ask questions such as what might healthcare look like, but everyone shouldn't be focused on the same thing within that context.

When I was so focused on how to make things better, I formed the Blue Sky Panel, a group of advisors. They looked back to see if a model exists. Diversity of tasks is so valuable. The Blue Sky Panel helped us identify our goals.

If you have the manpower, you should run a full-scale forecast. Look at the policy background and determine how you got from the policy of the past to the present. Running some general scenarios is always helpful. Thinking through what you would do if the economy goes up is very different from what you would do if the economy goes down. The same thing is true of changes in policy: think about what would happen if some key policy became more restrictive and how that would differ from what would happen if it were less restrictive. Many state governments don't have this luxury unless they have engaged in this process for a while.

If no agreement exists regarding data, the data mean nothing. In many organizations, especially in state government, roles change frequently and we often don't have a good system of retaining historical documents to trace people's thinking. When I worked in the 100th Congress, we were faced with the data that investing $1.00 for a pregnant woman resulted in $3.38 savings in maternal/child healthcare. Even though Congress received that report, they cut funding.

One really important thing is to think about the horizon issues, those that you can see but that aren't, so to speak, in your backyard. You have to think about fallback positions. Sometimes the idea of "no loss" is a win. Furthermore, sometimes the best you can do is help see how something is moving. However, the horizon issues are critical and should be addressed as soon as possible.

Chapter References

Alternative Futures. (2004, March). *2000 yearbook of medical informatics*. Alexandria, VA: Alternative Furtures Associates.

Bell, J. J. (2003, May-June). Exploring the "singularity." *The Futurist*, 18-24.

Bell, W. (2004, September-October). Humanity's common values: Seeking a positive future. *The Futurist*, 30-36.

Challenger, J. A. (2003, May-June). The coming labor shortage. *The Futurist*, 24-28.

Coile, Jr., R. C. (2003). *Futurescan 2003: A forecast of healthcare trends 2003-2007*. Chicago: Society for Healthcare Strategy and Market Development, American Hospital Association.

Davis, K. (2005, January). Transformational change: A ten-point strategy to achieve better health care for all. Commonwealth Fund. Retrieved January 21, 2005, from http://www.cmwf.org/usr_doc/Pres_Message_2004.pdf.

Forecasts for Management Decision Making (2003, November 26). *Kiplinger Letter*, Washington, DC: The Kiplinger Washington Editors.

Kaiser Family Foundation. Online health information poised to become important resource for seniors. Retrieved from KaiserFamilyFoundation@cme.kff.org. January 14, 2005.

Kiplinger Letter. (2003, November 26). *Benefit trends, Medicare, workers and pay.*

Laermer, R. (2002). *TrendSpotting*. New York: Penguin Putnam Publishers.

Manion, J. (2002). Emergence of the free agent nurse workforce. *Nursing Administration Quarterly*, 26, 5, 68-78.

Matathia, I., & Salzman, M. (1999). *Next trends for the near future*. Woodstock, NY: The Overlook Press.

Mironov, V. (2003, May-June). Beyond cloning: Toward human printing. *The Futurist*, 34-38.

Modis, T. (2003, May-June). The limits of complexity and change. *The Futurist*, 26-32.

Popcorn, F., & Hanft, A. (2001). *Dictionary of the future: The words, terms, and trends that define the way we'll live, work and talk*. New York: Hyperion.

Porter-O'Grady, T., & Malloch, K. (2002). *Quantum leadership: A textbook of new leadership*. Gaithersburg, MD: Aspen.

Stavely, D. J. (2003, September-October). The future of the book in a digital age. *The Futurist*, 18-22.

CHAPTER

7 Leaders and Development of the Self

Nothing happens without personal transformation. W. EDWARDS DEMING

This chapter focuses on how nurses develop themselves personally and professionally as leaders. The areas of development to be examined include characteristics of the leader; successful leadership behaviors, particularly appropriate for healthcare professionals; and additional factors that influence and facilitate leadership, such as attitude, motivation, failures, intentions, individual self-reflection, and emotional intelligence. Because no one is born a leader, the focus is on self-development and continued growth in all areas of leadership.

TO BECOME AN EFFECTIVE LEADER REQUIRES examination of strengths and weaknesses. This is not an instant process but part of a lifelong journey. In the Nurse Executive Competencies identified by the American Organization of Nurse Executives (AONE) (2005), an entire subsection discusses the leader's personal journey disciplines. The section regarding fundamental thinking skills stresses the importance of self-reflection and an understanding that all leadership begins from within. Areas are identified within which most administrators are working as they pursue

more effective leadership methods. Bennis and Nanus (1985), in their classic work on leadership, divide leadership into two major aspects: characteristics and behaviors. These two major aspects are discussed in addition to other influencing factors that constitute support for leadership development and knowing oneself.

CHARACTERISTICS

The characteristics of leaders are those aspects of leadership not immediately apparent. They are the qualities focused on "beingness" and how these leaders or chief nursing officers (CNOs) are present with other human beings. Five of these qualities—the character of the leader; the commitment these leaders have to themselves and their followers; the connectedness they maintain with their staff and the other stakeholders; the caring and compassion they exhibit for their followers, patients, and families; and the confidence evident in themselves, their staff, and the organization—are described below and appear in Table 7-1.

Character

Character is who a person is when no one else can see, when no one will discover what a person thinks, or, more importantly, what he or she does. Guinness (1999) says, "Character is the inner form that makes anyone or anything what it is...

Table **7-1** A SUMMARY OF CNO LEADERSHIP CHARACTERISTICS

Characteristic	Description	Example
Character	The core of a person's identity	Behavior in private when no one else will know
Commitment	A promise or a pledge	The passion for a goal; the fire in the heart; willing to do whatever it takes to meet the pledge
Connectedness	Being in relationship with others	Extra effort to be "in touch" with others
Compassion	Openness to human feelings	Being willing to cry or express sadness over a tragedy, pain, or sorrow that befalls someone
Confidence	A belief in a person's own abilities to handle whatever happens	Willingness to deal with conflict and difficult situations

whether a person, a wine, or a historical period." In leadership and administration, character makes a difference. If a nursing leadership team were asked to identify what constitutes character, the responses most likely would include integrity, honesty, moral accountability, reliability, trustworthiness, and a sense of responsibility. All of these would be accurate at some level, but to an even greater extent, "character is the major element of leadership" (Guinness, 2000, p. 4). Porter-O'Grady and Malloch (2002, p. 201), in exploring emotional intelligence, stated, "A person's character—the traits that form that person's nature—directly affects the person's ability to become emotionally competent." The foundation of this emotional competence is a strong character, uncompromising integrity, and a strong moral conscience.

Skills and tools are important at every level of leadership; yet in a crisis, lack of strong character is what leads to failure. Character is not created in a crisis; rather it is revealed or comes to light in the heat of the crisis (Bennis, 1999). Character is developed from the cradle. Furthermore, strong character, developed over time, is what creates trust in relationships; and trust is what allows leaders to lead. Nursing staff members tolerate mistakes in decision making or mistakes resulting from lack of experience; but lapses or "slips in character" are not forgiven readily. The manner in

which difficult situations are resolved demonstrates for peers, employees, and superiors the nature of a leader's character.

All human beings have done something in the past that they wish no one knew. Therefore character development fortunately is a continuously evolving process. Building on the base begun during a person's youth, character is created daily. Character essentially evolves with each decision that is made. As moral and ethical choices are made in a positive way, strong character is developed. Guinness (2000) believes that character can be cultivated or enhanced based on the following six essentials.

Character is based on the *standards or values* learned from family, faith, and a person's environment. Human beings assess their own actions and behaviors based on these standards and values. Any time the standard or value is violated, a small crack develops in the foundation of a person's character. Some people may have grown up with a belief that to keep a promise is essential. They believe character is defined by a person's word or promise. When people in leadership positions say they will do something, to follow through and keep the promise, or to *be* their word (their actions are critical), is critical.

An additional essential ingredient for good character is the *capacity for deep and lasting change.* Leaders must be open to changing thoughts, ideas, opinions, and behaviors when presented with new evidence or circumstances. For example, if people experience a dramatic change in life, they become so committed to the "new way" that it is an anathema to return to the old. This openness to change also could be seen as a paradigm shift, new evidence that completely alters how an issue is seen, a "light bulb" moment, or a flash of new understanding.

Moral accountability is essential to building strong character. Human beings were created to learn from mistakes, to experience the necessity of mid-course correction, and to be accountable for such correction. A major part of this accountability is recognition of when people have acted in violation of their own standards and acknowledgment of the wrong to the individual(s) involved. For example, a failure to keep a promise or agreement must be followed with an acknowledgment of the failure and an apology for the breakdown.

To cultivate strong character, a leader must be able to *recognize bad or destructive habits and say "No"* to them. Leaders can exercise the strength to shift behavior and refuse to participate in actions that do not serve them. This could be any habit or behavior that does not work: a vicious, uncontrolled temper; failing to meet deadlines; an unwillingness to work with others; or being "too busy" to make patient care rounds or spend time with faculty and students. Any of these habits may violate professed standards, and curtailing or stopping these habits creates an opportunity to strengthen character.

Forgiveness is essential to strong character. All aspiring leaders experience being hurt by others and actually hurting others. If leaders respond with resentment and the desire for revenge in the first instance, or smugness and glee in the second instance, the result is a lessening or weakening of character. In such circumstances, leaders are less human than they could be. Forgiving those who are hurtful is paramount to growing character. At the same time, asking for forgiveness after hurting someone is equally important.

A key aspect of forgiveness is self-forgiveness. When a hurtful act is committed toward another human being or a grievous error of omission or commission is made, personal growth in the leadership role requires the practice of self-forgiveness. Although to let go of self-condemnation is sometimes difficult, it is essential to continuing development as a leader.

Cultivating humility is the final key to building character. Leaders with strong character do not need public recognition; nor do they court awards or tributes. They do not need to laud or parade all their virtues. They do not need reassurances of being a great boss, how respectful physicians are of them, or how much staff members appreciate everything the leaders do. Rather, leaders know they are most effective when the followers say, "We did it ourselves."

> *As for the best leaders, the people do not notice their existence. When the best leaders' work is done, the people say "we did it ourselves."*
> LAU TZU

Developing strong character is a process. The key is to raise self-awareness and work proactively to increase strength of character. Perhaps Ruiz's (1997) work says it most simplistically by defining the "four agreements" leaders must make with themselves. They reflect the basic values of leadership:

1. **Be impeccable with your word.** As a leader, your word is the power you wield. Your "beingness" is manifest in the giving of your word or promise. True intentions are expressed in your words or promises. Your word is so powerful that it can change another's life.
2. **Take nothing personally.** Never take the actions or words of others personally. Whatever other people say or do, they chose the response. They chose the words or actions among hundreds of choices they could have made. Therefore it is about them, *not* about you.

3. **Make no assumptions.** Human beings make assumptions about most things and then proceed as though these assumptions are true. Wishing something does not make it so. A human frailty is to make assumptions about what others are thinking and feeling without checking for accuracy. Then it is the human condition to have judgments about the assumptions and the person.

4. **Always do your best, no more and no less.** Keep in mind that everyone's best changes from moment to moment, depending on emotions and mood. When you are tired and overwrought, the best you can do is different from when you awake fresh and ready for a new day.

These are inherent to solid character development. Everyone needs to work on these character development strategies and the four agreements every day.

Commitment

A part of strong character is the ability to make and keep commitments. To be successful in nearly any endeavor, leaders find it necessary to understand the concept of commitment, including when to make commitments and when and how to break them (Sull, 2003). When leaders make a commitment, they are bound to that specific outcome by a promise or a pledge. In the process, this pledge or promise is carried to some kind of action or outcome. Many humans, in the heat of the moment, make promises or commit to an action and are unable to follow through to the end. Maxwell (1999) believes that commitment is the will of the mind to finish what the heart has begun long after the emotion, in which that promise was made, has passed. This means that when the excitement of the initial phases of an idea or project give way to the long hours of focused detail and plain hard work, the leader remains committed to the promise. The difference between a successful person and those who are not so successful is not a lack of knowledge or skill but a lack of commitment.

Commitment can be demonstrated in different ways:

- *To the staff nurse,* commitment is being able to return, one more time, to a situation in which staffing and patient challenges are unrelenting.
- *To the nurse manager,* commitment is being able to "rally the troops" one more time.
- *To the educator,* commitment is being able to be as enthusiastic about content the tenth time as the first and to find something new and exciting each of those ten times (Kowalski & Yoder-Wise, 2003).

Colleagues frequently speak about being committed to quality patient care. However, *actions* separate those who are truly committed from those who merely speak about commitment. For the leader, commitment to quality care equals discovery of what occurs in delivering patient care, what is discovered when talking with staff and patients and when making rounds. If leaders want to make a difference in people's lives, they must demonstrate commitment to others. The exercise in Box 7-1 provides further clarification of the concept of commitment. This exercise can help explore what makes a person happy. Do leaders come to work because it pays well, because the status is important, or because it gives them a sense of control over their environment? Or does the leader care deeply about nurses? Does he or she want to enable staff members to grow and learn and give the kind of patient care the leader would give if he or she could care for every patient within the facility? The leader should understand why he or she has chosen a leadership position. As Bennis said in an interview with Harvard Management Update (Michelman, 2004),

Lack of self knowledge is the most common everyday source of leadership failure. A lot of gifted individuals I've known over the years who found themselves leading organizations aspired to that top position without knowing what it entailed and what was in store for them. They wanted to *be* a CEO but didn't want to *do* a CEO's job. (p. 4)

Box 7-1   Exploring Commitment

The key to finding your compelling mission or passion that will lead you to success and peak performance is to ask yourself the right questions. Your answers to these questions will tell you what you need to know about yourself. Read each question, then stop and think for a few minutes and answer each question honestly. Do not censor or edit out anything even if it seems impossible or unrealistic—allow yourself to be surprised. Let your imagination soar.

1. Am I deriving any satisfaction out of the work I am now doing?
2. If they did not reward (praise or pay) me to do what I now do, would I still do it?
3. What is it that I really love to do?
4. What do I want to pursue with my time and energy that is worthwhile?
5. What motivates me to reach out and do my very best, to excel?
6. What is it that only I can say to the world? What needs to be done that can best be done only by me?
7. If I won $20,000,000 in the lottery tomorrow, how would I live? What would I do each day and for the rest of my life?
8. If I were to write my own obituary right now, what would be my most significant accomplishment? Is that enough?

Repeating this exercise often will give you additional insights and information about what you really want and love to do. If taken seriously, the exercise should help you to have an understanding of why you selected this profession and whether or not you have the stamina to do whatever it takes to make a contribution and to make a difference in the practice of nursing.

Likewise, this occurs in nursing divisions. The nursing leader may want to *be* a CNO but may not want to *do* the CNO's job.

Connectedness

As important as character and commitment are, they are irrelevant without connectedness to people. Leaders make an effort to be connected to other people. These people may be staff members, colleagues, or members of a network. In many respects, being connected is about being in relationship with another human being; it happens on an individual, rather than a group, basis. Leaders develop credibility with people when they connect with them and show that they genuinely want to help. Understanding how people feel and think helps create relationships. On Boss's Day, 1994, a full-page newspaper ad appeared in *USA Today*. It was developed and paid for by the employees of Southwest Airlines and was addressed to the CEO, Herb Kelleher:

Thanks, Herb
For remembering every one of our names.
For supporting the Ronald McDonald House.
For helping load baggage on Thanksgiving.
For giving everyone a kiss (and we mean everyone).
For listening.
For running the only profitable major airline.
For singing at our holiday party.
For singing only once a year.
For letting us wear shorts and sneakers to work.
For golfing at The LUV Classic with only one club.
For outtalking Sam Donaldson.
For riding your Harley Davidson into Southwest Headquarters.
For being a friend, not just a boss.
Happy Boss's Day from Each One of Your 16,000 Employees. (Freiberg & Freiberg, 1996, p. 224)

Unquestionably, this group of employees felt connected to their leader. They knew what he had done for them and how he related with them.

Relationship Building: One Part of
Being Connected

A sensation of well-being and safety that results from the behavior of another is one aspect of being in relationship. Relationships begin with mutual interests, backgrounds, education, or professions. Often this fledgling connectedness expands into a deeper knowledge and a reciprocal understanding and commitment to support the other human being to learn and grow. One person might admire the other's sense of humor and the ability to reduce tension while restoring calm and purpose, whereas the second person might admire the first person's integrity, hard work, and creativity. Frequently, shared values, such as respect for others, patients, families, and co-workers, or dedication to the best quality of patient care, are held in common by both. Most human beings have a select number of people in their lives with whom they feel great pleasure, warmth, and comfort. These special relationships probably reflect character, commitment, confidence, and compassion in addition to connectedness.

Some of these relationships are deeply personal and last many years. Some are professionally or workplace based and possibly of shorter duration. In either case, these relationships can provide the "glue" that holds organizations together and establishes or maintains a culture. Similarly, relationships created or initiated by the leader are central to establishing and maintaining the group or team (see Chapter 10).

Communication: How Connection Is Created

A critical role in establishing relationships is the manner in which the leader communicates with peers, co-workers, and followers. Two aspects of communication are important: tools and attitude (tools are addressed in Chapter 9). Most would agree that words are the least important aspect of communication, whereas tonality and body language are the critical aspects and strongly convey an attitude. The Master Teacher story (Box 7-2) illustrates the importance of clear and accurate communication.

When things do not work out and leaders take responsibility for their own actions and behaviors rather than justifying mistakes or blaming others, they model the desired tools and attitude. When leaders hold team members and followers accountable for their communication, attitudes, skills, and behaviors in a nonjudgmental way and do *not* make people wrong, they demonstrate integrity in the work setting and their ability to connect to people in an effective and compassionate manner.

Leaders often communicate values, goals, and vision through the use of stories such as the Master Teacher story. Stories are a powerful communication method of conveying what is important. Stories are what are remembered and shared with others (Yoder-Wise & Kowalski, 2003). Connections can be made and relationships demonstrated through sharing stories about the organization and people. Leaders demonstrate connection and relationship through their empathy for others. In this empathy, leaders have a finely honed ability to find the very best in people rather than focusing on the worst in them. They do this by truly caring for people.

Compassion and Caring

Commitment and connectedness are important, and they are interwoven with compassion and caring. Dutton, Frost, Worline, Lilius, & Kanof (2002) identified the critical nature of compassion in the face of tragedy that can be demonstrated by organizational leadership. The leader's ability to demonstrate a compassionate response in times of disaster or trauma that affects employees elicits humanity in members of the organization. Further, it lessens the suffering of those affected by the trauma, decreases time needed for recovery, increases the potential for healing and the resiliency demonstrated in that healing, and increases attachment to peers and the organization. Co-workers gain two perspectives. They adopt the compassion exemplified by the leader, and they understand that they too would be

Box 7-2   Master Teacher

A master teacher uses an exercise to convey the message regarding tools and attitude. He leads the group in the childhood game of Simon Says. As the leader, the master teacher gets to be Simon and the group must do what he says to do. Usually, half of the group must sit down after the first round because they do not do what Simon says. Almost everyone, except for one or two people, is sitting after the fifth or sixth round. However, the learning from the exercise is in the debriefing. This master teacher has a great sense of humor and frequently considerable laughter ensues. He seeks to discover how people felt or responded when they had to sit down and the responses fall into three categories:

1. Many go to some form of **blame,** usually focused on the leader, with such comments as, "Your directions weren't clear," "You didn't speak loudly enough," or "You were purposefully deceptive."

2. Others focus on **justification:** "There was too much noise and confusion," "I'm too tired because I had to work late last night," or "I never liked that game anyway."

3. A few actually take **responsibility** for their actions. "I forgot that Simon Says is a listening game. I was supposed to do what Simon said rather than do what I saw Simon do."

In everyday communication, many people spend considerable effort in blaming others for mistakes or in justifying why they did something or did not do it. The master teacher helps the group to have an experience of this very human tendency and leads them to an "ah ha" or learning about how easy it is to blame and justify and how focused and clear one must be to take responsibility for the less-than-desirable outcome.

treated in a humane and compassionate manner, should some tragedy befall them or their family. Such behavior directly affects the organization's ability to maintain high performance in difficult times and fosters the capacity to heal, to learn to adapt, and to excel.

What does compassion look like in times of great stress? Dutton et al. (2002) suggest that leaders openly reveal humanness and express feelings. They cite New York City mayor Rudy Giuliani as an example of this behavior. When the events of September 11, 2001, unfolded, he demonstrated the honest expression of feelings while exhibiting a strong resolve to rebuild the city and restore confidence in the abilities of all New Yorkers. Second, Dutton et al. (2002) stress the importance of being physically and emotionally present to employees. They cite the example of one CEO who visited the home of every team member after the sudden death of a beloved colleague and

team member. He was present with people while they expressed their feelings. For many people, it is easier to avoid pain than to experience the resurrection of their own painful issues, which is the normal outcome of listening to the painful experiences of others. This CEO confronted his own pain with his employees. Then the CEO orchestrated the caretaking of the deceased's family with food, expenses, and support.

These are examples of behaviors that demonstrate compassion and serve as an example to other employees in the organization. As Porter-O'Grady and Malloch (2002) say, "Without feelings of deep sympathy and sorrow for others struck by misfortune and a genuine desire to alleviate suffering on the part of caregivers, patient care service would be no more than a robotic endeavor" (p. 195).

In their early research on leadership, Bennis & Nanus (1985) indicated that leaders simply care about more people. Furthermore, the leader's management and leadership philosophy and the culture created must match the nursing profession's core value of caring (Hocker & Trofino, 2003). Nursing leaders demonstrate this caring through knowing people and committing to help them grow personally and professionally. Kouzes and Posner (2002) believe that leadership is about people, and leaders must care about people. They find that expressing affection is pivotal to success and that human beings have a strong need for affection. In other words, everyone wants to be loved.

Likewise staff members love or care about a leader because of how the leader relates to them. A strong leader honors each person's possibilities: who the staff member can become and the hopes and dreams, as well as the possibilities, of each person. Effective leaders give people hope. They acknowledge each person's contributions, directly and specifically, in a timely manner and from the heart. Leaders give of themselves. They do not just talk to people (focusing on telling); they *listen* to what others have to say. When they interact with others, they focus completely on the individual with no interruptions.

Maxwell (1998) believes that caring is a way of thinking and acting, a way of approaching life. It is vital for leaders to care about people more than they care about their position, to be aware of people's needs while putting them ahead of themselves and their personal desires. Maxwell hypothesizes that being immensely secure in oneself is at the heart of serving people. How leaders treat others is a reflection of how leaders feel about themselves. Those with a strong sense of self, self-esteem, and self-confidence can lead and care about people in supportive, compassionate ways.

Confidence

To have the first four characteristics, leaders also must have confidence. Confidence, a belief in a person's own abilities, a reliance or trust in self, creates a boldness or self-assurance that enables

the leader to grow personally and professionally (Crane, 2002). This growth path encompasses the capacity for the leader to develop and improve skills. This is one distinguishing characteristic between leaders and followers: the inner drive to build on the previous day's progress and thus improve their abilities every day. As long as people do not know what they do not know, it is *not* possible to grow.

This ongoing process of growth and expanding confidence helps the leader develop an effective vision of the future for the department or organization. The ever-expanding confidence helps the leader to confront obstacles and difficulties. Just as strong leaders find the best in people, they focus on what they, themselves, do well rather than on their weaknesses. Buckingham and Clifton (2001) used the idea of building on personal strengths as the basis for gaining the most from work and life. This kind of focus enhances self-confidence. Furthermore, confidence conveys feasibility and workability (Zaccaro, 2001). The focus on positives conveys to the team that the leader can confront and successfully deal with difficult situations. On the other hand, low self-confidence leads to reward-based, autocratic, and coercive styles of management/leadership and a downward spiral in character development in addition to unhappy employees.

The greatest deterrent to confidence is fear. Fear is what limits a leader. Furthermore, leaders gain strength, courage, and confidence each time they stop and face their fears. Jeffers, in her classic work, taught that the core fear of all human beings is, "I can't handle what life brings to me" (1987, p. 15). Self-confidence is building continually on the belief that leaders can handle whatever life deals them, both the good and the bad.

One way in which leaders strive to grow and increase their self-confidence is to practice facing fears. Some may be afraid to write. Therefore they might take a writing course or force themselves to sit down at a desk and write. Some leaders fear confrontation with difficult people. To face such a fear requires sitting down with the person and talking to him or her, listening carefully, speaking from a caring and responsible position, and sharing what is true for the leader from a personal perspective. A helpful idea is to write down what needs to be said or to practice with a coach before confronting the difficult person. Such efforts to overcome fears constitute a major part of the growth path of a leader. Facing fears involves developing a "can do" attitude. An example of writing a character development story to be told from a personal perspective is found in Box 7-3.

One contributor to fear, which leads to a decrease in self-confidence, is negative self-talk. Negative talk includes such words as *stupid, dumb,* and *uncaring* and is directed toward oneself. With focus and concentration, each person can substitute the negative messages with more positive ones, which fosters learning and self-reliance.

Confidence can be misdirected into perfectionism. Frequently, those in healthcare can be obsessed with perfection. The need for care outcomes to be correct and right for the patient is easily translated into everything being *perfect*. However, perfection is an elusive, if not unattainable, quality. Human beings are learning continually and the goal must be to grow and learn, rather than to be perfect. Attending to self-esteem in others enhances the leader's own self-esteem. Being positive and demonstrating a positive attitude encourages others also to be positive. It is about an attitude of confidence.

The Interconnectedness of Characteristics

Each of the five identified characteristics just discussed is critical to the success of a leader. However, when the five characteristics interact to become a dynamic whole, leaders take on new abilities to connect with people and change their lives. Others know when leaders sincerely care and when they take risks on the behalf of staff. They know if leaders are trustworthy and confident in their abilities or whether they are superficial. A Personal Assessment Guide (Box 7-4) is designed

---

Box 7-3   A Story of Confidence

THE "CAN DO" BRIGADE AND CHARACTER DEVELOPMENT

Reviewing life events can help identify important or pivotal lessons learned. One life event that significantly affected me was the year I spent as an Army Nurse Corps officer in South Vietnam. This was the first time I remember an awareness and understanding of confidence in the face of incredible obstacles. I had spent the first 10 months of my nursing career in labor and delivery at Indiana University before volunteering for a guaranteed assignment to Vietnam. I went to Fort Sam Houston for 6 weeks of basic training, where they taught me really important things such as how to salute, how to march, and how many men in a battalion. I even low-crawled through the obstacle course, beneath live ammunition, with an M-1 carbine in my arms. However, no one asked me if I could start an IV or draw a tube of blood. This would have been an important question, because Indiana University had the largest medical school class in the United States at that time, and nurses did nothing that interfered with medical education. Therefore I had never started an IV or drawn blood.

When I arrived in Saigon, they put me in a sedan with another nurse and sent me up to the Third Surgical Hospital, which was located in the middle of the 173rd Airborne Brigade. Surgical hospitals are not unlike the one in the movie and television series *M*A*S*H*. We even had a Major Burns; that was not his name but it was his function.

Continued

Box 7-3 A Story of Confidence—cont'd

Surgical hospitals received only battle casualties; their purpose was to perform any needed surgery, stabilize, and then transport.

The primary mission of the 173rd Airborne Brigade was to defend the Bein Hoi Air Base, where all the sorties in the south were flown during the war. When we arrived, we were stopped at the gate by an MP, who stepped up and saluted very snappily. He knew that a staff car must contain either a very high-ranking officer or, if it was his lucky day, perhaps a woman. While I was in Vietnam, the male/female ratio was approximately 500 American women to 500,000 American men. The young MP looked in the window, saluted snappily, and said, "Afternoon, ma'ams!" He wanted to know where we were going; he talked to us for a few minutes and assured us that if there was anything he could do for us, we should just give him a call. He saluted us very snappily and said, "CAN DO." I was not sure I had heard him correctly because I did not know at that time that there are units with very high "esprit de corps," who attach sayings to the end of things such as salutes, phone conversations, and memos. The 173rd is the "CAN DO" brigade.

When we got to the hospital and met the chief nurse, she took us down to the mess hall and introduced us to all the doctors and nurses. We were sitting and having coffee when the field phone rang in the kitchen and the mess sergeant yelled out, "Incoming wounded." Everybody got up and started to leave for the Pre-op area. I just sat there until the chief nurse said, "Come on." I responded, "You don't understand, I deliver babies." She was not impressed! She took me by the arm and led me to Pre-op.

When we got there, we discovered the wounded numbered not just a few but more than 30, and some were very seriously injured. The chief nurse immediately told the sergeant to call headquarters battalion

of the 173rd Airborne and tell them that the Third Surg needed blood. She turned to me and said, "Lieutenant, you are responsible for drawing 50 units of fresh whole blood." I was shocked! I had never drawn a tube of blood! As I looked around, I noticed in the back section of "Pre-op" a Specialist 4th class, who was already setting up "saw horses" and stretchers, putting up IV poles, and hanging plastic blood sets. My first thought was that I was attaching myself to him because he looked like he knew what he was doing. I started to help and soon I heard trucks out back. I opened the door and looked outside. There were two huge Army trucks and jumping out of the back of them were kids, 17, 18, and 19 years old. They were covered with red mud from the bottom of their boots to the tops of their helmets. I looked at them and I looked at the clean cement floor and in an instant I thought of my mother. I put my hand on my hip and said, "Where have you boys been?" One PFC stepped forward and saluted me very briskly and said, "Ma'am, we just came in this afternoon from 30 days in the field. We've been out in the rice paddies chasin' 'Charlie' (Viet Cong). And Charlie's been chasin' us. We've not had a hot meal, and we haven't had a shower. But Sergeant Major said, 'The Third Surg needs blood!'" He saluted smartly and said, "CAN DO!" Although I was not clear about what my role was, they were very clear. After 30 days of chasing and being chased by the Viet Cong, giving a unit of blood was easy. They were confident. These were kids who had looked into the face of death. At that moment, I knew if they "CAN DO," I "CAN DO"! Fortunately, young men in this age group have veins like railroad tracks. I learned fast.

Life requires confidence, in doing things you have never done before and in whatever life brings to you. With confidence, you can handle adversity; you can make your dreams come true!

to help readers evaluate these five characteristics of leadership.

Leadership is cool—it's a glorious adventure that enables us to marshal the talents of others to a serious cause.
TOM PETERS

BEHAVIORS

In addition to characteristics, leaders demonstrate specific behaviors that enable them to marshal the forces of their staff and accomplish amazing goals in support of a motivational mission. Although leaders are individuals who demonstrate many

Box 7-4   A Personal Assessment Guide

The following questions are designed as a self-reflective strategy. In general, no single, correct response exists. Rather, this set of questions is designed to consider the five characteristics and the six behaviors described in this chapter in a way that allows people to understand their own specific abilities and how they are reflective of the five elements.

CHARACTERISTICS

Character (Core)

1. What have I done that I wish I had not? Did I apologize to the person? If not, what would it take to do it now?
2. Can I cite at least one example when I sided with someone in the face of adversity?
3. Can I describe an event that, or person who, could be described as changing my life? Have I held to that change?

Commitment (to Self and Others)

1. Would people say that I keep my word?
2. Can I honestly say that I have staying power to see things through after the "high" has passed?
3. Would I still be a nurse leader if I won $20 million?

Connectedness (with People)

1. What do I do on a daily basis to convey dedication to others?

2. Do I take accountability for my own actions?
3. Do I use stories to convey organizational values? To connect to my people?

Compassion and Caring (the Foundation)

1. How do I model caring behavior?
2. In the previous three conversations I had, how much of the time did I listen?
3. Can I name at least three staff or students and tell something distinctive or personal about each?

Confidence (Belief in One's Abilities)

1. Do I let fear paralyze me?
2. Do I capitalize on my strengths in working with others?
3. Can I describe how I muster courage to carry on?

BEHAVIORS

Visioning

1. What vision did I have for patient care or some change that needed to occur?
2. What strategies did I use to enroll others in this vision?
3. How successful were the vision and the enrolling?
4. What did I learn from the experience?

Building Trust

1. What have I done in the past week to build trust among staff and myself?

Continued

Box 7-4   A Personal Assessment Guide—cont'd

Building Trust—cont'd

2. How would I rate my reliability and accountability?
3. What recent experience demonstrated persistence?

Empowering People

1. What example(s) of a specific activity to empower another do I have?
2. When did I do something to support a staff member in his or her development?
3. What have I done to nurture further development of staff knowledge or skills?

Coaching

1. When was the last time I did one-on-one coaching with a staff member or peer?
2. Have I set periodic sessions with my direct reports to coach them for their own personal growth (not a corrective action)?
3. Have I encouraged my people to do peer coaching with one another? What was the outcome?

Getting Results

1. In what way have I focused on results?
2. Have I celebrated when results were positive?
3. Have I shared these results with those involved and acknowledged them?

Acknowledging

1. What did the last acknowledgment that I did look like?
2. Did I use the five rules of acknowledgment?
3. Did I check to see if the person received the acknowledgment and felt acknowledged?

Readers can take time with this exercise. They can talk about what they discovered with a colleague or classmate. It is possible to do this exercise alone and only for your own awareness. Remember, you never learn less. Learn from this tool.

Kowalski & Associates, 2003.

---

different styles and have their own eccentricities, successful leaders exhibit some common behaviors; among these are visioning, building trust, empowering, coaching, getting results, and acknowledging (Table 7-2).

Visioning

Creating a Vision

Effective leaders, regardless of their style or their strengths and weakness, have a guiding purpose, an overarching vision. In another classic work, Bennis and Goldsmith (1994) said leaders are more than goal directed, they are vision directed. These visions or intentions are compelling and pull people into the vision. For example, some CNOs may want their facility to become a Magnet hospital. Often these CNOs are intense regarding this vision, and when this intensity is coupled with commitment, it is magnetic. The intensity with which these leaders focus on the Magnet hospital vision is similar to the total absorption of a child building a sand castle. Thus, other key members of the nursing and administrative team are attracted to the vision. The leader first embraces the vision, and, partially because of magnetism in communicating the vision to the staff, they also embrace it. Most people want to be part of something special, some effort that is greater than themselves. The first task of the leader is to define the vision and mission with a focus on its uniqueness and ability to make a difference. Most people want to accomplish goals that make a difference for patients and their families. Visions that address this core desire generate passion and excitement.

Table **7-2** A Summary of the CNO's Leadership Behaviors

Behavior	Description	Example
Visioning	A guiding purpose or an overarching, compelling vision, in which the necessary people are enrolled	Wants the facility to become a Magnet hospital; talks among the directors and staff enthusiastically, pulling them into the vision of a Magnet hospital
Building trust	Being accountable	Accepts ownership of results
	Being predictable	Demonstrates consistent and known behaviors
	Being reliable	Can be relied on to keep promises
	Being persistent	Does not give in when obstacles appear
	Being an expert	Demonstrates a set of skills
Empowering people	Bringing out the best; encouraging and promoting a positive mindset	Is publicly appreciative for specific efforts of the senior leadership group in solving some of the problems related to acquiring Magnet status
Coaching	Asking questions and leading the coached through a process of discovery	Establishes specific times for coaching and supports the coached in personal and professional growth
Getting results	Focusing on the outcomes	Focuses on determining the cause of falls and builds interventions to reduce falls
Acknowledging	Staff are acknowledged for who they are and what they do by making the acknowledgment person to person, specific, from the heart, appropriately timed, and public when possible	Comes to the unit (even with the CEO), brings treats or rewards, speaks to each staff nurse individually, and thanks him or her for the work done on the plan to decrease falls; knows at least one specific thing that each person did; speaks to each staff nurse as soon as the results are known, and does it publicly

There is no more powerful engine driving an organization toward excellence and long-range success than an attractive, worthwhile, and achievable vision of the future, widely shared.
Burt Nanus

Enrolling in the Vision

A vision works only when people are willing to follow the leader. To achieve this, staff members must be inspired by a "brightness of the future."

Staff members must be able to see what in the situation will benefit them. This may look different for each person because most people are motivated individually. In addition, it is valuable to discover a common motivation for the group. Again, a story can be effective (Box 7-5). Analysis of this story reveals that to focus on shrimp was much more fun than to think about losing staff positions as a result of low volume.

Staff members needed to stay focused on the goal. This required the second aspect of enrolling

Box 7-5 THE SHRIMP STORY

When I was a new director, my assigned task was to save a new obstetric delivery system now known as LDRP (labor, deliver, recover, and postpartum care all in the same room). I was so busy working with cross-orientation to the new concept, I did not notice the bottom line. At the end of the fiscal year, it became clear that for the unit to "make budget," it would require doing 150 deliveries in the last month of the year. It had been 5 years since the unit had done 150 deliveries in 1 month. I was attempting to figure out a strategy for doing that many births, and all I could come up with was "visualizing" 150 births. Therefore stickers were put on all the phones that said "150 Births." It was talked up in unit meetings. I put up a large paper barometer next to the status board that had each day marked off, so that we had a daily visual of where we were in meeting the goal. After

the weekend off I found graffiti on the barometer. It did occur to me that the staff was not enthusiastic about the goal.

I sat down with staff at the morning change of shift and asked questions about their feelings. There was general silence, until finally a night nurse said, "So what's in it for us?" Thinking fast, I replied, "If we make 150 births, I'll bring in fresh gulf shrimp for all three shifts ... with all the trimmings." This was greeted with a thoughtful, "Hmmmmm." They actually did 165 deliveries that month.

So where did the deliveries come from? It happens that most of the physicians were "split admitters"; that is, they took patients to more than one hospital. So the staff enrolled the physicians in "shrimp." As everyone was sitting around the lounge, eating shrimp, one of the night nurses asked, "So what does it take to get lobster?"

in the vision, which is "frequency of interaction." In the early 1980s, Tom Peters called this MBWA, or managing by walking around. Although leaders often are so "busy" that they do not seem to find the time to walk about, it is still one of the most effective tools available for leading a department or a division. This frequent interaction with staff on various shifts allows for time to determine what staff members are thinking, if they are committed to the vision, what the problems are they confront, and what additional ideas they have.

A *believable alternative* must exist to enrolling in the vision. Obviously in the shrimp story, the alternative was no shrimp. However, staff members knew that positions most likely would be cut if the projected patient volume was not met. They understood the ramifications of not meeting budget projections. However, it was much more fun to think of the believable alternative in terms of shrimp.

Building Trust

Nothing happens without trust. Just as trust between the nurse and the patient has been documented to be the basis of keeping the chronically ill out of the hospital (Mays, 2004), trust has been demonstrated to be the key factor in holding the organization together. It is the lubricant that makes the organization run smoothly. To create trust, leaders make themselves known and understood by the staff. They make their positions clear. Trust is a very fragile commodity. It requires much more to heal broken trust than to gain it in the beginning. Therefore it is important to value and protect the trust the staff has for the leader. Five ways in which trust is developed and maintained follow.

Being Accountable and Responsible

Accountability is the act of accepting ownership for the results *or* the lack thereof; it is focused on outcomes. Responsibility is an obligation to accomplish a task or assignment; it is more specific. It is like the small sign that sat on President Harry S. Truman's desk in the oval office: "The Buck Stops Here." This meant he was responsible and accountable for what worked and what did not. Likewise, when an idea or plan does not work as anticipated, the leader cannot blame others for what did not work or justify what went wrong with all the reasons it did not work.

Being Predictable

Leaders must be predictable (Bennis & Goldsmith, 1994). They make themselves known and their positions clear. Their behavior, responses, and reactions must be consistent and known for most situations. Even if these responses are not what people want, they must be predictable so that a plan or approach can be developed. For example, if a supervisor asked the same question, "How much does it cost?" each time a clinical director had a "great idea" or creative solution to a problem, the repeated question would not be particularly supportive to the creative problem-solving process. However, before discussing a new idea, the clinical director could create a logical "ballpark" estimate to get past the cost issue and be able to discuss the idea based on its merits. Being predictably skeptical or negative is better than being unpredictable.

Being Reliable

Leaders must be relied on to do what is expected or promised. They are fully deserving of complete confidence in their honesty and good judgment.

For example, in one hospital, one of the projects undertaken was to create the labor, delivery, recovery, postpartum (LDRP) unit and to cross-train the nurses to scrub on cesarean sections. Naturally the leader experienced some resistance to learning operating room skills, so she refreshed her skills (she could remember all but one of the surgical instruments used in the case) and put herself "on call." Consequently when the unit was busy, she would go to the operating room and

function as the scrub nurse. The staff members knew they could rely on her. She left meetings or canceled them so that she could help. The first Christmas Eve she was in the facility, the nurse manager and the leader did three back-to-back "emergency" cesarean sections. It was a holiday and so many patients needed attention that adequate care could not have been given without the help of the leader and the manager. They were both reliable.

Being Persistent

The leader does not give in at the first obstacle or problem that arises when attempting to accomplish a goal or fulfill the vision. Rather, the leader keeps creating optional solutions until something works. This approach may involve just a bit of stubbornness. It also can be seen as believing in the goal or vision and continuing to find solutions.

> ### Drowning vs. Surviving
> *Two frogs fell into a can of cream,*
> *Or so I've heard it told.*
> *The sides of the can were shiny and steep,*
> *The cream was deep and cold.*
> *"O, what's the use?" croaked No. 1,*
> *"'Tis fate; no help's around.*
> *Good bye, my friends! Goodbye, sad world!"*
> *And weeping still, he drowned.*
>
> *But No. 2, of sterner stuff,*
> *Dog paddled in surprise,*
> *The while he wiped his creamy face*
> *And dried his creamy eyes.*
> *"I'll swim awhile, at least," he said*
> *or so I've heard it said.*
> *It really wouldn't help the world*
> *If one more frog were dead."*
>
> *An hour or two he kicked and swam,*
> *Not once he stopped to mutter,*
> *But kicked and kicked and swam and kicked*
> *Then hopped out, via butter.*
> EAST TEXAS COOKBOOK, ANONYMOUS

The moral of the poem is to persist, because circumstances can change. Strong leaders continue paddling until they make butter.

Demonstrating Expertise

The leader must be seen as having expertise. It does not necessarily mean that the leader is the best clinician. However, a set of skills is essential, such as excellent communication skills, great presentation skills, excellent coaching skills, good problem-solving skills, and expertise in working with budgets. Leaders must be seen as competent, which translates to being knowledgeable. Although the leaders' clinical skill sets are not as important as their clinical competence and understanding of clinical issues, the leader is the spokesperson for clinical issues.

Empowering People

When leaders empower their followers, they bring out the best in them. They encourage and promote a positive mindset. They support the staff with the belief that the staff can do what is required. They express positivism and confidence in their staff members' capabilities. They foster constructive thought patterns in the staff and nurture their development, particularly their self-development.

Coaching

Leaders establish a formal coaching process with people who report directly to them. The goal of this coaching is to support the personal and professional growth process. They share new learning and support the learning of the person they are coaching. Coaching is such an important aspect for leaders that some experts believe leaders need to devote nearly 40% of their time coaching their people (see Chapter 11).

Getting Results

Leaders are focused on results. They want to know and be responsible for the outcomes of decisions they make and the plans and policies they put in place. Measures are put in place to evaluate results, including measures of such outcomes as number of patient falls, medication errors, pain management, staff satisfaction, patient satisfaction, and financial measures or hours of agency nurses. Leaders are focused on qualitative and quantitative measures. They want to use benchmarks to compare themselves and their facilities with other comparable institutions. Leaders see these results as a measure of their personal effectiveness and of the effectiveness of all the programs they have instituted. At the same time, they would not sacrifice their staff for "results."

Acknowledging

One of the most powerful tools a leader possesses is to acknowledge followers. Everyone wants to be acknowledged for what they do and who they are as a contributing member of the team or the organization. It seems as though people frequently say, "Thank you." So why do most people not feel acknowledged? In actuality, the "thank you" often comes in a hurried, nonspecific manner. A few simple guidelines could greatly improve the quality and effectiveness of the leader's acknowledgments (Box 7-6). If all the guidelines are followed, staff members will feel acknowledged and appreciated for the work they do.

The primary behaviors demonstrated by effective leaders consist of these six behaviors (see Box 7-4). For the leaders who wish to assess their leadership behaviors, refer again to Box 7-4.

OTHER INFLUENCING FACTORS IN SELF-DEVELOPMENT

In addition to characteristics and behaviors, additional factors are involved in self-development. Focusing on improving skills in emotional intelligence is valuable. For staff members to understand the work style profile of the leader and for the leader to understand the profiles of the administrative team are beneficial in improving teamwork.

Box 7-6 GUIDELINES FOR ACKNOWLEDGMENT

1. **Person to person.** Acknowledgments must be said to the person to whom you are grateful. Look the person directly in the eye, take a moment, stop, and state the acknowledgment clearly. Acknowledgments also can be written. These can be kept, reviewed, and brought out whenever the person wants to remember the wonderful acknowledgment.

2. **Specific.** State exactly what the person has done that you appreciate. Do not just say, "Good job." Say specifically what he, she, or they did that was appreciated: "Thank you very much for completing the schedule for the next cycle. It looks fair, requests have been honored, and all the shifts are covered."

3. **From the heart.** Acknowledgments must be "real." If it is a mere formality, do not waste your time because people know when the gratitude is not sincere. When this is the case, it is almost insulting. To continue, "Had you not helped to finish the schedule, it would have been late coming out and staff would have been distraught. Your help was invaluable."

4. **Timing.** It is important to deliver the acknowledgment as close to the event as possible. The more time lapses between the event and the acknowledgment, the less sincere and heart-felt it seems.

5. **Public when possible.** Public acknowledgment has more power. It also lets everyone on the unit, for example, know what behaviors are valued by the leader.

Attitudes are (1) critical to the way in which an administrative team works together, (2) coachable, and (3) the precursor of behaviors for which team members are held accountable. What is the approach used with failures and mistakes? What motivates the leader and the team members? Does the group devote time or energy on self-development, personal and professional growth, or self-reflection for the purpose of learning? Do leaders have fun? Awareness of these factors can influence leadership development.

Emotional Intelligence

In the mid 1990s, Daniel Goleman (1995) presented the concept of emotional intelligence, which revolutionized the manner in which leadership is assessed. He organized somewhat scattered ideas regarding leader behaviors into a conceptual framework that identified and crystallized the thinking regarding the use of self in the leadership role. These ideas traditionally have been thought of as the "soft" side of leadership. Others such as Weisinger (1998) then began to specifically

actualize or apply these concepts to the workplace, and finally, nurses such as Porter-O'Grady and Malloch (2002) specifically applied them to nursing. This perspective is paramount to how leaders lead in a caring profession. The five pivotal aspects of this framework include *self-knowledge/self-awareness, self-mastery/self regulation, self-motivation, empathy/insight,* and *social arts/skills.*

Self-knowledge/self-awareness is the crux of this chapter and no doubt a cornerstone of leadership. The leader must be able to recognize and categorize his or her own emotions, moods, and the drivers that create the behaviors and the responses in the leader. At the same time, the leader must recognize the effect of these emotions on the people around him or her. For example, the leader can begin with self-reflection through analysis and honesty about his or her performance and note this through journaling (Johns, 2004). Through this process of self-observation, the intent of the leader is to learn, grow, and change behavior that differs from the idealized self or the vision of positive self-image.

Self-mastery/self-regulation refines the image and control of the leader's behavior. Reflection and self-awareness identify behaviors or attitudes the leader finds less than useful. The next step is being able to control and shift these undesirable or ineffective behaviors and strategies. The outcome of self-mastery is to display or evidence the appropriate emotional response in a given situation. This means to achieve balance between no passion in one's life and emotional excess. To have and show emotions is a human quality; the key is to be able to understand and manage them. For example, when upset or reaction occurs, effective leaders have strategies by which they soothe themselves and this emotional response. Such strategies could include reading a novel, hiking, painting, playing a musical instrument, or going dancing.

Self-motivation is a passion for the leader's work, for the nursing profession, for quality patient care, and for the growth of staff. These passions go far beyond the salary or the status of the leadership position. The focus is on the pursuit of goals related to these professional issues to the extent that the leader perseveres in the face of great obstacles, frustrations, or setbacks. The leader is enthusiastic, zealous, and confident about achieving these goals. The leader is willing to do whatever it takes to fulfill these achievements, including self-discipline and impulse control, the ability to think positively or have a positive attitude, and to overcome disappointment. Such leaders understand the power of positive thinking for themselves and for their staff.

Empathy/insight, or the ability to understand how another feels, is critical to the leader. Research (Goleman, 1995) describes the benefit in the ability to read feelings from nonverbal cues to include increased emotional adjustment, popularity, an outgoing demeanor, and sensitivity. Women appear to have more innate empathy than men do. This skill enables a leader to develop rapport with a broadly diverse group of people, from housekeeping staff members to physicians and board members. A critical link exists between empathy and caring, a core value of the nursing profession.

Social arts/skills constitute the effective dealings with others and allow the leader to shape and encounter, mobilize, and inspire staff members and colleagues; thrive in intimate relationships; and persuade and influence others while putting them at ease. On the other hand, a deficit in these skills leads to ineptness in the social world of work and repeated interpersonal disasters. A deficit in this area can lead even an intellectually brilliant individual to create difficulties in relationships while appearing arrogant, obnoxious, or insensitive. Such deficits can lead to a difficult leadership experience.

The skills that constitute emotional intelligence, like the other leadership characteristics, behaviors, and tools, can be learned and practiced through a commitment to reflection and learning from mistakes and successes (Freshwater, 2004).

Attitude

Attitude is an inward feeling expressed by behavior. It can be seen without a word being said, because verbal and behavioral expressions most often reflect inward feelings. These expressions become the "window of the soul." Because attitude often is expressed by facial expression and body language, it actually can be contagious. Most of us have noticed what happens to a group of people when one person comes into the setting who is very negative in both talk and actions. One person can bring the whole group down. Likewise when someone comes into the group who obviously loves and cares about the people in the group, the mood lightens, which is accompanied by smiles and laughter. Because people usually reflect on the outside what is going on inside, being aware of the internal feelings and their external reflections is important. What is attitude?

It is the "advance man" of our true selves.
Its roots are inward but its fruit is outward.
It is our best friend or our worst enemy.
It is more honest and more consistent than
our words.

It is an outward look based on past experiences.
It is a thing which draws people to us or
repels them.
It is never content until it is expressed.
It is the librarian of our past.
It is the speaker of our present.
It is the prophet of our future.
JOHN MAXWELL (2003, P. 4)

Attitude is the primary source that determines whether people succeed or fail. Attitude determines a person's approach to life. One way for a person to assess attitude is to answer the question, "Do you feel the world is treating you well?" And if a person's attitude toward the world is positive, the world will, for the most part, treat that person well. On the other hand, when people feel badly about the world, they perceive themselves to have bad experiences or primarily negative feedback. It is easy to see how this person would have a negative attitude. According to a psychiatric nurse colleague (who possesses a delicious sense of humor), "psychosclerosis" is hardening of the attitude. Leaders must be careful which way it hardens. They also must be aware of their primary attitude and approach to life in general and to make choices about what approach they will take every day. Attitude and the ability to be optimistic, based on reality, are critical to the approach toward mistakes and failures.

Failure Versus Mistakes

There is no doubt in my mind that there are many
ways to be a winner, but there is really only one
way to be a loser and that is to fail and not look
beyond the failure.
KYLE ROTE, JR.

The U.S. culture contains pervasive attitudes regarding failure. These perceptions regarding failure include an intense fear of failure, a lack of clear understanding of failure, and a lack of preparation for failure. Needless to say, this applies to nurses in leadership roles. Failure is an inevitable part of being human. However, in the drive for perfection, particularly pervasive in healthcare, the possibility of failure is denied and ignored. This denial comes in part from the perceived outcome, "If I fail, I could kill a patient." Clearly this is not just a possibility but a reality according to the research substantiating the number of deaths in institutions from medical and nursing errors (Institute of Medicine, 1999). Closer examination of failure would be helpful. What happens that creates so many mistakes in healthcare? What needs to occur to create the situation in a different way?

Fear of Failure

When Jeffers (1987) hypothesized the core of all fears as the belief, "I can't handle it," she translated that belief to mean whatever happens to human beings, they will not have the appropriate skills or the adequate responses to handle it. This is particularly true as people attempt to cope with failure.

Many healthcare professionals believe they cannot tolerate mistakes. Failure in healthcare can be so catastrophic as to engender considerable fear: fear of killing a patient, fear of losing one's job, fear of how the nurse or CNO will be perceived by others in the face of a significant failure, and fear of rejection or reprimand. Fear can be immobilizing to the extent that people can adopt the attitude, "At least I got through the day with no major faux pas." The problem with this approach is the lack of risk taking. Failure can produce such adverse painful results that people become fearful and guarded, which can lead to favoring the status quo. Thus fear can produce paralysis, the inability to move forward with programs or very good ideas, or immobilization. Paralysis leads to giving up. In addition, fear can lead to procrastination, which delays decisions that could jeopardize the leader's status and effectiveness. According to Maxwell (2000), procrastination steals time, productivity, and potential. Fear of failure also leads to lack of real purpose. To avoid the pain of failing, some people just put in their time, follow the rules, and do only what they are told to do. This purposelessness leads to self-pity and victim behavior and blaming others for poor outcomes or lack of results. Such a scattered approach to work reinforces a lack of focus, decreases results, and creates hopelessness or an inability to see the brightness of the future.

Some behaviors and emotional responses only exacerbate even a small failure. Anger as an emotional behavior is a natural human response to an undesirable outcome that leads to upset or reaction. Partially because of the fear of not being able to handle it, the person overreacts, taking frustration out on themselves and others. Angry responses often multiply or increase the problem, because the situation still needs to be fixed and staff or co-worker relationships need to be repaired. Next is a basic human desire to hide or cover up the failure. The result of hiding failures is the absence of learning from the failures.

> *It's okay to fail. If you're not failing, you're not growing.*
> H. STANLEY JUDD

One approach to stop the downward spiral of fear and negativism is to *view failures as major learning experiences* (Kowalski, Hayden, & Burck, 1996). Even in the most serious of circumstances, human beings make mistakes. The value in these mistakes is to be able to examine them and determine the multiple system problems that allowed the mistake or failure to occur. In healthcare, deadly errors frequently are produced by multiple system problems. If a punitive approach is taken toward the mistake, people are more likely to resist studying the situation and learning from it.

Working harder and faster is another ineffective approach to failure. When people stubbornly keep plowing ahead, it is most often in the same direction. This leads to repetition of the same mistakes or failures. This is also the definition of insanity, doing the same thing and expecting a different outcome.

Some people quit or give up in the face of fear and adversity. Leaders, on the other hand, have an instinct for perseverance. They can continue in the face of adversity.

> *Ninety percent of all those who fail are not actually defeated. They simply quit.*
> PAUL J. MEYER

Some leaders are able to persevere because they maintain their sense of humor.

Humor

Considering that the average American spends in excess of 70,000 hours of their lifetime working and more than 3 years in meetings (Buxman, 2001), would it not be healthier to have some fun and laugh during at least a portion of that time? The use of humor by the leader helps to solidify the group or team. The strongest leaders love to laugh and most often they laugh at themselves (Lyons, 2002). Laughing together helps establish a bond and support within the group or team. Humor can improve productivity and supports tasks that require intense concentration (Kehr, 1999). Humor is a powerful and persuasive form of communication, enrolling and holding the staff member's attention.

Leaders can create a more informal atmosphere, even in important meetings, by using humor. A playful work environment is supportive. An example is Southwest Airlines, where a sense of humor is a job requirement and the flight attendants vie for who can be the most humorous when making announcements about the safety aspects of the airplane (Goldsmith, 2002). The work environment can be supported through the use of humorous posters, memos, or signs in the break room. Some comic activities or theme days could be added to the calendar: a cowboy day (particularly in sections of the country that have rodeos or stock shows) or a joke of the day or daily humor rounds. Meetings could begin with a funny story about a patient or co-worker (with permission). A funny self-deprecating comment, a disarming remark, or light touch can make a positive difference for staff and patients. Humor does not work when it is forced or when it does not fit with the setting or the purpose. If the management meeting included some humor, people might arrive on time.

Motivation

Most people know what they need to do to achieve their goals and dreams. However, they have dozens of reasons why they cannot act on the knowledge, and thus the dreams and goals are unrealized. Motivation is a force that creates behavior to fulfill a need and is connected to acknowledgment (Huszczo, 2004); it is a powerful and complex force that causes people to act. Motivation has two basic levels: survival and achievement. Survival needs include safety, shelter, food, and procreation much as Maslow identified them. After the basic needs are satisfied, human beings begin to work on other areas such as achievement, emotional fulfillment, and personal growth. The motivation of a person to take action comes from knowing which need is most prominent in the moment.

According to Kim (1996), several key ideas help in understanding motivation:

1. Motivation is a force, positive or negative, that creates action.
2. Understanding the underlying motive that leads to taking action is the key to motivating people, including ourselves.
3. Every motive for taking action comes from a need and a desire to satisfy it.
4. Motives come in many forms and change throughout life.
5. Motives can change rapidly, even during a specific activity.
6. Motivation is the result of social conditioning and experience.
7. Motivation consists of the act of encouraging someone to do something they need to do but may be unable to initiate on their own. On the other hand, manipulation is the act of deceiving

someone into doing something they might not otherwise do.

Leaders frequently think about how to motivate employees. In reality, the primary way to motivate them is to give them challenging work for which they can assume responsibility (Herzberg, 2004). An example of this is keeping decision making and problem solving at the staff nurse level rather than being obsessed with policies and procedures that remove these important tasks from the bedside experts.

Intention

An *intention* is a strong purpose, aim, or goal accompanied by a determination, a commitment to produce a specific desired result (Dyer, 2004). Most of us have intentions and frequently these intentions are positive. From time to time, something gets in the way of intentions and obstructs the purpose. The fallout from these obstructions can be hurtful or destructive to other people. Frequently when mistakes are made, the intention was of the highest purpose and something intervened. When this occurs, what really matters is how the situation is handled. When the leader says or does something that did not fit with the intention, the most important approach is to apologize for the outcome or the incident and share what the real intention was: "That particular outcome was not my intention." It is also appropriate to ask for help and suggestions of other pathways toward the goal and the true intention. Focusing on intention, which is usually of the highest purpose and value, is helpful in resolution of mistakes or problems in interpersonal interactions.

TOOLS FOR SELF-DEVELOPMENT

Effective commonplace approaches exist for self-development as a leader. They include such concepts as creating balance in life and methods to achieve this, implementing some form of self-reflection, focusing on continual learning, and utilizing such tools as the personality or work style profiles that enlighten the leader and team members about their styles.

Personality or Work Style Profiles

Multiple assessment tools are available for use in identification of work style and personality styles of each leader and their key people. Such tools as the DISC Personal Profile System (DISC, 2001) or the Myers-Briggs can be helpful in discovering strengths and weaknesses. These tools can assist in assessment of co-workers or staff, not to put them in boxes but to help everyone learn how to work together more effectively and understand each other. Most tools make a point of emphasizing the value or strengths of every personality style. Each person has something important to contribute to the group. These tools also help with the coaching process and assisting staff members to identify strengths and weaknesses and personal and professional goals.

Another type of tool, referred to as a 360-degree assessment (Swain, Schubot, Thomas, Baker, Foldy, Greaves & Monteagudo, 2004), includes assessments of performance and feedback from subordinates, peers, and supervisors. Therefore the 360 degrees of feedback from each of the groups working closely with the leader benefits leaders in seeing how relationships change or remain the same with these different groups. It can pinpoint areas in which the leader could benefit from coaching to improve working relationships.

Learn and Role Model Balance in Life

Healthcare professionals are notorious for working many long hours and not taking care of themselves. Such work patterns lead to exhaustion and burnout. It is particularly critical for nursing leaders to take care of themselves and then to model self-care to staff members rather than modeling 60- to 80-hour work weeks. The following four areas in which imbalance frequently occurs are highlighted: *physical, intellectual, emotional,* and *spiritual.*

Physical

Caretaking of the physical aspects of the self is important to optimal functioning, being the best a human being can be. Excessive fatigue from long hours, too many shifts, and inadequate sleep leads to unclear thinking and reasoning. Other important physical aspects include a healthy diet (which rules out most fast food), adequate exercise (which could include regular workouts at a gym or at home), and regular massages or facials. The body needs exercise, which provides endorphin release and a sense of well-being. The important concept is taking care of oneself physically and even occasionally focusing on a special physical treat.

Intellectual

Activities that could support a leader intellectually include professional reading to stay current in the chosen field. A journal club among peers could combine the journal review with dinner. Continuously improving communication skills could include attending workshops or identifying a coach or mentor with whom clinical, administrative, or interpersonal issues could be reviewed and a plan developed. From an intellectual perspective it is critical to maintain a sense of humor. A leader might want to review the last week and look for the number of times situations evolved in which everyone had a "big belly laugh." Without laughter, physical and mental problems ensue.

Emotional

Attention to the emotional aspects of the self includes such activities as meditation and thinking about personal growth. A book on self-forgiveness may be helpful, because most human beings find it difficult to forgive their own mistakes. Journaling and actively pursuing self-reflection may be helpful. Reading a book such as Cheryl Richardson's *Life Makeovers* with a friend may be beneficial. After completing the weekly assignments, the friends could have dinner together and discuss what they learned. A favorite self-help TV show such as *Oprah* or *Dr. Phil* could be taped for later viewing. Attending the theater or a concert and dinner with a spouse or close friend may provide a lighthearted diversion from the daily routine. The objective is to free up the mind and emotions from the workplace and focus on something totally different.

Spiritual

Attending to the spiritual aspects of life can mean pursuing a religious belief system, including an active spiritual life. It might be focusing on improving unconditional acceptance of oneself and others. It should be something that replenishes the spirit; this does not necessarily mean religion. Enjoying nature or the outdoors or perhaps enjoying or entertaining family or friends may enhance a person's spirit. One of the best spiritual experiences may be a beautiful sunrise or sunset. The important aspect of focusing on spirituality is releasing all other worries and pain so that a level of peacefulness is attained.

These activities are not necessarily easy and many people claim, "There is no time!" In reality enough time exists for whatever each leader deems important, and care for the self is critical for all who must accomplish the goals and objectives in a high-stress job. Self-care is about personal restoration and coming to the job rested, refreshed, and refilled.

Meditation

Some people meditate on a regular basis. Meditation is a structured process that allows leaders to clear their minds and their thinking and provides a release from the stress of work. Many types of meditation exist, and many classes on meditation are available. Some people use yoga as an exercise and a meditation. Other people use prayer in one of its many forms to achieve the same result. For example, contemplative prayer or centering prayer is a way to open oneself to God or the Spirit. It is a 20-minute process of clearing the mind of all the business and the self-talk with a one-word mantra. Whatever form the leader chooses, meditation can be of great assistance in becoming more balanced and letting go of stress.

Continuous Learning

Reading, journal club, courses, national meetings, networking, and coaching are ways to stimulate learning and growing. One of the factors inherent in awarding Magnet (McClure & Hinshaw, 2002) designation is whether a learning environment is being created within the organization. This has evolved from the original work by Peter Senge (1990) regarding the importance of creating learning organizations for the twenty-first century. Such environments are important to support personal and professional growth and creation of a research-focused institution that desires to create best clinical practices. Nurse leaders should ask themselves the following questions:

- How many journals/magazines do I read per month?
- Do I have a structured way to discuss what I am reading/learning with a peer?
- Do I take any courses (adult education) just for the joy of learning something new, such as advanced computer courses?
- Do I surround myself with a network of people who expect more from me than I do and/or people who are supportive of my dreams?
- Do I have a professional coach who holds me accountable for my words and actions and supports me to discover what I have learned from any given situation and how I would like to do it differently in the future?

Self-Reflection

Leaders are supported in their growth by some form of self-reflection. The goal of self-reflection is to problem-solve in an intuitive yet systematic way that can transform future action and behavior (Freshwater, 2004). Learning through reflection is about finding the creative tension between understanding the current situation and its reality while attempting to reach a vision of the ideal (Hirt, 2004; Johns, 2004; Senge, 1990). Taylor (2004) defines reflective thinking as the review of thoughts and memories through methods such as thinking, contemplation, meditation, and any other form of attentive consideration. These are used to understand or make sense of the thoughts and memories and make appropriate changes in thinking and behavior. She divides the process into three steps: experiencing, interpreting, and learning. During the experiencing phase it is helpful to become silent and recall every aspect of the event, including sights, sounds, smells, the people, and any other aspects that were pivotal to the incident. When the image is clear, it should be described in writing or into a recording device. When this process is complete, the following questions should be addressed: (1) What happened? (2) When, where, and why did it happen? (3) Who was involved? (4) How were you involved? (5) What was the setting like? (6) What were the outcomes? (7) How did you honestly feel about the situation? (8) What worked well about the situation? (9) What did not work about the situation?

During the interpretation phase of the analysis, the following questions should be addressed: (1) What were my goals for the interaction? (2) To what extent did I achieve each goal? (3) How did my interpretation of the situation affect the other people involved? (4) What were the interpretations of the other people involved and how did this show up in the interaction? (5) What norms and values were at play, either enacted or avoided? (6) What influences and/or political relationships were in place that affected the outcome?

In the learning phase, the leader must be as honest as possible. This may require deep thought or, if the situation was particularly difficult, it could require a night's sleep before revisiting the situation with some of the following questions:

(1) What does the experience tell me about my expectations of myself? (2) What does it tell me about my expectations of other people? (3) What did I learn? (4) What would I like to change about my own actions or behavior? (5) How could I integrate this learning into my future actions and behavior? (6) How would I create the situation differently?

Reflection is enhanced by writing down thoughts and feelings about what happens in a day. A common form is to journal. An effective journaling method involves taking 10 to 15 minutes at the end of the day to note what has happened during the day and what was learned from these experiences. This is not for anyone else to see or evaluate; it is only for the leader. Any event with an undesired outcome can be examined during self-reflection to determine what might be done differently and what might be done about the situation. This process can be an extremely valuable learning experience that promotes growth.

SUMMARY

Although the characteristics, behaviors, and the additional tools provided in this chapter do not constitute an exhaustive list, they are examples of self-discovery and self-development. Cultivating these various aspects and elements benefits the effectiveness of leading. Each behavior, characteristic, or tool stands alone, yet each relates to and enhances the others. Investment in developing the self benefits the staff members with whom the leader works and the organization as a whole.

KEY POINTS TO LEAD

1. Analyze characteristics and behaviors of yourself as a leader.

2. Analyze where you currently are and what your goals are in the areas of humor, intentions, attitude, and motivation.
3. Evaluate the strengths and weaknesses you, the learner, possess in each of these three areas:

characteristics, behaviors, and additional influences.
4. Develop a plan for how you will continue to expand in your areas of strengths and what you would like to do with your weak areas.

Literature Box

Complexity science is based on holistic thinking, something at which women often excel. This article reports the research in which 50 women leaders in the United States, Canada, Australia, and the United Kingdom were interviewed. These women displayed "third possibility leadership" as depicted by the ability to hold masculine and feminine values and behaviors in balance. These women leaders were paradoxical, gathered people together, were holistic thinkers, and displayed well-developed "relational intelligence." In addition to the effectiveness of their leadership, they were often "invisible" and even demeaned for socio-cultural reasons.

Organizations guided by complexity science are found to be organizationally flat, place high value on diversity, and encourage open communication. As a result of interviews of multiple levels of employees in these 50 organizations, the authors found that relationships were the "bottom line" for business success for these complex business environments. They found that people had developed relationships grounded in mutual respect and interests and impact on each other. Genuine caring and connection existed between workers regardless of their position in the hierarchical structure.

Although the researchers see complexity science organizations as feminine, they acknowledge that it is a traditional view based on relationship-focused behaviors and a holistic viewpoint. They acknowledge that men who have these qualities can be just as successful as the women in these complex organizations. The majority of men in the nursing profession have such qualities partially as a result of the profession being focused on caring

as a core value. These third possibility leaders are gatherers; that, is they bring people together, even those who are disenfranchised. They are also paradoxical in that they are tough and empathetic. They are holistic in that they quickly see the whole picture in addition to the human and systems connections within the picture. These third possibility leaders exhibit rational intelligence as demonstrated by sensitivity to social context and individual needs. The authors highlight the traditional male factors that have influenced leadership such as a culture of greed, the obsession with obscene income levels for CEOs who believe they alone are responsible for the success of the company, the myth of CEO as hero, and the way in which hard-nosed (often male) business leaders devalue qualities such as nurturing and caring for their followers.

Women, who are often these third possibility leaders and often are gifted with the skills of "quiet leadership," have a skill set that is just now being recognized as the most powerful form of leadership. Women often are assumed to be incompetent, and when they quietly succeed, their success is attributed to blind luck. However, as more research emerges, it becomes increasingly clear that what creates successful businesses are positive relationships in which the people have healthy relationships with one another, and complexity science shows why this is true.

Regine, B., & Lewin, R. (2003). Third possibility leaders: The invisible edge women have in complex organizations. *The Learning Organization,* 10(6), 347-352.

Contemplations

- As the leader, how would you assess your character development? Where are you in relationship to your idealized character?
- What is your level of commitment in your current position?
- How confident are you in your current position?
- Think of a recent incident in which you demonstrated caring and compassion for an employee. What about your interaction was caring?
- What is your vision in your current job? Have you enrolled your people in that vision? What is the evidence that they are enrolled?
- What steps have you taken to build trust within your team? Be specific.
- What is the evidence or the outcomes that indicate you have been successful?

- How many of your people have you acknowledged this week? Have you checked with them to determine if they truly felt acknowledged?
- How often have you laughed this week? Was this laughter at the expense of another person?
- Describe your attitude yesterday. Would you have enjoyed spending time with yourself? Were you abrupt or curt with people?
- Did you take 10 minutes yesterday to review your day to see what worked, what did not work, what you could learn from the day, and what you want to change and do differently?
- Can you describe how you demonstrated the five components of emotional intelligence this week?

LEADER STORY

JOYCE C. CLIFFORD
PRESIDENT AND CEO
THE INSTITUTE FOR NURSING HEALTHCARE
LEADERSHIP

I look at leadership as a professional attribute rather than a role or job description. On the other hand, specific jobs demand strong leadership, which is why the selection of the person to fill such a position is so important. I have known clinical staff members who were tremendous leaders but did not necessarily have a leadership title. As nurse leaders we have tremendous responsibilities to design work environments in which safe patient care can be provided, and advancing the leadership of all nurses, clinical and managerial, is a wonderful strategy.

I did my dissertation on the role of the CNO and saw the role as having two important dimensions. At Beth Israel in Boston, I was Vice President for nursing and the Chief of Nursing. The VP title represented the organizational leadership role, which allowed me to be with other senior executives in the board room and other executive forums bringing the voice of nursing to the important organizational decisions and directions. As the Chief of Nursing, I represented the leadership of the clinical discipline of nursing, which put me on a par with the other clinical chiefs, such as the Chief of Medicine and Chief of Surgery. This position also facilitated the formation of collegial relationships with clinical staff and put me in forums in which clinical chiefs determined policy regarding patient care. These two dimensions of leadership are not always easy to keep in balance, especially when the pressures on the administrative role are sometimes so great that nurse leaders easily can lose track of the critically important clinical leadership role.

A great deal of emphasis has been placed on the financial aspect of healthcare leadership. Although it is important to understand the finances, I have said, "When the CFO is as effective in the clinical arena as I am, then I will strive to be as effective as he is with finances. We each have special areas of expertise and it is not necessary for me to understand every financial nuance." We did put the CFO on the clinical units at one point so that he would understand what occurred in the daily activities of patient care. At one point, I also was able to teach the CFO how to understand scheduling and he, in turn, did the same for me — helping me to understand more than a general ledger. It was important for me to realize that I didn't have to be a CFO but it was also important for me to have a meaningful working relationship with him.

To a large extent, understanding these two major aspects of the CNO role, administrative and clinical, and balancing the two is what makes the job challenging and satisfying. Some days when I was feeling overwhelmed with administration, I would go up to the units and talk to nurses or sometimes help them care for patients. Even more importantly, I would *listen* to nurses, and I was always comfortable doing so.

The most important aspect of developing yourself as a leader comes from Socrates, "Know thyself." Know what you are good at, what you need help with, what you should delegate, and what you should spend time developing. For me, my strength was the ability to relate to other people and convince them that they have unknown and untapped qualities and that they can accomplish things they never thought possible. I believe that staff members have marvelous potential and can do things that I cannot do. I merely help and support them to become good leaders and to know themselves at entirely new and deeper levels. Fear is what usually stops people, and my confidence in their ability could lead them to an entirely new level.

I will tell you a story about the nurse manager of the renal dialysis unit. Federal regulations and Medicare were in favor of replacing registered nurses with dialysis techs. So this nurse manager did a study that demonstrated the cost benefit of having an all-RN staff in the dialysis unit. I could have presented the study results to the board, but I thought it would be better to have the nurse manager come and make the presentation. It was her work, after all. A nurse manager had never presented to the board before. She was wonderful; she was passionate and confident. She had her data, and needless to say, the board members were very impressed. This situation demonstrated to me how important it is to support others to take the lead and to get the recognition that goes with the situation. It is important to learn how to help people fulfill the capacity that is within them. This is an important part of knowing yourself. One of my most valuable skills is motivation and encouragement of others. As the CNO, it was my responsibility to bring resources to nurse managers so that they could learn and grow and reach out to their staff, supporting the staff members as I had tried to support them.

I had regular face-to-face interactions with the nurse manager group. These monthly meetings were not held to talk so much about operational issues as they were to encourage communication and develop a commitment and understanding of the underlying philosophy and values. On one of these occasions, I asked a nurse manager what it was like to manage a primary nursing care unit. This manager (long before it was popular) talked about establishing a learning environment and the importance of mentoring and development of staff. By doing so, she modeled for other peers what the core element of the nurse manager role should be. Mentoring and development are so important, and these functions were key purposes of this meeting with the managers. In addition, I had the expectation that nurse managers would develop their staff just as they were being developed. Likewise, the directors were expected to coach and develop the nurse managers just as I was developing the director group. This approach should work today just as it did 25 years ago.

If a graduate student came to me for advice about a career in nursing administration, I would first need to know something about the person. I would ask several questions to assess how well the student could tolerate ambiguity. Is this person able to delay gratification and feelings of satisfaction? Is this person able to understand and enjoy vicarious recognition because he or she was involved by influencing the achievement of clinical nurses on the unit? Understanding oneself and the ability to accomplish goals through others is certainly as important as understanding the budget.

Nursing leaders need to be well educated and prepared. Three of my greatest concerns today are (1) Where are the mentors for upcoming nursing administrators? (2) Where are the nursing administration educational programs today? and (3) Where are the premier nursing administration educators? They do not seem to be as well known or recognized as they once were. Nursing administration preparation provides an opportunity for nurses to learn more about working in a cross-disciplinary way. My own preparation was through a master's program in medical/surgical nursing, but all my special projects in the program were directed toward administration.

I may have learned the most, however, through my professional association, which is now called AONE. My membership started in 1974 when the organization was called the American Society for Nursing Service Administrators (ASNSA). I became a member of the Board in 1978 to 1979, and I also became President of the organization and then Chair of the Task Force on Reorganization that led to ASNSA becoming AONE. This was between the years of 1981 to 1985. The colleagues and the contacts I developed through this work were and remain invaluable. Some of these nursing administrators were the wisest people I have ever known. The national meetings provided opportunities to network with role models and colleagues, and I learned a great deal from them in informal conversations and during committee work. Another essential is to be active in continuing education and be responsible for your own learning. If, upon self-reflection and self-evaluation, you feel some issues or areas of growth need attention, find an executive coach.

When I first went to Beth Israel, it was in an era when the nursing director never presented the nursing budget to the board. I was given the opportunity to do so, and one of the first things I taught the board about was NHPPD, or nursing hours of care per patient day. Later, I almost wished I had not taught them quite so well, because they held me to what they had learned. One of the earliest memories I have of working at the Beth Israel was helping people who worked in other departments to understand that they also were working for the benefit of patients.

Somehow, other departments were under the impression they were providing service for nursing, and I tried to reframe this thinking so that they thought more about providing service for patients. A great example is laundry. Does every facility not have issues with laundry? Enough linen is never available, and nurses tend to hoard it. I realized that somehow we had to break the cycle and stop the hoarding. I was attempting to help the nursing staff and other departments

establish what was acceptable and what was not. I told the nurse managers that even if they had to call me, we could not accept bad service because patients suffered. So the next day the fifth floor nurse manager called me and reported no linen was available. I made the call, "This is Mrs. Clifford, I'm calling about linen for the fifth floor." The response was, "We'll take it right up." After hearing a similar response a number of times, I finally told the laundry manager that whenever a nurse manager calls about linen, pretend her name is Mrs. Clifford. If you can find the linen for me, you can find it for the nurse.

The greatest thing you can do is respect the work of others. I am in awe of what nurses do every day. I would go up to the units, sometimes with my lab coat, and try to help in any way that I could. It helped me to get as much understanding as I could of the work. Furthermore, I could help nurses respect the work of others. It is helpful to know what a colleague's day is like. For example, a surgeon could go crazy, and I would ask the nurses to find out what patient had "gone bad." Almost always a reason existed for the surgeon to be so upset, and it was usually about a patient and less than desired outcomes. In this way, staff members began to think about and respect in a different way what goes on in the other person's world.

Chapter References

American Organization of Nurse Executives. (2005). AONE Nurse Executive Competencies. *Nurse Leader, 3*(2), 15-21.

Bennis, W. (1999). Lead with character. *Executive Excellence, 16*(4), 4.

Bennis, W., & Goldsmith, J. (1994). *Learning to lead.* Reading, MA: Addison-Wesley Publishing Company.

Bennis, W., & Nanus, B. (1985). *Leaders: The strategies for taking charge.* New York: Harper & Row, 1985.

Buckingham, M., & Clifton, D. (2001). *Now, discover your strengths.* New York: The Free Press.

Buxman, K. (2001). You can't be serious: Humor at work. *Training and Development, 55*(7).

Crane, T. G. (2002). *The heart of coaching: Using transformational coaching to create a high-performance culture.* (2nd Ed.). San Diego, CA: FTA Press.

DISC Classic. (2001). *Personality profile system 2800.* Minneapolis, MN: Inscape Publishing.

Dutton, J., Frost, P., Worline, M., Lilius, J., & Kanof, J. (2002). Leading in times of trauma. *Harvard Business Review, 80*(1), 55-61.

Dyer, W. W. (2004). *The power of intention: Learning to co-create your world your way.* Carlsbad, CA: Hay House.

Freiberg, K., & Freiberg, J. (1996). *Nuts! Southwest Airlines crazy recipe for business* (p. 224). New York: Broadway Books.

Freshwater, D. (2004). Tool for developing clinical leadership. *Reflections on Nursing Leadership, 30*(2), 20-26.

Goldsmith, B. (2002). Inside-out leadership: Learning to manage from the core. *Office Solutions, 19*(4).

Goleman, D. (1995). *Emotional intelligence: Why it can matter more than IQ.* New York: Bantam Books.

Guinness, O. (1999). *Character counts: Leadership qualities in Washington, Wilberforce, Lincoln, and Solzhenitsy.* Grand Rapids, MI: Baker Books.

Guinness, O. (2000). *When no one sees: The importance of character in an age of image.* Colorado Springs, CO: Navpress.

Herzberg, F. (2004). The best of Harvard Business Review. One more time: How do you motivate employees? *Harvard Business Review, 82*(1), 53-68.

Hirt, M. (2004, Jan-Feb). Capacity building: The self-reflective leader. *Public Management,* 12-16.

Hocker, S. M., & Trofino, J. (2003). Transformational leadership: The development of a model of nursing case management by the Army Nurse Corps. *Lippincott's Case Management 8*(5), 208-213.

Huszczo, G. (2004). *Tools for team leadership.* Palo Alto, CA: Davies-Black.

Institute of Medicine. (1999). *To err is human: Building a safer health system.* Washington, DC: National Academy Press.

Jeffers, S. (1987). *Feel the fear and do it anyway.* New York: Ballantine Books.

Johns, C. (2004). Becoming a transformational leader through reflection. *Reflections on Nursing Leadership, 30*(2), 24-26.

Kehr, N. (1999). Using humor in the college classroom to enhance teaching effectiveness in "dread courses." Retrieved January 8, 2005, from http://www.findarticles.com/p/articles/mi_m0fcr/is_3_33/ai_62839448/print.

Kim, S. H. (1996). *1001 ways to motivate yourself and others.* Hartford, CT: Turtle Press.

Kouzes, J., & Posner, B. (2002). *Encouraging the heart: A leader's guide to rewarding and recognizing others.* (3rd Ed.). San Francisco: Jossey-Bass Publishers.

Kowalski, K. E., Hayden, W., & Burck, R. (1996, Mar/April). Major learning experiences revisited. *The American Journal of Maternal Child Nursing, 20*(2), 76-79.

Kowalski, K. E., & Yoder-Wise, P. S. (2003). The five Cs of leadership. *Nurse Leader, 1*(5), 26-31.

Lyons, M. F. (2002). Leadership and followership—career management. *Physician Executive, 28*(1).

Maxwell, J. (2003). *Attitude 101: What every leader needs to know.* Nashville, TN: Thomas Nelson.

Maxwell, J. (2000). *Failing forward: Turning mistakes into stepping stones for success.* Nashville, TN: Thomas Nelson.

Maxwell, J. (1999). *The 21 indispensable qualities of a leader.* Nashville, TN: Thomas Nelson.

Maxwell, J. (1998). *The 21 irrefutable laws of leadership.* Nashville, TN: Thomas Nelson.

Mays, S. (2004, June 6). Trust, not technology, the root of managing healthcare. Retrieved June 8, 2004 from www.tennessean.com.

McClure M. L., & Hinshaw, A. S. (Eds). (2002). *Magnet hospitals revisited.* Washington, DC: American Nurses Publishing.

Michelman, P. (2004, February). What leaders allow themselves to know: Warren Bennis unveils some new thinking on the filters that govern decision making. *Harvard Business Update,* 4-5.

Porter-O'Grady, T., & Malloch, K. (2002). *Quantum leadership: A textbook of new leadership.* Gaithersburg, MD: Aspen.

Ruiz, D. (1997). *The four agreements.* San Rafael, CA: Amer-Allen.

Senge, P. (1990). *The fifth discipline.* London: Century Business.

Sull, D. (2003). Managing by commitments. *Harvard Business Review, 81*(6), 82-92.

Swain, G., Schubot, D., Thomas, V., Baker, B., Foldy, S., Greaves, W., & Monteagudo, M. (2004). Three hundred sixty degree feedback: Program implementation in a local health department. *Journal of Public Health Management Practice, 10*(3), 266-271.

Taylor, B. J. (2004). Improving communication through practical reflection. *Reflections on Nursing Leadership, 30*(2), 28-38.

Weisinger, H. (1998). *Emotional intelligence at work.* San Francisco, CA: Jossey-Bass.

Yoder-Wise, P., & Kowalski, K. (2003). The power of storytelling. *Nursing Outlook, 51*(1), 37-42.

Zaccaro, S. (2001). *The nature of executive leadership.* Washington, DC: American Psychological Association.

Developing a Culture of Caring, Learning, and Service

To achieve all that is possible, we must attempt the impossible. To be all we can be, we must dream of being more. To reach our dreams we must reach out to others. JOHN C. MAXWELL

This chapter focuses on an important element of the chief nursing officer (CNO) role: creating the culture in which staff members can flourish. That culture has to support people and convey a sense of genuine caring about them as individuals. It has to provide sufficient learning opportunities for staff members to feel nurtured intellectually so that they remain competent in providing care. The culture also needs to engender the enthusiasm to provide service to the community and the profession. Creating the culture for being the best possible is the ultimate outcome of investment. Shared governance is one example of the efforts of creating the culture of caring, learning, and service. This chapter provides information about moving the culture toward exemplary status.

A KEY EXECUTIVE FUNCTION IN NURSING IS creating the culture in which the whole nursing team functions. The culture conveys how sincere the workplace is and whether it is safe to trust and

sets the tone for how other disciplines come to think of nurses and nursing. The culture conveys whether employees are valued and if care is the core value. This work takes careful, deliberate consideration. To optimize the presence of a positive environment, the CNO must support learning and service to the team and to the larger community. Many organizations have not integrated this kind of attitude into the essence of the organization; therefore creating such an environment is a challenge. It is paramount to creating excellence.

CULTURE

Organizational culture comprises a set of values, conventions, behaviors, and attitudes that create the sense of an organization. These elements, in one sense, create the "persona" of the organization. The culture is how an organization is known. Muller (2004) suggests that corporations can be viewed as living entities. They reflect society and often form local communities within themselves. Just as in society, norms and practices are inherent in the cultures present.

Organizations operate in cycles. As society has moved from the industrial age to the informational age, we have changed metaphors for organizations. The industrial age referenced production lines and often spoke of people as "cogs" in the whole operation. The refocus in the age of information has been to relationships and personal and organizational growth. This change in terminology within organizations reflects the change in society as it moved from one era to another.

A Time Perspective

Immediacy of action also is reflective of today's organizations and society. No longer does someone write a letter and wait a month for a reply. Instead, a person sends an e-mail and then checks the inbox every few minutes for the response. Waiting more than 24 hours for a response results in frustration. Of course, organizations still write letters and wait, but they also are sending e-mail and wanting instant response.

This focus on immediacy works against creation of an organizational culture, which is a time-intensive, prolonged activity. In other words, culture does not happen overnight. "Many of the crises facing organizations (non-profit and for-profit) are identity and values problems that emerge and manifest in the financial and competitive arenas" (Muller, 2004, p. 4). Muller suggests that organizations must answer the questions in Box 8-1. These answers reinforce and build on corporate/organizational identity. They help prevent (or at least clarify) the crises that manifest in many organizations.

Culture is created by reality, not by ideas or promises. When someone says, for instance,

"We are already a Magnet facility," people respond by thinking of 14 forces of magnetism or looking for the obelisk and Magnet pins. They do not think that statement means someday in the future; they are looking for the reality of the moment. Therefore immediacy relates to reality in that what is experienced right now is what the organization is at that moment.

Further, the entire organization and its culture is a result of choice. Were salary increases delayed to keep all employed? Were professional development benefits eliminated to purchase a piece of equipment? These choices convey the culture more clearly than any document or motto can. The choices are the reality of the culture. Choices that are made for the short term (immediacy) can affect organizational culture for long periods of time.

"Understanding the past affects how the present is lived and affects the choices made in the present and future" (Muller, 2004, p. 7). This is one view of time in an organization. It determines how the organization evolved to its current status. Another view of time is length of employment. Newly hired staff members have a limited understanding of the culture. They see the culture from a limited exposure. One of their tasks becomes learning the culture and determining their fit with it. More longevous employees have participated in creating the existing culture. They have stories to share and exemplars to cite. They understand culture on a different level because they have been exposed to it for a greater period of time. A third view is generational. Older employees expect commitment and value of traditions; they helped form them. They tend to be loyal to the organization. They have upheld the organizational culture. As Grayson (2005) points out, the baby boomers (yes, the same ones who were the protesters and hippies of the 1960s) are currently described as workaholics. Now the "new generation" will have the opportunity to evolve. In the meantime, just as the baby boomers—and every other generation before—did, the new generations want to change the organization and the work. They challenge

---

Box 8-1   CRITICAL QUESTIONS ABOUT ORGANIZATIONAL CULTURE

Who are we?
What is our business and purpose?
What is our role as good corporate citizens?
What is our uniqueness and what values drive our decisions?
What is our passion?

From Muller, R. (2004). Time, narrative and organizational culture: A corporate perspective. *Journal of Critical Postmodern Organization Science, 3*(1), 4.

the past and the present to change the future. This cultural clash, like any other, must be managed so that both groups leave work feeling they are part of a valued workplace.

Organizational Culture

Organizational culture is composed of four categories (Waters, 2004). These are symbols, heroes and heroines, rituals, and values.

Symbols

Symbols are found in words used (and avoided), in the physical environment, and in codes of behavior. Words may be "coded" for insiders to exclude outsiders of the group. What a "red alert" comprises at one hospital may be very different from that at another. Words suggest the level of formality at which the organization functions. Similarly, the physical design conveys the culture through visual presentations. For example, is the wall art limited editions or originals of professional artists, or is the art children's drawings about hospitalization experiences, or is it a mixture? Geary (2003) describes a cultural shift to a healing environment. The described organization went so far as to create healing gardens replete with soothing fountains, a nurses' lounge that promotes comfort, and numerous strategies to incorporate the outside into the hospital. Each of these is an example of the symbols of the culture. Codes of behavior convey such practices as casual Fridays and the type of work attire. They are visible to other employees and to the public. Experience with codes of behavior may dictate whether someone confronts an issue or quietly stands by.

Heroes and Heroines

Heroes and heroines are the people who convey the stories of the culture and who model what it is like to be a certain employee. They often are introduced to others through a corporate story illustrative of some value. These individuals may not be known outside their organization. On the other hand, they also may be acknowledged in the local or national press because of the exemplary way in which they lived out a value.

Rituals

Rituals are the standard practices that occur in various interactions. They are seen in how meetings are conducted and how business is managed. They are evident in how the organizational founder is treated and how the homeless patient is received. Rituals are even evident in how someone is announced to the group. Rituals that are aligned with the organizational mission exemplify the mission and translate as the common, everyday examples of the culture. Routine celebrations are often a form of rituals.

Values

Values derive from the ingrained beliefs about the organization. They frequently can be found in the mission statement. Aligning the subcultures that exist in an organization can create a strong view of the organization as a viable entity. Finding the "commonness" among the various subcultures allows for various groups to see how different work in different areas contributes to the overall organizational values.

Wooten and Crane (2003) identify three valuable features of organizational culture. The *collective mission* creates a feeling of oneness with the organization. As groups work, they see how they contribute to the whole. This view creates an organizational synergy that propels the organization to new levels. If one group believes that another is treated in a more special way, the collective mission view is diminished. Clarifying how each group contributes to the whole is an important element of a leader's role.

Keeping culture alive through human resource management means that people and their values are emphasized. This emphasis can begin at recruitment and last through retirement. For example, when people know that an organization will invest in their personal and professional development so that they are more valued citizens and employees, they are more committed to the organization.

The culture of the organization makes this value clear. *Constructive culture equals patient-centered cultures* suggests that creating the "right" cultures helps people focus on the real purpose of healthcare organizations—the care of patients. Therefore using this feature of culture means that employees must be clear that patients are the number one concern and that employees are also highly valued.

How then do CNOs and others help members of the organization be culturally competent? Earley and Mosakowski (2004) suggest that developing and using cultural intelligence helps members of the different or new cultures assimilate. Cultural intelligence refers to one's ability to interpret unfamiliar and ambiguous gestures and words in a way that would be understood by the presenting culture. Like using emotional intelligence, using cultural intelligence allows the person to pause to think and reflect on meaning before acting. Earley and Mosakowski identify three sources of cultural intelligence. They are head, body, and heart. Table 8-1 provides an example of each source. Cultivating these sources helps people assimilate into a new culture. Culture is learned, as Kramer, Schmalenberg, and Maguire (2004) say, when individuals "connect behaviors with consequences" (p. 45). Thus incorporating the culture has its rewards. Because each clinical area has its own subculture, nurses who work on more than one unit have an enormous amount of talent. They have become bicultural and know how to thrive in two or more settings.

Culture is a complex concept with numerous facets. It is evident in daily work and in long-range decisions. Each choice an organization makes further refines or reinforces the culture of the organization. It is the context of the culture in which care is delivered. The focus of tenured people in the organization has to be to help new members come to know and value the organization for its rich history and its culture. To do so requires promotion of caring, learning, and service. These three elements interact as illustrated in Figure 8-1, while having distinct contributions.

Table 8-1 THREE SOURCES OF CULTURAL INTELLIGENCE

Source	Example
Head	Rote learning about the beliefs, customs, and taboos of foreign cultures, the approach corporate training programs tend to favor, will never prepare a person for every situation that arises, nor will it prevent terrible gaffes. (p. 141) Focus on learning strategies!
Body	By adopting people's habits and mannerisms, you eventually come to understand in the most elemental way what it is like to be them. (p. 141) Remain visually alert!
Heart	If they [people] persevered in the face of challenging situations in the past, their confidence grew. Confidence is always rooted in mastery of a particular task or set of circumstances. (p. 142) Believe in self and persevere!

From Early, P. C., & Mosakowski, E. (2004, October). Cultural intelligence. *Harvard Business Review,* 139-146.

THE CONCEPT OF CARING

The concept of caring and its association with the profession of nursing is rooted deeply in history. Long before Florence Nightingale, the ministry of nursing (often derived through support from the churches) was based on care. Nightingale advanced this concept and modern theorists built on that concept. Watson (1999), for example, developed a Model of Human Care based on the relationship of the nurse and the patient. She emphasizes the need to see patients as individuals with distinctive needs.

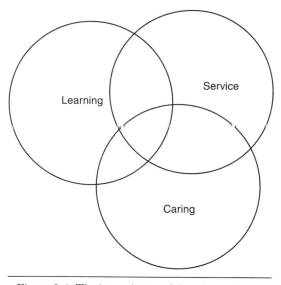

Figure 8-1 The interrelation of three key cultures.

The way to determine those distinctive needs is to be in a caring relationship with the patient. She emphasizes that the nurse and the patient are interconnected. What affects a member of that dyad affects the other, because the relationship is altered when one member is refocused on some other aspect of care, work, or life. Her key concern, of course, is that caring is what happens to the patient so that the patient has sufficient resources to regain wellness.

Caring "influences the way patients and their loved ones respond and heal. It influences the morale and subsequent efficiency of the healthcare team" (Felgen, 2004, p. 290). "Caring and healing cultures are those in which there is palpable, visible regard for the dignity of human beings, and where relationships between the members of the healthcare team and the people they serve are built on mutual respect and a shared commitment to healing" (p. 290).

This means that caring is critical to an organization's culture. The first concern is placing value on patients and the relationship of nurses to them. Valuing the way in which the team of nurses and others works together to achieve safe,

quality patient care is also important. When pervasive in an organization, caring can be felt. It is evident in touch, with patients and with colleagues. Caring is evident in words communicated in ongoing conversations and in moments of great tension. It creates a sense of acceptance and value.

Although nurses have historically and consistently claimed caring as the service they provide, many nurses have not used that same word to describe their work environment. Caring, in terms of a workplace value, suggests that nurses in official leadership positions act so that followers understand the nature of the distinct service they provide to the organization, that followers believe in and trust their colleagues, and that followers "sense" the support for them as they integrate their personal and professional lives. How the CNO works to influence all other administrators within nursing presents opportunities to model how others can work with their respective staff members.

Felgen (2004) suggests four general areas that support care. Each is applicable with the organization and with patients. Therapeutic relationships, the first area of support, in patient care refer to development of such aspects as trust and security. Proactive communication supports the development of therapeutic relationships. In organizational work, relationships between and among members of a team also focus on development of trust and security. Similarly, proactive communication contributes to the development of such trust and security. Systems that support therapeutic relationships, the second area of support, involve the ways in which decisions are made, or who is assigned to care for a patient, or what is required of communication. Each of these areas is also important in organizational work. Making decisions that involve others in the decision or making a clear commitment to communicating with others is just as valuable when focused on workers as it is when focused on patients. Practice innovations, the third area, obviously support the quality of patient care. Further, innovations keep nurses engaged in the desire to improve the work they do and the need to see changes enacted.

Finally, process improvements maximize the outcomes of care and the outcomes of organized services. Using these elements strengthens nursing practice and also strengthens the nursing organization.

Caring related to the staff embodies concern for the staff as a whole and for staff members as individuals. Thoughtful attention to what people are experiencing in their full lives, and especially the events related to work, is an example of how CNOs convey their concern for others.

> *We lead by being human.*
> *We do not lead by being corporate,*
> *By being professional or*
> *By being institutional.*
> PAUL HAWKEN

Creating the culture that supports caring, learning, and service is serious work. If the CNO does not truly care about others and their welfare, words and actions will not appear sincere. In the 1990s, for example, considerable dissatisfaction existed within nursing practice. Staffing was less than desirable, and in some cases, downright dangerous. Nursing staff members often were discounted in their attempts to provide input and solutions to the problems besieging the profession. It was difficult, if not impossible, to maintain positive relationships with other departments and disciplines when nurses felt so undervalued themselves. Fortunately, that situation changed for many organizations. Nurse leaders realized that the actions of the late 1980s and early 1990s related to downsizing, layoffs, fairly static wages, and uninspired benefit packages that contributed significantly to the poor view of the workplace.

Turkel and Ray (2004) suggest that the first step to reestablish trust and to enhance the organization is to facilitate the creation of caring. In other words, making clear that the organization is focused on caring is important. The changes implemented by leading CNOs showed this value and reversed the negativity of the work environment for many staff members. This commitment took some organizations on a journey to Magnet status. Many CNOs, Magnet coordinators, and staff nurses in Magnet organizations say that the reversal of the negativity in the workplace helped an organization become a better place to work and also encouraged further creativity in approaching problems.

Some of the beginning elements of creating caring relationships derive from organizational values. Lencioni (2002) suggested that four types of values exist and that they need to be clearly differentiated so that people in an organization have a sense of belief and concurrence. Table 8-2 summarizes the four types of values. The key is to make certain that core values are those that exist and that create distinctions between and among healthcare organizations. If quality, as an example, is designated as a core value, everyone must be able to describe how quality is demonstrated on a daily basis. If quality is not exemplified in daily practices and is indicated as critical to the organization, or if it is a value an organization wants to integrate but has not done so yet, it is an aspirational value. The problem is that if these two are not delineated clearly, some employees will distrust the organization because quality is espoused as a core value and yet the staff knows that quality does not exist. As a result, the organization is viewed as not living up to its values. Permission-to-play relates to *minimum* standards. For example, the command to children, "No hitting," reflects the minimal expectation. Honesty might be a minimal standard unless it is well integrated into—and practiced—on a regular basis. So, for example, if a nurse is honest about a mistake and then is punished, honesty becomes a false value.

Accidental values arise when something happens spontaneously. For example, patriotism was accidentally reactivated after September 11, 2004. In the workplace, if a co-worker is being stalked or a sudden rise in attacks on employees in the parking facilities occurs, a new camaraderie forms. This new relationship may be another example of accidental values.

Table **8-2** Lencioni's Types of Values

Type of Value	Meaning	Example
Core	Deeply ingrained— evident	Within nursing, the value that is most expressed as "core" is caring. This term is used to justify requests, to convey what services an organization provides, and the attribute the public perceives as most reflective of nurses.
Aspirational	Desirable (goals)— not evident	One important aspirational goal for nursing would be work-life balance. It is seen as an aspirational goal because currently many nurses focus intensely on work without the companion focus on personal life.
Permission-to-play	Minimal behaviors	Because these values tend to be common across organizations, they reflect basic issues such as attendance, appearance, and procedural adherence.
Accidental	Spontaneous that take hold over time	As organizations addressed cultural diversity and the need to celebrate differences, new values about recognition of cultural differences began to take hold. When a risk is taken to incorporate other ways of celebrating a holiday into the traditional approach, the potential exists that the broader, encompassing approach becomes the new tradition over time.

From Lencioni, P. M. (2002, July). Make your values mean something. *Harvard Business Review, 80,* 113-117.

Caring relationships do not just happen. Rather, relationships have to be developed, nurtured, tested, and celebrated. Reviewing personnel files provides facts and often creates a perception about a person. However, it is not until a relationship is established with that person that true synergy occurs. Being in relationship with others creates a mutually beneficial exchange that contributes positively to the whole nursing enterprise. Box 8-2 contains an exercise that can be used to help others see the importance of interpersonal relationships.

Developing a caring relationship takes specific effort. As an example, the CNO must walk the halls and interact with nurses and others frequently. Authier (2004) calls this "being present." In addition to the idea of being present for one's own benefit, he points to the need for others to know that leaders are "there" for them. Presence conveys this quickly if it is fully engaged. This means that being physically present is not sufficient. Mental connectedness also must be evident. In addition to learning about people who work within the organization, the CNO who interacts with the staff on a regular basis also conveys that this interaction is a valued part of administrative practice.

Having met everyone in the organization at least once does not create a relationship. Deliberately nurturing the relationship is a process that has to be incorporated into administrators' daily work. Stopping by or calling to see how some previously discussed problem has turned out can take a relationship to a different level. Or, as some new idea is being advanced, stopping by or calling to gain that person's perspective can nurture the beginning of a relationship. Obviously, it is not sufficient to have mere dialogues. The other person needs to know what comes next. For example, if a staff nurse has offered a suggestion about managing the transfer of patients, he needs to hear back

Box 8-2   MAKING A DIFFERENCE IN PEOPLE'S LIVES

Write answers to the following items as quickly as possible. If you do not have an answer, go on to the next item.
1. Name the most highly rated, worker-friendly organization for the prior year.
2. Name the Nurse of the Year selected by your organization for the prior year.
3. Name the Speaker of the U.S. House of Representatives.
4. Name the prior governor of your state.

Now write answers to these questions as quickly as possible.
1. Name one nurse who helped you in a difficult situation.
2. Name one friend you could count on in difficult situations.
3. Name one person who taught you something that you will never forget.
4. Name two stories that inspire you.
   Your list of answers for the last four items is likely to be more complete because we are most affected by people and events that directly affect us. Many of those people and events stem from a workplace.

Modified from the Charles Schultz Philosophy (http://www.rb-29.net/HTML/03RelatedStories/03.10.FunStuff/05.fschashltz.htm).

why the idea cannot work or why it can and what will happen next. That ongoing interchange with the sincerity of intent creates true relationships.

The best part about this commitment to each other is that the relationship can be tested. Testing, however, is not done just to see how someone reacts; it means that at some point, people in relationship may not be in agreement. The questions are as follows:

- Are we sufficiently connected so that we can tolerate the strain of disagreement on something that might be important to both of us?
- Can we come back to another dialogue with a willingness to converse openly and honestly?
- Do we trust in the participants in the relationship sufficiently so that we believe we can still be colleagues and move forward?

These kinds of tests strengthen a relationship and convey positive messages to reinforce commitment to caring about each other even when viewpoints differ. It is almost incomprehensible to think about every nurse in an organization having such relationships with other nurses. However, how will we know if we do not try? The whole point is to become well connected with each other.

This results in a better understanding of common goals and exertion of specific energy to make relationships work. This kind of synergy moves organizations forward in unusual ways. It is partly what fosters transformational changes.

The final element of work relates to celebrating the relationship. Celebration does not necessarily mean a party or dinner or flowers. Celebration may be as simple as a note from one person to another about valuing the relationship or support in a specific situation. It may be some small organizational recognition (e.g., the designation of "champion" on effecting change about a specific practice), or it may be a surprise such as a quote in the organizational newspaper. It may even be something so simple as a sincere thank you, especially when a difficult problem was resolved or averted. Most nurses want to know that they contribute positively to others' lives. They do not want to operate in a vacuum.

John Yokoyama, the owner of the World Famous Pike Place Fish Market, described how he applied the concepts of creating caring for his employees (Yokoyama & Michelli, 2004). Yokoyama would be the first to tell how controlling and authoritarian he was before he engaged in a new leadership style. This is an important point: Any leader can learn new ways of working with others to be effective in creating a culture of caring. In fact, the term *shared governance* could be ascribed to the way in which he approached his organization's work.

Caring as a Leadership Value

Just as the concept of caring is at the heart of nursing, the same is true for leadership. Caring about others and the values of the organization is expressed in many ways. If these ways of expression are not sincere, belief in the value of the organization and the concern for each other diminish. Each time belief in the values diminishes, the organization is prevented from moving ahead. Caring, then, has to be at the heart of the motivation to be in administrative positions. Caring, as described by Watson (2005), involves connecting with people in numerous ways, which is also true from an administrative perspective. These connections may involve caring for difficult patients, making certain all are all right after a particularly difficult death, or asking about family and their well-being. Caring takes relationships to new levels of connections, helps everyone know that the challenge of nursing's intensity is valued, and helps emphasize that the outcomes of the nurse are equally important.

Numerous stresses occur in any work situation, but in healthcare, those stresses are magnified by the intensity of the nature of the work. Downsizing, for example, in healthcare is traumatizing, just as in other work, and it is further complicated by concerns about patients' care. Terminations are always traumatic, and deaths among colleagues are usually devastating. Few other work groups see a co-worker who is ill and have the expectation of care for that person. Illness is a major challenge where caring can be evidenced. Many stories were told about the way in which employers whose businesses were located in the World Trade Center responded on September 11, 2001. The opportunity to embrace each other, provide support, and experience the humanity of each other can be a defining moment in an organization's history.

In the lives of those for whom events unfold, any experience can take on the intensity that September 11, 2001, took for the majority of the United States.

How the CNO and other administrators respond is highly influential for the person experiencing anguish. This is the opportunity to shape people's perspectives about their workplace. The Literature box identifies the importance of compassion during times of trauma. Exhibiting true compassion not only helps the leader but also supports employees. Citizens of England who lived through World War II remember fondly that the Queen (Queen Mother of England) and the King remained in London and encouraged citizens to be strong. This level of role modeling affected the commitment of the whole country.

If the movement of caring occurs from some other level than the CNO, the CNO's role is to support that movement. As an example, staff nurses may choose to create a project to support the work of the children's unit. How full-heartedly the CNO embraces the effort sets other commitments in action.

Kowalski and Yoder-Wise (2003) indicate that one of the five Cs of leadership is compassion. The ability to laugh and cry and worry together exemplifies compassion. The culture that supports true expression of emotions without limitations or punishment, no matter how mild, for compassionate care allows staff members to connect with their patients and with each other. When in compassionate relationships, people connect as a team on a different level than when they do not express emotions.

Shared Governance as a Cultural Support

If the CNO has made strides in connecting with the staff at various levels of the organization and in various clinical areas, advancing those relationships to a formal process is a natural evolution. Shared governance consists of various strategies designed to ensure that the staff nurses who implement direct care are supported in their communications and strategies to resolve issues that diminish the interchange between patient and nurse or that distract the nurse from focusing on patient care. One example is the idea of transferring patients. Transfers from one unit to another are not solely a nursing issue. Transferring is still seen as a way to "control beds," and the effort may not have been made to see the problem from multiple perspectives. Such activities greatly increase a nurse's workload. In other words, staffing does not relate only to the 30 patients on the unit, it is how many total patients (how many times each bed has been emptied and filled) that more accurately represent the workload. Encouraging involvement in a formal relationship to resolve such issues is a great way to foster shared governance.

Rather than focusing on abstract issues that may eventually influence practice, focusing on a current issue allows all employees to see that nurse leaders are serious about resolving difficult problems and that the solution is not going to be an edict. Knowing that a formal protocol is in place for all voices to be heard honors the value of each of us within the organization.

Walking and Talking at the Same Time

That may seem like a strange heading, but it has a clear message. It is not sufficient to be out walking around and hearing what others have to say. Nurse leaders have to be talking, too. And the talk and the walk had better match! (Another way to think about this is the saying, "Put your money where your mouth is.") If the CNO really believes in shared governance, the nurses with administrative titles cannot "trump" the offerings of other nurses. Being able to demonstrate on a consistent basis the action that reflects the statements of mission and values is important. Words cannot merely appear on a piece of paper or be iterated at various meetings. Words have to be reflected in action. For example, if the environment truly values caring, several individuals should be able to tell stories about their experiences in which

support and concern were shown to them when they needed it. Telling someone, for example, that she should leave work to be available to a dying parent conveys more about caring than any document possibly could.

Changes coming from the grass roots of the organization frequently connect more quickly within the organization because they are seen as "ours" and because they often are tested in a peer group before they arrive at a place where decisions will be made. Although proposed changes may not be perfect, they have to be heard and considered if the influence of shared governance is to be honored. Discounting any idea before it is heard conveys a totally different message than that which is meant to be conveyed by shared governance. Even something that has failed before may now be the successful idea because the organization in which the failure occurred is not the present organization. Valuing people's suggestions is critical to conveying that governing the practice of nursing is a shared experience.

LEARNING

Although Senge (1994) was the first to describe what learning organizations were and their value to the viability of the organization, many others have subscribed to the concept and expanded it. Creating a culture of learning requires a significant investment of time and energy. It is more than creating educational services; it is also fostering the value of, and expectation for, continued learning. This continued learning enhances clinical practice and whetting the appetite of learners to be engaged in their own development. With the advent of the concept of best practices, in which we are constantly striving to do the newest "best," a culture of learning is critical to the success of an organization. The goal of a culture of learning is to practice from the best, most relevant position. In a blame-free culture, the intent is to help everyone learn from a mistake so that others do not make the mistake, and the maker of the mistake helps solve what is usually a system problem.

When Patricia Benner (1984) created the publication *From Novice to Expert*, she documented what nurses had said for a long time. She gave credibility to intuition and she provided a framework for looking at learning development. Her work, in essence, is about the culture of learning. It is the movement of nurses from wherever they are on the continuum of novice to expert to higher levels. The culture of learning is the reason why various learning activities are provided internally and externally to the organization; it is the journey toward excellence. Benner (2000, p. 99) stated, "A growing practice involves engaging others in ongoing dialogue about research and the implication of science in everyday care." This statement suggests that the ongoing dialogue contributes to nursing's body of knowledge and to individual personal growth. Learning as an organization and learning as individuals is the essence of thriving in the future. In a 2005 survey reported in *Hospitals and Health Networks* (2005), 43.7% of nurse respondents under the age of 32 said that a source of dissatisfaction was insufficient development opportunities. Although this factor was far surpassed by concerns about work and personal life balance and the organization not being focused on patient needs (96.3% and 91.7%, respectively), the number of responses related to development suggests that learning opportunities are a major concern for nurses who are younger in the profession. Numerous issues surround learning in organizations. Two key issues are the financial aspects and the strategies for providing for diverse learning needs.

Financial Investments in Learning

Two key factors relate to budgeting for learning. The first is the organizational work toward addressing learning needs internally; the second is the organizational work toward addressing learning needs externally.

Internally, a departmental, or organizational, accountability is designed as the "continuing education" service. The organization provides for anticipated learning needs. The service may be central or based on units, patient populations, or roles, or it may be clinically based. So, for example, a hospital in Vail, Colorado, anticipates orthopedic patients from the local ski areas and provides for the continuing competence of the staff in managing musculoskeletal injuries. Similarly, a hospital in New Orleans with a focus on diabetes wants to employ the best practitioners in this clinical area. Another hospital in Los Angeles may focus on the aging population. In each of these settings, some specific clinical or patient population is the determining factor for ongoing needs of educational programs to promote learning for the staff. That is unlike the small rural hospital in Arkansas, where every nurse must be ready to handle the full range of patients and their needs that present for care. Each of these organizations needs to support staff members within the organization to maintain current knowledge and clinical skills. In the first three examples, the task is easier because of the focus of their client base. The small rural hospital may eliminate the need for complex tertiary practices, but the scope of their client base and their geographic remoteness dictate that they have to be experts at diagnosis and stabilization of patients regardless of age or diagnosis.

External learning opportunities abound. The skilled CNO is certain to have a policy regarding priorities for payment for external activities that defines what is included in any payment/reimbursement. Typically, it defines appropriate learning topics and whether national and international travel is permitted. Some hospitals assign this money to units for their more decentralized decisions, whereas others maintain the money in a central resource. Some hospitals use a first-come-first-served approach, others expect each case to be considered on its own merits, and others delegate funds per capita so that each employee has the same amount allotted.

Typical learning organizations external to the healthcare organization are those providing formal, degree-granting learning and offering continuing education credit. Although the continuing education credit approach is the most familiar, the need for formal degree granting learning is equally great. Whether the organization's commitment is played out through tuition reimbursements or through bringing an educational program to learners, the critical factor is to move the formal preparation of the staff to higher levels. If research by Aiken, Clarke, Cheung, Sloane, and Silber (2003) is correct, increasing the educational level of nurses to those with baccalaureate and higher degrees is critical to patient safety. This array may begin with moving nursing assistants through practical/vocational nursing educational programs and end with providing registered nurses with graduate educational opportunities. For example, Texas Health Resources provides the full array for employees within its various hospitals in the area around Dallas-Fort Worth. Choice is not just attractive. Choice is relevant to the future of the quality of service.

Embracing the idea of the workplace as a learning organization fosters the ambiance of being inquisitive and knowing that the goal is to be the best that can be, not just the best that one can be. This commitment engages others in the idea of learning. The availability of information influences how easily new information is incorporated into practice.

Strategies for Diverse Learning Needs

Providing learning opportunities in a meaningful way and at the right time is a challenge. "In a survey of several hundred nurses we discovered that nurses are quintessential learners…they have a thirst for knowledge because of their sincere desire to give quality care. Unfortunately, shortages and complexity have reduced the amount of time free to attend refresher/update classes" (Knapp, 2004, p. 286). Knapp found that scenario-based simulations were critical for learning.

Another solution can be found from a well-known business. At Dell Computers, every technician is able to build any model of computer. When a customer places an order, robotics locate all of the necessary component parts. The technician is now ready to assemble the computer. But how would technicians keep all of that information in their heads? In fact, technicians do not keep those details in their heads. Rather as they receive the order, the specifications direct the technician to an overhead screen that drops down in front of the work area. The technician enters the specifications information and a step-by-step tutorial appears to guide the technician through the "just-in-time" information.

What if healthcare used such an approach? Although a few very sophisticated systems exist, they are not the norm. Currently practitioners are expected to retain complex linkages of information and procedures in their heads. In some cases, no computerized documentation systems are in place, so the idea of patient care on-site learning is really removed from reality. The impact of such an approach could be great. Davenport and Glaser (2002) described what Partners HealthCare in Boston did to change the way in which clinicians in medicine could remain current with learning. First, they designed a system based on the medical record to create a relationship between knowledge and the specifics for a particular patient. "No matter what the industry, knowledge workers often can't keep up with the knowledge being generated" (p. 108). Because the knowledge is imbedded into the system, prompts are made when, say, a physician wishes to order a medication in a dose that exceeds normal dosages or uses. Although an override is possible, the point is that a physician could not err based on out-of-date knowledge. To achieve this quality, "only clinicians at the top of their game can create and maintain the knowledge repository" (p. 110). In other words, the top experts create and maintain the prompting information and responses. What would happen if nursing used its best experts to create the knowledge in such a timely and useful manner?

A Culture for Change

In essence the purpose of a culture of learning is to foster a culture for change. New ways of practice are impossible if knowledge lags behind current practice. And too often the educational endeavor is focused on the wrong strategy. Livingston (2004) indicates that using logic as a strategy when an idea was not gained by logic initially is difficult. How much of the internal offerings are based in the cognitive domain? However, often the affective domain moves people to action.

Being able to remain current in knowledge is a component of creating a culture for change. The focus of the culture for change is to answer the following question: "How can we make it happen here?" Part of the movement for this is based on the true desire to be the best possible and on the commitment to eliminate as many organizational obstacles as possible, but another part is related to how nurse leaders help the whole organization advance to becoming well informed. Without the information being available to all who need to know, the organization is unlikely to advance.

Considering the rapidity of change affecting current healthcare, nursing leaders must be creative in the way they each share what they know and influence others in their learning. In addition to the rapidity, the complexity makes learning an ongoing challenge. Rapidity and complexity provide increasing pressure for more learning to be done in Internet formats in which content is readily available and an individual learner can take as little or as much time as necessary to master critical content.

SERVICE

In creating the "right" culture within an organization, nurse leaders face the challenge of the concept of service. Many already believe they are engaged in service from 8 to 12 or more hours per day. Why volunteer to take on something else? Clearly, the amount of time someone can commit to "extra" endeavors is limited. Therefore creating the culture for service is valuable.

Many staff nurses believe they are deeply immersed in providing service to patients, even as they feel underappreciated and unserved. Service *to* nurses is as important as valuing nurses to *serve*. Simons (2004) points out that caring for patients is emphasized, but staff members may have demanding needs too. Although nurses do not function in an organization for the service to other nurses, providing a supportive environment serves nurses well as they work to resolve their personal challenges and concerns. If a staff member's mother died recently, providing coverage for work may not be needed, but it is appreciated. That kind of support conveys that distinctive services are available to help individuals.

The Baylor Health System created a staffing pattern several years ago known as "the Baylor Plan." Some nurses were employed on weekend-only schedules (12-hour shifts) to provide care for patients. This approach was a service to nurses— weekends off for some and weekdays off for others. Baylor also created the Baylor Butlers. This service is available at low cost for any employee. The Butlers perform many tasks, such as picking up laundry and scheduling appointments that normally distract nurses from their day-to-day care. Sometimes, to accomplish these tasks, nurses needed to take time off and were not present to provide care. This service helps them concentrate on providing care and yet be assured that the errands and tasks of normal life are accomplished. Services such as this support nurses so that they can devote their professional talents beyond the employment setting. Regardless of whether that professional talent service is in a clinically focused voluntary community organization, such as the American Heart Association, or is in a professionally focused voluntary organization, such as the state nurses association, support to eliminate concerns about everyday life helps nurses focus on their external work, which reflects in a positive manner on the organization.

Whether the service is what nurses provide to the community or to the organization or what is provided to nurses to support them in their roles, the focus is on the culture of service, the attitude—and execution—of valuing the community at large and feeling valued. Both of these exemplify how a culture of caring is a lived value. Similarly, a culture of learning exposes learners to opportunities to relate to the community. Furthermore, promoting learning exemplifies a culture of caring as a lived experience. The interrelationship of these elements contributes to each subelement and enhances the entire organizational culture (see Figure 8-1).

SUMMARY

Each of the elements described here—caring, learning, and service—provide a way to create the culture of an organization. The belief in the organizational values can be real only when the values are clear and executed. Saying what is valued and then living it through various ways is critical to creating quality organizations. Caring must be evident in everyday activities. Learning provides a mechanism to enhance individual abilities and the organization as a whole. Supporting service involvement beyond the organization contributes to the community and the profession.

KEY POINTS TO LEAD

1. Value the importance of a culture of caring, learning, and service.
2. Evaluate strategies that convey such a culture.
3. Critique an organization from a high-level assessment on its culture of compassion.

Literature Box

Research from the University of Michigan and the University of British Columbia revealed a major difference between situations in which the formal leaders showed compassion and those in which they did not. This research focused on tragic situations. The researchers found that compassion is universal; the difference is whether it is shared within the organization. First, the researchers made a clear distinction between empathy, which does not engender a broader response, and compassion, which can permeate the workplace. Compassion, these researchers found, helped people deal with the current issue and created a base from which to work to recover from future situations. "Unleashing compassion in the workplace not only lessens the immediate suffering of those directly affected by trauma, it enables them to recover from future setbacks more quickly and effectively and it increases their attachment to their colleagues and hence to the company itself" (p. 56). Where leaders were detached in situations in which workers were suffering, employees grew more distant and in some cases left the organization.

Organizational compassion has two contexts: meaning and action. The context for meaning allows for expression of feelings; context for action leads to ways in which individuals and the organization can help alleviate suffering. Leaders in organizations can facilitate a culture of caring by modeling humanness. For example, when leaders express their angst about a situation, the culture supports others sharing in a similar manner. A second strategy for creating meaning that the authors suggested is "just being present." A third strategy consisted of specific examples of how to provide personal support. These could include such endeavors as providing food or transportation. "The meaning-making process can also be supported by communicating and reinforcing organizational values—reminding people about the larger purpose of their work even as they

Literature Box—cont'd

struggle to make sense of major life issues" (p. 59). The context of action begins with role modeling activities. The authors suggest that leaders could reallocate resources to support people, help generate ideas to deal with the issue, and coordinate groups.

The authors also offered a high-level assessment based on four dimensions. *Scope* of compassionate response refers to breadth of resources. For example, in what multiple ways does the organization respond to tragic situations? *Scale* of compassionate response focuses on the volume of efforts. Scale refers to the amount of resources, time, and effort. *Speed* of compassionate response addresses

how quickly the organization responds in times of need. The last element, *specialization*, relates to how the organization can customize responses so that the response fits the need.

Leadership in the organization supports the culture of caring through the context of meaning and action. "This is a kind of leadership we wish we would never have to use, yet it is vital if we are to nourish the very humanity that can make people—and organizations—great" (p. 61).

Dutton, J. E., Frost, P. J., Worline, M. C., Lilius, J. M., & Kanov, J. M. (2002, January). Leading in times of trauma. *Harvard Business Review,* 55-61.

Contemplations

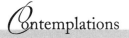

Consider the amount of effort the organization exerts on behalf of employees' continued learning.
- Is there a staff development/professional development department/service?
- How much work-related education is available?
- What types of personal development education are available?
- How is education promoted as a value within the organization?

- Is there an expectation that employees in the organization are involved in the work of their professional association?
- How is this evident?
- What would be one example (story) that illustrates a culture of caring?
- Would the organization pass the high-level assessment described in the Literature box?

LEADER STORY ✒

JANE LLEWELYN
VP NURSING SERVICES
RUSH UNIVERSITY MEDICAL CENTER
RUSH UNIVERSITY
CHICAGO

I've been at Rush since I was a young nurse. The greatest influence on my professional career, without question, was Luther Christman. He was a wonderful example of a caring mentor who liked to take on "mentees," particularly when they were young nurses and, as he put it, "hadn't established bad habits but were approaching nursing care and patients with 'fresh eyes.'" In this spirit I came on as a new faculty member. I learned so much from Luther. He was masterful at setting out a vision and *not* micromanaging. One example is the practitioner-teacher model, which he developed and moved into national prominence. A major part of this model was the equality set out between nursing, medicine, and administration. This created positive relationships with physicians. They are not the enemy. Nursing and medicine have more in common than they have different because they have the same values and the same goals and share the same science. If nurses had education and knowledge and demonstrated it, they were colleagues with physicians. Consequently, nursing could embrace physicians in their plans and create joint practices and joint projects. Nursing had to be willing, then and now, to contribute in this way to the science and be full partners with medicine.

Another example is primary nursing. Luther set out the principles of primary nursing but didn't tell nurses how to do it. Consequently, one unit constructed it in one way and another unit tried a slightly different model. It wasn't necessary to have all the details worked out so the best practices rose to the top.

He was an example of the axiom, "A leader is one who knows the way, goes the way, and shows the way." Luther walked the walk just as our current CEO is doing. He is a true practitioner-teacher. Over the years, since Luther's retirement, I watched the practitioner-teacher model gradually slip away to be replaced with "silos."

When I was asked to take the VP position, it was like being given a precious jewel that was old and tarnished, a gift, to polish and return to its former luster. So we began the Magnet journey, which reached back into the history of Rush. The hospital-within-a-hospital model has wonderful advantages and some significant disadvantages, such as different standards for each hospital (silo). Staff and leadership rallied behind the Magnet Vision. We worked very hard and it was unifying in how everyone came together. Then, of course, we got to *celebrate* when we were awarded Magnet status in 2002. It felt, in many ways, like all of the good aspects of the "old days."

It is very special to be on such a great senior administrative team. In an attempt to get costs under control, we observed that unit service managers were essentially taking the place of engineering and materials management, particularly for the specialty units. So I enrolled the VPs in this area. Parts of the patient care areas are more than 135 years old. Consequently, there are multiple issues to handle with such an old structure. Rather than maintenance and engineering handling these issues, it had fallen to unit service managers.

We decided to eliminate this position and have the appropriate departments handle the problems. As you might know Rush is a relationship-driven organization, and the VPs decided to attend all the task force meetings for this project, and it has worked. *We* asked the question, "What if engineers inspected the rooms instead of unit service managers?"

Engineering identified one of their own who is outgoing and great with patients and families. He makes rounds on every unit and finds out which rooms are too hot or too cold, he discovers what furnishings and equipment aren't working, *and* he sets the priorities for all the patient units as to what is worked on first. He loves this new aspect of his job and the units don't need a unit service manager for every unit. It is great to do problem solving and to create change in this way.

If I were giving advice to nursing administration graduate students, I would suggest they examine their personalities first...to see if they can tolerate or work with delayed gratification in job satisfaction. Because change is very slow and someone who needs instant positive feedback and reward won't do well in administration. It is important to tolerate a lot of ambiguity and uncertainty. However, it is very rewarding to influence the nursing work environment. It is a job I love in a setting that warms my heart and brings together the past, the present, *and* the future … for nursing and for Rush.

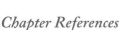

Chapter References

Aiken, L. H., Clarke, S. P., Cheung, R. B., Sloane, D. M., & Silber, J. H. (2003). Educational levels of hospital nurses and surgical patient mortality. *Journal of the American Medical Association, 290,* 1617-1623.

Authier, P. (2004). Being present—the choice that reinstills caring. *Nursing Administration Quarterly, 28*(4), 276-279.

Benner, P. (2000). The wisdom of our practice. *American Journal of Nursing, 100*(10), 99-105.

Benner, P. (1984). *From novice to expert: Excellence and power in clinical nursing practice.* Menlo Park, CA: Addison-Wesley.

Davenport, T. H., & Glaser, J. (2002, July). Just-in-time delivery comes to knowledge management. *Harvard Business Review, 80,* 107-111.

Dutton, J. E., Frost, P. J., Worline, M. C., Lilius, J. M., & Kanov, J. M. (2002, January). Leading in times of trauma. *Harvard Business Review,* 55-61.

Earley, P. C., & Mosakowski, E. (2004, October). Cultural intelligence. *Harvard Business Review,* 139-146.

Felgen, J. (2004). A caring and healing environment. *Nursing Administration Quarterly, 28*(4), 288-301.

Geary, H. (2003). Facilitating an organizational culture of healing in an urban medical center. *Nursing Administration Quarterly, 27*(3), 231-239.

Grayson, M. (2005, March). Generation X, Y, Zzzz. *Hospitals and Health Networks,* p. 8.

Hospitals and Health Networks. (2005, March). What nurses want. *Hospitals and Health Networks,* pp. 34-42.

Knapp, B. (2004). Competency: An essential component of caring in nursing. *Nursing Administration Quarterly, 28*(4), 285-287.

Kowalski, K.E., & Yoder-Wise, P. S. (2003, September-October). Five Cs of leadership. *Nursing Leadership,* pp. 26-31.

Kramer, M., Schmalenberg, C., & Maguire, P. (2004). Essentials of a magnetic work environment, part 4. *Nursing 2004, 34*(9), 44-48.

Lencioni, P. M. (2002, July). Make your values mean something. *Harvard Business Review, 80,* 113-117.

Livingston, G. (2004). *Too soon old, too late smart.* New York: Marlowe & Company.

Muller, R. (2004). Time, narrative and organizational culture: A corporate perspective. *Journal of Critical Postmodern Organization Science, 3*(1), 1-13.

Senge, P. M. (1994). *The fifth discipline: The art and practice of the learning organization.* New York: Doubleday.

Simons, M. (2004). The cycle of caring. *Nursing Administration Quarterly, 28*(4), 280-284.

Turkel, M. C., & Ray, M. A. (2004). Creating a caring practice environment through self-renewal. *Nursing Administration Quarterly, 28*(4), 249-254.

Waters, V. L. (2004, January). Cultivate corporate culture and diversity. *Nursing Management*, 36-37, 50.

Watson, J. (2005). *Caring science as sacred science*. Philadelphia: F.A. Davis.

Watson, J. (1999). *Postmodern nursing and beyond*. Edinburgh: Churchill Livingstone.

Wooten, L. P., & Crane, P. (2003). Nurses as implementers of organizational culture. *Nursing Economics, 21*(6), 275-279.

Yokoyama, J., & Michelli, J. (2004). *When fish fly: Lessons for creating a vital and energized workplace*. New York: Hyperion.

Communication and the Leader

I know that you think you understood what you heard me say, but I'm not sure you realize that what I said was not what I meant. UNKNOWN

This chapter focuses on recognition of specific aspects of communication, including developing specific skills that change and enhance communication, improving written communication, and addressing special situations requiring unique communication skills.

THE ONLY THING HUMANS DO MORE THAN communicate is breathe. People also seem to think that communication is as natural as breathing. So how can something so natural go so wrong? When people are taught to sing, they often are "retaught" how to breathe. Singing requires deep, abdominal breathing, and as they mature, many humans use shallow, chest breathing. Just as a person needs to relearn to breathe when learning to sing, a human being also needs to relearn how to communicate. This chapter builds on basic communication skills.

So how does communication break down so quickly? Each day, numerous models of poor communication abound. Extremely poor communication is evident on television, in movies, in families, and in professional interactions. These poor communication patterns are a reflection of a lifetime of unconscious communication techniques. Few people actually study communication, and most

are unaware of the lack of skill exhibited. In actuality, communication is a habit (albeit a lifetime habit) that can be changed.

The importance of communication is emphasized in the first nurse executive competency described in the American Organization of Nurse Executives (AONE) Nurse Executive Competencies (2005). This competency stresses the importance of effective communication as it relates to managing and resolving conflict, making oral presentations to many different audiences about nursing healthcare and organizational issues, and producing cogent and persuasive written communication.

SPECIFIC ASPECTS OF COMMUNICATION

In everyday communication, leaders can facilitate clarity and understanding through awareness of some of the key aspects that exist. Everyone has filters through which they receive or send communication. Reviewing these and being aware of what creates breakdowns in communication help avoid serious problems.

Communication Filters

Communication is almost always a challenge, whether it is personal or professional. As Patterson, Grenny, McMillan, and Switzler (2002) convey, the need of human beings to connect with one another is paramount. They do this intellectually, emotionally, spiritually, and physically through the process called communication. This process is complex because the least important part of the message is conveyed with words. Greater than 90% of the message comprises voice tonality and facial and body language. Humans are experts at saying one thing and reversing the meaning with tonality and facial expression.

In addition to this complexity, each person has created an interpretation of the world based on his or her own reality. This reality evolves from life experiences, socialization, genetic heritage, and life choices. Each of these aspects can transform into communication filters through which people interpret the world and other human beings. Because the world of each person is different, distortions in communication are common. These distortions, or filters, affect how people speak and how they hear the messages of others.

Crane (2002) identified several primary communication filters such as mental state, assumptions, hidden agendas, belief systems, judgments of self and others, emotional states, and the current state of the relationship.

Mental State

Mental state also is known as a frame of mind that exists during an interaction and includes positive and negative attitudes. This mental state affects the ability to focus and be aware of the many nuances and messages signaled by the other person. A clear mental state with no upset reaction facilitates a focus on the communication sent by the other person. Even with distractions, it is easier to shift gears and be present with the person when in a clear mental state. When human beings feel overwhelmed and stressed, it is much more difficult to shift into a clear mental state.

Assumptions

One of the most significant issues in relationships is failed expectations. Often expectations are based on assumptions and not clarified. To become conscious of assumptions and expectations requires constant self-examination and reflection. It also requires frequent contact with the other person to identify any expectations and/or assumptions. Nothing should be assumed.

Hidden Agendas and Intentions

Human beings are not always aware of what motivates behavior. Therefore habits, conditioning, and underlying needs and desires actually may control behavior. Habits and unconscious needs and desires can dictate a person's reaction to a situation rather than creating an appropriate response or an effective assessment of the communication interaction. Hidden agendas can be either positive or negative.

Beliefs

Belief systems comprise personal values acquired throughout life. These belief systems expand or limit thinking, actions, and responses. Most people seem to operate from a positive perspective of "live life": learn, laugh, and love. On the other hand, some people consistently see life from a negative perspective; they feel they must protect and defend from all the terrible events in the world. Those who approach life positively are open to change, easy to communicate with, and receptive to others. At the same time, staff members like to be around positive people, and such people function well in leadership positions.

Judgments of Self and Others

Human beings often use their cognitive ability to make judgments about others. It is convenient and saves time to categorize and stereotype others. If human beings feel "less than" others, the evolution of defective and deficient attitudes is easy to understand. Thinking of oneself as better than others breeds arrogance, feelings of self-importance, and a condescending manner. The judgments each person has of others are reflective of personal internal self-talk and self-esteem. Because the mind cannot readily hold two opposing thoughts simultaneously, a person with low self-esteem discounts positive input and feedback.

Emotional State

Emotional states significantly affect the thinking process. Consequently, emotions of upset, anger, and hurt affect the ability to think clearly and logically. Negative feelings such as insecurities, threats, stress, fear, needs to be right or perfect, and unhealed interpersonal "wounds" affect a person's ability to communicate and think clearly. Conversely, positive emotions such as delight, joy, hopeful expectations, and humor affect communication and thinking in a positive way, which could cause a person to overlook issues that require attention.

An example of problems with emotions can occur when a team member or staff member brings negative information or "bad news." It is critical that emotions are not inflamed when the message is not what the leader wants to hear. For a more in-depth discussion, see the Literature box.

Current State of the Relationship

Any nurse who has been in a nurse's station and listened to the conversations knows how important relationships are within the work setting. These relationships affect the team and the performance of the individual and thus the organization. As Crane (2002) indicates, negative feelings and interactions, unfinished business, unresolved conflicts, and emotional residue are poisonous to communication, relationships, and team functioning.

To compensate for these communication filters, it is helpful to practice becoming centered and self-aware and to work at being less reactive. Communication breakdown can be avoided by listening carefully to others and striving for awareness of these filters. The goal is to neutralize them as much as possible. This is a process or journey in communication growth and improvement, requiring time and energy.

LANGUAGE TO AVOID

Language choice can make communication more or less effective. The following is a helpful reminder of what language works and which words create negativity and defensiveness.

Finding the Best Words

The language used in communication flavors everything in life and certainly affects how others perceive a person, a critical aspect of leadership. Without a doubt, certain words and phrases convey emotional energy and affect the ability to connect with others in positive and constructive ways. A single word can change an entire interaction in addition to specific attitudes (Patterson et al., 2002).

Jargon

Few professions have more jargon, abbreviations, and acronyms than those in healthcare. The use of jargon creates unclear communication that leads to confusion and prevents some colleagues, patients, and families from understanding the message. In addition, its use establishes a sense of exclusivity by establishing the "in group," who knows and understands the unique usage, and the "out group," who have no idea what is being discussed. This creates dissonance and discontent. Few people enjoy being on the outside attempting to discern meaning. This is a time when humans begin fabricating and ascribing negative meaning.

Although jargon is common to most groups, whether they are airline pilots, government workers, the military, or physicians and nurses, no substitute exists for common, ordinary words when discussing subjective thoughts, feelings, and ideas that arise during the normal course of work. This is especially true when talking with persons not knowledgeable about these special "languages." Specific attention is required to convey messages in common ordinary language.

Word Choices

Crane (2002) identifies several word choices that create communication problems. The use of some words can upset people and create communication breakdown and lack of understanding.

These choices can activate communication barriers. Examples include the following:

You vs. I or We: The use of *you* potentiates judgment, blame, and defensiveness, whereas the use of *I* connotes self-responsibility and personal ownership of a specific point of view or of specific feelings. Further, the use of *we* is inclusive and implies teamwork and working together. Building positive relationships requires the use of inclusive language.

Should vs. Could: When *should* is used, it implies control and often results in feelings of guilt that are not helpful in building relationships. Using the word *could* implies options and possibilities in thinking, acting, and cooperating.

But vs. And: When *but* is used after expressing any thought, it cancels or discounts the statement that has gone before it and creates an argumentative tone in the discussion. The use of the word *and* implies connection and possibilities or alternatives.

Try vs. Will: When people say they will *try*, it can imply a built-in excuse for not succeeding or doing whatever it takes to succeed. It leaves a back door open for failure. *I will* is much stronger and implies a commitment to take action and fulfill the promise. In the movie *Star Wars,* the Jedi master, Yoda, says, "Do or do not; there is no try."

Always/Never vs. Sometimes: Hardly anything is always or never and using those words implies exaggeration that can lead to judgment and defensiveness. The use of *sometimes* or *often* avoids the extreme position and decreases opportunities to be judged and found wanting.

Can't vs. Won't: Most of us are able to do most things requested of us. When we say, "I can't," we really mean, "I won't" for whatever reason, and we are attempting to be "nice" in the refusal. *Can't* is less truthful and negates honest, direct communication. *Won't*, on the other hand, is clear and honest.

Additional clarity results from elimination of certain words from daily vocabulary such as *it*. People usually can be more specific than such a general term. This usage implies not taking the time or creativity to describe *it* more clearly.

The use of *they* or *them* in a blaming way separates and excludes people and judges those who are referred to in this manner. Language is critically important and creates breakdowns and defensiveness in others. Many misunderstandings can be avoided by elimination of the use of certain overworked and commonly used words and tonality.

COMMUNICATION BREAKDOWN

In complex situations such as those encountered in hospitals, multiple stressors feed communication breakdown. Communications are more apt to break down in cases of multiple different roles and multiple players interacting with one another, particularly when patients are very sick and too much work must be accomplished. As discussed above, in these intense situations, the tendency is to have a more muddled mental state; to make assumptions; to have old, unresolved issues with co-workers; to judge and blame others; and to have negative emotions. All of these lead to the downward spiral of relationships. When these stressors exist, it is easy to see how people can react to anything that does not work and to blame others, judge others, and make demands. Sometime this looks like a temper tantrum. Most people know what physical responses occur when these situations arise. Some yell, some turn red in the face, and some withdraw from the situation. The Awareness Model (Senge, Kleiner, Roberts, Ross, & Smith, 1994) depicted in Figure 9-1 demonstrates the difference between conscious responses and unconscious reactions to stressful interactions. Regardless of how difficult situations are, each human being has a choice about how he or she will respond. No one "makes" a person feel anything. Each person chooses various responses. It is possible to work toward a communication interaction that produces a positive constructive outcome.

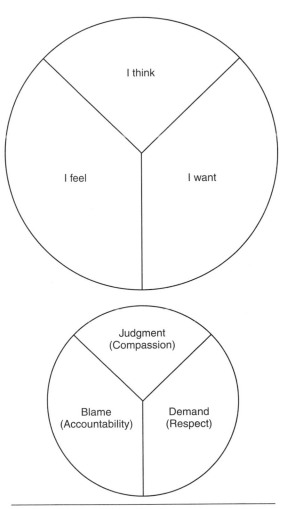

Figure 9-1 The Awareness Model: differentiating between conscious and unconscious responses. (Modified from St. Charles Medical Center. [1993]. *People centered teams.* Bend, OR: The Author.)

When a person is in reaction to a situation at the feeling level, he or she focuses on blaming others for whatever has happened. "If the night shift had given a decent report before leaving, I would have known that patient was supposed to be in radiology." By taking responsibility for at least part of the breakdown, the communication shifts: "I feel confused and disappointed because I didn't ask the night shift for additional information about the patient's test schedule for today."

Likewise, when a person is caught up in reaction at the thinking level, it is easy to make a judgment: "The night shift made a big mistake." Thinking compassionately about the situation allows a person to surpass judgment and be more reasonable: "Both of us missed something in this situation; now how do we reschedule the patient's tests?"

Finally, in this stressful, out-of-control situation, making an unreasonable, angry demand is a natural progression: "The nurse manager better write those incompetent nurses up!" This type of response is motivated by fear that something negative will happen to the patient and the nurses will be blamed or that the family will be upset and heap retribution on the nurses. When it is possible to breathe deeply and become calm, a respectful way to make a request becomes possible: "I want patients to have tests done in a timely fashion and it would help me if I'm given an alert at report about the tests scheduled for the day. Would you be willing to support me in this way?"

Most broken relationships, whether they are with co-workers, physicians, or family members, are focused on blaming another person, judging them as wrong, and insisting that something mean and hurtful happened. Accountability, compassion, and respect in interpersonal interactions are much more likely to create situations in which each person's needs are met and the work is done. This leads to positive feelings about one another and units operate more smoothly.

SKILLS THAT ENHANCE COMMUNICATION

Improving communication is a goal most of us have. Although many of us focus on what to say and how to say it, the key skill is listening.

Listening

Many human beings rarely feel "heard." In other words, many people are so busy talking and attempting to convey their story or point of view, they seldom take the time to listen attentively to the other person. A colleague once shared that her 6 year old crawled up on a chair and took her face between his hands, looked into her eyes, and said, "Calling Mom, this is Kevin calling Mom." She was embarrassed that she had not been listening to him but instead was focused on making dinner and reflecting on a key problem at work.

> *Listening is a rare happening among human beings. You cannot listen to the word another is speaking if you are preoccupied with your appearance or with impressing the other, or trying to decide what you are going to say when the other stops talking, or debating about whether what is said is true or relevant or agreeable. Such matters have their place, but only after listening to the word as the word is being uttered. Listening is a primitive act of love in which a person gives himself to another's word, making himself accessible and vulnerable to that word.*
> WILLIAM STRINGFELLOW, PHILOSOPHER

One of the greatest gifts given another human being is to focus 100% on what that person has to say. Active listening is defined as listening in a way that the listener can feed back accurately the emotional content of a speaker's message.

Initial guidelines for active listening are found in Box 9-1.

The purpose is to demonstrate to the speaker that (1) the message has been heard, (2) the intensity of the speaker's emotions is understood *and* accepted, and (3) he or she should continue to share even more deeply. Actively listening requires the following actions:

- Listen to what the speaker says and distinguish between the content of the message and the underlying emotional and nonverbal aspects of the message.
- Assess the intensity of the speaker's emotions, selecting a word or phrase that describes the feeling and its intensity.
- Paraphrase the emotion and thoughts and be able to convey these to the speaker. Actively listen for the response to the feedback and clarify a second time if necessary to be accurate in the interpretation of the message.
- Check for accuracy and the other person will confirm or deny and more than likely clarify or elaborate on the interpretation or redescribe the situation and emotions.
- Continue to empathize and clarify. The emotion or the upset of the speaker often decreases and the listener can continue with reframing and paraphrasing.

Box 9-1   GUIDELINES FOR ACTIVE LISTENING

Slow down internal processes and seek data. Do not interrupt the speaker.

Listen carefully. The more information acquired through listening, the less interpretation (making up the missing pieces or motivations) is needed. The less information the listener has, the more interpretation occurs.

Realize that the first words from the other person are not necessarily representative of inner thoughts or feelings. Refrain from making assumptions. Be patient.

Suspend beliefs, views, and judgments, at least temporarily, while listening.

Attempt to understand the perspective of the other person, particularly if it is different.

Realize that any judgments or "labels" strongly influence the manner in which listening occurs.

Appreciate the difference between understanding other peoples' perspectives and agreeing with them. First strive to understand. Then agreement or disagreement can occur.

Learn about the person. Effective listening is based on an inner desire to learn about another's unique experience of the world.

Some barriers to active listening come from the physical aspects in the presentation of the message such as the words themselves, the verbal and nonverbal cues, stereotyping and judgments, emotions, self-concept, and individual differences. See Box 9-2 for more details about physical and emotional barriers and related exercises. Some barriers come from behaviors surrounding active listening events. See Box 9-3 for strategies that help prepare the leader for active listening.

Listening is critical for leaders and therefore it is helpful to review the five behaviors that are key to active listening. The first is *attending behavior*, which communicates that the receiver of the message is listening and paying attention to what the speaker is saying. The physical behaviors associated with attending include maintaining eye contact, leaning forward, and stopping all other activities such as phone calls, pagers, shuffling papers, or anything that could be construed as disruptive. This means no computer work and no interruptions. These activities are distractions that could be interpreted by the listener as devaluating. These activities could also be construed as the leader's elevated self-importance compared with the listener/follower's lesser importance.

The second is *encouraging behavior*, which includes nodding the head affirmatively, comments such as "uh huh," a positive or upbeat voice tone, or positive comments such as, "Yes, I see what you mean," or "I understand." The purpose is to convey interest in what the other person is saying and to encourage further conversation.

The third behavior is asking *facilitative questions*. These questions are open-ended and support and clarify the content of the message. Questions are

---

Box **9-2**   PHYSICAL BARRIERS TO ACTIVE LISTENING

- **Words:** Regional expressions (e.g., "fixin' to"), lingo, jargon, or the use of acronyms make communication to outsiders more difficult and influence their ability to listen actively. Listeners can be confused in an attempt to understand the words.

    Exercise: Notice in a 5-minute timeframe within a conversation with a co-worker how many slang or local expressions are used. Also notice how many abbreviations or acronyms are used during the time (this is particularly true in the healthcare industry).

- **Nonverbal cues:** These include body language, posture, gestures, and facial expressions. Look in the mirror to discover how you look when listening intently. You may furrow your brow, which could be misperceived by a speaker. It may be interpreted as being concerned, angry, or frustrated.

    Exercise: (1) Observe yourself in a mirror. Pretend anger, confusion, frustration, or concentration. Note the

corresponding facial expressions. Is this what you would like to convey to staff or co-workers? (2) Notice in a conversation with a co-worker what body language, gestures, and facial expressions are used and check out the message that was sent. Was it what was intended?

- **Verbal cues:** Tone of voice, pacing, and volume can interfere with communication. Think about what you do when someone raises his or her voice or talks loud or fast. The reaction could be defensive. A monotone might be considered boring. Fast talking might even confuse the listener.

    Exercise: In conversation with a co-worker, notice the response when the other person raises his or her voice, talks very fast or very loud, or even talks in a monotone. Notice the same thing in yourself. When voices are raised, how do people react? If they back away or react, share the exercise and ask for feedback.

Box 9-3   EXERCISES THAT IMPROVE THE ABILITY TO LISTEN ACTIVELY

Clean off your desk. If loose papers are around, the computer is turned on, or phones are ringing, it is easy to begin to fiddle with papers or interrupt a conversation to take a call. This interrupts your focus and prevents active listening.

What is the color of the other person's eyes? Train yourself to notice eye color at the beginning of the conversation. It ensures eye contact and reassures the speaker of an attempt to connect. At the same time, do not overfocus on eye color and create discomfort in the other person.

Ask questions rather than making statements. Talking excessively prevents listening.

Learn to "lubricate" conversations. Phrases such as "I understand" show that you are listening. Encourage the other person to keep talking, and keep your attention focused on the speaker.

Take time to respond to the speaker. If questions are blurted out as soon as the speaker is finished, it appears as though you were not listening. Before asking questions, paraphrase what you just heard the speaker say. This decreases the chance of miscommunication.

Smile only occasionally. It is not reassuring for a person to smile the whole time. It can be interpreted as mental absence or a sign that you do not take the speaker seriously. Save smiles for humorous remarks or clear expressions of pleasure.

---

so important in communication that they are discussed in a separate section. They elicit discussion or help the person clarify the problem or thinking. They also can help people hear what they are saying and how it sounds to others.

The fourth behavior is *paraphrasing*, in which the listener, to determine accuracy, uses his or her own words to rephrase what someone is saying. This process helps the other person feel heard and encourages the person to expand or clarify the intent of the message. It allows the listener to assess understanding before responding or reacting to what was said. Helpful guidelines for paraphrasing include the following: responding in a way that neither adds to nor subtracts from what the other person said, keeping comments brief, using one's own words rather than saying exactly what the other person said, and refraining from conveying agreement or disagreement. The listener might begin with a phrase that indicates what he is attempting to do, such as "Let me see if I understand you correctly."

The last active listening behavior is *reflecting feelings*. This skill goes beyond paraphrasing and detects and observes how the speaker feels.

The advantage in the use of this skill is to help the person feel understood, reduce defensiveness in the speaker, and diffuse emotions in a situation. Although some of these skills were learned as a part of therapeutic interventions with patients and families, they are used infrequently with peers, physicians, or staff members. Few situations demand more use of reflecting feelings than with co-workers or in personal family situations.

QUESTIONS

It is better to know some of the questions than to know all of the answers.
JAMES THURBER

Questions are the most powerful tool a leader possesses. Several reasons exist for leaders to use questions. The first reason is to *stimulate the brain* to engage. Questions are like the "power on" switch on a computer. When the brain is asked a question, it goes in search of an answer. Questions also *create an information exchange*. When a question is asked, the answer is given and an effective exhange occurs. Next, questions permit the leader to *discover what others know* by prompting them. The leader can also find out what problems others are experiencing. In addition, questions allow the leader to *listen to others* and, even more important, these questions allow the leader to *acknowledge others* for what is learned from them and for their willingness to interact with the leader. The last key purpose that questions serve is to *provide a vehicle* for the leader to encourage and support a staff member through the process of discovery. By asking a series of questions, the staff member can be more enlightened than had the leader merely given an answer.

> *The leader of the past was a person who knew how to tell. The leader of the future will be a person who knows how to ask.*
> PETER DRUCKER

Asking questions requires knowing and understanding the purpose of the question. Possible purposes include the following:

- To generate the cooperation of the staff
- To help the leader garner resources
- To gain important information
- To acquire commitments from staff members
- To acknowledge improved performance

These questions can be asked of nursing staff members, clerks, housekeeping personnel, pharmacy personnel, or physicians. Leaders should put themselves in the shoes of staff members. What might their goals be? The question needs to be phrased in a way advantageous to both parties.

When asking questions, nursing leaders need to speak clearly, calmly, and directly. The interaction with staff members is important. It helps to be positive and refrain from communicating any underlying negativism or disapproval. The question can be stated simply to avoid obscuring its meaning. The nursing leader must display interest in the answer and listen actively and intently.

When receiving the response to the question, nurse leaders must practice all the active listening skills. Evaluation of the answer is important because question clarification may be appropriate, and a follow-up question may be necessary. Last, the leader must take some action with the information discovered. For example, the staff member should be acknowledged for the response. If questions were related to performance and the performance improved, acknowledgment is mandatory.

When questions from staff or from "listeners of the message" are handled appropriately, thoughtfully, and effectively, regardless of the manner in which they were asked, the perception is that the leader is effective (Weissman, 2005). Effective translates to positive or good leadership. Therefore the ability to ask meaningful questions and respond effectively to difficult questions creates a positive impression of leadership ability.

Situations in which it is useful to question are limitless. Questions often indicate interest in the other person (Porche & Niederer, 2001). Reminders of when leaders can use questions are found in Box 9-4.

WRITTEN COMMUNICATION

Leaders write on a regular basis. Written communication is received daily. The challenge is to understand the most effective ways to communicate in writing. Today, via computer, communication is nearly overwhelming. For that reason it is critical to know the most effective way in which to construct and write memos, business and professional letters, executive summaries, and perhaps most importantly, e-mail messages.

Memoranda (Memos)

Writing memos within the facility is an important process and can be crucial to career progress. A memo is a written document that stays inside the facility or system. Even though they are small or short, they instigate big headaches to everyone

Box 9-4 When to Use Questions

- **Persuading people:** The leader wants to persuade someone to her point of view or gain support for an idea. Questions help discover what would concern the other person or what the objections might be. Such questions could be as simple as, "What do you think?" or "How does this idea strike you?" or "What doesn't work about this idea?"

- **Gaining information:** This is the most obvious use of questions. A leader must be well informed, and incomplete information can be a disaster. "Is there anything else I need to know?"

- **Planting ideas:** Plant an idea and then let the other person run with it. At a meeting the leader might ask, "What do you think about using plan A (describe it) or plan B (describe it briefly) to improve how we deliver care?" Once the discussion starts, let the people expand the idea and give them the credit for it.

- **Clarifying thinking:** Questions can be used to clear up "fuzzy," or ambiguous, thinking. Asking questions implies thinking things through completely. It requires expanding how the leader thinks. Do not only ask, "How is it you plan to proceed with care for this patient?" but also follow up with, "How specifically will you handle this new procedure?"

- **Motivating staff:** Use questions to encourage staff to solve their own problems. For example, when someone comes to you with an idea, do not immediately dismiss it or OK it, ask, "How much time do you think it will take?" or "What do you estimate the cost will be in both time and money?" or "Does that make sense to you?"

- **Solving problems:** Questions help identify problem areas. Talk to staff and ask them what is going on. Then ask them, "What solutions do you see?"

- **Taking the sting out of feedback:** When critical feedback is given, most people become defensive and no longer hear the observations. Rather than saying, "You're always late," try, "How do you think lateness affects the unit?" (co-workers? patient care?) This stimulates thinking, discussion, and the ability to obtain a commitment.

- **Reducing mistakes:** When assigning a task, ask, "Can you summarize what we have just discussed and what your plan is?" Instead of a head shake to indicate understanding, describe specifics to clarify and avoid errors.

- **Overcoming objections:** When giving directives, staff often say, "Yes, but...." To defuse this situation, use a question such as, "What are your major concerns about this idea (project)...?"

- **Obtaining cooperation:** When attempting to acquire help or support from another department, facility, or entity, and you meet resistance, ask questions such as, "Have you ever made an exception to that rule or policy?" or "What would it take to create an exception in this case?" or "Is there anything else I can do to facilitate the process?"

- **Clarifying statements:** Questions are critical in obtaining clarity. When someone says they want to change a policy, it is good to ask, "How would you like to change it?" Lack of clarity has had serious implications for organizations. One CEO informed his staff that they needed better communication. Shortly thereafter he had a proposal and cost estimate for a new phone system. That was not what he meant.

- **Defusing a crisis:** When conflict begins to escalate, it can be handled with questions rather than direct confrontation. "Can you tell me more about what's happening here?"

Modified from Leeds, D. (1987). *Smart questions: A new strategy for successful managers.* New York: Berkley Books.

from unit clerks to the chief nursing officer (CNO). They are difficult to construct quickly or clearly. Some of them "are like *War and Peace* to read, require Miss Marple to figure out, and if written in the wrong tone of voice, can make the nicest people sound heartless" (Chesanow, 1987). The following are some helpful tips for effective memo correspondence.

A memo is a short document, maximum two pages and preferably two paragraphs, and is written to encourage someone to take some action or to understand something (e.g., meet a deadline, explain a project, give feedback). It should be personal and written in the first person and in the active rather than the passive voice. Memos are conversational and use contractions. Jargon, scholarly words, and esoteric phrases such as "per your request" obfuscate the message. At the same time words can be "smothered" by adding fancy or effusive endings to short, clear words (e.g., "issuance" rather than "issue" or "prioritization" rather than "priority"). Spell-check functions are helpful but will not check the accurate spelling of names and the appropriate dates or numbers. This is where errors are most likely to occur and require double-checking. Triteness tends to irritate people, for example, "We're sorry for any inconvenience" or "Please don't hesitate to call." Rather, the following sentence works much better: "If you need help, call me."

English Works at Gallaudet University (2002) suggests that imagining a face-to-face conversation with the reader of the memo is effective. Then, the memo is written from the reader's point of view. The reader will have to do something with the memo when it is received, so clarity is essential. The action the reader needs to take must be identified clearly in the first sentence or the first paragraph. This explanation must be short so that the message is not lost in too much verbiage and explanation. Each paragraph should be limited to five or fewer lines, and each rationale should be placed in a separate paragraph. Finally, the memo is closed with a call to action, particularly if a deadline is required. It further helps if the

deadline is boldface or underlined so that the reader sees the timeframe more clearly. Memos can be a valuable communication tool when constructed wisely.

Business and Professional Letters

Business Letters

Leaders are responsible for corresponding with businesses, other healthcare facilities, community leaders, and patients or family members. This is an acquired skill, which includes a few rules and guidelines that support constructing good business letters. Some useful web sites have excellent tips for constructing business letters (Business Letter Writing, 2003; Colorado State University, 2005) in addition to examples of letters.

Effective letter writing essentials include being clear as to why the letter is being written, understanding the recipient's needs, and speaking clearly to the needs. Furthermore, in Business Letter Writing (2003), seven Cs are emphasized, which encourage the writer to be clear, concise, correct, courteous, conversational, convincing, and complete. Business letters are written when a permanent record is necessary of a response to a letter or inquiry or information that was sent.

The general format begins with a letterhead or return address; inside address of the recipient; attention line; subject line; salutation; body of the letter, which includes an introductory paragraph, one or more "body" paragraphs, and a concluding paragraph; and the complimentary close and signature. The following suggestions are tips for writing effective letters.

First establish the right tone for the letter by writing as if you are in an actual conversation. Refrain from using stilted languages such as, "Please be advised"; rather use such language as, "I'd like to explain." Use personal pronouns such as *I, we, you,* and *yours* and contractions such as *it's, doesn't,* and *I'm.* Use active verbs (the committee agreed) rather than passive verbs (It was agreed by the committee), which tend to be longwinded, ambiguous, impersonal, and dull. Edit the business letter ruthlessly because unnecessary words and phrases clutter the letter and obscure the meaning. Avoid using jargon and abbreviations by imagining yourself as the recipient. Do not assume the reader knows or understands the jargon or abbreviations. Write a strong opening and closing paragraph. For the opening, ask or answer a question, explain action taken, express pleasure or regret, or give information. Avoid clichés such as, "I am writing," "I refer to my letter dated," or "I write in reference to." In the closing paragraph, avoid clichés such as "Thanking you for" or "Hoping for a prompt reply." End the letter positively and politely without leaving the reader in mid-air. Instead, explain or repeat what action is expected.

For the business letter, *keep it short* by cutting needless words or information and delete repetitive things such as references to previous or future correspondence. *Keep it simple* by using familiar words, short sentences, and short paragraphs; using a conversational style; and keeping related information together. *Keep it strong* by answering the reader's question in the first paragraph, then explaining why, and using concrete words and examples. *Keep it sincere* by answering promptly, being human and friendly, and writing the way you talk (Business Letter Writing, 2003).

Letters of Recommendation

Leaders frequently are asked to write letters of recommendation for employees, peers, or even superiors. These letters may be about returning to school, a promotion, a new position, or an award or honor. Possible subject areas for these letters include personal attributes, job performance, strengths, limitations, capabilities, and career/leadership potential. Examples that demonstrate the reasons for the candidate's evaluation are important. In the opening, the writer can explain the relationship with the candidate, including the length of time of the relationship. In addition, means of contacting the writer for additional information should be included, such as address, phone number, and e-mail address (University of Wisconsin-Green Bay, 2004). The letter should convey knowledge of the candidate, especially in relation to competencies and potential. The respectability of the leader's position increases the credibility of the letter (Luthy, 2005). If the leader cannot write an exemplary letter, he or she must talk with the employee about what the letter will say and what existing issues prevent writing an outstanding letter. This situation could even be used to coach or counsel the employee or peer.

According to Verba at the Derek Bok Center at Harvard University (2004), the contents of the letter should make a statement of support for the candidate, be well documented, include supportive evidence and information, and address the specific purpose for which it is written. It can be helpful to have a copy of the candidate's resume or curriculum vitae to assist with accurate dates and activities in addition to a copy of the guidelines used for the application. These letters should be one to two pages, because anything shorter indicates either lack of interest or little knowledge or familiarity with the candidate. The letter must sound sincere, unlike a form letter, and the best, polished prose must be employed. Jargon or other terms not understood by people in professions other than healthcare should be avoided. A sincere and personable approach is important in business and recommendation letters.

Executive Summary

An executive summary could be used for a business proposal, a large project, or a research project. It is a brief overview or guide to an extensive report or business plan, which gives the reader a quick preview of the contents of the long document and consolidates the major points of the report. The following guidelines may be helpful:

- Explain the purpose of the report or proposal; emphasize the conclusions, recommendations, and any essential supporting data.

- Follow the sequence of the full document.
- Ensure the length of the summary corresponds to the full document, usually no more than 10% to 15% of the report. Most summaries are one to three pages.
- Use key words and phrases from the full report in the summary.
- Employ conciseness and clarity in the description of how the conclusions were reached.
- Include only the information contained in the full report.
- Spell-check and proofread the document. (Guidelines for Writing an Executive Summary, 2004)

The executive summary is written for people who do not have time to read the complete report. See Box 9-5 for the steps in constructing a summary. The Harvard Business School (Clayton, 2003) offers several tips for executive summaries. The summary is crafted with the audience firmly in mind and focuses on "bottom line deliverables." If the CEO likes the summary, it will be given to an assistant so that the entire report is studied. The need or the problem must be established quickly as something worth an intervention. A solution is recommended and its value explained. The benefits or value must be the focus. Why does the writer (or his or her department) have the best answer or response? The key reasons must be provided and substantiated with evidence. Headings and bulleted or numbered lists enable easier, faster reading. A well-chosen graphic, if possible, is an effective tool.

E-Mail and Its Corresponding Etiquette

E-mail helps workers in the ability to communicate quickly and easily with colleagues, peers, administrators, and others in the workplace. Leaders are overwhelmed by dozens of e-mails that need to be read or answered, and many of them are inappropriate. Most forms of communication can have problems or create misunderstandings regardless of good intentions. Face-to-face communications or even telephone conversations allow for assessment of communication breakdown from either tonality or body language and repair of the breakdown before the conversation is ended. However, e-mail does not offer any additional information beyond what is written. Therefore problems can ensue. The following guidelines have been extracted from suggestions

---

Box 9-5   STEPS FOR CONSTRUCTION OF AN EXECUTIVE SUMMARY

1. Plan to write a summary for each report that exceeds four pages. It can be written after the main report is finished and should approximate one-tenth the size of the report or less.
2. List the main points the summary will cover; they should correspond to the full report.
3. Write a simple declarative sentence for each main point.
4. Add supporting or explanatory statements as needed but avoid jargon.
5. Read the summary critically to be sure it conveys the purpose, key message, and recommendations.
6. Read for errors in style, spelling, grammar, and punctuation. Have a colleague proofread and edit also.
7. Ask a nontechnical person (e.g., a parent or spouse) to read the summary to be sure it is clear to them. If it confuses or bores them, it needs to be rewritten.

Modified from eHOW. (2004). *How to write an executive summary.* Retrieved August 29, 2005, from http://www.ehow.com/how_16566_write-executive-summary.html.

by the staff at the Yale University Library (1999) and other sources:

- Send the right message.
- Create single-subject messages whenever possible and stick to that subject.
- Think through clearly what you want to say and be succinct.
- Make use of bullets and short paragraphs.
- Be careful with the "send button" because any message you send is permanent and cannot be recalled.
- Use a subject line for e-mail that is clear and relevant so that it can be easily found.
- Think about the audience for the message. The audience shapes the way the message is constructed, or how formal or informal it is.
- Separate opinions from factual material.
- Limit the length to 65 to 70 lines.
- Identify yourself and your affiliations clearly.
- Take the time to proofread and use spell-check.
- Refrain from responding to an e-mail when upset or reactive.

Flaming/Blogging

The most important problem with e-mail is the phenomenon called *flaming*. E-mail is the most easily misunderstood form of communication *and* the most likely to result in a hasty, ill-conceived response from the recipient. The expression of extreme emotion or opinion in an e-mail is referred to as "flaming." In contrast to direct interactions or telephone conversations, e-mails can be saved in files, "forwarded," or printed out and circulated, which can create a level of upset that was never intended.

An additional prospect for misunderstanding is *blogging*. Blogging is a web-based source of opinions. When bloggers are negative about people and organizations, problems ensue. Clearly, such situations must be avoided. A person should not write or respond to e-mails or post comments in a blog when upset. Allowing sufficient time to pass or making personal contact with the individual

are helpful tools to resolve the situation, using the differentiation/awareness model (see Figure 9-1), questions, and active listening skills.

WORKING WITH THE MEDIA

Interviews

Increasingly, the media want to talk with someone on the administrative staff of the hospital. Reporters and broadcasters are looking for a "local" angle on national or state stories. They want to find someone who is knowledgeable and articulate. The following information summarizes media interactions and interviews and how the CNO can use them to his or her advantage.

The Message

The message is constructed from the total communication. The relationship of voice tone and body language to the words is important to remember. If tonality and body language are not used effectively, very little of the content gets through. The TV sound bite is only about 5 seconds, although the local news may use longer bites. That is the equivalent of one solid sentence. So, that sentence better be dynamite!

Constructing the Message

It is better to have three key messages and restate, rephrase, or repeat them three times than to have nine separate messages. So, it is important to think in advance of any interviewing situation (or potential situation) about what those messages are. No matter what the CNO is asked, he or she needs to address that point *briefly*. Then, using a bridging technique, the CNO moves to one of the key points. This is called "staying on message." Bridging is accomplished with words such as *however, so,* and *therefore*. It may include phrases such as, "Even more importantly," or "Let me give you an example." Bridging words signify transition to something else.

The interview may be divided into four parts (Figure 9-2). The first part is the *headliner*, which

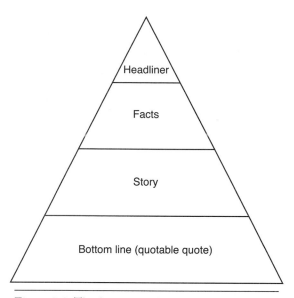

Figure 9-2 The four parts of an interview.

consists of the key message on which the leader wants to stay focused. The next part consists of the *facts*. The leader must focus on the knowledge and facts he or she has to support any of the key points. The third part is the one that makes a message come alive. It is the *story, analogy, anecdote,* or *example.* It "puts a face" on the facts. The final, and most important part, is the *bottom line.* What quotable quote can be created that the interviewer will want to use? This bite needs to be memorable.

Before an Interview

The CNO does not need to take a "cold call" interview. Rather, the leader can ask what the interviewer is looking for and what kind of help is needed. The CNO may say, "Let me get back to you" and set a prompt, specific time for the interview. This added time allows the CNO to discover with whom the interviewer has talked already. This could help to clarify further what the interviewer is looking for, and it could provide clues about the type of interview being conducted.

If time permits, it is useful to go to the related web site (newspaper, journal, television, or radio station) or to a search engine to see what the interviewer is known for or the general tone of material produced by the interviewer. Setting a time limit, especially with telephone interviews, facilitates remaining focused on the key messages.

Once the interview focus is clear, a sheet of paper or file cards can be created for each of the three major points. (Again, the idea of emphasizing messages is critical.) The known facts are listed; words to trigger the interest points (e.g., story or analogy) are jotted down; and the bottom line, "quotable quote" message is written down. On another sheet of paper or file card the anticipated key negating statements are listed. Beside each negating statement, a bridging statement is identified and then the positive answer. Positive responses, in this sense, mean reinforcing the key messages the leader wants the interviewer to remember. The negative words or message an interviewer might use must not be repeated, because invariably those are the words that are included in the sound bite.

During the Interview

Unless the leader is "on camera" and required to have a specific posture, he or she should stand or lean forward. This body position energizes the message and keeps the leader alert. One important rule for being "on camera" is appropriate attire. Solid colors (not patterns) that will not reflect or absorb a lot of light are best; black and white should be avoided. Minimal accessories avoid distracting audiences by a great scarf or tie instead of listening to the message. Even though it takes longer to say the names of organizations, procedures, or equipment, doing so prevents the sense of exclusivity that jargon conveys. Many people outside of healthcare think professionals use jargon to show off or to make a message more complex than it really is. Above all, *nothing is "off the record."* The leader must stick to the key points even if the interviewer does not. The goal is to get the message out, not to answer specific questions.

After the Interview

The interviewer should be given additional information on the topic or on other important topics. Keeping promises is important to an ongoing relationship and thus following up with materials or information is essential. Analyzing the interview as a basis for feedback and subsequent improvement is also useful. A quiet place is conducive to thinking about how the interview proceeded and whether the key message was clear. The leader should obtain a copy of the videorecording or print media if possible. What did the interviewer think was important? Was it the key message? (TTUHSC Nursing: #5371 Syllabus, 2005).

PRESENTATION SKILLS

The skill with which interviews, presentations, and staff meetings are conducted is critical to the listener's appreciation of the information and affects whether the content will be retained or remembered. These skills are also important in telling stories, which is discussed later in the chapter. Simmons (2001) describes key aspects of presentation that facilitate the listener receiving and being open to the information. These include the following:

Oral language: The words must show action, feeling, and even passion about the topic. Using a word such as *roared* conveys a different emotion than merely saying *laughed*. Although it may or may not work for the speaker to memorize a presentation, being *very* familiar with the content is critical.

Tonality: Presentations usually work better, particularly when given at hospital meetings (even board meetings), if they are informal. The speaker needs to share the experience or the perspective of whatever the topic is. Presentations that sound like reports usually are not effective.

Facial expressions: These expressions can help emphasize various points and are crucial to convey a message about what happened in the facility or on a specific unit. Eye contact is also important because it draws the listener into the topic.

Body language: Whenever people speak, they use their bodies, including hands and head movements, to convey messages and stress an idea. These movements are used particularly when stories are told.

Senses: Employing the use of senses descriptively in conveying a patient's condition, a chaotic situation, or a confrontation helps convey messages. Appealing to multiple senses through tactics such as use of sound effects enriches the description.

Details: Using details to create a mental image and then to enrich the image enhances communication. With an in-depth mental image, the listener can imagine being in a specific situation and the imagination is captured. Engaged listeners are more apt to be interested and receptive to the goals of the presentation.

Presentation tools: Many presentation tools are used to enroll the listeners, such as experiential learning activities, games, and exercises; audio visual tools; stories; skills such as creating set, closure, anticipation, permission, participation, stable datum, humor, acknowledgment; and the use of questions (Kowalski, 2004; Kowalski, 2004a; Kowalski, 2004b; Kowalski, 2005a; Kowalski, 2005b). Selecting strategies to fit the purpose and audience is crucial. In the role of nurse executive, the leader who feels deficient in some of these skills could find an appropriate learning opportunity. Many of these skills and tools are best learned at workshops, where videotaping of practice sessions occurs. Learning and changing behavior occurs more quickly when the necessary changes are visible on videotape.

STORYTELLING

One of the most important communication skills for leaders is the ability to convey ideas, organizational vision, goals, and objectives. Many nursing staff members have experienced monotonous presentations that fail to ignite their spirit or passion about what needs to be accomplished. Nurses have experienced management meetings in which pages of financial data or "information" were shared that easily could have been communicated in writing and then discussed at the meeting. According to McFee (2003), an excellent alternative to such dry, boring approaches is telling a story that conveys the message.

The word *story* comes from the Greek language and means to know or to have knowledge or wisdom (Gill, 2005). Stories help people gain knowledge about situations, institutions, and values. Employees are much more receptive to stories than to data and do not become defensive when hearing a story. In addition, stories provide insights into the self, roles, and values. Professionally, they help convey the organizational vision, objectives, and values in an exciting and challenging way. To facilitate this, stories must be powerful, astutely selected, and told with considerable thought and skill.

Although most people tell stories every day, ranging from the incident on the highway coming to work to a powerful life event such as the death of a loved one or a time when a powerful lesson was learned, they often do not analyze a story or how it was told or what happened as a result of telling the story. As leaders become more conscious of stories, they actually can begin collecting stories and categorizing them. Based on Simmons (2001), the following can serve as a framework.

- The presenter and the purpose
- The presenter's intention
- Stories that convey a vision
- Teaching stories
- Stories about values
- A nursing story

It is helpful to consider each of these categories and find an example in each from the leader's own experience.

The Presenter and the Purpose

If listeners suspect that the goal is to influence them, they want to know who the storyteller really is and the agenda. This concern is true regardless of whether the leader is speaking to small groups of staff members or presenting to a large group at a formal meeting. According to Ibarra and Lineback (2005), this is true in the business world and is a very human trait. A story about the leader helps staff members see what the leader wants them to know about her or him.

An example of such a story follows:

When I was a new graduate student, I was fortunate to have Dr. Ingeborg Mauksch as my professor for the "Issues in Nursing" course. Because the class was so large, she broke us into groups of 8 to 10 and had us come to her apartment for wine and cheese. She asked each group a different question, and for our group it was, "Why are you here in graduate school?" My fellow students responded with many altruistic reasons for coming to school. When my turn came, I spoke my truth: "I'm here for more money and better hours." Inge was taken aback at my brashness. She paused, was thoughtful, and then said, "Nursing is in desperate need of leaders. If the ONLY reason you are here is for more money and better hours, you had best reconsider."

I spent the next 18 months reconsidering. I took a leadership position after finishing my master's degree and have spent the remainder of my career learning and focusing on additional skills related to leadership.

One could also use such a story whenever the discussion is about leadership, for example, introducing a new leadership development program in the institution.

The Presenter's Intention

Providing a plausible reason and the goals for the leader's meeting with the group is important.

If reasons are unclear, people will fantasize about an imagined or suspicious reason. Worse yet, if the leader comes across as manipulative or insincere, trust dwindles significantly. However, if the leader has genuinely good intentions and goals and is honest and up front about those, staff members will be willing to listen, and the leader has the opportunity to enroll them in the vision. If the leader wanted to bring in consultants to increase the effectiveness of staff communication skills, voluntary stories of communication breakdowns can set the tone for sharing. The story can convey how consultants can help build communication skills for better patient outcomes.

Stories That Convey a Vision

Whenever attempting to convey a vision and enroll others in that vision, the leader must identify "What's In It for Me," or the WIIFM, as it is known in the business community. The chances of staff members becoming engaged in a new vision increase considerably when their potential gain from the effort is clear. President John Kennedy's 1962 speech to Congress about landing a man on the moon before the end of the decade is an example of a speech about a dream or vision. At that time, the space scientists knew 10% of what they needed to know to land a man on the moon. Even after the assassination of Kennedy, the dream continued. All the workers were part of a dream that had captivated men for hundreds of years: humans going to the moon. Vision can be a powerful motivating tool, regardless of the focus of the vision.

Teaching Stories

Regardless of what needs to be taught, teaching stories are very helpful. The technical skills are probably the easiest part. How professionals intervene for a patient is the most important and the more difficult intervention to teach. If the leader wants to teach staff members to be flexible and creative regarding patients' requests, a story

about a time when staff members demonstrated these traits works best.

An example of such a story follows:

In the "old days" in Labor and Delivery, fathers were not allowed in the delivery room. This was true even for fathers who had gone to all the prenatal or Lamaze classes and stayed with their spouse throughout labor. In an attempt to change this "rule," physician acceptance of spouses in the delivery room was paramount. In a somewhat subversive manner, we began with the most sympathetic physician and worked toward the toughest by listing all the physicians who allowed fathers in the delivery room. The epitome of the staff's success came when a mother was transported from a Native American reservation in South Dakota and arrived with eight women of her tribe. The staff convinced the physician to allow all the women to attend the birth with their feathers and other holy objects and to chant in support of the patient. It was a huge success! And everyone present learned something about support of the patient and about the culture and values.

Stories about Values

Role modeling or setting the example is the best way to teach about values. Staff members must understand that mistakes are learning experiences and are not punished.

An example of such a story follows:

When I was a new Director of Women's and Children's Services at a private tertiary center, I wanted to convey to staff that I considered mistakes to be learning experiences and staff would not be punished for mistakes. Within 90 days after I started the job, three night nurses made a life-threatening error with a high-risk perinatal patient. The outcome was grave. All three nurses came to my office with the nurse manager. I asked them what they had learned, and they were speechless. With assistance from the nurse manager, they were able to identify at least three things they had learned. I thanked them for coming in to talk with me but they just sat there. I excused them, and with stunned expressions on their faces, one finally asked, "Aren't you going to fire us?" I indicated that I wasn't. Then I asked, "Could you guarantee that I could find replacements for you who have had the same learning experience and wouldn't make the same mistake you did?" With that they understood that I was serious about mistakes being major learning experiences. (Kowalski, 1996, p. 77)

A Nursing Story

A strong statement is to share a story about how nursing has affected the leader's life and what it means to model for the staff the importance of the profession. By the time a nurse reaches a leadership position, staff members fail to see that this person was ever a "real nurse" and consequently discount or reject observations, suggestions, or objectives based on the leader's "not knowing what it's really like." At these times it is important to be able to draw on some clinical practice stories that highlight having spent time taking care of patients and dealing with issues. The leader can collect several of these stories.

An example of such a story follows:

When I was serving as a 2nd Lieutenant, Army Nurse Corps in Vietnam, we worked whatever hours were needed. The first 3 months of my tour, I was the triage nurse. I was on-call for the pre-op area 24 hours per day, 7 days a week. My hospital received only battle casualties. It was situated next to a helicopter gun ship base. Helicopters that have heavy machine guns sound different from medical evacuation helicopters that have no guns. After a few weeks, I could hear the difference between them as far as 2 miles away from the hospital. I would sleep through the approaches and landings of the gun ships but would hear the "med-evac chopper," wake up, and have my combat boots on and laced by the time the field phone rang to call me up to the pre-op area. It is amazing how the mind can be conditioned to respond in critical circumstances.

Collecting Stories

Stories are more powerful when they relate to the listeners, such as the staff members (Yoder-Wise & Kowalski, 2003). Often they can be humorous or poignant and emphasize teaching or motivating or inspiring or caring. Stories bring meaning to a situation. They can demonstrate that the leader understands exactly what staff members are experiencing. Conscious thought is necessary to create stories. Interesting or funny experiences with staff members, patients, physicians, administrators, or unique family members provide fertile ground for storytelling. A storytelling journal may be helpful, in which notes can be made about experiences that can lead to a good story. This is a tool that facilitates reflection, a critical process for leaders. Guidelines for creating stories are found in Box 9-6.

Developing Stories

In developing stories, leaders consider their own experiences or may use a well-known public figure's experience or stories. Stories from literature, movies, or plays are also an excellent source for creating stories. Dennehy (1999) identifies five steps to develop a story to use with staff members and students (Box 9-7).

SUMMARY

Oral and written communication skills are some of the most powerful tools to create a positive constructive work environment. Better yet, they are learnable and teachable. A leader must identify personal communication filters and refine language, eliminating jargon, poor word choices such as "you" statements, and words such as *should*, *but*, and *try*. To avoid communication breakdown, regardless of stress, leaders can focus on what they feel, what they think, and what they want rather than focusing on frustration, blame, judgment, and demand. Leaders can help people with written communication by teaching how to construct memos, executive summaries, and appropriate e-mails. The CNO can lead the executive group in creating stories and using them in meetings to enroll employees in patient care and in the mission of the facility. Investing the time, interest, and feedback can produce dramatic results.

Box 9-6   GUIDELINES FOR CREATING STORIES

- **Look for themes**. Look for repetitive themes or situations in life, particularly those that represent values, priorities, interests, and experiences. Themes also can evolve from overcoming adversity, securing scarce resources, or creating change and overcoming obstacles.
- **Look for consequences**. Reflect upon the cause and effect of choices. It can be helpful to review aspects of your life chronologically. A specific thing happened or you met a specific person who shaped your choices and thus influenced your life. Think about it from the perspective of the meaning in life rather than merely reciting a specific incident.
- **Look for lessons**. In the process of reflection, ask, "What did I learn from this experience or incident? How did this learning influence me? Was there a flash of insight?" When sharing this incident as a story, others learn much more than when material is presented didactically.
- **Look for what worked**. Personal and professional successes also can be shared in story form. Scrutinize these successes for hidden meanings or principles. The meaning is what is transferable to listeners. Be sure to outline specifically the events that led up to the success such as timing, human and material resources, strategies, and goals.

- **Look for vulnerability**. Be clear about personal imperfections. Do not be afraid to identify them and share them publicly. Some of the best stories are about mistakes, failures, and distractions or derailments that occur along the way. Talking about these with staff conveys to them that you are human too, and it builds trust. Telling such stories conveys both vulnerability and resiliency and also provides balance. No one is perfect and the important thing is what was learned from the experience.
- **Look for humor**. Being able to find the humor in situations emphasizes your humanity. For you to be able to laugh at some crazy event that deteriorated out of control models the ability to laugh at yourself and not take life too seriously. Being funny can lighten the mood of the group and increase productivity. It can build rapport with staff.
- **Build for future experiences**. Often sharing experiences can help others imagine what they would do in a similar situation at some point in the future. Your listeners can extrapolate from what you've learned.
- **Explore other resources**. Stories can be found in many media, such as classic literature, movies, or professional books and journal articles.

Modified from Kaye, B., & Jacobson, B. (1999, March). True tales and tall tales: The power of organizational storytelling. *Training and Development*, pp. 362-371. Reprinted with permission of American Society for Training & Development.

KEY POINTS TO LEAD

1. Identify at least three communication filters you have used in the past month.
2. Analyze at least one communication breakdown that has occurred for you in the past month, including the following: whom you were blaming,

what the judgment was about, what the demands were, and how you would reframe the incident.
3. Review five e-mails you have sent in the past 2 weeks for e-mail etiquette.
4. Describe preparation for a television interview.
5. Construct a letter of recommendation for one of the nurses reporting to you.

Box 9-7   Five Steps in Story Development

1. **Establish the setting**. Describe the time, place, participants, and the setting. If possible, connect the listener with the story by creating a sense of familiarity or identification between the characters and the listener. This process should create a visual picture of the action in the story.
2. **Build the plot**. As the story progresses, create a sense of anticipation or what will happen next. This anticipation and excitement engage the limbic system and increase the memory and learning.
3. **Resolve the crisis**. When bringing the situation in the story to resolution, readers often experience a sense of enlightenment that emphasizes learning or a different perspective. It becomes obvious why the story was told.
4. **Describe the lessons learned**. This description creates a link to the key message. Even though the lesson may seem obvious, listeners may be thinking along a different path. Therefore make your intent clear, because frequently, stories have multiple messages.
5. **Explain how the main characters changed**. The further clarification of what happened to the main character of the story reinforces the ability of the listener to acquire new behaviors or change old, ineffective behaviors.

Modified from Dennehy, R. F. (1999, March). The executive as storyteller. *Management Review*, pp. 356-361.

Literature Box

Institutions that do not welcome disagreement and that punish truth tellers may pay a high price in patient safety and satisfaction. At an unconscious level information may be actively suppressed within the ranks. Policies and processes must be in place that encourage middle managers and employees to relay "bad news" or to voice dissent. Otherwise, the institution is encouraging its people to keep vital information to themselves. Creating a culture that rewards straight talk about problems is essential. To be effective, leaders must have information.

Some of the reasons the information does not reach leaders include their resistance to hearing "bad news," the reluctance of staff members to speak up and deliver the message, staff members covering up problems and mistakes, and organizational structures that discourage information exchange. The author identifies NASA and the Columbia disaster as an example of a culture that discouraged the free flow of information or dissent. The engineers requested a TV view of the wing that would have revealed the 10-inch hole in the tiles, but senior management squelched the request. Organizational barriers existed that prevented effective communication of critical safety information and stifled key differences of opinion. So how would such policies be constructed?

1. *Promise not to kill the messenger, then don't.* This could include adopting a policy of "honesty above all." Deliver the message that staff members will not get into trouble for telling "bad news" to the leaders, but they will get into trouble for not telling the truth, which results in the leadership being "blindsided" by bad news. When the truth is told, the leader and the employees can strategize how to deal with it. Anger and upset on the part of the leader toward the employee (messenger) blocks communication, just as ignoring the message discourages employees in giving bad news in the future. The leader must not only "not kill the messenger" but also must develop relationships in which the leader trusts the staff and they trust the leader. Some of the ways to establish this trust are to

Literature Box

share performance and financial numbers with the staff and to empower staff members to make decisions (such as implementing a shared governance model). The leader can tell staff members when a mistake has been made and what is being implemented to correct it. If the problem is unit-based, the staff can help create strategies to address the situation. Share organizational strategic plans with staff.

2. The leader must create options for *bridging hierarchic gaps*, particularly when a power imbalance exists between the leader and the staff member. The possibility of embarrassment, humiliation, or serious damage to career advancement creates gaps. Significant status differences, such as those between nurses and physicians, contribute to communication problems and breakdown. Staff members are not always comfortable confronting physicians with possible errors. Furthermore, all situations or problems must be debriefed or assessed with a process such as "root cause analysis."

Optimally, an assessment would occur at the midpoint of a process or project.

3. *Avoid communication drift.* Frequently processes are established only to be abandoned when the unit gets busy or people are stressed and pressed for time. Rather, ask questions such as, "What are the implications here?" This can create more openness and understanding between professional groups and between units.

4. *Do not lose sight of the ultimate beneficiary of good communication, the patient.* Communication and even "bad news" can be framed around creating value for the patient and family. The question, "What's best for the patient?" works to bring down barriers to communication.

Bielaszka-DuVernay, C. (2004). How to get the bad news you need. *Management Communication Letters.* Reprint No. CO401A.

Contemplations

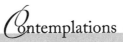

- What communication filter(s) appear the most often in daily interactions?
- How often is jargon used, how many "you" messages are sent, and how many times do *you, but,* or *should* appear in a discussion?
- What happens when a communication breakdown occurs?
- How is blame, judgment, and demand evident in clinical and managerial situations?
- Are you able to paraphrase what another person says?
- Consider having someone teach a class on constructing memos, executive summaries, and e-mail etiquette.
- How can stories be used to increase the effectiveness of the monthly managers meetings?

LEADER STORY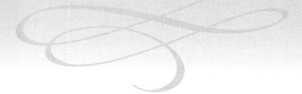

MARGRETTA MADDEN STYLES[†]
2005 CHRISTIANE REIMANN AWARD RECIPIENT
PAST PRESIDENT, INTERNATIONAL COUNCIL OF NURSES
PAST PRESIDENT, AMERICAN NURSES ASSOCIATION
PAST PRESIDENT, AMERICAN NURSES
CREDENTIALING CENTER
FORMER DEAN, UNIVERSITY OF TEXAS HEALTH
SCIENCE CENTER, SAN ANTONIO; WAYNE STATE
UNIVERSITY; UNIVERSITY OF CALIFORNIA,
SAN FRANCISCO

In at least five professional roles communication has played a major, even decisive, part in my career.

The first is teaching, especially doctoral students. I offered seminars on "self-presentation," including all settings and all modes of communication: one-on-one, meetings of small groups, as participant and as leader, ranging from interviews to addressing large audiences. I learned as much about communication from teaching students as I did from reading on the topics.

A second role in which I learned a lot about communication was that of administration. I asked my former assistant dean at UCSF about what stood out for her about my style. She said two things: no surprises and don't write a memo when an issue is on the burner. The first has to do with informing people, including the dean, well in advance on any emerging issue so that they wouldn't be caught unprepared. The latter admonition refers to putting things on the record prematurely and/or when emotions are running high. If you do feel compelled, write it and then tear it up. Do not escalate flaming communications. In other words, there are times not to communicate. Knowing when to remain silent is as important as knowing what to say when you speak up.

Also within the realm of administration I learned that some things about communication are real and others are symbolic. For example, an open office door conveys a message. Making rounds to talk with people, in a sense coming to them, is important. Additionally, retreats can create reflective conversations conducive to strategic planning. In faculty meetings, I would often open with questions and remarks and then we would just talk. Often a number of topics arose that would not be expected. That format was effective and created a bond with and within the group, I believe.

I was very active in interdisciplinary situations with other deans and with top administration. Many times I was the only female. I found it very important to establish through my communication the importance of nursing and mixed genders in leadership. First I had to gain respect for myself and my contributions. In one instance, I challenged the chancellor on a gender issue. From that point on, the women in the other disciplines on campus asked me to speak to their groups. I think they saw me as an advocate for the women and also as a person experienced in dealing with high-level administration.

A third role in which I attempted to promote professional communication was that of author. For example, I was co-author with Pat Moccia of *On Nursing: A Literary Celebration,** a compendium of creative literature, interspersed with commentaries. The purpose was to encourage nurses to use literature widely in reflecting on their

---

*Styles, M. M., & Moccia, P. (1993). *On nursing: A literary celebration: an anthology.* Elkins Park, PA: Jones & Bartlett.
[†]Deceased.

profession and in communicating about nursing. Through this experience I came in contact with colleagues from other countries where nurses seem more likely to reach out through creative writing. Australia and Iceland stand out in my memory.

The fourth role, one in which my communication skills were most challenged, was that of service in elective and appointive positions in professional associations. Consensus building is a major function of such positions, and communication is the foundation of diplomacy. Representing organizations (i.e., serving as the public face and voice of the membership) draws heavily upon a person's ability to communicate to broad and diverse audiences, groups of multiple cultures, norms, and expectations. Other key responsibilities of such positions involve motivating the members to pursue worthy objectives followed by strategic planning toward achievement of such goals. The first requires the ability to inspire with vision; the second demands massive attention to detail and different forms of communication. Above all, communication is two-directional; listening is critical.

Finally, one additional role stressing communication skills was leadership within the credentialing movement, which is my area of expertise, if I could be said to have one. I had first chaired the ANA credentialing study; then I wrote the original International Council of Nurses (ICN) position papers on regulation, which, without amendment, were accepted as the official position of ICN. Having produced these guidelines, we then proceeded to conduct workshops in all the regions of the world. In this manner, representatives of the (then) 120 national nurses associations viewed the "ideal" and then developed projects within their own countries to improve regulation as a form of quality improvement. The sequence was an example of how organizations move from vision to achievement. Currently, I am involved in the definition, education, and regulation issues in advanced practice nursing in the United States. I am building on the book on specialization that

I did some years ago,* by updating and adding the advanced practice component. To continue with the vision to reality theme, I could point out that this book first proposed the formation of the American Board of Nursing Specialties, now very active today in the credentialing movement.

Each of those roles represents an area in which I thought communication was critical. They served as sources of many lessons and perspectives.

My ultimate lesson in communication is preparation, preparation, preparation. Whether it is for an interview or a committee meeting or a presentation to 10,000 people, the key is preparation. I am an absolute detailist. What I mean by this is gathering information on the background of the issues. Also, organizing thoughts, assessing the audience, and setting goals are really important. These strategies apply whether the group is small or large. After determining my goals, I outline the content and then rehearse. I try to anticipate all contingencies. For example, with respect to auditorium presentations, if the podium is too low, I slip off my shoes; if it is too high, I ask for any box that would be sturdy enough to stand on. I tell students not to turn pages, if using notes. Slipping pages from one side to the other is less noisy and less visually distracting.

Although words are the smallest part of communication, I believe key phrases are most inspirational and memorable. Words can be symbolic of a whole line of thought. For example, in 2003 I spoke to the ANA House of Delegates and used the phrase, "the house of nursing." I proposed to delegates that they not think of the assembly as the house of delegates, but the house of nursing. In the debate that followed, several speakers used the phrase "house of nursing" in their appeals for unity. Words are symbolic of a whole line of thinking or a whole philosophy.

Another example of using symbols in speaking to inspire and instill vision took place when I spoke

*Styles, M. M. (1989). *On specialization in nursing: Toward a new empowerment.* Kansas City, MO: American Nurses Foundation.

at the Acropolis in Athens, as president of ICN. That ancient Greek setting was both intimidating and inspiring. The audience was diverse and included lay people, local dignitaries, and nurses from various countries. I thought about the audience and envisioned this speech. I wanted to be simple and clear. The goal was to create a dream for nursing that nurses and lay people would understand. My theme was Seven Ultimate Victories for Nursing. Each point began with using a "V" sign and the phrase, "Victory will be declared and celebrated, the day that…." The victories were in education, practice, research, management, socio-economic welfare, ethics, and policy. For example, the one on policy was worded: "Victory will be declared and celebrated the day that a nurse, backed by a unified and respected profession, occupies the position of Director General of the World Health Organization." As I traveled around the world from that time on, nurses would remind me of the seven victories. Words create dreams and visions. They create hope. Actions create success.

ICN established the practice of the president creating a watchword to set the tone for the 4-year term of office. I adopted that same tradition at ANA. My word was "March," both with ANA and ICN. It was derived from an admonition attributed to Florence Nightingale, "No system shall endure that does not march." I was fascinated to discover that I was the only ICN president who selected a verb as the watchword, which demonstrates my passion for activism.

Consensus building requires considerable skill and planning. I probably have had more experience in such formal processes than most nurses. I have found it is useful to be "within" and not preside over the group. It is also important to ascertain what everyone wants, in other words, the bottom line for all. I think it is effective to lead the group in devising a set of principles and goals and then to develop and adhere to a framework for the discussion. After reaching accord, next steps must be addressed.

Two forms of interpersonal communication have worked for me, although they are seemingly contradictory. The first is humor. I have found that humor assists in connecting with someone or turning the tide in a stressful situation. I have an irrepressible, but dangerous sense of humor. It has taught me, as ICN president, that one must be very careful in using humor with other cultures. It essentially could undermine what one is trying to do. The other form, of a very different nature, is that of the short, direct answer, such as "no way," "never," or "absolutely not." This type of message has to be delivered very, very carefully. I convey these messages with a facial expression that intends to say I want you to understand where the borders are and that I respect you and trust you with this understanding. This clarity facilitates the expectations of others. When they respond similarly, I am pleased.

Communication is very, very personal. This is a lesson not mentioned in many writings on the subject. Developing someone's own style is the secret to success. People often come to me if they are very, very stressed. I usually tell them that life is like eating an elephant. You have to size it up and then eat one bite at a time. Pace yourself but continue to eat.

I also am often asked for career counseling. The words I use to sum up my philosophy on career building are, "Build it and they will come," from the movie *Field of Dreams*. Develop yourself as an expert within a field that is in need or demand. People will come. Opportunities will unfold. The career will flow.

Chapter References

American Organization of Nurse Executives. (2005). AONE Nurse Executive Competencies. *Nurse Leader, 3*(2), 15-21.

Business Letter Writing. (2003). *The secret to effective business communication.* Retrieved November 9, 2005 from http://www.business-letter-writing.com/writing-a-business-letter-examples.

Chesanow, N. (1987, September 17). Quick, take this memo. *The Washington Post,.* Retrieved November 14, 2005, from http://rcw.raiuniversity.edu/management/bba/Business Comm/lecture-notes/lecture-22.pdf.

Clayton, J. (2003). Crafting a powerful executive summary. *Harvard Business School, Working Knowledge Newsletter.* Retrieved November 9, 2005, from http://hbswk.hbs.edu/item.jhtml?id=366094=career_effectiveness.

Colorado State University. (2005). Writing@CSU: writing guides. Retrieved November 9, 2005, from http://writing.colostate.edu/guides.

Crane, T. G. (2002). *The heart of coaching: Using transformational coaching to create a high-performance culture.* (2nd Ed.). San Diego, CA: FTA Press.

Dennehy, R. F. (1999, March). The executive as storyteller. *Management Review,* pp. 356-361.

eHOW. (2004). *How to write an executive summary.* Retrieved November 9, 2005, from http://www.ehow.com/how_16566_write-executive-summary.html.

English Works at Gallaudet University. (2002). *How to write memos?* Washington, DC. Retrieved November 9, 2005, from http://depts.gallaudet.edu/englishworks/writing/memowriting.html.

Gill, P. (2005). *Once upon an enterprise: The ancient art of storytelling emerges as a tool for knowledge management.* Retrieved November 7, 2005, from http://www.destinationcrm.com/km/dcrm_km_article.asp?id=823.

Guidelines for writing an executive summary. Richard T. Farmer School of Business. Miami University. (2004). Retrieved August 26, 2005, from http://www.sba.muohio.edu/hwi/executivesummary.htm.

Ibarra, H., & Lineback, K. (2005). What's your story? *Harvard Business Review, 83*(1), 65-71.

Kaye, B., & Jacobson, B. (1999, March). True tales and tall tales: The power of organizational storytelling. *Training and Development,* pp. 362-371.

Kowalski, K. E. (1996). From failure to major learning experience. *The American Journal Of Maternal Child Nursing, 21,* 76-79.

Kowalski, K. (2004). Powerful presentations. Castle Rock, CO.: The Author.

Kowalski, K. (2004a). Teaching tips: The use of set. *The Journal of Continuing Education in Nursing, 35*(2), 56-57.

Kowalski, K. (2004b). Teaching tips: The use of closure. *The Journal of Continuing Education in Nursing, 35*(4), 152.

Kowalski, K. (2005a). Teaching tips: Keeping participants enrolled: Use of anticipation. *The Journal of Continuing Education in Nursing, 36*(1), 16.

Kowalski, K. (2005b). Teaching tips: Keeping participants enrolled: Use of gradient. *The Journal of Continuing Education in Nursing, 36*(5), 195-206.

Leeds, D. (1987). *Smart questions: A new strategy for successful managers.* New York: Berkley Books.

Luthy, M. (2005). Recommendation letter tips, tricks, and advice. WriteExpress. Retrieved Jaunary 12, 2005, from http://www.writeexpress.com/recommendation-letters.html.

McFee, R. (2003). Storytelling that moves people. *Harvard Business Review, 81*(6), 51-56.

Patterson, K., Grenny, J., McMillan, R., & Switzler, A. (2002). *Crucial conversations: Tools for talking when stakes are high.* New York: McGraw-Hill.

Porche, G., & Niederer, J. (2001). *Coach anyone about anything: How to help people succeed in business and life.* Del Mar, CA: Wharton.

Senge, P. M., Kleiner, A., Roberts, C., Ross, R. B., & Smith, B. (1994). *The fifth discipline fieldbook: Strategies and tools for building a learning organization.* New York: Doubleday Dell.

Simmons A. (2001). *The story factor: Secrets of influence from the art of storytelling.* Cambridge, MA: Perseus Publishing.

Texas Tech University Health Sciences Center. (2002). Nursing 5371. Syllabus. Lubbock, TX: The Author.

University of Wisconsin-Green Bay. (2004). *Writing letters of recommendation.* Retrieved November 9, 2005, from http://www.uwgb.edu/careers/recommendation_letters.htm.

Verba, C. (2004). *GSAS guide for teaching fellows on writing letters of recommendation.* Derek Bok Center for Teaching and Learning, Harvard University. Retrieved November 9, 2005, from http://bokcenter.fas.harvard.edu/docs/Verba-recs.html.

Weissman, J. (2005). *In the line of fire: How to handle tough questions . . . when it counts.* Upper Saddle River, NJ: Pearson Education, Inc./Prentice Hall.

Yale University Library. (1999). *Email etiquette.* Retrieved November 9, 2005, from http://www.library.yale.edu/training/netiquette.

Yoder-Wise, P., & Kowalski, K. E. (2003). The power of storytelling. *Nursing Outlook, 51*(1), 37-51.

10 Leadership and Creating Teams

It marks a big step in your development when you come to realize that other people can help you do a better job than you could do alone. ANDREW CARNEGIE

This chapter discusses the role of the chief nursing officer (CNO) in mastering the concepts and tools with which to create, lead, and maintain a smoothly functioning team. The CNO's role of important team member in the senior leadership team also is addressed.

MANY AREAS OF A LEADER'S LIFE REQUIRE working in a smooth and efficient manner with other professionals, including the development of collaborative partnerships. A healthcare team can include physicians, nurses, administrators, allied health professionals, and support staff such as housekeeping and dietary. Most people recognize a smoothly functioning team such as a *rapid response team,* which is called for in patient emergencies. Even healthcare professionals do not necessarily analyze what constitutes the effectiveness of such teams. How much practice occurs to have a flawless resuscitation? What are the relationships between the team members? What motivates them? What values are in place? Do they have team meetings?

Rapid response teams are not the only teams in a healthcare facility. Having a smoothly functioning nursing leadership team is reasonable. Striving for a functioning senior management team also is reasonable. However, some differences exist between

leading a team and participating as a team member. The first part of this chapter focuses on how the CNO can create an effective and efficient leadership team. Most nurse leaders have at one point in their career been a member of a team that was exciting, wonderful, effective, and memorable. Some of these memories can serve as a starting point from which to create, maintain, and troubleshoot a nursing leadership team.

> *Coming together is a beginning*
> *Keeping together is progress*
> *Working together is success*
> JOHN C. MAXWELL

DEFINITION OF TEAM

The word *team* seems to be used loosely in healthcare, particularly in the past 10 years. In the 1990s, everyone was focused on building teams. It was the "in thing" to do. Managers and administrators didn't adhere to the concept and then wondered why the results were borderline at best.

Teams require work and preparation. Teams are inhibited by the need for quick decisions, the ongoing technical and social training required to create smoothly functioning teams, the high level of skill in the team leader required to deal with interteam and intrateam conflict, the logistics of meeting times, and the expense of releasing team members from regular duties (Billington, 1997; Ray, 1999). Teams do not exist because they are mandated by the nurse leader. They take work, thoughtfulness, focus, problem solving, and acknowledgment. Thoughtful consideration is necessary for choosing and developing or building teams (Box 10-1).

For purposes of this chapter, a team is defined as a small group of individuals that achieve higher collective results or outcomes through cohesiveness, cooperation, consensus, collaboration, focus, commitment, and hard work, including empowerment of one another, togetherness, and effective use of small group dynamics. For famous, effective examples of such teams, see the work of Bennis and Biedermann (1997), which is discussed in the Literature box on p. 209. According to Huszczo (2004), the word *team* comes from the Latin root *deuk*, which means "to pull." In other words, a team pulls together to reach a common goal.

Nurse executives may lead groups of nursing directors, or if they work hard, may lead a team that has specific purposes such as quality patient care or obtaining Magnet status. If the facility has approximately 200 beds, a team will probably be a nursing director group. If the facility is much smaller, the team may be a group of managers.

The American Association of Critical Care Nurses (2005) created Standards for Establishing and Sustaining Healthy Work Environments. Rather than address the issues in terms of teams, they addressed the importance of collaboration, especially in the many ways in which teams were formally discussed. True collaboration is defined as an ongoing process rather than an event. This process results in communication and joint decision making between nurses and other professionals, particularly physicians, and among only nurses. In true collaboration, the unique knowledge and abilities of each professional group are respected to achieve safe care of the highest quality for patients and their families. This true collaboration requires skilled communication, trust, knowledge, shared responsibility, mutual respect, optimism, and coordination. Many of these behaviors and activities also are required for smoothly functioning teams.

Box 10-1 Guidelines for Team Building

1. Form teams for their value in creating answers and accomplishing goals, not because they are in vogue.
2. Assess each team member in terms of his or her relationship skills and abilities for the task.
3. Commit openly to honest, direct discussions.
4. Use a guide to ensure that elements of team success are incorporated (e.g., the activities on pp. 190-191).
5. Build each team based on its distinctive abilities. Fill in missing skill sets (see pp. 190-191) necessary for achieving the team's goals.
6. Support the team by removing or reducing organizational barriers.
7. Create an esprit de corps, which may include creating and using mottos, logos, signals, and symbols.
8. Be present...physically and mentally to determine the mood and status of the team.
9. Value the ongoing process of building a team.
10. Invest in the growth and activities of the team.
11. Value continuous improvement in the team.
12. Share the power of the leader.
13. Celebrate accomplishments
14. Encourage team members to lead the other teams.

Based on Huszczo, G. (2004). *Tools for team leadership*. Palo Alto, CA: Davies-Black.

Authors seem to agree that teams that achieve excellence have common key components (Brounstein, 2002; Huszczo, 2004; Katzenbach, 1998; Katzenbach & Smith, 1993; Maxwell, 2002a, 2002b). These elements of success include such activities as the following:

1. **Developing clear goals and a sense of direction:** The purpose of the team is clear, the goals are challenging and stated in ways that can be measured, and all members are committed to the goals.
2. **Identification of talent:** The leader determines what talent exists on the team and whether it is being fully utilized and continuously developed.
3. **Clearly defined roles and responsibilities:** Each member knows his or her role and how it will lead to success for the team.
4. **Consensus regarding procedures:** These are established for planning, making decisions, completing the tasks, holding meetings, and solving problems.
5. **Positive interpersonal communication and relationships:** Members demonstrate respect for one another, differences are celebrated, and conflicts are resolved.
6. **Active internal and organizational team-oriented behaviors:** Members are recognized for living up to their responsibilities and for helping teammates.
7. **Positively evolving external (to the team) relationships with other segments of the organization:** The team nurtures relationships with other teams, particularly as they support the primary purpose of the organization: The Patient Comes First.

The attributes identified above are not easy to achieve. According to Huszczo (2004), although he tried his best to deny it for more than 20 years, leadership is the key to achieving excellent results. In most of his research, he found that in reality, even in successful teams, most often one or two people carried the team. Leaderless teams do not work (Davis & Sharon, 2002). If the nurse leader is to support the creation of truly effective teams, it requires that every member of the team must work toward the goal. Consequently, it is better for the team to have some insight into how this group functions both separately and together. Several skills are required of the leader of a team if optimal team functioning is to be achieved:

1. Help the team to take an honest look at itself. This honest look includes an accurate assessment of its actions and its structure. Smoothly functioning teams may look like magic, but a supporting foundation and structure allow them to be successful. When it succeeds, the question to pursue is, "Why do things go well?" And when it is struggling, "What, specifically, are the problems?" As the leader, you can support the team to identify patterns. The first step to becoming more effective is for the team to understand its strengths and its problems. See Box 10-2 for an example of how to assess a team.
2. Support the generation of options. With teams, more than one way always exists to generate excellence. Rather, the role of the leader is to stimulate, usually with questions, multiple options for addressing issues. The excellence of teams evolves from the diversity of available viewpoints. One way to free up the thinking of team members is to use brainstorming to achieve additional strategies and tactics. Early in the evolution of the team, one role of the leader is to guide members in first expanding their thinking about strategies and then focusing them on the action(s) to be taken.
3. Plan for success. Often teams are so pleased when they arrive at a solution that they fail to ensure the implementation of the solution. The team must operationalize the solutions they derive.

When leading a team, several factors are important to remember. First, the leader must strive to influence rather than control the team. The goal is to create collaborative partnerships while helping others help themselves (Weiss & Hughes, 2005).

Box 10-2 Team Assessment

A team is only as good as it becomes. To determine whether a team is currently functional and is moving forward in its operational effectiveness, review the following questions. This tool can be used by the team leader, a team member, or the whole team. Circle the number on the form to reflect your assessment of each item. The ratings are from1 (the team has problems) to 5 (the team functions extremely well).

	Low...............High
1. Members of the team value the organization's values.	1 2 3 4 5
2. Members of the team value the work of the team.	1 2 3 4 5
3. Members of the team are committed to the organization.	1 2 3 4 5
4. Members of the team are committed to each other.	1 2 3 4 5
5. Members of the team are committed to improvement.	1 2 3 4 5
6. Members of the team are willing to take risks.	1 2 3 4 5
7. Members of the team commit to the truth.	1 2 3 4 5
8. Members of the team hold open, honest communications.	1 2 3 4 5
9. The ambiance of the team meetings is such that disagreement is encouraged and welcomed.	1 2 3 4 5
10. Members of the team would say they trust each other.	1 2 3 4 5
11. Members of the team engage in difficult conversations.	1 2 3 4 5
12. Members of the team take no criticism personally.	1 2 3 4 5
13. Members of the team see their interdependence with other members of the team.	1 2 3 4 5
14. Members of the team are present (psychologically as well as physically) for their team members.	1 2 3 4 5
15. Members of the team actively engage in conversations and the work of the team.	1 2 3 4 5
16. Members of the team keep promises made to each other and to themselves.	1 2 3 4 5
17. Members of the team commit to the execution of decisions made by the team.	1 2 3 4 5
18. Members of the team are supportive of each other and hold each other in high regard.	1 2 3 4 5
19. Members of the team ask for, have, or obtain the necessary resources to be effective in executing their work.	1 2 3 4 5
20. Members of the team move easily between the roles of leader and follower.	1 2 3 4 5

SCORE TOTAL ————

Total all circled numbers. That is the team assessment score. The higher the score, the more likely that the team is more positive and effective.

90 to 100 The team is working well.

80 to 89 The team is working fairly well, but has some potential to improve.

70 to 79 The team is minimally functional and needs to address issues that prevent its best work.

69 and below The team is in trouble and needs considerable work, including restructuring the team, consultation, facilitation, or refocusing on the relevance of the team.

Leaders are created, not born. No DNA leadership traits exist. Rather, some people develop their skills through formal or informal education and nurture their opportunities, making the best of each situation, whereas other people squander both. Nurse leaders must be willing to apply themselves to learn the skills and to develop their talents. This process involves an important aspect of self-reflection in this approach.

In the spirit of self-reflection, several aspects of leadership with teams follow (Brounstein, 2002; Davis & Sharon, 2002). *No specific characteristics or behaviors predict leadership success.* Some team members or nurse leaders have technical or business skills but no people skills. Others have people skills but lack technical and business competencies. Team functionality is facilitated when the leader approximates the same intellectual level as the team members. That is, the leader should neither be excessively smarter than team members nor significantly less smart than other members of the team. What is needed is for the leader to simultaneously be *both task and people oriented.* To accomplish this goal requires total dedication to getting the job done while demonstrating full respect for team members. Although getting the job done well is critical to the overall success of the organization, relationships matter very much. Effective nurse leaders request input; they listen, they encourage, and they celebrate success.

The nurse leader's *style must correlate to both the work to be accomplished and the members of the team.* Usually the most appropriate style is participative because it gains commitment rather than compliance. Although a crisis may indicate the *temporary* use of a more directive style, its excessive use can destroy a team. The leader must be flexible yet wise.

Credibility is the key. The team members must believe in the leader. This belief comes from trustworthiness, which is a function of the leader being reliable and dependable. Actions must be consistent with the words of the leader, who must be careful about promises. Leaders keep promises small; they do not promise too much or exaggerate, and they always follow through on any promises made.

Credibility also requires knowledge and competence about the administrative tasks, operations, the organization, and the people involved. (In other words, the nurse leader models expertise in the administrative role.) Bluffing results in a major learning experience and usually is not effective. What is required is a commitment to continuous learning regarding professional knowledge and skills. Credibility also requires enthusiasm in what the leader says and does with the team. The goal is to generate energy in the team, and that is unlikely without great enthusiasm from the leader.

The leader knows how *to focus* on the problem or issue. With all the ongoing issues and activities in addition to leading the team, the only way for the nurse leader to accomplish all these tasks and outcomes is to remain focused. At the same time the leader must be open to feedback to improve his or her leadership of the team. Strong nurse leaders are aware of their strengths and their weaknesses. They model continuous improvement in their leadership skills through working on one or two weaknesses at a time. They focus on what they can improve in the moment. They do not attempt to be all things to all people; they focus on developing specific skills (Box 10-3).

From another perspective, a skill set in team construction and maintenance is recommended for nurse leaders. These skill sets are in the areas of knowledge, behaviors, and personal qualities. The knowledge set needed for success in leadership consists of understanding the organization's plans, including the roles, responsibilities, procedures, and expectations for team development. The team leader also needs to know and understand the overall company rules, including any union contracts. Next, the leader needs technical knowledge of the clinical area and particularly the product, which in this case is quality patient care. In addition, the leader needs to know the organizational culture and politics and to understand the formal and the informal information structure in addition to who can provide access to the information. Finally, the leader needs to have an understanding of people and individual personalities. The behavioral skills

Box 10-3   Areas for the Development of the Team Leader

1. Recommit to the servant leader role. Everyday, effective leaders ask what they have done for someone else and have examples they can site.
2. Learn from personal experience and self-reflection to ensure that future mistakes are new ones and lessons learned from errors are incorporated into personal development.
3. Ponder what effective leadership means, using research, journals, publications from other fields, and conversations with "experts" to form a personal view.
4. Evaluate skill sets as they relate to leading an effective team, including clear goals, well-defined roles and responsibilities, effective team-operating procedures, positive interpersonal relationships, well-developed team talent, and mutually established accountability within the team.
5. Compare personal strengths with the characteristics of an effective leader, and focus on self-development as well as complementing these strengths and personal growth areas with team members that complete the skill set.
6. Perform ongoing assessments of the participative leadership skills that are proven effective in a team environment, such as preparing, planning, organizing, motivating, monitoring, and building commitment.
7. Access, understand, and utilize personality and work-style profiles for the leader and the team members, capitalizing on identified strengths and working to understand differences and how these predicts the interactions of team members.
8. Identify and develop conflict resolution strategies for the team with a focus on a win/win approach while recognizing the advantages and the disadvantages of conflict and developing strategies for dealing with particularly difficult people.
9. Recognize the importance of the change process within organizations, and develop approaches to communicating organizational change within the facility.
10. Understand how to identify symptoms of stress in self and in team members while acknowledging the possible consequences of stress and implementing stress reduction strategies.
11. Focus on a specific plan to use any and all team training received, especially the assessment of the current state of the team, problems within the team, and how to constructively cope with the problems.
12. Be ready to let go; allow team members to develop and enhance personal skills through learning from their own successes.
13. Identify strategies to develop team members for leadership of future teams.

Based on Developing Team Leaders from Huszczo, G. (2004). *Tools for team leadership*. Palo Alto, CA: Davies-Black.

that support a nurse leader working with teams include the following (Davis & Sharon, 2002):

- Communicating
- Listening actively
- Solving problems
- Facilitating meetings
- Facilitating discussions
- Facilitating decision making
- Giving group presentations
- Speaking publicly
- Holding people accountable
- Motivating
- Planning
- Organizing
- Managing time
- Writing reports

- Resolving conflict
- Using diplomacy
- Networking

Examples of the personal qualities needed by the nurse leader include the following:

- Approachable
- Committed
- Compassionate
- Creative
- Direct
- Fun loving
- Honest
- Humorous
- Nonprejudicial
- Nonjudgmental
- Open to new ideas
- Patient
- Persistent
- Respectful
- Responsive
- Resourceful
- Sincere
- Trustworthy

The Management Research Group (1998) in Portland, Maine, has created the Leadership Effectiveness Analysis instrument, which includes the following six sets of behaviors. This tool can be used by organizations to determine appropriate fit with their organization, as well as by the individual to perform a self-assessment to determine strengths and weaknesses for team leadership. These sets of behaviors were derived from work with some 30,000 leaders.

1. *Creating a vision.* The nurse leader needs to be able to help the team create a vision that will orient their efforts. If it's a collaborative effort with the team, and McKenna and Maister (2002) firmly believe it should be, it can be facilitated by asking questions, actively brainstorming, and then using some type of modified Delphi process to prioritize the brainstorming items. Both a short-range and a long-range vision are possible, depending on what the focus of the team is.

2. *Developing followership.* Some nurse leaders use persuasion to convince the team of their point of view. This connection also can be created through being friendly, informal, and outgoing. Many leaders display great enthusiasm and energy for the motivation of the team, whereas others attempt to calm the team members and minimize any potentially destructive emotional displays (perhaps a high-energy critical care unit). It is valuable for the leader to assess the group and her or his own level of skills to choose the approach that will work best.

3. *Implementing the vision.* The next step beyond creating the vision is the implementation, which requires another skill set. One team may require a systematic, organized approach, including step-by-step processes to accomplish the goal. Another team may require considerable time and clear communication concerning expectations and a continuous flow of information. Yet another team and leader may use delegation because the team includes a very talented nurse who wants to be turned loose on the project. Is the leader able to select any of these approaches or is it better to select one approach that fits the leader's style?

4. *Following through.* In this process, the nurse leader needs to focus on control and feedback. Can he or she set very clear deadlines with specific outcomes at each point in time? How closely does the leader feel a need to monitor? Does it depend on the team? What kind of feedback is needed and when should it be given? (For more information on feedback and coaching, see Chapter 11.)

5. *Achieving results.* Strong leaders seek to exert influence through their position and authority. They take charge, lead, and direct the team. They tend to be somewhat dominant, pushing vigorously to achieve the desired results. They tend to be quite competitive. They hold high expectations of themselves and of all the members of the team.

6. *Team-Playing.* Successful leaders are cooperative and accommodate the needs and the different characteristics of team members. They value the ideas, perspectives, and opinions of other team members, using this input as part of the decision-making process. They are loyal to the organization and respect their administrative superiors who are viewed as sources of information and direction. They form close and supportive relationships with other team members.

CREATION OF THE TEAM

Selection of the Team

Because several types of teams are in a hospital, clarifying with which type the leader is working is important. For example, if the team consists of a given shift on a unit, selection occurs when the nurses are hired. If the team is a group such as the rapid response team, members will come from across disciplines, and the composition needs careful consideration (Box 10-4). If the team is within the nursing division and its purpose is organizing to obtain Magnet status, careful consideration is necessary to include nurses from such areas as quality improvement, nursing education, and shared governance councils.

The Stages of Teams

Tuckman and Jensen's (1965, 1977) work on the stages of small group work has survived into this century and is still being used by those focused on the development of teams (Davis & Sharon, 2002; Huszczo, 2004; Outhwaite, 2003). According to Tuckman, teams tend to go through various stages as they develop.

Forming

This is the stage at which individuals begin to see themselves as team members. This period can include confusion, testing of behaviors (both

Box 10-4 Guidelines for Team Member Selection

- The goal is to have the right people as part of the team. Be clear about the purpose of the team as well as what talent, knowledge, and personal qualities are needed. Are there protocols or organizational politics that should be considered? (Davis & Sharon, 2002)
- Should certain leaders in the organization give suggestions regarding the composition of the team?
- What criteria for involvement have been developed (e.g., are any physicians needed)?
- What skills and qualities are needed on the team in addition to subject matter expertise? For example, have any nurses participated in a Magnet effort before?
- Should any categories of membership be identified (e.g., resource people who only attend when needed)?

- How should team members and their managers be notified?
- Because team responsibilities will require time away from previously assigned duties, how will priorities be clarified? Who will replace a team member for the time in which the person is dedicated to the team project, and how will the costs be covered?
- How will activities of the team members be evaluated in performance reviews?
- How does a system-wide team or an interdisciplinary team relate to the rest of the organization? Who ensures alignment and integration?
- Could membership on such teams be part of succession planning and leadership development? If so, how would this be coordinated?

oneself and the other members), and getting to know how each member fits in with the rest of the group. While attempting to understand the political undercurrents and the dynamics of the group, team members often depend significantly on the team leader for direction, information, and vision.

Leader's Role in This Stage. The leader needs to begin with a team purpose, which would include goals, responsibilities, procedures, and ground rules or norms. (See Box 10-5 for an example of rules.) These rules or norms must be clear so that each member feels respected and valued for his or her contribution (Laing, 2003). The team purpose is about why the team has been formed and what the goals are. For example, the team might be the Magnet Organizing Committee, and the purpose might be exploration of what is needed to meet Magnet criteria and assessment of what actions are necessary to meet the criteria.

Storming

This stage is characterized by "jockeying for position," infighting, challenges among group members, defensiveness, and competition. Team members have emotional responses and resist demands. Fault finding and blaming can occur among members.

Leader's Role in This Stage. A key benefit to teams is differing points of view. These differences can lead to competition for influence and thus to conflict. The leader must support the team in learning how to handle conflict constructively and help them understand that disagreements are normal. These competitive urges must be channeled toward the team goal. The more specific the goals, the easier this task is to accomplish (see the following section/sections for specifics about conflict).

Norming

This stage is characterized by calm and effective working together. The rules for how the team will cooperate and work together have been defined and

accepted. Members embrace the responsibilities, establish harmony, and achieve their goals.

Leader's Role in This Stage. The best teams choose how they will organize group actions, including meeting structure, problem solving, and decision making. They discuss options and reach agreement. Holding people to their agreements helps build belief in the team and creates trust. Overachieving team members may be reluctant to rely on the rest of the team, thinking they could do it better themselves. The leader can step in to update and reconfirm the team's purpose, facilitate team member learning regarding problem solving and decision making, and run effective meetings. Then the leader holds members accountable for what they learned. The leader also can support through providing awareness and feedback about the processes in addition to facilitating a short debriefing at the end of the meeting.

Performing

The team is fully functioning and accomplishes tasks according to the team rules and goals. Each member knows his or her roles and responsibilities. Accountability, responsibility, and authority have been clearly defined (Box 10-6). The team has established high performance, including high-level problem solving and decision making. They seem to have a high level of personal insight and have grown and changed since beginning with the team. When changes occur, the focus is on what is best for the team, the project, the company, and the employees.

Leader's Role in This Stage. The leader must help team members know if they are accomplishing the goals. Regular feedback on team goals or outcomes is provided. The team must be allowed to do work and then be given feedback about progress against expectations. Guidelines for debriefing and feedback are in Box 10-7.

Closing

When the task is completed, the team disbands.

Box **10-5** AN EXAMPLE OF RULES FOR TEAMS

These "rules of the game"* were adapted from a San Francisco real estate broker who was the founder and president of Hawthorn-Stone.† Karren Kowalski adapted these rules to nursing practice. She proposes that nurses use the rules for themselves and with each new person who joins the organization. Those using the rules should be asked if they are willing and able to do the very best they can to support the rules.

1. **Be willing to support the organization's purpose, games, rules, and goals.** By first asking if people will support the rules, we have their agreement that they can be held accountable for times when they violate the "rules of the game."

2. **Speak supportively.** If it does not serve a purpose, do not say it. If it does not support others, do not say it. Do not make other people wrong. You may choose not to say negative things. This means no swearing. Language either empowers or limits people in terms of achieving their potential. How we speak about such topics as a colleague, the institution, our job, or the workplace does make a difference.

3. **Correct supportively.** Make corrections without invalidation or correct without crucifixion.

4. **Acknowledge that whatever is being communicated is true for the speaker at that moment.** Most of the time people make comments because they truly believe them. Therefore it is important not to judge what is being said and misinterpret it but to listen so that we can understand what is being said. The emphasis is on active listening.

5. **Complete your agreement.** Only make agreements that you intend to and are willing to keep. This is especially important for those who (a) procrastinate and (b) say "yes" to everything. If one must break an agreement, communicate this information ASAP.

6. **If a problem arises, first use the system for corrections, then communicate the problem with optional solutions to the person who can do something about the problem.** This is another way to eliminate gossip, judgment, and self-righteousness.

7. **Be effective and efficient.**

8. **Optimize every event—create more with less.** Items 7 and 8 go together. Look for value in every event. Focus on what can be learned or done; use "lateral thinking" to create effective options.

9. **Have the willingness to win and to allow others to win.** "Win/lose" is a "zero sum game," so someone must win and someone else must lose. Effective problem solving allows everyone to win or for their needs to be fulfilled.

10. **Focus on what works.** The converse of this concept is to relinquish what is not working. Be willing to try something new. When something about the workplace or system is broken, fix it!

11. **When in doubt, explore feelings.** When communication or progress seems to be blocked, it often is related to how people are feeling. Explore these feelings by talking to the person or people in question. Get the feelings out in the open, where they can be addressed.

12. **Agree to disagree until reaching a consensus.** Commit to working together toward mutually agreeable solutions. This keeps things in a forward motion without judgment. It keeps things hopeful.

13. **Tell the truth from the point of view of personal responsibility.** Always begin with the assumption that you are willing to assume 50% of the responsibility. This eliminates "you, you, you" messages and allows you to work with others toward a solution, not toward blame.

Modified from Kowalski, K. E., Burton, L., & Rehwaldt, M. (1997). Re-visioning, re-educating, re-generating and re-committing: Nursing in the 21st century. *Nursing Outlook, 45*(5), 220-223.
*"Rules of the Game" for Women's and Children's Hospital, Rush-Presbyterian–St. Luke's Medical Center.
†Marshall Thurber, Hawthorne-Stone, San Francisco, CA.

Box 10-6   CRUCIAL CONCEPTS WITHIN TEAMS

RESPONSIBILITY

Reponsibility is the legal, moral, mental, and ethical obligation to fulfill one's job or role. This encompasses reliability, which means keeping promises in addition to reliability in behavior, actions, accomplishments, and any failures or mistakes. Responsibility must be accepted so that the responsible person can then be held accountable.

ACCOUNTABILITY

Accountability means to hold someone (or a team) accountable or to hold responsible or to have one person or team commit to an obligation. Accountability is the core of a successfully aligned organization. Accountability is the way in which an identified person is held responsible for a specific job or task. It eliminates confusion or doubt on an individual level in addition to how the organization will measure effort based on promises by individuals who commit to the goals of the facility.

AUTHORITY

Authority is the right and freedom of the CNO to use management power and to ultimately enforce compliance with organizational policies and procedures. CNOs must deploy corporate resources and authority and effectively delegate to directors, and managers must have a span of control to implement compliance appropriately.

From Hellen Davis, CLU, Author and CEO of Indaba, Inc. *The 21 laws of influence.* (2004). St. Petersburg, FL: Indaba, Inc.

Leader's Role in This Stage. In this instance, the goal is to facilitate positive closure for the team. The team needs to feel appreciated for its efforts and also recognized by administration. Members will want to be assured that the ideas and outcomes of the team project will be utilized. It will be valuable to the organization to identify the lessons learned to improve future team projects. The members also may identify bigger system problems over which they have no control and over which feelings of frustration occur. As the team is closing down, some members may experience separation anxiety. A sense of "loss" often occurs as the team is dissolved. The leader remains alert to the process of loss while creating a genuine celebration for the team.

LEADING THE TEAM

Communication

Most teams, at least at some point in the process, complain about communication. Consequently, the team leader's communication skills are paramount to helping the team with their communication skills. The first priority is the ability of the team leader to communicate clearly the team's purpose, any current or up-to-date organizational information that would affect the team, and any changes in the expectations that will influence the team. The skills that are basic to the team leader and the team members in communicating are sharing information, listening effectively, and providing feedback (Brounstein, 2002).

Sharing information means providing facts in a meaningful and useful manner. (For more information regarding expanding skills in sharing information, see Box 10-8 and Chapter 9.)

Listening effectively is more important than sharing information. For the leader, listening is key to understanding, relationship building, problem solving, and learning or gathering information. As discussed in Chapter 9, many adults have not learned to listen. Few adults can describe what they have heard before evaluating and judging the message. When team leaders demonstrate that they heard the message, it is a powerful way to show respect. Active listening is a way to connect to team members.

Box 10-7   DEBRIEFING SESSION
            AND FEEDBACK ON THE
            ACTIONS TAKEN

After each meeting and each significant
action or event the team has implemented, a debriefing needs to occur
that documents the outcomes and lessons learned from the process. The
following questions support this debriefing process.
1. How did this meeting go? What about
    the meeting process worked or didn't
    work?
2. What specific events or actions were
    taken?
3. What actually happened in each
    instance?
4. What was learned from the meeting?
5. What are the next steps considering
    what was learned?
6. What is the specific plan for putting
    what was learned into action/practice?
7. Who should know about what was
    learned and the resulting plan, and
    how should the information be shared?
There should be a specified way in which
closure is structured for each meeting.
Some groups use "check in" and "check
out." Check out could be structured to
include any of the above questions or a
general assessment of whether the team
members believed their goals for the
meeting were met.

Providing feedback is completion of the loop
of effective communication. The team cannot
proceed with its work if the members cannot
give feedback. Within the team, feedback entails
stating what the other person said or did and
verifies that the message or actions were received
and understood. This is an opportunity to provide
an acknowledgment. Leaders also need the
courage to give constructive feedback. Guidelines
for giving feedback to the team are found in
Box 10-9.

Team Meetings

Clearly the team must have meetings to work on
the project. However, meetings can be the source
of problems. Certain strategies help leaders to deal
with issues that frequently arise during meetings
(Gary, 1997; Huszczo, 2004; Laing, 2003).

Sometimes the meeting turns into a complaint
session. The members complain about management, equipment, and each other. The leader must
shift this complaint session to a problem-solving
session about the things over which the team has
control.

Meetings can become demand sessions. This
usually is focused on demanding that management take care of the problem. These sessions
evolve into an alternative to negotiation. Although
administrative support is important, the team has
to be refocused on issues they control. The leader
must redirect the team to what they can do to
make things better, things over which they have
control.

From time to time, team members do not
participate. This is problematic to a highly functioning team because synergy and collective
wisdom are missing. If further acting out occurs,
such as reading other papers during the meeting,
the other teammates will become resentful and
cynical. One of the rules (team member responsibilities) could focus on active participation by
each team member. And the team leader can
encourage involvement.

Sometimes in a team, everyone participates
and no follow-through occurs between meetings.
Talk is great, and it must be followed by action.
The leader must be clear about this up front and
be certain everyone is in agreement. Sometimes
team members share whatever is in their heads,
having given the thought or comments little or no
consideration. Such problems can be minimized
by beginning with and adhering to an agenda.
The agenda should be sent out in advance of the
meeting so that people will have an opportunity
to consider the agenda items prior to the meeting.

Box 10-8   Communication Tools Used with Teams

1. **Remember to use personal greetings.** Always say "Hi" or "Good morning" to each person. Even with the multiple problems leaders have on their minds, personal greetings are a form of recognition. When staff or team members do not receive a greeting, they can imagine problems or difficulties in the relationship that do not exist. Remember the importance of acknowledgment and recognition and do so whenever the opportunity presents itself.

2. **Speak the truth.** Truthfulness builds trust. When the truth is compromised, credibility suffers and the leader has to remember what was said to whom. Such situations stimulate communication breakdown and distrust.

3. **Ask many questions.** Rather that the leader telling everyone his or her point of view, ask questions about what team members think. Questions can be used to lead team members to a process of discovery of the answers. Demonstrate with team members that sharing information and responding to questions is valuable. Questions can lead to a dialogue, and information sharing becomes two-way.

4. **Practice storytelling.** When sharing information, bring the information alive by delivering it in the form of a story or an analogy. Help people visualize important information. Connect with them on a personal or humorous level through these stories and analogies.

5. **Repeat—Repeat important information.** Human beings learn through repetition. It is advisable to summarize main points or outcomes so that the rest of the team hears them a second time. It also can help anyone who is taking minutes for the meeting.

6. **Distinguish facts from rumors or opinion.** Facts are valuable, and it is important and helpful to know with what issues the team must cope. It can also be helpful to share a point of view both on the part of the leader as well as team members. It is critical to squelch rumors with the facts.

7. **Group data and information.** Human beings have difficulty remembering lists of facts or information. Three or five key points are relatively easy to remember. If there are more than seven, find ways to group the information. One apprach is share major points and use the fingers on the hands to "tick them off." This helps in visualizing the data.

From Hellen Davis, CLU, Author and CEO of Indaba, Inc. *The 21 laws of influence.* (2004). St. Petersburg, FL: Indaba, Inc.

Domineering team members can be a problem. Some people are more talkative than others, and the quiet ones often do not assert themselves. The team is not functioning optimally if only two or three members are doing all the talking. To gain the full wisdom of the team, most all of the members need to give their ideas. The leader can suggest such options as silent brainstorming or round-robin participation to ensure that all members have an opportunity to contribute.

Coping with Conflict

Conflict is inevitable in a team. By definition conflict is merely individuals or groups having different perspectives on a specific subject. People who care about their work speak out. This conflict is infused with energy. People can talk endlessly but until they are truly invested enough to do whatever it takes to meet the goal, no change will occur. Conflict creates energy that actually can move

Box 10-9   Guidelines for Providing Feedback

1. **Timing is critical**. Give the feedback as close to the behavior or the action as possible. This timing is as important for the recipient as for the feedback provider so that the memory is fresh for what was said or done and what was intended. Assess instantly the listener's reaction and receptivity. Be prepared to suggest a time when the feedback might be better received. Be sensitive to the feelings of the recipient.

2. **Describe behaviour**. Describe the facts as closely to what was said or done as possible. Check to see if the person experienced the event as described. When evaluating or judging the behavior in the event, praise the positive aspects before offering constructive criticism. Positive feedback should be given regularly and not only when constructive feedback is given.

3. **Be specific**. Be clear and detailed about the actual behavior the leader would like to see changed or to reinforced and give specific examples. For example, speaking privately with the team member, the leader might say, "I feel concerned about comments made in the meeting." "I noticed that you said, 'Yeah, right' each time a team member demonstrated enthusiasm or made a promise. Am I correct in thinking you don't believe there will be follow through on the commitments that were made?" "Can you see how negative comments can be damaging to the team and to the project?"

4. **Focus feedback on what is changeable.** Focus also on behaviors that matter to the team and the project. The purpose is not to change general behaviors but the ones that affect the team, the project, and the leader. As the leader, reflect on relative importance, "Does this really matter?" Give the receiver an opportunity to identify options. The goal is to help the receiver to help him- or herself.

5. **Focus on evaluating behavior rather than the person.** Refrain from any form of attack, discounting, or demeaning of the person to whom feedback is being given. Focus on behaviors, not personalities. Be clear that the issue is what was said, not the person. If there is upset around the situation, schedule another time for the feedback, after tempers have cooled.

6. **Third-party feedback.** It can be a significant problem when one person describes the problem behavior of another. It is natural for people to inquire as to who said what or who complained. Be cautious when using this information. The leader can use the information as a corroborating example of behavior he or she has observed, or the leader can support the person who shared the issue/concern in speaking directly to the team member.

7. **Summarize the interaction and the agreements.** If the interaction leads to an agreement, summarize *who* will take *what* action and *when* it will be completed. Offer assistance to ensure a successful outcome. If the only agreement is to continue the discussion, be sure to arrange both a place and time. Be certain to follow through on these meetings and agreements.

8. **Receive feedback.** Ask for feedback on how the interaction went and how effective your leadership was when providing feedback. Ask for specifics regarding both what leadership behaviors helped and what can be improved or handled better. It is an opportunity to model a non-defensive approach to feedback. Demonstrate how it can be learning experience rather than a defensive experience.

Based on Communicating Feedback from Huszczo, G. (2004). *Tools for team leadership*. Palo Alto, CA: Davies-Black.

important issues forward (Huszczo, 2004). When conflict is handled well, it can be constructive. It can enable people to confront issues openly and to clarify them. When disagreements are allowed and encouraged, communication and team involvement are increased (Ray, 1999). As Weiss and Hughes (2005, p. 97) said, "Clashes between parties are the crucibles in which creative solutions are developed and wise trade-offs among competing objectives are made."

One outcome of eliminating conflict can be "groupthink," in which all team members think alike. This would be boring and would defeat the purpose of a synergistic team. More than likely, the purpose of the team would not be met. It is the responsibility of the leader to recognize conflict and facilitate resolution of that conflict.

Causes of Conflict

Clearly, the sources of conflict are as varied as the number of human beings. However, Huszczo (2004) groups these areas of conflict into competition, misunderstandings, and historical events. Individual and team competition in this society is emphasized at every level of interaction. Therefore competition logically would be found within a team. It can be focused on the limited resources within the organization, which is applicable in nearly every healthcare facility. Some organizational cultures hold rewards or acknowledgments in scarce supply, which creates competition. Human nature dictates a desire for events to happen in an individual's favor, which may conflict with the desires of another individual. This desire may stem from a strong need for control of the work environment. It also may be that the values of various team members are different. For example, one nurse may be working primarily to support a family and the work is "just a job." By contrast, another nurse may have a strong professional identity, love taking care of patients, and see nursing as a career. Consequently the values and goals of these two people could be in competition.

Many people are surprised to discover that other people do not share their thoughts and beliefs. Rather than accepting that people are all different, some individuals become very frustrated about these differences and do not seem to be able to discover ways to understand. These differences can be in backgrounds, professions, education, age, ethnicity, gender, or life experiences. One team member may have a difficult time understanding another because they have not had the same life experiences. If a team member broadens the dissimilar life experiences into stereotypes, the attempt at understanding is further complicated. Lack of understanding inflames many of the conflicts experienced in organizations.

Many feelings, opinions, or judgments brought to the team are based on the history or past events team members have with each other. Because an extensive amount of time is spent with co-workers, people who may otherwise never have a relationship or interact with one another are forced to interact. Because of these significant differences, people have many opportunities to hurt and disappoint one another in these interactions. It is human nature to remember particular actions or comments that were hurtful or disappointing. Memories of these old, or historical, events can put people on guard or make them defensive, and these events show up as lack of trust and even lack of respect. Any of these areas of conflict can appear to varying degrees in the team process.

Conflict and the Stages of Team Development

Conflict can occur at any of Tuckman's stages of team development. However, in the forming stage, avoiding and accommodating are the behaviors most often seen. This is a time of learning about one another, and team members are prone to be "nice" to one another. What is most likely to facilitate the team in this beginning phase is a clear purpose and rules focused on personal interactions. The leader must be certain every team member participates in these processes.

Much of the overt conflict occurs during the storming phase of team development. Deciding how things are to be done can lead to conflict. This is a time when the leader ought to focus on non-verbal behavior and facial and body language. The quieter team members may attempt to gloss over conflict and take the path of least resistance, which does not serve the team. The leader should look for signs of withdrawal from team members who lost "battles" early on in the discussions of "how to accomplish the goal." Pulling each team member into the discussion is the goal of the team leader. Because the opposite of conflict is apathy, not peace and harmony, the leader must deal constructively with these conflicts.

Successful navigation of the storming and norming phases of development usually leads to team cohesion. Within the performing phase, the team usually closes ranks and the conflict may be external to the team. Here the leader's task is to develop bridges between the team and the rest of the organization, particularly administration, so that the good work being done can be acknowledged and appreciated. Likewise, in the closing phase, when the team begins to dissolve, conflict can arise in place of being able to share feelings and reach closure through discussion of what the team experience meant to each member. Again the team leader must be aware of the pitfalls in this final phase and facilitate confrontation of feelings rather than other destructive behaviors such as sarcasm or false jocularity. The leader can facilitate the debriefing or analysis of the team efforts and refocus the team on the positives.

Approaches to Conflict

One of the most unproductive areas of conflict is the blame game. This game focuses on pointing fingers or finding someone or some group to blame for the problem and determine who is "one up" on the others. When the team leader recognizes this approach, the response could be, "Let's move on to problem identification rather than argue about who is to blame." Brounstein (2002) identifies

additional destructive approaches used by groups and the constructive behaviors that work through the conflict and maintain respectful team relationships (Box 10-10). Although some of these may seem familiar, the team leader benefits from holding these at a conscious level in all team meetings so that the responses and interventions are immediate.

Another helpful way to think about conflicts is using the model developed by Thomas and Kilmann (2002), which identified five basic approaches to handling conflict: avoiding, accommodating, competing, compromising, and collaborating. Although each coping strategy has advantages and disadvantages, the real key is to match the conflict situation with the approach. When the issue is minor and the need for harmony is great, it may be best to *avoid* certain behavior, remembering that behavior that is not reinforced or is ignored tends to diminish. The work of the team may be structured in ways that significantly decrease the time the conflicted members are together. If the issue is not very important, avoidance may work.

If the issue is important to one person and not to the other, *accommodation* may work, especially when the need for harmony is high. Either the person or the situation is accommodated. The team member for whom the issue is unimportant may be able to acquiesce and say something such as, "Obviously, this is more important to you. We can just do it your way this time." Or, as so often works, the leader could use some humor and say jovially, "We've been through too much together to allow this issue to create bad feelings." If none of the above works and the situation is deteriorating, the leader could request a "time out."

Both sides should be given a chance to cool off. This request is accommodating the situation by providing some time to the parties. The leader must be sure an agreement is made regarding when the parties will talk again to attempt to resolve the issue. They may want the leader to support the conflict resolution process at a later time without the other team members present. Accommodation should not be used excessively, because the team

Box **10-10**   RECOGNIZING DESTRUCTIVE ACTIONS AND CONSTRUCTIVE BEHAVIORS

DESTRUCTIVE ACTIONS

Finger pointing: Finding fault and blaming does nothing to solve problems and builds unhealthy tension.

My way or the highway: When someone insists on his or her point of view and considers no one else's, the volume of the debate increases and obviates any resolution.

Insults: Name calling and personal insults negate resolving conflicts.

Verbal threats and ultimatums: Outbursts are intimidating and fail to promote teamwork.

Defensiveness: Justifying actions rather than listening builds walls between team members and negates agreements.

Avoidance: Running from issues and hoping they go away seldom resolve anything.

Beating around the bush: Rambling or talking around the point, clouding the issue, results in the fact that it remains unaddressed.

Not taking issues to the source: Complaining to others about what a third party has done rather than talking to the person with whom you are upset is not helpful. "Take the mail to the right address."

Flaming e-mails: Blaming and complaining electronically and copying the disruptive e-mail to others in the organization, or responding in a critical, verbally abusive manner, is counterproductive.

CONSTRUCTIVE BEHAVIORS

Staying in control: Begin by controlling your own emotions. Sarcasm and anger show you are out of control. Cooperation is best.

Being direct, factual, and sincere: Express concern clearly and constructively. Speak with candor and respect. Ask the person to talk about your point back to you.

Going to the source: Conflict is best resolved by going to the person and speaking face to face to resolve the conflict. A direct face-to-face talk is the best method for resolving conflict, no matter how uncomfortable it is.

Active listening: Showing that you care and working to understand the other person, both what they say and what they mean, are important. These actions are even more important in conflict situations and when working out issues and concerns.

Brounstein, M. (2002). *Managing teams for dummies.* New York: Wiley.

may have the impression that the leader cannot tolerate conflict or stand up for his or her own views.

For strong team members not easily threatened by conflict, the *competing* approach may be used, including such tactics as convincing, debating, and voting. Use of this method requires an open and fair debate of the issues. The facts must be clear, and the remainder of the team needs to also be clear when facts are presented versus opinions. Facts can be reviewed by each party in a respectful way, and it

must be clear who is making the decision and how the decision is being made. The leader must be certain that for the person whose viewpoint was rejected, some graceful and face-saving strategy exists to support the person and allows him or her to remain enrolled with the team and the project. However, if it becomes clear that the differing opinions are based on values rather than facts, the competitive method should not be supported.

In some instances *compromise* can be used. In some situations a middle ground can be found, and the team leader can ask, "What is the halfway point between these two positions? Would you be willing to consider this point?" In compromise both parties gain something and the stalemate is broken. It can promote the possibility that team members can work together. However, compromise has a down side. In a compromise, something is gained but something is also lost. Each team member must give up a position or an idea to which he or she was committed. That translates as neither party "won" or got what they wanted. Often compromises must be reworked later, and the two parties have negative feelings about what was relinquished. For example, the Missouri Compromise delayed the Civil War by 12 years when the 38th parallel was established as the dividing line. All states coming into the Union north of the line were free states, whereas all states coming into the Union south of the line were slave states. In the 12 years the war was delayed, innovations in weaponry enabled the killing of three times the number of men than would have been killed in 1850. Compromise is not necessarily a good thing.

If both the issue and the development of good relations are critically important, *collaboration* is the best approach. This includes creative problem solving, principled interest-based negotiation, and a "win-win" approach. This differs from compromise in that the solution derived is something neither party could think of on their own. The emphasis is on creation of a new way as opposed to "your way," "my way," or "let's meet halfway." Rather than being stuck on a position, the approach is focused on creating and gaining new insights to the issue. When a win-win solution is reached, both sides feel extremely positive, as though they could accomplish anything together.

This approach, which was first identified by Fisher and Ury (1981), who were members of the Harvard Negotiation Project, is presented in depth in the classic book, *Getting to Yes*. The four major principles of the process are summarized in Box 10-11. This process focuses on the issues rather than on the person arguing the issues. In this process, the blame game is transformed into constructive problem solving. No solutions are

---

Box **10-11**   THE FOUR PRINCIPLES OF WIN-WIN NEGOTIATIONS

1. **Focus on the issues, not on the personalities of the people involved.** Identify the subject to be discussed, not the person who is presenting the discussion. Be willing to accommodate for people but be firm on issues. Listen to the words and refrain from interpretation and judgment. Do not blame either party; help both parties feel respected and preserve their dignity. Do not present a solution; involve both parties in creating a plan or solution.

2. **Focus on interests instead of positions.** Look for true interest and a direction to take and discourage score keeping between parties. Carefully identify interests that are shared, those that are in opposition, and those that are only different. Continue to focus on whatever interests, goals, and objectives are shared between parties.

3. **Appeal to mutual interests.** Create options that focus on mutual gain. Suspend all judgment and use brainstorming to create options. Find ways to use and adapt the differences. Look for trade-offs that are equal but different opportunities, perspectives, or options as they relate to situational wins.

4. **Use standards to evaluate options.** Apply objective rather than subjective criteria. Find external criteria or standards to use as comparisons.

Box 10-12   Seven Steps for Dealing with Difficult People

1. **Decide, "Is it worth it?"** Is it worth the time and energy to deal with the person? Working with someone who is in upset or reaction is hard work and emotionally draining. However, dealing with the person may be worthwhile because the leader must work closely with the person, the person has some intriguing characteristic, or the leader could learn a great deal in the process. If the person leaves the team and minimal future interaction is necessary avoidance may also work.

2. **Observe and be prepared.** Observe the person's behaviors. Attempt to give up preconceived notions and judgments. Treat these observations as a scientific experiment. Be clear about why it is important to proceed. Prepare in writing a session planning instrument that could include (1) stating your case with the opening statement; (2) hypothesized listening for understanding, including the possible topic, tonality, and emotion of the team member; and (3) estimating the negotiations and possible agreements, including desired behavior change and possible options. When these are written on the session planner, it is less likely that the leader will be surprised and speechless or in reaction.

3. **Initiate the confrontation and declare the importance of the issue.** Choose a time and place that is private. The opening of the conversation should include the following: (1) "I feel concerned." (2) "I think it is because we seem to have difficulty working together." (3) "I want us to have a better working relationship—one in which we are respectful and supportive with one another." (4) "Are you willing to sit down with me and brainstorm different ways we could work together better?" Then be quiet and wait for a response.

4. **Use active listening skills and reflection.** Whatever the person says in response, repeat it to be certain of accuracy. Practice the best active listening skills possible that signify respect. Hear, verify, and clarify what the person is saying. If the person is angry and makes broad general accusations, merely repeat what was said and the corresponding implications. Do not counterattack or become defensive.

5. **Ask questions. Jointly identify three options each can agree to improve.** Emphasize that the purpose is *not* to assign blame. Rather, ways can be created to work together better. Do not argue about values. Role model patience and understanding. If the person seems willing to work, agree to generate options (each person must come up with at least three) for improving how to work together. Find a time when both parties can reconvene. Both parties must commit to agreed-upon options and to their implementation.

6. **Do no react or express anger.** If the person refuses to discuss the options or walks away, say in a nice tone of voice, "I still want to work this out with you, and I will see you tomorrow at X time to discover what you're thinking is." Always follow up. The next day be sure to keep the time agreement and check to see if it is a good time and convey willingness to listen and negotiate.

7. **If the interaction fails, restate the goals and the willingess to negotiate.** Be clear about what the desired outcome is. Repeat the goal (it may be specific behavior or certain information required to complete the job). Continue active listening and repeat everything the person says. If this does not work, state the consequences of failing to meet the goal. Be clear. If behavior changes, acknowledge it enthusiastically. If the behavior does not change, invoke the consequences. Repeat again the goals, the willingness to negotiate, and the consequences. Know that the relationship may further degenerate. As the leader, be consistent.

Modified from Huszczo, G. (2004). *Tools for team leadership.* Palo Alto, CA: Davies-Black.

given at the beginning of the process. The focus is on issues rather than the bottom line. The goal is to reframe the competing interests in such a way that it is possible to brainstorm creative alternatives, looking for those that satisfy mutual interests. To effectively use collaboration, skills such as diplomacy, good communication, and effective problem solving must be employed. If the team or the team leader are not experienced in these skills, support from outside the team may be needed. This could be an external consultant or a human resources person experienced in these skills.

Dealing with Difficult People

A few people, perhaps less than 10%, do not respond to any of the skills previously discussed in this chapter. These are the truly difficult people. First, leaders need to think about who these people are for them: Is it the "know it all," the person who holds a grudge, or the person who is chronically negative or angry? Perhaps it is the person who lies or is unreliable. The intriguing piece of this identification process is that the difficult person is different for every leader. It becomes clear that the most difficult person for each leader is the person with whom the leader's usual methods of coping with conflict do not work. The leader probably cannot change this person; however, to alter behavior in specific instances might be possible. Huszczo (2004) has identified a seven-step process for leaders to use in dealing with difficult people, which is found in Box 10-12. The leader must decide if he or she is willing to attempt to cope with this difficult person.

CNO as Team Member of the Senior Executive Team

Without question the CNO needs to be part of the senior executive team. The question is, How successful in the team will the leader be? In reality,

CNOs who use the skills suggested in this chapter, coupled with relationship-building skills, can be successful. A helpful tactic is to review each team meeting and significant interactions with other team members in a reflective way to determine whether any interactions could be altered. This fosters ongoing growth in the process of building additional skills.

The nurse leader has a knowledge base essential to the decision-making process for the organization. In addition, if he or she is practiced in leading teams *and* being a team player, the ability to function effectively in the senior executive team is ensured.

SUMMARY

True teamwork is an exciting, stimulating process that requires a considerable amount of hard work. Clarity regarding the team, its structure, and its purpose is important. The most rewarding exercise for nurse leaders is to carefully examine their skill sets for the skills needed to grow a team and create a synergistic outcome for issues that could not be achieved in any other way. Attempting to build a group into something that is not a team in name only requires risk taking by both the leader and the team members. However, the advantages to nursing service and the organization make the process worthwhile.

KEY POINTS TO LEAD

1. Analyze the team leader role in working with a team.
2. Compare the team leader characteristics identified here with your own leadership characteristics.
3. Reflect on the team leader's role during the five stages of teams.
4. Compare the three reasons for conflict given here with your experience in working in a team.
5. Evaluate destructive and constructive behaviors with the conflict you have seen in teams.

Literature Box

This interesting book looks at some of the truly great teams in the past 70 years, such as the Manhattan Project (which made the first atomic bomb), the Walt Disney team that made the first feature-length cartoon, Xerox's Palo Alto Research Center (which made the first personal computer but did not market it), Apple computers (who refined this idea, took it to market, and created the Macintosh), and the Clinton 1992 presidential campaign. Bennis and Biederman look at what made these teams successful, how team members were recruited (the leaders went for the best and the brightest in their field), the leadership component and what it was like (it varied from team to team), the working conditions of the teams (mostly grim) and the daily length of time they worked (14 to 16 hours), and how their lives outside of the project (many divorced) were affected.

These team members were rogues and yet found ways to work together constructively. Furthermore, they were young; many were in their early twenties. And the leaders occasionally would select someone who was less than brilliant if they had great interpersonal skills. These teams all believed the leaders who told them they were very special and that they were creating something that would change the world. They were outrageous and synergistically creative. They did accomplish goals that changed the world, from the atomic bomb to the personal computer to some of the best entertainment ever imagined. For the most part, these teams knew that they were part of something they could not recreate someplace else and stayed on the team because they were clear it was the best job they would ever have in their lifetime.

Although few nurses fit the criteria for such teams, and it would be difficult to attract them all to the same place, lessons may be learned about teamwork from this book, most of which already have been outlined in this chapter. The mutual respect and the willingness to collaborate within the team are highlights that we could attempt to recreate in nursing.

Bennis, W., & Biederman, P. (1997). *Organizing genius: The secrets of creative collaboration.* Cambridge, MA: Perseus Books.

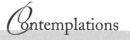

Contemplations

- What do you see as the problems currently facing your team?
- What are the current strengths of your institution? Of the leadership team?
- What are you currently doing well?
- Does your boss do anything that prevents you from being as effective as you would like to be with the team you are leading?
- What would your team say about you as a leader?
- What are your overall strengths and weaknesses?
- Does anybody else in this group do anything that prevents you from being as effective as you would like to be?
- What would you like to accomplish at your upcoming team-building session?
- What changes would you be willing to make to create a smoother-functioning team and accomplish the team's goals?
- What organizational problems prevent you from growing your team?
- What is working well in the senior management team?
- What tools could you use to improve the outcomes and the relationships on the senior team?

LEADER STORY

ANGELA BARRON MCBRIDE
DISTINGUISHED PROFESSOR AND UNIVERSITY DEAN
EMERITA
INDIANA UNIVERSITY SCHOOL OF NURSING
INDIANAPOLIS, IN

I believe that the same principles generally apply regardless of whether leadership is being exerted in the academic setting or the service setting. I would recommend to leaders that they reflect on what their own philosophy and values are and how these influence their "world view." The organizing framework from which I proceed as a leader is "creating a learning organization," meaning by that phrase always assuming change is the order of the day and success will depend on being prepared to meet new challenges. Because I'm committed to creating a learning organization, my intention is not being bogged down in completing 300 separate activities; instead key developmental goals are articulated and moving forward is conceptualized as everyone learning how to achieve them.

I take very seriously the core competencies identified by the Robert Wood Johnson Foundation's Nurse Executive Program under the leadership of Shirley Chater and others.

The first competency is that the leader has *self-knowledge*. In part, this knowledge of self comes from life experiences and the ability to understand how one responds to challenges and demands. In reflecting on these experiences, the leader can build on strengths and use others to shore up limitations, hopefully, without spending precious time or energy in always making sure any weaknesses stay hidden from everyone else. At this point in my career, I know what I know and what I do well. At the same time, I know that it's OK not to know everything. Through networking, you get to know the skills of others and begin to see that using others effectively is another form of being effective yourself.

The leader has *strategic vision*. This is the ability to connect the various changes in the world

(e.g., economic, scientific, social, political) to the home institution. Being strategic requires a clear understanding of what is going on in the local community, the state, and the region as well as nationally and internationally. I often volunteered my school to be involved in the university's pilot projects, particularly if I sensed that the work of the pilot was probably going to become mandatory over time. "Pilot" status usually came with additional resources and provided the opportunity to influence what would subsequently happen. Strategic vision is the ability to see the direction of change and apply it to the task at hand in your own institution.

Risk taking and creativity are critical to leadership. Leaders can transform themselves as well as their organizations by moving out of the traditional ways of looking at issues. This is critical because leadership is about persistence and continuing to make progress. I often get ideas, with some of them being downright "silly," yet out of all the ideas there are almost always a couple of really good new directions. I often have a conversation with myself when I'm feeling "stuck." I "pretend" I can do something about an issue then try to figure out what that would look like.

Effective interpersonal communications are essential to the leader. Do you know how to see the big picture and communicate it in ways that motivate others? As the leader, do you even know what is going on in the institution? When I was dean, I would deliver annual state-of-the-school addresses; this was a way of linking the achievements of the previous year to our key goals and of articulating the major objectives for the new year. When I listened to the concerns of others, I discovered that colleagues on the smaller campuses

(Indiana University has nursing programs on eight campuses) were annoyed because I talked so much about the health sciences campus where most of the faculty and students were located that my remarks weren't heard as pertinent to them. So I responded by giving two annual addresses—the state-of-the-school address focused on where we were going as a total school and had a particular emphasis on excellence in undergraduate teaching, a goal we all shared; the second address focused on the special concerns of the two research-intensive campuses. It is critical that all faculty and staff be able to understand the key goals and accomplishments of a school (and the same is true for health systems). Such activities can affect change without the leader appearing to steam roll. In my case, I used these annual addresses to insinuate new directions without saying, "I'm the dean and you better do this."

Last, leaders *inspire and lead change*. Leaders inspire and create forward movement or progress in a continuous manner. The leader, hopefully, inspires people to "see" the direction of things to come. The leader represents the institution to many stakeholders and thus tends to have the broadest perspective, then helps her colleagues understand future trends and incorporate them as they plan to meet challenges and opportunities. The "how" of implementing needed changes is worked out as a shared process. As the leader, my role was to listen to my colleagues' discussions and decision making then comment in ways that added value. I asked questions or made suggestions about other ways they might think about an issue or how they might rethink using available resources. It was not a question of ordering people to "take that hill" but of getting accomplished individuals to understand that the old ways of doing things will not work in new circumstances, then encouraging them to figure out needed changes.

For me, creating teams begins with my philosophy about a learning organization. It includes an approach, "We're all in this together to create cutting-edge responses to the issues of the day." These issues come as a result of the current economic and societal conditions. These issues are sufficiently complex that no one person can address them effectively. This complexity requires an array of viewpoints and talents that none of us can meet by ourselves. When there are team members who are highly defended, it is very difficult for them to say they don't know all the answers. The notion that we are all in this together, is the beginning of team. There is a "dance" in the team that involves moving the issue or problem forward.

A range of things can happen when there is someone on the team I might not like. The first question I ask is, "Why?" It could be that the person sees the world differently than I do. Several years ago we had an administrative retreat in which we all did the Myers Briggs. What I discovered was that the people who annoyed me the most were the people who were the least like me. There were people who annoyed me regularly, but I learned that I could not ignore them because they actually raised the important issues that I would rather ignore but couldn't afford to ignore if we were to be successful. We worked together much better after the retreat because we understood that we just saw the world differently. In another instance, I had difficulty with an administrator who reported to me because she defined leadership as able to take command and give orders, so she didn't see me as a leader when I didn't act that way and she thought I should instruct others to do what she proposed. One day I just asked her to pretend I had just given the best speech of my life in behalf of her ideas and then asked her if she thought my words would really make any difference in terms of subsequent actions. She admitted that it wouldn't, which provided me with an opportunity to say that's why I wasn't giving that speech. Then we talked about our different perspectives and reached some new understandings. Sometimes there are people who simply aren't effective. It is important to give those people feedback, in the moment if possible. It is also possible that people who are not effective in one situation might be effective in another one. It is important to play to people's strengths if at all possible;

they need to find a job that matches their skills, and the leader can often facilitate that.

If a graduate student asked me about a career in administration, I would say truthfully that I never set out to have a career in administration. Rather, I sought to prepare myself to be competent in whatever I did. Leadership is about facilitating other people in their growth and learning and you don't necessarily have to have a formal administrative title to do that. For example, the full professor is supposed to do that in a way that the assistant professor has not yet mastered. For me, orchestrating a career means getting prepared (Stage I), then making independent/interdependent contributions (Stage II), after which you increasingly work to build the home institution and mentor junior colleagues (Stage III).

When you work in a professional association to build the profession and shape healthcare, you work beyond your home setting (Stage IV). My belief is that building the home institution and shaping the field are obligations all nurses must shoulder as they move from competence to expertise. As one progresses, one may need to go back to school and get another injection of education because formal education is one way to improve the ability to "see the lines" and learn what needs to be done to achieve desired goals. Experience, by contrast, may be the best way to "see between the lines" and acquire the political savvy to get needed changes embraced by the institution as a whole. Both "knowing what to do" and "getting things done" are important, but they are not one and the same.

Chapter References

American Association of Critical Care Nurses. (2005). *AACN standards for establishing and sustaining healthy work environments: A journey to excellence*. Aliso Viejo, CA: American Association of Critical Care Nurses.

Bennis, W., & Biederman, P. (1997). *Organizing genius: The secrets of creative collaboration*. Cambridge, MA: Perseus Books.

Brounstein, M. (2002). *Managing teams for dummies*. New York: Wiley.

Davis, H., & Sharon, B. (2002). *Cutting edge team dynamics workbook*. Malvern, PA: Indaba Press.

Fisher, R., & Ury, W. (1981). *Getting to yes*. Boston: Houghton-Mifflin.

Gary, L. (1997, January). Managing a team vs. managing the individuals on a team. *Harvard Management Update*, pp. 11-13.

Huszczo, G. (2004). *Tools for team leadership*. Palo Alto, CA: Davies-Black.

Katzenbach, J. (1998). *The work of teams*. Boston: A Harvard Business Review Book.

Katzenbach, J., & Smith, D. (1993). The discipline of teams. *Harvard Business Review, 71*(2), 39-48.

Laing, K. (2003). Teambuilding. *Gastroenterology Nursing, 26*(4), 156-158.

Management Research Group. (1998). *Leadership effectiveness analysis: LEA resource guide*. Portland, ME: Management Research Group.

Maxwell, J. (2002a). *The 17 essential qualities of a team player*. Nashville, TN: Thomas Nelson.

Maxwell, J. (2002b). *Teamwork makes the dream work*. Nashville, TN: J. Countryman.

McKenna, P., & Maister, D. (2002). *First among equals: How to manage a group of professionals*. New York: The Free Press.

Outhwaite, S. (2003). The importance of leadership in the development of an integrated team. *Journal of Nursing Management, 11*(6), 371-376.

Ray, R. (1999). *The facilitative leader: Behaviors that enable success.* Upper Saddle River, NJ: Prentice Hall.

Thomas, K., & Kilmann, R. (2002). *Thomas–Kilmann conflict mode instrument.* Palo Alto, CA: Xicom.

Tuckman, B. (1965). Developmental sequences in small groups. *Psychological Bulletin, 63,* 384-399.

Tuckman, B., & Jensen, M. (1977). Stages of small group development revisited. *Group and Organization Studies, 2,* 419-427.

Weiss, J., & Hughes, J. (2005). Want collaboration? Accept— and actively manage—conflict. *Harvard Business Review, 83*(3), 93-101.

CHAPTER 11

Leadership and Coaching

To create a high-performance team, we must replace typical management activities like supervising, checking, monitoring, and controlling with new behaviors like coaching and communicating.
RAY SMITH, CEO, BELL-ATLANTIC

This chapter examines the essential nature of administrative and peer coaching to enhance the professional and personal growth of the nursing leadership team and thus the professional staff.

LEADERS WHO ARE FOCUSED ON THE development of their followers use several different methods to encourage or support their growth. These could include meetings, team building, external and internal conferences and speakers, support for advancing their educational/academic preparation, and specific educational activities. So why would an experienced manager or director need a coach? According to Zemke (2004), experienced organizational development professional and editor of *Training Magazine*, even experienced administrators can gain invaluable help from a coach, because evaluation of a person's own performance in difficult situations may be challenging. Consider top athletes such as Tiger Woods (golf) or the Williams sisters (tennis); they still have coaches who are on continual alert for any "bad days or bad habits" that might creep into their game. Likewise, each nurse in a leadership position can have difficult situations where performance could be improved.

One of the most valuable activities is coaching the people who report to the leader in their personal development and in the ways they, in turn, encourage the development of those who report to them. Estimates suggest that 30% to 40% of a leader's time needs to be focused on some form of coaching (Hargrove, 1995). This coaching can be for individuals or teams, people who report directly, or "bosses," secretaries, or peers. Coaching is a constructive, positive, and enabling process that supports those nurses who report to the leader to learn, grow, and solve current and future healthcare delivery problems. This process facilitates communication skills that improve relationships among members of the healthcare team and between professionals, patients, and families. Coaching is about challenging, stimulating, and supporting people by giving them the gift of the leader's time, concern, and presence.

ORIGINS OF COACHING

The use of the term *coaching* appears to have its origins in the traditional English university, where coaching was used to improve academic performance. Another perspective associates the term with the multitasking skills required to control the team of horses in a horse-drawn coach (Wikipedia, 2004). Sometime later, after the 1880s, American college sports teams began using "coaches" to improve performance. This role was separate from the team managers, who focused on the business aspects of the team. During the twentieth century, sports coaches acquired significant status.

They are now perceived as motivators and builders of character, a concept that has taken considerable time to transfer into the business world.

In the current age of coaching in the business world, some authors and researchers have been critical of the pre–coaching era, the time before the 1990s, in which the emphasis was on management. Gilley and Broughton (1996) were critical of the lack of coaching and adequate leadership skills that were evident in the business world, calling it *managerial malpractice*. The main problems came as a result of recruiting and using and maintaining "managers" who were unqualified, poorly trained, misguided, or inadequately prepared. This included such deficiencies as the lack of interpersonal skills required to enhance employee commitment and improve organizational performance. Gilley and Broughton (1996) identified three areas in which managers can fail, including attitude, skills, and behaviors.

These concerns also apply to healthcare. In the area of attitude, some managers can be indifferent to staff, other professionals, and sometimes patients and their families. Some of the poor skills exhibited by managers include poor listening skills, inadequate or poor delivery of feedback, and poor interpersonal skills. These managers also demonstrate inadequate performance appraisal, little or no employee development, lack of patience, and criticism focused on the person rather than behaviors, thus creating a poor work environment. These nurses are not "bad people." They simply have not been adequately selected, trained, or coached. How many units and areas in healthcare facilities today have managers and directors in this same situation?

Sometime in the past 25 years, non–sporting coaches who offered generalized motivational or inspirational advice began to appear. These coaches did not necessarily have expertise in the specific technical field (e.g., would not necessarily know a lot about healthcare) but worked on more general issues thought to contribute to success.

Evered and Selman (1989) define coaching as a means to convey a valued colleague from where he or she is to where he or she wants to be, much like the horse-drawn coaches carried people. Whitmore (2002) describes coaching as unlocking a person's potential to maximize his or her own performance, helping the individual to learn rather than "teaching." Outstanding athletic coaches help the player reduce or remove obstacles that affect success or to reshape experiences that happen to all of us when we have a really bad day, whether in basketball, golf, tennis, or healthcare. In the Managerial Era of the 1970s and 1980s, the primary concern was in controlling behavior (mostly negative behavior), and it was expected that "professionals" functioned at an optimal level with little clarity regarding expectations and negligible amounts of either positive or negative feedback.

On the other hand, successful coaching adopts an optimistic view of the dormant capability of all people and reframes people in terms of their potential rather than their current performance. Robinson-Walker (2005) believes that coaching helps people change, can be applied at any level of the organization, is different from friendship, does not guarantee a happy ending, and is definitely *not* therapy. Clearly the content of the coaching relationship is confidential and it is a safe haven for exploration and discussion and an opportunity to try on new behaviors.

Because of the excessive stress healthcare organizations are enduring, new strategies and approaches must be developed to support people in expanding their skills in the never-ending process of leading organizations into the next phase of healthcare development. To this end, it is logical for a specific intervention to replace "trial and error," or learning by osmosis, which has often marked the development of clinical managers in the past. Coaching in the healthcare arena has come down through the sports world and the business world and proven successful. It is a people-based "art" that is at the heart of leadership and occurs within a relationship that is action based and results oriented while focusing on the individual. Such relationships consist of (1) enhancing the intellectual capacity and the skills of the novice "leader," (2) facilitating the implementation of healthcare and leadership innovations through coaching, (3) working effectively as a team member, and (4) developing positive, effective, interpersonal relationships (Costa & Garmston, 1994). In addition, coaching develops leaders in the context of their current jobs without removing them from their day-to-day responsibilities (Michelman, 2004).

DISTINCTIONS SURROUNDING COACHING

Multiple aspects and distinctions are applicable to coaching. These distinctions include differing aspects of interpersonal relationships related to coaching and serve differing functions such as mentoring, tutoring, counseling, and confronting. Sometimes a service needed by a peer or subordinate is mentoring by a wise and trusted advisor. The *mentor* has vast experience of the situation and could include such areas as how to "get ahead" in the organization, which people to contact, what the career path might look like, how to network with individuals who could help, and important aspects such as what and where the "land mines" are in any organization. Mentors are usually not involved with the mentee in the day-to-day functions. For example, a nurse might want to find a mentor if he or she desires to become active in professional associations and needs advice about what committees to join and with whom it is helpful to network.

On the other hand, a *tutor* is a person charged with the instruction or guidance of another and would be responsible for helping the individual fill in any gaps in information, knowledge, or behavior needed for a specific purpose. It usually involves giving one-on-one instruction that increases understanding, builds confidence, or enables the individual to achieve a level of mastery in a designated area of performance. For example, if the decision is made that all RNs will function as scrub nurses and circulating nurses on cesarean sections in the labor, delivery, recovery, postpartum (LDRP) unit, nurses might need to be tutored to fill in the gap in operating room knowledge and skills. A tutor with extensive experience in the operating room would be most helpful in closing the gap.

Counseling is a one-on-one method of advising a nurse on how to deal with specific situations. Counseling could occur around interacting with certain "difficult" patients or family members. Likewise, it might be appropriate in helping a nurse achieve balance between personal and work life. Another aspect might be focusing on time management and how to prioritize workload, or even something as straightforward as personal appearance.

Confrontation is used in cases of a performance gap between how the individual is performing or behaving and the unit-based or hospital-based standards for that same performance or behavior. Performance gaps could include such things as personal appearance or body odor or interpersonal relations. It could be a behavioral issue such as a negative attitude or approach to peers, patients, or physicians.

COACHING EXERCISE

Many examples exist regarding what works about coaching. An experiential game that facilitates learning about the power of coaching appears in Table 11-1.

The game of darts in Table 11-1 is like many new jobs: Sometimes there is no feedback, sometimes the only feedback is negative, and other times it is irrelevant. When coaching occurs, however, people in new jobs feel supported and learn what knowledge and behaviors are most important. The effects are identified for each round.

This game is an experiential learning tool highlighting the power of coaching. Table 11-2 outlines the expected outcome of various coaching strategies in the workplace.

Table 11-1 THE GAME OF DARTS AND ITS APPLICATION TO COACHING

In a coaching seminar taught recently, participants were enrolled to play several rounds of the game of darts. One participant volunteered to be the person up to play, and while out of the room, the leader gave the following directions to the remainder of the group.

Directions	The Effects
Round 1: The group was to be absolutely silent, regardless of whether the player hit the dartboard or not.	**Round 1:** Often little or no feedback is given while a new job is learned. People are busy and they do not take the time to make observations, which places the new employee in a vacuum with no feedback regarding successes and failures during the learning process.
Round 2: The group was to "boo and hiss" when the player missed the dartboard and be absolutely silent if the player hit the dartboard.	**Round 2:** In new positions, it is common to receive negative feedback when something is performed incorrectly and little or no feedback when the learning process is proceeding well and many aspects of the job are learned and performed well.
Round 3: The group was to give unrelated positive feedback that had nothing to do with whether the player hit the dartboard or not (e.g., "Great shirt [or shoes or haircut, etc.]").	**Round 3:** Sometimes indiscriminate and unrelated feedback is given, which cannot be connected to the skills and tasks in the new job. And although it may be nice to receive, it is little help in the process of learning the job.
Round 4: An additional volunteer was to coach the player about how to increase the likelihood of hitting the dartboard. *And,* the player was blindfolded for all four rounds.	**Round 4:** Personal, individualized coaching, which includes job-specific positive and negative feedback, is a powerful tool to use in these situations. It supports the "new employee" to learn more quickly and achieve positive outcomes and more consistent results. Contrast these coaching behaviors with the process that frequently occurs: unsupervised trial and error.

Table 11-2 EXPECTED OUTCOMES OF COACHING STRATEGIES USED IN THE WORKPLACE

Application of Strategies to Workplace	Expected Outcomes
No feedback	No behavior change
Negative feedback	Increased negativity/anxiety about the work and the team
Unrelated feedback	Social connections but no behavior change
Coaching	Specific behavioral and technical improvements plus the added benefit of positive feedback

THE COACHING RELATIONSHIP

Remember that existence consists solely in its
possibility for relationships.
MEDARD BOSS

According to Flaherty (1999), the coach does not need to have chemistry with the coachee. Especially, they should not be best friends or dinner companions. However, a workable relationship is necessary for the coaching work to be completed. Sometimes people attempt to hide behind roles such as chief nursing officer (CNO), parent, or boss and use the power of the role in place of an effective relationship. It does not work. Roles may provide the structure, but it takes a meaningful relationship to provide the foundation for coaching.

The Values of Coaching

The nature of a meaningful coaching relationship is focused on the "being" aspects of a person rather than the "doing" aspects. It is about who the person is and who he or she wants to be rather than a rush to do things in an attempt to fix whatever is not working. Establishing a coaching relationship involves a shared or mutual commitment between the coach and the coachee. Craumer (2001) believes this mutual commitment is usually based on mutual trust, mutual respect, and mutual freedom of expression. Notice that the emphasis is on mutual, which means the relationship must go both ways, the coach and the coachee trust and respect each other, and each feels free to express themselves. These might be thought of as "the basic coaching values" needed in the relationship.

Mutual Trust

Trust may, in fact, be a gift we give each other. Trust is an internal quality as much as an external effect of, "Do I trust someone?" It is more appropriate for a person to ask, "Do I trust myself to handle whatever comes my way?" Someone may not be able to keep their word, but the underlying issue is, "Do I trust myself to cope with a person who has difficulty keeping agreements?"

Trust involves two more aspects. One is the ability to keep a commitment, or take action to fulfill promises and commitments. Does the person tell the same version of an event to several different groups? Does the person bend the truth to fit the group or situation, or does the person maintain consistency in speaking to different people, clearly displaying his or her values? Another element of trust is competence. Rarely is trust of a particular person required in every aspect of life. Instead the question is, "Does the person display competence in specific areas?" Levels of competence are seen in an entire range of skills and tools.

Mutual Respect

This begins with liking and agreement, at least in a specific area of life, and ends in admiration in which the person could be held up as a model. In assessment of the area of respect, past behavior is considered and a decision is made about respect based on whether that past behavior is tolerable. The assessment of past behavior must be objective and impartial, and sometimes that is difficult for a coach. It seems to come down to judgment (an imposition of the coach's values on the other person's behavior), which essentially is a choice. The effective coach chooses to refrain from judging the coachee.

Mutual Freedom of Expression

This approach comprises openness, listening, and confidentiality. Communication within institutions and families is shaped by many forces that significantly affect the individual. Some of these forces are hidden or unspoken. No openness exists. A local facility has used an approach developed by Argyris (1990), called "Uncovering the undiscussable," in which a line is drawn down the middle of a page of paper. In the right column, each person writes down what he or she says. In the left column, everyone writes down what they are thinking, the "undiscussables." When this is done in a safe atmosphere with adherence to agreements about how information is shared, it can be very valuable, because issues are addressed that otherwise would never be discussed. This creates true freedom of expression. Obviously listening is a critical component of the coaching relationship (see Chapter 9). When the coachee realizes that whatever he or she is saying is being heard, it enhances and solidifies the coaching relationship. Another aspect to freedom is confidentiality. All that is discussed in a coaching session is private and not to be shared with anyone in the organization.

Creating a working coaching relationship begins with an invitation for the coachee to speak openly, and conversely the coach is open to receive this information. The coach uses no arguments or defensiveness; rather the focus is on asking clarifying questions. The coach must model the behaviors being taught to the coachee. "Be the change you wish to see." Relationship is the foundation of coaching and if it is solid, any mistakes made by the coach will be accepted by the coachee for exactly what they are—mistakes.

Characteristics of the Coaching Process

Coaching is a profession of love. You can't coach people unless you love them.
EDDIE ROBINSON,
FOOTBALL COACH,
GREMLING UNIVERSITY

Crane (2002) and von Hoffman (1999) believe that coaching is not mystical but rather has identifiable characteristics and beliefs that are part of the process. The following characteristics are needed in the coaching process:

Data based: A coaching session must be based on as objective a description of the situation as possible. If those involved in the situation are upset about it, objectivity usually decreases.

Performance based: The process must be focused on behaviors and the effect they have on patients, the other individuals, the team, and the facility.

Relationship focused: The coach must have a quality relationship with the coachee and a willingness to work together.

Slow vs. fast process: This process requires people to slow down, listen deeply, learn, and decrease the reactivity.

Dialogue: Coaching is not based on "telling, telling, telling" but on asking questions, sharing feedback, and exploring options.

Positive regard: Coaching requires Carl Roger's unconditional positive regard for the other person. Valuing and showing high esteem for other people establishes openness, compassion, vulnerability, and humility. Caring about more people improves the quality of the human connection.

Humility: The process is based on mutual dialogue with the intent to eliminate arrogance while fostering mutual understanding.

Balance: The intention is to improve the balance between head and heart, performance and relationships, and the known and unknown, in addition to mind, body, and spirit.

Self-responsibility: This process encourages full accountability on the part of both the coach and the coachee for how their behaviors affect others. It also encourages ownership of thoughts, feelings, and desires/actions.

Beliefs That Inhibit Coaching

One of the most important jobs for a coach is to convey the message that the staff is doing important work and making a difference. However, attitudes and approaches limit the ability to coach, including the belief that not enough time exists. Many leaders have said or heard the following statements made: "The unit is so busy, it takes too much time to coach." "Some managers and administrators believe that staff only need to know about mistakes because their errors are all they need to know."

"When people get too much praise, it decreases in value and doesn't mean anything." "The best learning is trial and error." "No news is good news." "It's not my job, so why should I offer to help?" "I might hurt someone's feelings if I gave them feedback." "I didn't have coaching and I did OK."

If the people involved are not strongly committed to the process, many reasons can be found to avoid coaching.

How to Coach Employees

Craumer (2001) believes that coaching is a method by which the manager can produce the most effective outcomes. The focus is first on what is right about the employee and avoids manipulation or coercion. Some basic steps can work:

- **Build mutual trust and respect.** As discussed previously, trust, respect, and freedom of expression are essential aspects of the process. The leader, as coach, must be honest, objective, and fair. It is not necessary to "like" someone to develop a coaching relationship with that person.
- **Ask permission to coach.** Approach the coachee from a perspective of, "May I offer a couple of suggestions?" This constitutes an offer to share control with the coachee and minimizes the likelihood of a defensive response.
- **Rethink performance goals.** Develop and encourage what the coachee does well naturally. Look for areas in which he or she can be a superstar, and present him or her with the opportunity to really make a difference. Look for ways to leverage the coachee's strengths.
- **Rethink "weaknesses" into strengths.** Look at the flip side of the perceived weakness and see if you can find a strength. Perhaps "wimpiness" is actually a very sensitive side of the coachee and can be strengthened in great patient care service or counseling.

- **Be objective and fair.** Always link feedback to specific examples of witnessed events. Do not consider third-person reports. Before jumping to conclusions, double-check observations and conclusions and ask lots of questions.
- **Be fully present.** Focus attention completely on the coachee. This is not a time for multitasking. Clear the desk, and hold calls. Use active listening skills.
- **Build confidence.** Nurture the coachee's self-image and self-confidence. The goal is to develop self-awareness in the coachee, which can lead to self-correction.

The focus is to support the nurses to grow and learn and feel valued and respected. These are the employees who become committed to the coach/leader.

Identify the Situation, Issue, or Problem

If a major performance issue must be confronted, it is valuable to identify the situation, issue, or problem (SIP) clearly before a managerial coaching session. Before the session it is helpful to create a plan for handling the session (see the Administrative Coaching Session section). A situation is a condition or circumstance that needs to be altered for better functioning of the unit, the nurse, or for quality patient care. Table 11-2 illustrates how a coach uses events witnessed, personal ownership, possible outcomes, and insight.

Using the Coaching Format allows coaches to have open, honest communication that improves behaviors. Being consistent in using this approach reinforces the core elements for the coachee.

ADMINISTRATIVE COACHING SESSION PLAN

Administrative coaching occurs between the leader and his or her direct team members or staff members. All of the discussion about coaching applies equally to administrative coaching. Leaders coach because they are committed to the

Table 11-3 COACHING FORMAT

Statement Lead In	Core Element	Example
COACH'S OBSERVATION		
"When I observe that…"	Action the person has/has not taken	"When I observe escalating or argumentative behavior between you and Nurse Sally from the night shift…"
COACH'S REACTION		
"I feel…"	Your feeling or reaction	"… I feel concerned and somewhat alarmed…"
IDENTIFIED CONSEQUENCES		
"Because…"	Consequences for person, other team members, the unit/the facility	"because anger, upset, and serious disagreements between team members are destructive to team cooperation, harmony, and unity."
THE CONCLUSION		
"Can you see how…"	The Tie Down: Seek agreement from the coachee concerning outcomes or consequences of behavior	"Can you see how arguing, particularly at the nurses' station where many people can observe, is harmful to team relationships and team goals?"

Used with permission from Walker Kowalski, President, BreakThroughs, Inc., Castle Rock, CO, a leadership, coaching, and management development company working with Fortune 500 companies.

growth of their followers. Leaders care about others and want them to succeed. Leaders want others to provide care to patients just as they would give it, if they could care for each and every patient. Specific steps can create an effective session.*

Step 1: Decide on the Coaching Approach

Based on the SIP (the situation, issue, or problem), decide on the coaching approach. If it is a counseling or a confrontational situation, use the Coaching Format (see Table 11-3). The focus

*Modified from work done by Walter Kowalski, President, BreakThroughs, Inc., Castle Rock, CO.

must be on the behavior and the consequences of that behavior to the person, the team, or the institution—*not* on the person.

Step 2: Set the Stage for the Session

- Establish rapport.
- Consider how you would start the conversation to establish rapport.
- Determine what specific feedback you have for the person.
- Decide what you will say to let the person know you value him or her as an individual and appreciate the contributions he or she has made. (Remember words to be avoided, such as *but*.)
- State your intentions.

- Ponder how you will communicate your intention to discuss something that will prove helpful and enable the person to learn, grow, and improve his or her performance.

Step 3: The Session and Description of SIP

- Describe the SIP.
- Give feedback on the current performance.
- Describe specifically (in behavioral terms) the area in which the person needs to focus or improve behavior.
- Gain agreement with the coachee that the SIP exists.
- Consider what questions you will ask to determine if the person is aware of the situation.
- Consider what you will do or say to convince the person that the SIP exists.
- Consider what you will say to ensure that the person understands the consequences of the behavior to himself or herself, the team, and the facility or to patient care.
- Identify your plan to confront the behavior or to identify the next step if "push back," denial, or justification results.

Step 4: Discussion of Problem/Issues

- Discuss what the causes are for the SIP, focusing on asking questions to discover what is going on for the coachee, and mutually decide on solutions and identify benefits.
- Ask the person to identify what needs to occur and be prepared with your ideas if the person is not forthcoming.
- Identify the words you will use to describe what needs to be done.
- Determine what questions you will ask to involve the person in the discussion, to obtain his or her participation in identifying the cause of the SIP in addition to potential solutions.
- Decide how you will lead the coachee through a process of discovery (using questions) so that he or she sees the situation differently.
- Consider what you will ask the coachee in order to obtain agreement on the action plan to correct the SIP.

- Ask how you will anticipate the coachee will react to your suggestions.
- Decide what benefits are to be derived from addressing the SIP.

Step 5: Agree on Actions

- Set definite goals.
- Establish goals that will assist in evaluating the effectiveness of the solutions. Example: Plan of action.
- Prepare a written plan of action, along with a timetable for implementing agreed-upon solutions. Make sure the person receives a copy of the plan (electronic or hard copy). The plan must include a specific date and time for a follow-up session.

Step 6: Follow-Up

- Set a date and time for the follow-up.
- Thank the person for his or her willingness to participate and learn.
- Express confidence in the person's ability to address the SIP.

Step 7: Follow-Through

- Inspect what you expect.
- Check to determine the following:
  Whether the solution has been implemented and in a timely manner
  Whether the solution is working
  Whether the goals have been met

Recognition
- Determine how you will reward or recognize the improvement in a positive way.

Consequences
- Implement consequences for achieving or failing to achieve the plan, solutions, and/or goals.

Reminders

- Give the coachee advanced notice of the time and place of the meeting.
- Allot a minimum of 30 minutes for the session.

- Remove all distractions (e.g., phone, visitors).
- Remove physical barriers between yourself and the person being coached (e.g., don't sit behind the desk).
- Complete the Coaching Session Plan. Keep your notes in front of you during the session to stay on track.
- Plan to take notes to document the session and to develop a record of the corrective action plan and performance improvement.

FEEDBACK

Giving feedback is crucial to the administrative coaching process (Craumer, 2001). Remember, whenever possible, feedback must be given based on direct observation. Furthermore, even with this approach, giving feedback is still a subjective interpretation. It helps for the coach to be as clear and unambiguous as possible. Rather than judging or evaluating the behavior, the coach must describe it. Then follow-up questions are beneficial, such as, "What would happen if…?"

The coach must be clear in his or her purpose for coaching—to be helpful rather than manipulative or controlling. Feedback must occur as close to the event as possible, even in the same moment. Without this kind of timing, the feedback is not very helpful. The coach can use dialogue to create mutual understanding while being honest. The appropriate tone is to demonstrate care, respect, and concern. Things are not always what they seem; so innocence should be presumed.

Topics for feedback are nearly limitless and have changed significantly over the years. A couple of decades ago, "soft" subjects were not discussed, and staff members were not held to account for issues such as attitude. Today Crane (2002) reminds us, "attitude and morale top the list for areas to discuss in coaching sessions when giving feedback." In addition, areas such as being aligned with organizational values and behavioral expectations are very important. Strong communication skills, openness, and rapport with peers are vital to working together

as are collaboration and teamwork. Areas such as flexibility and adaptability are coachable. Feedback, regularity, honesty, and integrity are essential. Obviously, more objective aspects are evaluated such as organizational and technical skills. Peer coaching skills are important, as are creativity and openness to change.

From a different perspective, as much as the leader fears confrontation and giving feedback, the nurse fears receiving feedback. According to Jackman and Strober (2003), employees are terrified even of performance reviews, let alone a formal administrative coaching session. Most leaders, at least in the beginning, also are fearful that the nurse will close down and be unable to hear. The fear exists that even the mildest of criticism will evoke an angry outburst or a flood of tears. Such reactions create discomfort and anxiety, resulting in avoidance of any future situations. It may be one reason that most hospitals have maintained annual evaluations. This entire thinking process is unfortunate because most people need help figuring out how they can improve their performance and meet their goals. Hopefully with the use of tools and skills described here, all participants can become more comfortable with feedback.

PEER COACHING

Many leaders need support in accomplishing goals: someone who will help stretch our boundaries and find a deeper understanding of who the leader really is and what motivates him or her. Leaders need someone who gives them a sense of their own power to change. This is someone who is not administratively superior to them, who advocates for them, and gives positive feedback. As Waddell and Dunn (2005) describe it, what is needed is a volunteer who is nonevaluative, a partner with whom mutual benefits are created. Because peer coaching builds on prior knowledge and skills, this coaching dyad usually self-selects and coaches each other on the basis of attempting to grow in the areas of a specific set of skills and tools. For example, if a group of staff members have just learned about using the communication tool The Awareness Model (see Chapter 9) to improve their interpersonal skills, they could use peer coaching to continue to learn from each other while practicing the model.

The following guidelines could be used to support the use of the new communication tool, I think, I feel, I want.

A coach reflects to the coachee what he or she says is wanted—mirroring. Coaching is not advice giving or fixing.

1. Coaching utilizes questioning rather than telling. The basics are as follows:
   What are you feeling?
   What are you thinking?
   What do you want *for yourself* (not for the other person) right now?
2. A coach is someone other than the supervisor. This prevents confusion between coaching and managing.
3. A coach is outside the immediate team, or the people who work together daily. This enhances objectivity and reduces low-level bonding and alliances.
4. Coaching is best done on a regular basis vs. in crisis mode only. This provides consistent opportunities to "mirror" wants and focus on progress or revision of goals.
5. Multiple coaches are helpful. This increases immediate accessibility to a coach and provides expertise in specific areas.

COACHING FOR THE CHIEF NURSING OFFICER

At first glance, nursing leaders may be somewhat anxious about having an executive coach but with further information, many discover coaching has significant advantages. Many executives consider other options to one-on-one coaching such as mentoring, training seminars, good supervisors, or self-help books. The shortcoming of these methods is they do not provide an objective assessment of current behavior. Neither do the previous methods offer a confidential option for working out specific issues or problems from the workplace.

In addition, Smeltzer (2002) reports that the primary benefits of coaching include improved profitability, increased respect of peers, improved performance, and the opportunity to grow and develop additional skills that can advance the executive in his or her organization. One CNO reported marked anxiety at the start of the process but shifted her thinking after the coach emphasized the many strengths she had demonstrated, and she discovered the opportunity to increase her skills and tools and improve weaknesses. Her coach served as a sounding board for problems in addition to supporting her with suggestions and additional tools in such areas as communication and delegation. Once she was clear that the organization provided her with a coach to help groom her for a higher position, she was able to appreciate the investment and use it to facilitate her professional growth.

Coaching can help leaders to expand their skills in multiple areas from finance to creating change in patient care models and from reallocation of resources to retention and recruitment of professional staff. A professional external coach can assess strengths and weaknesses, create a plan for growth and improved performance, and implement the plan.

More importantly a coach can support the leaders to know themselves better, live more consciously, and contribute more richly to their facilities, their families, and their communities (Sherman & Freas, 2004).

SUMMARY

Coaching can support every level of the nursing team from the CNO to the staff nurse. Administrative coaching is essential, and peer coaching is an additional tool to support ongoing continuous improvement, particularly in more subjective areas. This approach creates an entirely different work environment, one that will improve patient care and retain staff members.

$\mathcal{O}$KEY POINTS TO LEAD

1. Value the evolution of coaching.
2. Compare and contrast aspects of administrative coaching versus peer coaching.
3. Describe examples of tools to be used in coaching sessions.
4. Analyze the underlying philosophy of administrative and peer coaching.
5. Explain the purpose and intent of tools such as the ARC Statement and The Awareness Model questions to the coaching process.
6. Explore advantages and disadvantages of coaching for the CNO and the nursing leadership group.

$\mathcal{L}$iterature Box

Not just individuals benefit from one-on-one coaching; employees can gain immensely, too. However, in an industry without universally accepted standards, all the parties need to be clear about their goals and how to reach them. Although insufficient evidence and inadequate or inconclusive research exist regarding the benefit or the return on investment (ROI) of coaching, the business world is spending an estimated excess of $1 billion annually on training and coaching.

This growing popularity is a response to compelling needs. The move into the Knowledge Age has created considerable contradictions and separations between organizations and their leaders. Developing more fruitful ways for leaders to interact with their people has become a priority. In some respects the more fruitful way began with the rehumanization of leaders in the 1970s. With the concurrent rapid and radical change in the workplace, clearly and emotionally intelligent leaders were needed to work constructively with workers who were now perceived as "intellectual capital."

WHY EXECUTIVE COACHING WORKS

This process engages people in constructive ways to know themselves better, live more consciously, and contribute more richly. Coaches serve as sources for candor and objective feedback. Surprisingly, relatively smart, highly motivated leaders often do not pause to reflect on their own behavior. Coaching helps them to slow down and to become aware and conscious of the effects of their words and behaviors. They can move from reaction to choice.

Coaching is a form of action learning that transfers these new or refined behaviors through the rest of the organization.

Executive coaching is focused on improved performance that leads directly to the bottom line. The authors believe a triangle comprises the coach, the coachee, and the client who pays for the service (this could be the coachee's boss or corporate leader). They use an extensive 360-degree feedback tool to begin the coaching process. The triangular nature of the relationship should be acknowledged up front, and honesty and openness are important.

Qualifications of the coach, the client, and the coachee are critical to the coaching process. The client must understand what objectives he or she desires to accomplish. How will coaching advance the goals of the organization? The process needs top-level support rather than for it to be a "really good idea" from the human resources department. At the same time, a good coach grounds the process in the environmental relationships of the coachee and the agreed-upon values, goals, and dynamics of the client. A good coach fosters independence. Good coaches ask great questions, those that are penetrating and thought provoking.

Qualifying the coach relies primarily on experience and success with other executives or organizations. There is no widely accepted body of knowledge or universal standards with high barriers for entry for coaches. However, the client should be clear about the outcomes, including measurable goals or objectives. Most choose to have coaches work with successful leaders rather than unsuccessful, problem leaders.

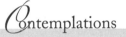

Literature Box

The process is based on contracting the goals and having agreement from all three entities in the triangle. Making all aspects explicit seems to work best. Early and frequent contact is necessary between the coach and the coachee. Assignments can be specific. If the relationship does not work for any reason, it is best to terminate the relationship, and the coach exits.

The authors recommend coaching of the entire senior executive group to accelerate lasting change and have the maximum impact on the organization.

Such programs need enthusiastic support of the group being coached. Starting with this top group has an advantage. Once senior people have changed their behavior, it is easier for them to influence change in the people reporting to them. Even fraught with problems, businesses can profit from creating more positive relationships with the human beings who work in them.

Sherman, S., & Freas, A. (2004). The WILD WEST of executive coaching. *Harvard Business Review, 82*(11).

Contemplations

- As the leader, how open are you to personal coaching? Do you believe that coaching could support your growth as much as it does for top athletes?
- Have you ever wished you had some assistance in coping with a difficult interpersonal interaction?
- Have you had a mentor or tutor at some point in your career? In what ways was this relationship helpful?
- The next time you are doing a performance appraisal in which constructive feedback must be given, notice the sensations in your body and how you approach the situation.
- Are some interactions more stressful for you than others? If so, what are the topics, the situations, or the people that lead to the feelings of anxiety?

- Review, in your mind, the last person you hired or promoted. How helpful were you in coaching the person into his or her responsibilities? What feedback did you give?
- Do you meet with all of your direct team members at least weekly?
- Do these meetings include discussions of how they are doing with difficult situations or interactions?
- Do you ask open-ended questions in these sessions?
- In retrospect, have you seen considerable growth in your direct team members over the past year, and to what do you attribute that growth?
- How do you give and receive feedback? What aspects cause you to feel uneasy?
- Reflect on what you would like to do differently as a result of what you have learned from this chapter.

LEADER STORY ✒

RHEBA DE TORNYAY
DEAN AND PROFESSOR EMERITUS
UNIVERSITY OF WASHINGTON, SEATTLE

I believe leadership is extremely important because it sets a climate for the organization. My leadership background is in education, and I like to think of the dean's role as that of an orchestra conductor. All of the participants in an orchestra are excellent musicians. They can play well even without the conductor. But it is the conductor who keeps them on the same page, keeping them playing all together in harmony. As in academia, the conductor doesn't choose members of the orchestra himself; they are chosen by a group decision. The conductor creates balance so that the orchestra can provide the full spectrum of its music. In much the same manner, the academic leader creates balance within the faculty in order to create forward progress toward the goals of offering rich and varied content for students and enrich research programs. Both the conductor and a leader negotiate any problems or issues that may arise within the group.

The dean is a leader among peers. In thinking about this leadership or administration, the good administrations are often more conspicuously noticed by their absence rather than their presence. When faculty begins to talk about the dean, there may be a major problem brewing. When the administration is functioning well, no one really thinks about the dean. I believe that communication is a major component in a smoothly running organization. Any time the dean makes decisions without clearly communicating why they were made and what the consequences were or would have been, there are going to be problems.

I was fortunate to have very good working relationships with the senior administrative team in both of the deanships I held. Those were the days when I was the only female dean. It's important for the dean to believe strongly in what she is doing but to also be a team player. Sometimes, as a member of that team, it is important to give a little in order to gain a lot. It is a major mistake to create adversarial relationships (especially with medicine). It is critical to choose battles wisely. Being right is not the important issue. That old adage of sometimes it's more important to win the war instead of the battle holds. I tried hard to focus on the long-term goals that I wanted to accomplish.

One main problem I had in the deanship was difficulty gauging faculty views or the intensity of reactions. As the dean, you can become very insulated and alone. People don't always tell you how they feel. Sometimes in this situation, it isn't easy to discern what people are upset about. I remember only too well walking into a faculty meeting with a Dean's Report, thinking it was all quite innocuous and finding the faculty reactive to something that seemed very benign to me. At these times, it could be that the real issue is something else and the benign topic served as the trigger for the upset. Much of what happens in the workplace is like what happens in families. All families have their dysfunctional times and each member plays on the feelings of its members. So leadership and administration is about "knowing and understanding how to work with people." If there were not people problems, they wouldn't need a leader.

My husband, Rudy, helped me more than anyone else in my leadership roles by giving me a different and needed perspective, most notably that of a male. When I was at UCLA, it was my first experience working with a dean of medicine. At times from my perception, I felt he was ignoring a written request. I would write a memo about something I wanted and he would simply not reply. So I would send another memo. Rudy told me that he actually liked me and didn't want to send a memo saying "no" or telling me something that would upset me. So he didn't respond. Rudy also pointed out that in business no response was negative. So his advice was, "Stop bugging him by sending memos."

When I was the director of the Robert Wood Johnson Fellowship Clinical Nurse Scholar program, I mentored 62 scholars over a 4-year period. I was a coach for these nurses. In addition to monitoring their progress, I attempted to support them in analyzing job prospects at the end of their program to help them find the right match for their new talents and aspirations. I did most of this by asking questions such as, "Describe your ideal job. What would you like to do now?" I remember one scholar wanted to take a job mainly because it offered the best opportunity for her husband but, unfortunately, her opportunities were limited and didn't fit her research interests or long-term goals. I just kept asking her questions such as, "How will you handle being in a place that doesn't appreciate your research? What alternatives might there be for you? What strategies could you

use to overcome the discrepancies between your 'ideal' job and what this job may be?" I still hear from many of these scholars, now 15 years later.

I have done and am continuing to do some coaching with new deans. What I have done is to contract with them for a year. Because we don't live in the same locale, much of our work is done through telephone and e-mail. I talk to them and serve as a sounding board. They bounce ideas off of me and I ask questions about the ideas. I ask them to look at some options and we talk about those. I ask them to consider the consequences of any action they want to take. I attempt to provide another perspective based on my experiences. I share both positive and negative things I have done. Most of all, I am their cheerleader. I give them positive acknowledgment when they accomplish tasks or goals. They are not likely to get acknowledgment from other places, which makes it even more important. I have gained so much, personally, from being a coach. Even better, the people I have had the privilege of working with have remained my friends. At the end of the year, I assure them they can continue to call me any time (no fee) for the rest of their lives because we are friends and friends help each other.

Chapter References

Argyris, C. (1990). *Overcoming organizational defenses.* Boston: Allyn and Bacon.

Costa, A. L., & Garmston, R. J. (1994). *Cognitive coaching: A foundation for Renaissance schools.* Norwood, MA: Christopher-Gordon.

Crane, T. G. (2002). *The heart of coaching: Using transformational coaching to create a high-performance culture* (2nd ed.). San Diego: FTA Press.

Craumer, M. (2001, December). How to coach your employees. *Harvard Management Communication Letter,* p. 5.

Evered, R., & Selman, J. (1989). Coaching and the art of management. *Organizational Dynamics, 18,* 16-32.

Flaherty, J. (1999). *Coaching: Evoking excellence in others.* Boston: Butterworth-Heinemann.

Gilley, J., & Boughton, N. (1996). *Stop managing, start coaching.* New York, NY: McGraw-Hill.

Hargrove, R. (1995). *Coaching: Masterful extraordinary results by impacting people and the way they think and work together.* San Francisco: Jossey-Bass Pfeiffer.

Jackman, J., & Strober, M. (2003). Fear of feedback. *Harvard Business Review, 81*(4), 101-107.

Michelman, P. (2004). Do you need an executive coach? *Harvard Management Update,* p. 4.

Robinson-Walker, C. (2005). Reflections on executive coaching. *Nurse Leader,* pp. 24-27.

Sherman, S., & Freas, A. (2004). The WILD WEST of executive coaching. *Harvard Business Review, 82*(11).

Smeltzer, C. H. (2002). The benefits of executive coaching. *Journal of Nursing Administration, 32*(10), 501-502.

von Hoffman, C. (1999). Coaching: The ten killer myths. *Harvard Management Update,* p. 4.

Waddell, D. L., & Dunn, N. (2005). Peer coaching: The next step in staff development. *Journal of Continuing Education in Nursing, 36*(2), 84-89.

Whitmore, J. (2002). *Coaching for performance: Growing people, performance, and purpose* (3rd ed.). London: Nicholas Brealey Publishing.

Wikipedia, The free encyclopedia, coaching. Retrieved August 25, 2004, from http://en.wikipedia.org/wiki/coaching.

Zemke, R. (2004, September). The need for coaching. *Training,* p. 8.

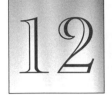

CHAPTER

12 Advancing with Technology

Roy Simpson

A computer does not substitute for judgment any more than a pencil substitutes for literacy. But writing without a pencil is no particular advantage. ROBERT MCNAMARA

This chapter explores the increasing importance of information technology (IT) to nursing in general and nursing administration in particular. It outlines key applications of IT for nursing and nurse managers and examines the critical role of the chief nursing officer (CNO) in system implementation and the key competencies needed to fulfill that role. Finally, this chapter describes emerging technologies with applications for nursing.

IN THE FACE OF WHAT MANY REGARD AS A care crisis in healthcare, nurse leaders have grown increasingly vocal about their concerns that cost cutting, restructuring, downsizing, and overall focusing on the bottom line have gone too far.

Unfortunately, no simple solution exists. Nurse leaders must approach the problems from all angles, from finding ways to stem the tide of nurses leaving the profession to attracting a whole new generation to the profession. At the same time, nurses must not lose sight of patient care, safety, and satisfaction.

Fortunately, one thing can help nurses do all these things—IT. IT will elevate and change practice. However, if IT is to be fully effective for

nursing, nurse leaders must fully engage in the process of implementing it. An entire section is devoted to information management and technology in the Business Skills Competency in the American Organization of Nurse Executives 2005 Nurse Executive Competencies (AONE, 2005). This competency reflects the need for basic knowledge of word processing, e-mail, spreadsheets, and Internet programs. Another aspect for CNOs is to recognize the relevance of nursing data to improving practice and the utilization of hospital database management, decision support, and expert system programs to analyze various sources of data to use in planning for patient care, both processes and systems. The CNO is pivotal in the data system changes and the analyses of what the limitations are in addition to what these systems can offer in the future.

THE STATE OF NURSING TODAY ... AND TOMORROW?

Ironically, the constituencies shaping tomorrow's healthcare—global leaders, healthcare chief information officers (CIOs) and chief executive officers (CEOs), vendors, and patients—really do not care about full engagement in the process; they just want their problems solved. However, these groups are key players. They influence and exert tremendous control over the use and abuse of technology. Nursing, which has traditionally ignored or severely criticized the process, must now refocus and take control of its future by grappling with current informational challenges.

Three major issues are having an impact on the workplace, the profession, and the future of both. These issues are the following:

1. The nursing shortage
2. Increased demand for patient safety
3. The need for visibility

Together, these three issues have created a wealth of opportunity for nursing to capitalize on the use of IT. At the same time, they have created a challenge: When faced with limited time, personnel, and financial resources, should nursing pursue its mission to provide care or should it concentrate on mastering emerging technologies? Given today's industry-wide demands to increase the quality of care while decreasing its cost, the answer is both.

The Nursing Shortage

The worsening nursing shortage will reduce the supply of working RNs to 20% below requirements by the year 2020 (Buerhaus, Staiger, & Auerbach, 2000). Three primary factors are contributing to the current shortage:

1. **Steep population growth and an aging population, which increase the need for healthcare services.** The U.S. population age 65 and over is predicted to reach 82 million in 2050, a 137% increase over 1999. Between 2011 and 2030, the number of elderly could rise from 40.4 million (13% of the population) to 70.3 million (20% of the population) as "baby boomers" begin turning 65 (U.S. Census Bureau, 2000).
2. **A diminishing pipeline of new students in nursing.** Although enrollments in entry-level baccalaureate programs in nursing increased by 16.6% in 2003, this increase is not sufficient to meet the projected demand for nurses. Because the number of young RNs has decreased so dramatically over the past two decades, enrollments of young people in

nursing programs would have to increase at least 40% annually to replace those expected to leave the workforce through retirement (Buerhaus, Staiger, & Auerbach, 2003).

3. **An aging nursing workforce.** 40% of all RNs will be older than age 50 by the year 2010 (Government Accounting Office, 2001).

Unfortunately, the nursing shortage has no simple solution. Nursing must approach the problem from all angles, from finding ways to stem the tide of nurses leaving the profession to attracting a new generation to the profession, all while maintaining high standards of patient care, safety, and satisfaction. IT clearly has some of the answers. The Literature box at the end of the chapter identifies a way one school is attempting to transition students to the emerging practice environment.

Increased Demand for Patient Safety

Patient safety is an international issue. In 2001 in Britain, more than 10,000 recorded medicine errors resulted in 1100 deaths (O'Farrell, 2002). The United States recorded 750,000 medical errors with a death rate of between 44,000 and 90,000 (O'Farrell, 2002). According to international statistics, 1 in every 300 errors will result in a serious, and possibly fatal, adverse effect (O'Farrell, 2002).

Spurred into action by the impending nursing shortage and the rise in medical errors, the federal government, state legislatures, payer and provider groups, and accrediting organizations are authoring new policies and standards faster and more cooperatively than ever before. Consumers are now more discriminating and vocal about what they want, and healthcare organizations are increasingly called upon to be accountable for the results they achieve.

In light of these startling numbers, managed care companies, the Joint Commission on Accreditation of Healthcare Organizations (JCAHO), and business coalitions such as the Leapfrog Group increasingly expect organizations to demonstrate their effectiveness and quality of patient care services. The National Quality Forum (NQF) continues to create measures of quality, some of which have direct implications for IT purchases and strategies.

The Need for Visibility

In healthcare, what is not documented is not done. If nursing cannot establish its contribution to patient outcomes, nursing becomes invisible. In a fiscally tightened market, invisibility can mean expendability. Nursing must have a way to substantiate its role in the healthcare process and its vitality to outcomes. In many organizations today, the documentation system comprises paper and pen and multiple entries (handwritten) of data.

NURSING INFORMATICS: A DEFINITION

To understand the symbiotic relationship between nursing and informatics, one must first understand the two. The definition of informatics is person and situation dependent.

The "textbook" definition is, "Medical Informatics is the rapidly developing scientific field that deals with the storage, retrieval and optimal use of biomedical information, data and knowledge for problem solving and decision making" (Blois & Shortliffe, 1990, p. 20). Collen (1997) provided a more utilitarian, or working, definition of medical informatics. Collen said that it was the use of computer technology in all aspects of medicine including medical care, medical teaching, and medical research. Finally, the classic, short-answer definition is that medical informatics relates to healthcare delivery issues of information—its acquisition, analysis, and dissemination (Levy, 1977).

In summary, medical informatics is about obtaining, reviewing, dispensing, and using information to solve medical problems and make medical decisions. Nursing informatics therefore is about obtaining, reviewing, dispensing, and using information to make *nursing* decisions and solve *nursing* problems. Making nursing decisions and solving nursing problems compose the core of nursing practice.

Together nursing informatics and IT can help change practice—for the better—in several areas, including the following:
- Patient care and patient safety
- Care outcomes
- Nursing visibility
- Nursing accountability
- Evidence-based practice (EBP)

How Information Technology Changes Patient Care

As a result of the intensive work of the Institute of Medicine (IOM), healthcare completed the decade of the 1990s with some of the most chilling news: Patients were not safe. The 1999 report of the IOM, *To Err is Human: Building a Safer Health System*, shocked the industry when it attributed thousands of deaths each year to medical errors engendered by failures in the healthcare delivery system.

According to state and national disciplinary records, RNs long have been responsible for more patient deaths and injuries each year than any other healthcare professionals because they spend the most time with patients (Berens, 2000). Therefore, in some respects, nursing errors are no great revelation. However, the increasing number and frequency of these errors are significant, as is the number of patient deaths and injuries resulting from these errors. The best explanation for the situation can best be summarized in the following equation:

Nursing shortage + Rampant cost cutting = Overworked, underpaid nurses prone to error

Today's information systems, however, have the power to make a difference. Informatics tools help nurses make better decisions faster. Some of the most promising developments include the following:
- **Point-of-care computing**. This refers to the availability of computers where care is delivered. Most clinical documentation comprises clinical records and physiologic measurements.

Clinical records, which document encounters between healthcare professionals and patients, usually include descriptive text, diagnoses, treatment protocols, and nurses' notes on charts and forms. Physiologic measurements are what nurses, therapists, and other practitioners periodically read from monitors and transfer to the patient record. Although clinicians and other end-users of patient records may be held legally responsible for the quality of clinical data, they typically do not enter it until the end of the shift. In many cases, they delegate the task to a nonclinical transcriptionist. When they delegate or postpone clinical data capture, they increase the risk of error. Point-of-care technology addresses this problem by capturing clinical data at the site of care as it is generated.

- **Clinical decision support**. This term refers to large storehouses of information that relate to patient-specific information. Clinical decision support or clinical expert systems improve care by automating care management across the continuum—from abnormal clinical findings to routine dietary requirements. Clinical experts customize the systems to know what information to look for, when to look for it, and what to do when they find it. By keeping a constant watch for potential problems and notifying nurses when they arise, clinical expert systems help improve the quality of care.

- **Pharmacy information (PI) systems**. Because so many errors in healthcare relate to medications, using a system that tracks a person's medication usage across settings and practitioners (a PI system) provides greater safety. To reduce medication errors, pharmacy information systems provide a single, longitudinal solution for managing medication therapy. Information on a patient's health condition and medication history can flow seamlessly to each new setting, making service delivery more efficient and eliminating redundant and potentially inaccurate data collection. The care team can assess a patient's health status; place and evaluate medication orders; and dispense, administer, and document medication more accurately.

- **Telemetry**. Telemetry measures patients' vital signs—from heartbeats to respiration and glucose levels—from a distance. As telemetry becomes more prevalent, its devices become more sophisticated, and the lines between medical devices and clinical information systems (CISs) begin to blur. Telemetry devices are becoming part of hospital information systems, for example, through integrated data input. Together, they will help to streamline care and improve patients' quality of life.

Care Outcomes

Managed care has fueled a growing uneasiness that providers are more concerned with the bottom line than individuals' health. As a result, consumers are now more discriminating and vocal about what they want, and health organizations are increasingly called upon to be accountable for the results they achieve. Results are evaluated based on outcomes.

Standards focusing on the patient's well-being cut across all models of care, categories of disease and health conditions, and types of providers. Simply put, when healthcare organizations do the right things, they are most likely to have good outcomes, which translate into improved quality of care for patients, in addition to improved outcomes for providers and payers. If quality is the goal, how is it best achieved?

Many vendors promote the "right" software as the key to any effective outcomes measurement initiative. They paint a picture of an application that captures information at the point of care and distributes it instantly across the enterprise to the clinical, administrative, and financial users, who then "mine" or search each episode for data to apply against the system's quality targets.

However, decision support systems, which are the crux of this aspect, evolved from the financial arena. As such, they do a reasonable job of allowing managers to assign value to services and identify business opportunities by analysis of data and past performance (Marietti, 1998). Unfortunately, although these systems are great for financial departments, they often fail to capture the full range of data the *clinicians* need for effective decision making. The financial "bottom line" is important, and healthcare organizations need to understand costs and how to assign resources to patients properly. Nevertheless, they also need to track outcomes, and few of today's decision support systems facilitate clinical assessment and decision making.

Increasingly, the IT software solution is a hybrid one, adding clinical data to existing, functioning financial/administration systems to generate the risk-sharing and profiling information that is invaluable for effective outcomes systems (Marietti, 1998). This approach is resource intensive. Before systems can exist, standards must be in place for the systems to follow. Table 12-1 details some of the information initiatives currently being considered as requirements for the nation's regulatory agencies.

JCAHO has focused on establishing uniform, minimum expectations for all organizations providing care to federally funded health programs. This evaluation encompasses all aspects of a managed care organization's operations regarding quality of care, including the following:

- Patient-focused, performance-based standards
- Periodic on-site evaluations, performed by qualified reviewers who are independent of the organization, to determine quality of care at the sites where services are actually delivered
- Routine gathering and reporting of performance measurement results, including clinical outcomes, enrollee health status, administrative/financial practices, and enrollee satisfaction with care

- Understandable reports for the public on organizations' performance

So what prevents any or all of these initiatives from improving the quality of care? Several factors affect this progress toward quality, including the rules and patient guidelines that vary significantly by facility, which make rules-based programming virtually impossible. In addition, physicians are reluctant to adopt tools and are wary of technology. Another factor is the lack of a standardized clinical vocabulary. Furthermore, outcomes are expensive to measure, in actual financial costs and human resources.

Part of the challenge of measuring outcomes rests in defining exactly what an outcome is. An outcome must be described in sufficient detail so that two (or more) evaluators can be clear about what is desired and its relationship to healthcare provider actions. Outcomes measurement can relate to any of these areas: organizational performance, clinical effectiveness, patient satisfaction, service quality, appropriateness of care, patient responses to treatments, cost of services, and efficiency of services delivered (Matthews, Carter, & Smith, 1996).

Once the standards-setting organizations decide on the "what" and "why" to measure, they will need IT leadership to suggest the best ways to use hardware and software for the "how," "when," and where." IT can also help with the following:

- Tools with easy-to-use features and robust functionality that simplify organizations' transition to outcomes measurement
- Systems with the speed and bandwidth to supply current (or even real-time) information in multiple locations without unwieldy load times
- Data security
- Improved information access

If you cannot name it, you cannot control it, finance it, teach it, research it, or put it into public policy.
NORMA LANG

Table 12-1 Information Standards Initiatives

OASIS	Targeting home health agencies, the Outcome and Assessment Information Set (OASIS) is a group of data elements compiled by the Centers for Medicare & Medicaid Services (CMS) that represents the core of comprehensive assessment program for the care of adult home care patients and forms the basis for outcome-based quality improvement (OBQI).*
QISMC	The Quality Improvement System for Managed Care (QISMC) is CMS's plan to strengthen managed care organizations' efforts to protect and improve the health and satisfaction of Medicaid and Medicare enrollees. It was developed in 1996 to target effective use of quality measurement and improvement tools. With approval of the Balanced Budget Act in 1997, it took on the additional goal of providing a timely and "best practice" approach to implementing the Act's quality assurance provisions.[†]
HCQIP	In the Medicare arena, the Health Care Quality Improvement Program (HCQIP) is CMS's effort to ensure the quality of care for beneficiaries by concentrating efforts to improve the mainstream of care received.[†]
ORYX	This "Next Evolution in Accreditation" from the JCAHO is an initiative to integrate performance measures into the accreditation process. On July 1, 2002, accredited hospitals began collecting data on standardized—or core—performance measures. JCAHO identified four initial core measure sets for hospitals in the following areas: acute myocardial infarction; heart failure; community-acquired pneumonia; and pregnancy and related conditions. JCAHO is currently developing new measure sets that address surgical infection prevention, ICU care, pain management, and children's asthma care. More core measures will be identified in the future. Beginning in 2004, core measure data will be used by JCAHO to assist in focusing on-site survey evaluation activities and will be publicly reported on the JCAHO web site.[‡] ORYX is intended for hospitals; long-term care facilities; and network, home care, and behavior healthcare organizations.

*Centers for Medicare & Medicaid Services web site: http://www.cms.hhs.gov/oasis/obqi.asp
[†]Centers for Medicare & Medicaid Services web site: oasis/obqi.asp
[‡]JCAHO web site: http://www.jcaho.org/accredited+organizations/hospitals/oryx/

Despite the inherent limitations of most information systems today, the marketplace continues to demand outcomes data. Managed care companies, JCAHO, and business coalitions such as the Leapfrog Group increasingly require organizations to demonstrate their effectiveness and quality of patient care services. The pressure is not just external; outcomes measurement is a critical part of internal business requirements for continuous quality and process improvement activities.

How Information Technology Changes Nursing's Visibility

Traditionally, nursing work has been "invisible" because care and nurturing are highly subjective and difficult to measure, and nursing services are not separate charges. The challenge is to position nursing work visibly within the informational world. The world of IT has excluded nurses from the equation. IT posited nurses should remain excluded because nursing is invisible to IT because the work is not measurable, finite, packaged, or accountable (Huffman, 1990). IT can help nursing quantify and substantiate its value, which is even more critical today.

Nurses are indispensable to healthcare. After all, with millions of practicing nurses, they constitute the largest group of healthcare providers. However, in a healthcare environment in which a specialty is only as viable as its billability, nursing has yet to reach consensus in the development of a working set of language standards by which to describe its unique role in healthcare. Nursing has little representative language with which to define and elucidate its best practices and patient outcomes. Without such explication to demonstrate its contribution to patient care and outcomes, nurses risk becoming generic healthcare workers.

The difficulty in settling on a singular language lies in nursing's multifaceted nature. Healthcare has diagnoses, procedures, and outcomes; nursing has all of these plus interventions, joined by specialty practices and specific populations. All have their place and each has unique value. However, the most widely used healthcare standards have such administrative terminologies as ICD-10 and CPT codes, which meet reimbursement and regulatory requirements (Buerhaus et al., 2000).

One key question is, "Can nursing define itself in a coded structure?" With all that nursing does, from the tangible to the intangible, winnowing out what must be coded from what might be coded is no easy task. As a result, most languages attempt to include everything. For example, when the Nursing Interventions Classification (NIC) System added dozens of new interventions, it dropped only one. Those codes may have been critical definitions, but they must be coded into the existing software. The cost of changing software or developing a new release is astronomic. The only viable solution is that updates must be coordinated systematically nationwide. This calls for bridging the gap between research and economics in the business world.

Nurses need to be able to relate what they do with costs and benefits to patients and populations. Standardized nomenclatures make abstracting possible. Table 12-2 lists the 13 standardized languages approved by the American Nurses Association (ANA).

In the data-to-information-to-knowledge continuum, precisely defining the data is crucial. Linking knowledge to clinical processes for decision support and aggregating data to develop new knowledge both require standards (Ozbolt et al., 1999). An overabundance of data elements makes it impossible to develop the mapping structures necessary to achieve this. The lack of standard clinical terminologies and codes has handicapped vendors, limiting their ability to develop the systems nursing really needs.

How Information Technology Changes Nursing's Accountability

Current technology has a downside. Data do not lie. This was not always the case. At one time, physicians thought nothing of giving verbal orders to nurses while passing in the hallway, a practice that resulted in the organization having no accurate record of who said what or when. Handwritten documentation also left much to be desired in terms of accountability. Issues of legibility, timeliness, and accuracy still haunted hospital corridors. Next came the computerized workstation, with specialized login procedures, identifiers, and system checks. Did that indicate that everything was secure? Not completely—the occasional borrowed password or lost smart card sometimes confused matters.

Currently, the trend toward accuracy continues, however, with information systems that rely on biometrics (e.g., fingerprints, iris scans) to authenticate user access. For the time being, these new tools generate, by definition, an irrefutable record of who did what and when. Passing the buck is thought to be impossible; attempting to "cover up" for someone, futile.

Table **12-2** ANA-Recognized Standardized Nomenclatures

Name	Description	Type	Category	Organization	Scope	Established
North American Nursing Diagnosis Association International (NANDA-I)	Data elements describe patients' reactions to a disease. The structure is organized around nine "human response patterns."	Diagnoses	Taxonomy	NANDA-I; Original developers: Gordon, Kim, Carpenito, et al.	All	1973
Nursing Interventions Classification (NIC) System	This comprehensive, standardized language describes treatments nurses perform in all settings and all specialties, including the physiologic and the psychosocial. The system includes 486 interventions for illness treatment and prevention, as well as health promotion. The interventions are organized in 30 classes and 7 domains.[a]	Interventions	Nomenclature	University of Iowa; Original developer: McCloskey-Dochterman	All	1991
Nursing Outcomes Classification (NOC) System	This comprehensive, standardized classification of patient/client outcomes was	Outcomes	Nomenclature	University of Iowa; Original developer: Mass et al.	All	1991

	developed to evaluate the effects of nursing interventions. The 260 outcomes are grouped into 29 classes and 7 domains for ease of use.[b]					
Nursing Management Minimum Data Set (NMMDS)	The purpose of the NMMDS research is to identify, define, and clinically test basic elements that would constitute an NMMDS. Seventeen elements have been identified and defined.	Outcomes	Taxonomy	University of Iowa; Original developers: Delany and Hubert	Management	1989
Home Health Care Classification (HHCC) System	Two interrelated taxonomies, HHCC of Nursing Diagnoses and HHCC of Nursing Interventions, comprise 21 care components of patient care.[c]	Diagnosis, interventions	Taxonomy	Sabacare; Original developer: Saba	Home health and ambulatory care	1991
Omaha System	This system is designed to generate meaningful data following usual or routine documentation of client care.	Diagnosis, interventions, outcomes	Taxonomy	Visiting Nurse Association (VNA) of Omaha; Original developer: Merrick	All	1993

Continued

Table 12-2 ANA-Recognized Standardized Nomenclatures—cont'd

Name	Description	Type	Category	Organization	Scope	Established
	It consists of three components: problem classification scheme, intervention scheme, and problem rating scale for outcomes.[d]					
Patient Care Data Set (PCDS)	This set of standard terms represents and captures clinical data for inclusion in patient care information systems. It contains a data dictionary and sets of terms and codes representing specific values of patient problems (363 terms), patient care goals (311 terms), and patient care orders (1357 terms).[e]	Care processes	Nomenclature and taxonomy	Vanderbilt University Medical Center; Original developer: Ozbolt	Inpatient clinical services and emergency departments (acute care)	1994-1995
Perioperative Nursing Dataset (PNDS)	This addresses the perioperative patient experience from preadmission until discharge.[f]	Outcomes	Nomenclature	Association of Perioperative Registered Nurses	Operating room	1996

Name	Description	Content	Type	Developer	Setting	Year
Systematized Nomenclature of Medicine Reference Terminology (SNOMED RT)	This concept-based clinical reference terminology supports the integrated electronic medical record for nursing. It includes terminology models appropriate for nursing diagnoses, interventions, and outcomes.	Diagnoses, interventions, outcomes	Nomenclature	College of American Pathologists	All	1974
Nursing Minimum Data Set (NMDS)	This minimum set of items of information has uniform definitions and categories concerning the specific dimension of nursing.	Nursing care, patient demographics, service elements	Taxonomy	University of Iowa; Original developers: Werley, Lang, et al.	All	1983
International Classification for Nursing (ICNP)	The terminology describes nursing practice.[9]	Diagnoses, interventions, outcomes	Nomenclature	International Council of Nurses; Original developer: Coonen	All	1994
Alternative Billing Concept codes (ABCcodes)	These are used in alternative medicine, nursing, and other integrative healthcare interventions. They describe healthcare interventions CPT	Interventions, outcomes	Nomenclature	Foundation for Integrative Healthcare	Alternative medicine	1996

Continued

Table 12-2 ANA-Recognized Standardized Nomenclatures—cont'd

Name	Description	Type	Category	Organization	Scope	Established
	codes cannot address because of conventional physician practice focus.[h]					
Logical Observation Identifier Names and Codes (LOINC)	These standard codes and nomenclature are used for identifying laboratory and clinical terms.	Outcomes	Nomenclature	Regenstrief Institute for Health Care	Laboratory	1995

[a] The University of Iowa College of Nursing, Nursing Interventions Classification. Available online at http://www.nursing.uiowa.edu/centers/cncce/nic/nicoverview.htm.

[b] The University of Iowa College of Nursing, Nursing Outcomes Classification. Available online at http://www.nursing.uiowa.edu/centers/cncce/noc/nocoverview.htm.

[c] HHCC system introduction. Available online at http://www.sabacare.com/introduction.html.

[d] The Omaha System, Omaha System overview. Available online at: http://www.omahasystem.org/systemo.htm.

[e] Ozbolt, J. The patient care data set: Profile. Available online at http://ncvhs.hhs.gov/990518t3.pdf.

[f] Perioperative nursing data set. Available online at http://www.aorn.org/research/pnds.htm.

[g] International Classification for Nursing Practice ICNPR, April 2002. Available online at http://www.icn.ch/icnp.htm.

[h] An overview of ABCcode design and functionality. Available online at http://www.alternativelink.com/ali/abc_codes/default.asp.

The Critical Aspect of Trust with Information Technology Implementation

Here is where the issue of accountability becomes problematic. When caregivers know any error they make will be easily traced back to them, their ability to trust the organization becomes crucial. To build a trusting organization, administrators must do away with the culture of blame that existed previously, adopting instead attitudes and policies that encourage rather than punish open reporting of errors. In other words, good leaders do not allow technology to become "Big Brother."

A tendency to play the blame game is an unfortunate aspect of human nature, one that is proliferated in healthcare. The increasing number of malpractice suits filed each year has reinforced the practice of assigning fault. By fostering the notion that someone must always be blamed when a medical error occurs, healthcare professionals have also supported the idea that someone "must pay." A scapegoat, too often a nurse, is then portrayed as being culpable and system issues are not addressed. Further, many educational programs instill in students the perception that they could practice perfectly.

However, assigning blame is not so easy. Only a fraction of medical errors stem from the actions of a single individual. Furthermore, in more than a third of the cases studied, it was impossible to assign blame to one person (Krizek, 2000). Repeatedly, findings demonstrate that the majority of errors result not from carelessness but from a breakdown in the healthcare delivery system. Often fragmentation is the problem; a lack of integration still exists between primary caregivers, specialists, and ancillary systems, such as the laboratory.

The ANA actively supports the position that nurses should feel safe to report medical errors and near misses, without fear of punitive actions. It makes sense: if you can identify something that *almost* went wrong, you can probably identify ways to keep it from actually happening. In addition, the ANA has taken a systems approach to improving

patient safety, citing that one of its major concerns is adequate and appropriate staffing (American Nurses Association, 1999). The ANA has identified the following troubling trends in nursing staffing:

- In some areas, a nursing shortage has resulted in vacant nursing positions being left unfilled or in greater numbers of unlicensed personnel on hospital units.
- Although aware of staff attrition, hospital administrators have reasoned that because hospital admissions and lengths of stay have been reduced, fewer numbers of nurses are needed. They fail to take into account that hospitalized patients today tend to be more seriously ill and require more care.
- Several surveys of nurses reveal that inadequate staffing often leads to medication errors. Inadequate staffing was defined by the report as too few RNs, lack of unit-specific training for nurses, or inappropriate use of unlicensed personnel (American Nurses Association, 1999).

Until the nursing shortage can be reversed and national staffing standards implemented, nurses need to feel that technology is working for them, not against them. Fortunately, in many ways, technology can do just that.

Technology alone cannot solve problems that result from staffing shortages. However, it *can* help prevent errors by giving already-harried nurses a system of double-checks. Systems such as decision support help catch adverse events before they happen, including drug interactions, inappropriate doses, and potential side effects. Computerized provider order entry (CPOE) can replace verbal orders and handwritten orders, both of which can be easily misinterpreted. In addition, nurses who have such tools as bar codes and other patient identifiers are less likely to make mistakes. Point-of-care technologies that allow caregivers to document interventions at the bedside are useful for streamlining the workflow, freeing up time, and helping reduce errors caused by rushing.

Timeliness of data is another consideration related to patient safety. When all members of the care team can access the same data in real time, they can base their care decisions on up-to-date lab tests, vital signs, and other criteria. Essentially, they sidestep the fragmentation for which healthcare has been criticized. Knowing such systems are in place fosters an environment of trust between colleagues in different departments and eliminates second-guessing.

How Information Technology Changes Evidence-Based Practice

The University of Minnesota defines evidence-based practice (EBP) as the process by which nurses make clinical decisions using their own clinical expertise, the best available research evidence, and patient preferences. Three main areas of research competence include interpreting and using existing research, evaluating clinical practice, and conducting new research (University of Minnesota, 2004).

In simple terms, evidence-based nursing (EBN) is caring grounded in investigation, intuition, and reaction. These EBPs are based on proof, professional experience, and response to patients. Think about the description of the three main areas of competence in the preceding paragraph. We cannot seem to master research competence. However, the problem is not competence; it is research—or, rather, the lack thereof. The competence part of the capability is a simple four-step process:

1. Identify the issue or problem by analyzing current nursing knowledge and practice.
2. Search the literature for relevant research.
3. Evaluate the evidence in the research using established criteria.
4. Act and validate the action with the best available evidence.

Each step assumes evidence-based research exists. However, in many areas of nursing care, research in the desired form of random clinical trials does not exist.

Unfortunately, two things, an increasingly critical nursing shortage and the lack of a nursing-specific language, make it difficult for our profession to accumulate the research it needs for evidence-based care. To have a body of current research, enough people with enough time and enough expertise to conduct it are necessary. To use research, structured, standardized ways to aggregate it and access it are required. Despite this, several EBP models exist. Box 12-1 highlights some key models. One of the biggest challenges facing us is how to evolve the models and the research into EBN, and how to convert the information into practical, accessible data that can inform practice. The answer is IT.

Most healthcare organizations acknowledge automated clinical documentation is the only way to reduce nurses' administrative tasks. It improves accuracy and interdisciplinary communication. It gives nurses more time for patient care. Clearly, all these things improve care indirectly.

EBP improves care directly. It puts actual knowledge, elements of practice that have been proven to work, in the hands of nurses. However, for EBP to become a reality, we cannot expect nurses to go to the evidence. Rather, we must bring the evidence to nurses. This requires collaboration between those who have the knowledge and those who can deliver it. It is happening with the help of universities and IT vendors.

The globalization of healthcare, escalating healthcare costs, and the nursing shortage demand consistent practice based on effective, proven, documented practice. Continuing challenges, such as the need to validate the importance of nursing, call for structured documentation of practice. EBP is a way of thinking and practicing that requires discipline and practice. It demands continual assessment of the question, "Where's the evidence for procedures, protocols, or traditional practices?" EBP consistently demands weighing the validity and reliability of the activities nurses do every day.

ENSURING DATA SECURITY

The Health Insurance Portability and Accountability Act (HIPAA) mandates that the CIO implement strong policies and procedures to ensure the confidentiality of patient health data. Although

Box 12-1 EVIDENCE-BASED PRACTICE MODELS

THE HARTFORD MODEL

The Capitol Alliance is a formal collaboration of various clinical and academic settings. Their annual conference and "afternoon with an author" series promotes more rapid adoption of evidence. Research roundtables are focused on teaching EBP skills. In addition, a clinical nurse leader is responsible for integrating research utilization skills into daily practice.

BETH ISRAEL MEDICAL CENTER (NEW YORK CITY)

The CNO acts as a key facilitator for a large group of advanced practice nurses. The director is proficient in research utilization and EBP models and uses this expertise to continuously develop and direct the practice behavior of the advanced practice nurses. Systematic steps of EBP help clinicians answer questions with external and internal evidence. The CNO directs them to published guidelines and helps them analyze findings.

THE CONDUCT AND UTILIZATION OF RESEARCH IN NURSING (CURN) PROJECT

The CURN project is a model for using research-based knowledge in clinical practice settings. It views research utilization as an organizational process. It accepts the fact that change is essential to establishing research-based practice on a large scale—and therefore integrates change into the process.

THE IOWA MODEL OF RESEARCH IN PRACTICE

The Iowa Model of Research in Practice ties research to quality. Like CURN, it views research utilization as an organizational process. It uses planned change principles to integrate research and practice. It also uses a multidisciplinary team approach.

THE STETLER MODEL OF RESEARCH UTILIZATION

The Stetler Model of Research Utilization applies research findings at the individual practitioner level. This six-phase model emphasizes critical thinking and decision making through preparation, validation, comparative evaluation, decision making, translation and application, and evaluation.

---

few would argue the importance of HIPAA's mandates, they pose a dilemma: How can organizations implement procedures that protect patient privacy yet facilitate patient care?

As originators, managers, and users of patient data, nurses can—and should—play a key role in resolving this dilemma. For example, nurses know exactly what data are needed. So why could nurses, rather than the CIO, not suggest and implement procedures that allow staff to see information only on patients currently assigned to their duty station? In addition, nurses could evaluate the systems they use to make sure they include the following:

- Encryption software for any health data transmitted over the Internet

- Authentication that validates the identities of senders and receivers of information
- Authorization (e.g., unique user IDs and passwords) to ensure the right access to the right data by the right people
- Audit trails to track who accessed what information

Even though HIPAA compliance may be delayed, it will be a reality soon enough. When it is, keeping data secure may not be nursing's primary job, but it will definitely be everyone's problem. By helping solve this problem, nurses can further confirm its contribution to healthcare and the healthcare IT bottom line.

FINANCING INFORMATION TECHNOLOGY

Few would argue the value of IT for nursing. However, as healthcare organizations struggle to strike the critical balance between increased costs and decreased reimbursements, justifying the cost of even the most helpful technology is no easy task. Box 12-2 lists some of the funding sources available in August 2005.

Nurse leaders must be prepared to defend nursing's need for systems and IT tools. Return on investment is measured in such tangibles as the savings gained by employing IT to eliminate costs and manage scarce resources and such intangibles as using knowledge-driven applications at the point of care to improve patient safety. Nursing administrators must know how to prove nursing's need for IT objectively.

In financially challenging times, organizations may need to jettison some things. With only a surface review, they may see nursing information systems as possible candidates. The nursing leaders' responsibility is to make sure organizations understand the value of these systems. Furthermore, despite what organizations may say about nursing systems, they can and do have value in the new equation. Indeed, although they require an initial outlay, they often can help an organization save money through gains in productivity, outcomes, and patient satisfaction.

Nursing information systems can do the following:

- Maintain outcomes and demographic and health-related data to help organizations better manage what care they provide and to whom
- Eliminate routine manual documentation and optimize human resources
- Improve accuracy and completeness to ensure timely reimbursement
- Support practice decisions aimed at providing higher quality care at a lower cost (Fitzgerald, 1996)

Advocacy for such systems does not occur at the bedside, however. Today, a CNO's place is in the boardroom, or wherever the high-level systems decisions are made. If nursing is to have the systems it needs for continued viability, then nursing will have to make sure that organizations understand the contribution to the bottom line of nursing systems and the work they support. The survival and continued development of nursing informatics rest on nurses.

NURSING ADMINISTRATION'S ROLE IN INFORMATION TECHNOLOGY IMPLEMENTATION

Installing a system simply to automate manual processes is a serious error. Computer programmers use the term GIGO (Garbage In, Garbage Out) to explain that computers will unquestioningly take the most nonsensical input data and process it into nonsensical output. The same problem exists for processes: Automating a bad process produces a faster bad process.

Technology can, should, and does change things. Often it makes some things seem worse before they become better. However, that is because introducing technology means introducing change: changes in the processes and changes in the culture.

In the earliest stages of an implementation, it is important to make the right assumptions up front. Specifically, most technology initiatives require the following three components in addition to the system:

1. A well-defined strategy
2. A process design that remains focused on meeting the business objective
3. Recognition of the impact of process and technology changes that will inevitably affect the people involved

Evaluation of several successful and unsuccessful clinical system implementations proves one thing clearly. Those that succeed remain in harmony with the organization in three ways:

1. Technologically: The system software works with currently installed hardware.

Box 12-2 Sources of IT Funding

The Agency for Healthcare Research And Quality (AHRQ) supports three grants for planning, implementing, and demonstrating the value of health IT to improve patient safety and quality of care.

TRANSFORMING HEALTHCARE QUALITY THROUGH INFORMATION TECHNOLOGY (THQIT): PLANNING GRANTS

- Supports: These grants support community-wide collaborative partnerships among acute care hospitals, clinics, healthcare providers, and other health delivery organizations (e.g., public health) aimed at providing effective IT tools for immediate access to complete and timely healthcare information in diverse healthcare settings. AHRQ seeks to support collaborative planning processes that will result in standards-based data sharing across multiple care sites and lead to measurable and sustainable improvements in patient safety and quality of care.
- How funds may be used: For planning development of important infrastructure components including, but not limited to, computer networks, hardware, software, personnel, project management, and quality improvement and research capacity. Grant amount: $7 million for up to 35 grants.
- Who may apply: Domestic institutions, public and private nonprofit institutions, units of state and local governments, tribes and tribal governments, or faith-based organizations.
- More information: http://grants.nih.gov/grants/guide/rfa-files/RFA-HS-04-010.html

TRANSFORMING HEALTHCARE QUALITY THROUGH INFORMATION TECHNOLOGY (THQIT): IMPLEMENTATION GRANTS

- Supports: These grants support organizational and community-wide implementation and diffusion of IT and assess the extent to which IT contributes to measurable and sustainable

improvements in patient safety and quality of care. Research should inform AHRQ, providers, patients, payers, policymakers, and the public about how IT can be successfully implemented in diverse healthcare settings and lead to safer and better healthcare.
- Grant amount: AHRQ will provide up to 50% of the total costs in matching funds, not to exceed $500,000 per year, for each project.
- Who may apply: Domestic institutions, public and private nonprofit institutions, units of state and local governments, tribes and tribal governments, or faith-based organizations.
- More information: http://grants.nih.gov/grants/guide/rfa-files/RFA-HS-04-011.html

DEMONSTRATING THE VALUE OF HEALTHCARE INFORMATION TECHNOLOGY

- Supports: These grants support projects that will increase our knowledge and understanding of IT's value, which include clinical, safety, quality, financial, organizational, effectiveness, efficiency, or other direct or indirect benefits that may be derived from the use of IT in the delivery of healthcare. The findings should provide these stakeholders with information needed to make better and more informed clinical, purchasing, and other decisions regarding the use of IT in their environments. The other objective of this RFA is to support the development of models or other tools that can be used to help demonstrate the value of IT or to advance the adoption of IT.
- Grant amount: $10 million for up to 20 grants.
- Who may apply: Domestic institutions, public and private nonprofit institutions, units of state and local governments, tribes and tribal governments, or faith-based organizations.
- More information: http://grants.nih.gov/grants/guide/rfa-files/RFA-HS-04-012.html

2. Socially: The system's features and functions replace the current formal and informal communication networks.
3. Organizationally: The system supports the organization's mission.

The dilemma is this: The system is expected to change the organization and thus by definition cannot be totally aligned with the current environment. Therefore change management is a must, and the CNO has key administrative accountability.

To effectively manage IT and clinical systems, the CNO must develop an IT-specific approach and competencies.

First, the CNO must *understand* CSIs. No matter how basic it may seem, a CNO cannot manage what he or she cannot understand. Few would disagree that the primary job of the profession is care. Unfortunately, nurses sometimes use this argument to justify technology avoidance. Because of the total focus on patient care, CNOs and nurses are often uninvolved in decision making for key IT systems. This is where the cycle begins: Nurses avoid the technology, which diminishes their learning, which keeps them from trying newer technology, which leads to little or no input into the development of the next generation of technology, and so on. The CNO has a critical role to play in stopping this cycle. The CNO is not required to know the intricacies of program development. It is not a requirement to be an "IT nerd." However, the CNO can take the leadership role only if he or she understands the general principles of the system.

The CNO must be able to *navigate the political environment*. Often the people making the decision about IT—administration, the board, the IT department—are not really thinking about what nursing needs. Is nursing leading or being led by the IT plan? Is nursing a political pawn in the overall process? Whatever the case, the CNO must have a clear understanding of the game and how to play it so that nursing acquires what is needed for quality patient care.

As the nursing leader, the CNO must *think beyond reporting structures*. The nurse informatician

is a hybrid breed. As such, it is sometimes difficult to know to whom he or she should report, nursing or IT. In actuality, it all depends on the contract with the vendor and the budget. Regardless of the nurse informatician's reporting responsibility, the CNO must make sure nursing information is included in all systems. The only way to do that is by mandating the use of standard taxonomies and nomenclatures. With them, nursing can document its truly important role in the healthcare equation. Without this strong leadership, nursing effectively disappears. CNOs must focus less on reporting structures and much more on what informaticians can and should do. If they help ensure nursing's visibility, and thus its viability, it is less important where the position appears in the organizational chart.

One of the most important battles to be led by the CNO is the *fight against duplicate charting*. Maintaining manual and automated systems simultaneously can increase administrative costs threefold. However, despite the mandate to slash costs, eliminating manual processes is one of the hardest things to convince a group to do. The CNO can and should serve as the dissenting voice in discussions to maintain manual systems. After all, nurses are the epicenter of the charting process. Only with complete automation can organizations ever hope to reap true return on their investments from IT.

A strong nurse leader *develops keen financial insight*. The wisdom to evaluate the annual reports of specific companies under consideration supplying IT systems is critical. It is particularly important to access the research and development (R&D) disclosure. In this segment the CNO can discover the value and emphasis placed on specific systems and products. It takes money to create, develop, and maintain IT systems. If the company is not allocating dollars to a certain system, it is highly likely they are planning to eliminate it.

The CNO must *maintain a realistic perspective on CPOE*. Even though CPOE is about providers entering orders, it has a significant downstream effect on nursing and other departments. The CNO must determine the potential impact of CPOE on nursing to ensure proper human and clinical resource utilization.

A *commitment to education* by the CNO is critical in a knowledge-based organization. At the same time, one of technology's most valuable uses remains as a tool for education. The CNO must understand the value of training to the ultimate success of any CIS implementation, and, with this understanding, make it a priority for nursing. Given the current and impending nursing shortage, making education a reality will mean the CNO has to think of other ways to provide it. From virtual classrooms, to distance learning, e-learning, and interactive training programs on CD-ROM, technology can help the CNO teach technology in addition to clinical and professional education.

In addition, the CNO must understand that an IT system is usually ahead of the organizational curve, but if it is too far ahead, the organization will find it too difficult to catch up. Nursing administration's job is to help ensure the beneficial change that technology affords is not lost amid the challenges such change brings. Even more important, nursing management must provide a vision for change, a revelation of nursing and patient care in a technologic environment.

EMERGING TECHNOLOGIES

Several critical trends, from globalization to the culture of change and the rise of the information age, will fuel development and deployment of future IT.

For nursing, technology is a solution to short-term problems and the foundation of a long-term vision. In other words, technology is critical. Nursing can either embrace technology and bend it to the profession's purposes or continue to wait in the wings, watching other industries and constituencies prosper and grow. Or, even worse, nursing can find itself replaced by the very technology it avoids in the name of patient care. Technology is the key to ensuring that nursing remains present and able to continue contributing to healthcare.

Key emerging technologies include those detailed in the following sections.

Mobile Technology (mHealth)

As information and telecommunication infrastructures converge to create mobile health systems, and mobile technology improves in terms of availability, miniaturization, performance, and communication bandwidth, we can expect to see a host of cost-effective technologies that powerfully affect the way healthcare organizations deliver care. Wireless local area networking and personal digital assistants (PDAs) are the foundation for mHealth. With wireless computing, caregivers use radio signals to access, update, and transmit critical patient and treatment information. By providing and documenting care where they provide it, caregivers can eliminate the human error that happens in translation. Rapid developments in the areas of wireless communications are coming in the next few years. This growth will rest on advances in Universal Mobile Telecommunications System (UMTS), a third-generation (3G) broadband, packet-based transmission of text, digitized voice, video, and multimedia, that transmits at data rates up to 2 megabits per second (Mbps).

Pervasive Computing

Pervasive computing uses machines that are not personal computers but very tiny (even invisible) apparatuses, either mobile or embedded in almost any type of object imaginable, including medical devices. They all communicate through increasingly interconnected networks.

Single Sign-On

Single sign-on (SSO) is a session/user authentication process that allows a user to enter one name and password to access multiple applications. The SSO is requested at the session initiation and authenticates the user to access all the applications the user has rights to on the server, which eliminates future authentication prompts when the user switches applications during that particular session.

Artificial Intelligence

Artificial intelligence (AI) refers to rapidly evolving computational intelligence. Fuzzy logic, neural networks, and genetic algorithms dominate the research.

Computerized Provider Order Entry

CPOE systems are designed to catch and prevent potential errors at the earliest possible point in the treatment process. With CPOE, the provider enters the order into a computer, and then the system checks the order for incorrect dosages and/or drugs, drug-allergy interactions, drug-drug interactions, drug-food interactions, and other possible causes of error. The system monitors the treatment process to ensure that nurses administer the right drug to the right patient at the right time and issues an alert if the patient's condition changes. For nursing, such technology removes the guesswork from medication administration, which reduces stress levels, improves clinical effectiveness and productivity, and allows nurses to focus on patient care rather than paperwork.

Virtual Reality

Virtual reality uses computers and multimedia peripherals to produce a simulated clinical setting of the future, which better prepares today's students for everything from remote-controlled robotic surgery and nanotechnology, to voice-activation documentation and telehealth kiosks.

Electronic Healthcare Records

Electronic healthcare records (EHRs) are a critical way for nursing to document its contribution to healthcare.

SUMMARY

In every sphere, nurses must work to bring practice and education firmly into the twenty-first century. Clearly, nursing needs a major restructuring from within, rather than something imposed by external forces.

The first step in this restructuring is to embrace informatics as a solution to the many challenges the profession now faces. From educating new nurses and easing the strain of the nursing shortage, to helping practicing nurses improve the safety and ensure the rights of patients, informatics and nursing's acceptance and advocacy of it will play a key role in the evolution and elevation of the profession. Indeed, informatics may be the difference between ultimate success and total extinction.

KEY POINTS TO LEAD

1. Examine the current and future state of nursing in light of the nursing shortage, increasing demand for patient safety, and nursing's need for professional visibility.
2. Define nursing informatics.
3. Examine how IT changes patient care, care outcomes, nursing's visibility, nursing accountability, and nursing best practices.
4. Discuss data security.
5. Delineate sources of IT funding and discuss the importance of ensuring it.
6. Value nursing administration's role in IT implementation.
7. Delineate emerging technologies.

Literature Box

PROBLEM OR PURPOSE

As healthcare evolves inexorably into an electronically mediated environment, nurses must become comfortable with and knowledgeable about IT. Nurses' exposure to IT must happen before they enter the profession. It must happen in nursing school. That means a radical educational change. The partnership between University of Kansas School of Nursing and the Cerner Corporation and the study detailing it represent the first use as a simulated teaching tool of a live-production CIS designed for care delivery. The purpose is to teach the basic nursing curriculum, while helping students develop the requisite skills (e.g., using clinical decision supports to access reference databases, conducting Internet searches in the context of doing assessments, care planning, and documentation) to operate as knowledge workers.

This new approach contrasts dramatically with the informatics programs and computer labs currently in place in programs for healthcare professionals. Simulated e-health delivery system (SEEDS) is designed to provide teaching and learning tools that help professional students develop the competencies necessary to participate in an information-age healthcare environment. The main teaching strategy employed by SEEDS is problem-based learning through the use of virtual case studies. Students access a virtual patient's record in the system and document his or her assessment and plan of care exclusively with the system's ordering and documentation tools. The student learns by trial and error in a controlled environment.

SEEDS has five objectives:
1. To enhance the development of critical thinking and problem solving
2. To integrate online patient assessment, problem identification, treatment, and evaluation
3. To demonstrate the impact of structured data and information on patient care
4. To provide the information infrastructure for evidence-based clinical practice
5. To promote dissemination and evaluation of knowledge and research

METHODOLOGY

The faculty and informatics team developed database content to teach health professional students conceptual and practical applications of electronic health records. The faculty and vendor partner adapted case studies for the system, creating virtual patients within a virtual healthcare system. In the classroom and clinical seminar groups, students used these case studies for problem-based learning experiences that simulated a real-time practice environment.

Using the case studies and a vendor-created electronic medical (health) record (EMR), students documented assessment data and a subsequent plan of care for the patient. As appropriate, the system triggers a request for additional data that are important elements for clinical decision making. The student then easily navigated to evidence or knowledge bases to support clinical decisions. The instructor could display all student documentation to share responses among the students. Such mechanisms provide the student immediate feedback and just-in-time learning.

Initial implementation began with a pilot group of 34 typical undergraduate nursing students. These students were assigned according to the seminar groups: two groups in the summer and two during fall semester.

The partners introduced all 120 students in the baccalaureate program to the system, but only students in the pilot group had hands-on training with the automated system. They learned nursing practice and clinical documentation using traditional methods and paper documentation systems.

Approximately 5 months later, the partners extended the project to the second-level nursing curriculum, introducing electronically mediated medication management. Students were required to produce clinical course assignments via the system as opposed to the traditional paper medium.

About 7 months later, critical care and population-based CIS management techniques were added. The system was expanded for use by all students in the program, in addition to the Schools of Medicine and Allied Health.

Literature Box

CONCLUSIONS AND IMPLICATIONS

According to an on-line evaluation study, students reported a greater sense of collaboration with peers and faculty, enjoyed timely feedback about their work, and found assignments interesting.

Preliminary results indicate students and faculty are satisfied with the new teaching and learning strategies. Faculty have found it harder to change.

They, too, had to gain familiarity with the system to adjust their teaching techniques to allow for more data-driven case presentations and to rework familiar case studies and teaching strategies.

From Connors, H., Weaver, C., Warren, J., & Miller, K. (2002, September/October). An academic-business partnership for advancing clinical informatics. *Nursing Education Perspectives, 23*, 5-7.

Contemplations

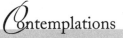

- What skill sets and organizational culture issues help or hinder the change processes that computerization demands?
- Do staff and management understand the change process? Have they received sufficient opportunity to make personal and organizational preparations for the change?
- What existing workflow processes require change? Are there, for example, potential redundancies in documentation, discrepancies between work practice and policy, or unclear or undefined processes?
- How, exactly, should these processes be changed? What is not working? Is the ideal process the existing one? How can automation improve a manual process?
- How are the capabilities of a new system evaluated (e.g., at a national meeting exhibit)?
- In what way is the potential of the new system evaluated in terms of what the current system can or cannot do?

- Does a sufficient difference exist to warrant a new purchase?
- Are major clinical problems traceable in the new system?
- What new data are provided?
- Does a reason exist to pursue more information about cost?
- Does the system address the projected needs of the patients, staff, and facility 5 years from now?
- Does the CNO understand how asking such questions may allow understanding of what the issues and concerns may be?
- What can be done to ensure that potential users are and continue to be engaged in the project?
- Are nurses able to express their expectations and concerns and identify their roles?
- Are they encouraged to make suggestions?

LEADER STORY

Karlene Kerfoot
Senior Vice President, Nursing and Patient
Care and Chief Nursing Officer
Clarian Health Partners
Indianapolis, IN

I work at the corporate level of a multi-hospital system, which adds to the complexity and ambiguity of a leadership position in healthcare. You have no choice but to lead by example and influence rather than by command and control in these positions. We have made excellent progress in terms of establishing a sophisticated leadership team in the 4½ years that I have been at Clarian. We have been able to retain and promote from within talented leaders and recruit nationally to fill openings. With a supportive internal development program, excellent clinical nurses have been promoted to managers and been able to learn the required skill sets and leadership abilities well.

Moving from a clinical staff position to manager, director, and hospital/systems CNO requires planning and development. The requirements for strategic thinking change within each of these positions. Managers need to be able to think 3 months out, directors need to think at least 1 year ahead, the CNO for a hospital needs to think 3 years into the future, and the system CNO needs to think and plan 5 years into the future. The broader your span of control in the system, the more proactive long-range thinking is required. However, the operational parts of these positions are as equally important as the strategic. Many people fail because they do not have the abilities to operationalize the strategic plan they develop. Failure comes from the inability to balance the requirements of being operational and strategic in a mix that is appropriate for that level of position within the organization.

To illustrate this kind of thinking, I tell a story about three modes of travel. From an airplane at 30,000 feet you can see the "big picture." When you fly over the Rockies, it is very clear, there are many mountains, and they are huge. In a helicopter, you fly much closer to the ground and you can see a few mountains that surround you, but you have little appreciation for the massiveness of the mountains that you cannot see. In a car at night, even with the high beams on, you can see only one small hill at a time and you have little sense of how these hills and turns are part of an enormous mountain that is part of many other mountains. Managers are responsible to operate at the level of the car with the headlights on and the directors and facility CNOs at progressively higher levels of the helicopter. The system CNO must see around many mountains from the 30,000-foot level to chart the course of the organization for the next several years.

If we convert this thinking to the world of IT, we can see similar patterns. With the headlights of the car at night, we can see that a specific IT system would be good for the operating rooms or even the ICU. From the helicopter, we can see that a specific IT system would be good for the hospital and we can begin to see how the various systems would or would not work for the hospital from this height. From the 30,000-foot level, we can see how a specific IT system would or would not link an entire system of facilities and perhaps even the community. It takes this kind of thinking and vision to conceptualize decisions about choices in IT.

The strategy for selecting a system for Clarian was an airplane strategy but we also looked at the opportunities from the helicopter and car. We were interested in how many nurse thinkers were in the company. We wanted a system in which nurses and other clinicians were thinking and designing clinical systems 5 and 10 years out rather than just

253

for today. For today and for the future, the CNO must possess as a core competency informatics and the application to clinical systems. Otherwise, you can end up with a system that doesn't meet the needs of your facilities. Decisions and leadership around IT involve a very long-term commitment and many downstream consequences that can be good or bad. The CNO must surround himself or herself with bright nursing informatics people who can translate clinical knowledge into clinical applications that work for the front-line user and also for the researcher who needs to access information in the future to measure clinical outcomes. I am very concerned about the lack of nurses prepared in nursing informatics. Consequently, Clarian improvised to train their own. As a pilot, we sent two nurses to the vender for a 6-month "boot camp" to learn everything they could, which included system implementation projects. We anticipate that when they return, they will be turbo-charged with information and skills that would take them years to acquire if their only learning experience was Clarian.

There needs to be serious in-depth thinking about IT for the future. IT doesn't necessarily solve all safety problems and can create some new problems if we are not *very* careful. For example, with all the pharmaceuticals in use, we can potentially create a whole new set of problems. If drugs are programmed inappropriately, we can hurt 100 patients before the error is discovered, whereas in the "good old days," we would only harm one patient. We are now working with Rolls Royce on building a culture of high reliability into our hospitals. We have to look at other industries who have years of experience in high-reliability systems and learn from them how easy it is to "muck up" a system. It is important to create a system where the least-prepared person can reliably handle a procedure or routine every time. We must simplify our systems for the future. IT can be tremendous for healthcare but it can also be horrendous. If the system goes down and you have to go to manual processes for a period, there is an entire

generation of nurses who have never done manual procedures and are clueless as to how to handle it.

The work of leaders is to change things while managers keep the status quo. Managers are important, but for the most part they are not charged with the responsibility of developing new knowledge. When a leader leaves a position, the staff should say, "I'm better as a person and a professional for having worked in the culture this leader created."

Leaders should be attracted to the improvement of the professional practice as a given. Rather than focusing totally on the business side, nursing leaders must have both business and advanced clinical training. They must be able to do business plans as well as to know *what* needs to be changed in clinical practice. Nursing leaders don't have to have degrees in both business and nursing, but they must have both skill sets. CNOs are usually hired by nonclinical people. Unfortunately some are looking for someone with business savvy as the prime prerequisite. It's more difficult for nursing to articulate for them the importance of clinical savvy. Schools of nursing need to capitalize on offering both skill sets. Of course there are programs like Johnson & Johnson's Wharton School for Nurse Fellows and the opportunities exist for schools to create similar programs. One is never finished learning as a nurse administrator. I attended Wharton school in 1987 and religiously return for the 3-day update whenever it is offered. Leaders must be held accountable for evidence-based administrative practice as well as clinical practice. And now we have the Magnet Hospital criteria and clinical program development that is as important as the financial outcomes.

If a graduate student came to me for advice, I would tell that person to first go for diversity of background. There is much to be learned in areas outside of clinical nursing. In my experience, the people who have been the most creative and innovative have had a diverse background, which includes different specialties, and different professional and organizational experiences. They read in many diverse areas such as the *Harvard Business Review*, IT literature, nursing, healthcare and policy literature, and current events. A nursing leader must not be wedded to only one way of doing things and must have a wide variety of experiences from which to draw. For example, when I was mentoring a young man, I asked him to do all manner of things that he thought he didn't like to break down the walls of his preconceived ideas. I asked him if he liked the symphony. He replied that he didn't. I then told him to go anyway and to analyze how the symphony works and what he could learn about leadership from the symphony. After several sessions, he became aware that there are many opportunities to learn about leadership and to stretch your mind absolutely everywhere. People who experience a diverse set of experiences are less afraid to change, to think outside of the box, to think with a more open mind, and to take risks. Second, I would tell this individual that an effective nursing leader has to be passionate about making a difference for nurses and for patients and

their families. And finally, I would tell this person that it is important to choose a mentor who is very different from you as well as those you want to emulate and that you should have many mentors. It is very true that we can learn as much and sometimes more from negative examples of leadership than we can from positive. So it's important to be exposed to all types.

As a nursing leader, I have had incredible highs and incredible lows. I believe I have lasted longer than many others because of what my grandmother told me, "Don't get your bowels in an uproar over something you won't remember when you're 85 years old." So I do my best to prioritize and not get emotionally in an uproar over what will be inconsequential many years from now. It is very important to have balance in my life. When I'm here, I work, and I love it. When I'm home, I'm home, and I love being there. The abilities to compartmentalize and not get myself worked up have been effective survival strategies for me.

Chapter References

American Nurses Association. (1999). *Principles for nurse staffing*. Washington, DC: The Association.

American Organization of Nurse Executives. (2005). AONE Nurse Executive Competencies. *Nurse Leader, 3*(2), 15-21.

Berens, M. C. (2000, September 10). Nursing mistakes kill thousands injured. *Chicago Tribune*.

Blois, M., & Shortliffe E. (1990). The computer meets medicine: Emergence of a discipline. *Medical informatics: Computer applications in health care*, p. 20.

Buerhaus, P. I., Staiger, D. O., & Auerbach, D. I. (2000, June 14). Implications of an aging registered nurse workforce. *Journal of the American Medical Association, 283*(22), 2948-2954.

Buerhaus, P. I., Staiger, D. O., & Auerbach, D. I. (2003, November-December). Is the current shortage of hospital nurses ending? *Health Aff (Millwood), 22*(6), 191-198.

Collen, M. (1997). Preliminary announcement for the Third World Conference on Medical Informatics, *MEDINFO*, p. 80.

Fitzgerald, J. M. (1996). Application of computers in nursing: A position analysis. Retrieved August 17, 2004, from *The Nursing Resource* home page.

Government Accounting Office. (2001, July). Nursing workforce: Emerging nurse shortages due to multiple factors (GAO-01-944).

Huffman, E. (1990). *Medical record management*. Berwyn, IL: Physician's Record Co.

Krizek, T. (2000). Surgical error: Ethical issues of adverse events. *Archives of Surgery, 135,* 1359-1366.

Levy, A. (1997). Is informatics a basic medical science? Proceedings of MEDINFO, p 979.

Marietti, C. (1998, March). *Operations or outcomes?* Healthcare Informatics.

Matthews, P., Carter, N., & Smith, K. (1996, Spring). Using data to measure outcomes. *Journal of Healthcare Information Management,* 10(1), 3-16.

O'Farrell, M. (2002, October 11). Bar codes urged to halt hospital errors. Retrieved May 8, 2003, from http://archives.tcm.ie/irishexaminer/2002/10/11/story218097572.asp.

Ozbolt, J., Beyers, M., Button, P., Bakken, S., Simpson, R., Warren, J., & Zingo, C. (1999). The 1999 Nursing vocabulary summit conference: process and outcomes. Available on-line at http://www.amia.org/pubs/symposia/D005369.PDF.

University of Minnesota's Evidence-Based Nursing page. Retrieved October 6, 2004, from http://evidence.ahc.umn.edu/ebn.htm.

U.S. Census Bureau. *Census Bureau projects doubling of nation's population by 2100.* Retrieved January 13, 2000, from http://www.census.gov/Press-Release/www/2000/cb00-05.html.

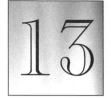

CHAPTER

13 Building the Business of Nursing Services: Marketing to and for the Community and the Profession

Many of life's failures are people who did not realize how close they were to success when they gave up. JOHN MAXWELL

This chapter focuses on an organizational service, marketing, from the nursing perspective. Marketing to the community, the prospective consumers of healthcare, is the common focus of marketing. Marketing to the profession, being concerned with the affiliations of professionals with the service entity, is equally important in achieving success in an organization. Both aspects build the business of nursing services within the organization. This chapter explores both of these aspects.

ONE OF THE KEY BUSINESS FUNCTIONS OF a nursing service is to create the right environment for patients and the profession. However, if that creation is not marketed to and for the community and the profession, growth and improvement will be difficult at best. Andrew Jackson and Mark Twain are noted for saying people weren't very creative if they couldn't spell a word more than one way.

Although that concept is humorous, it applies to marketing the work of a healthcare organization. If an organization has only one way to tell the message, it is limited in its impact. Multiple messages may need to be developed, all focused on the same product or service and with the same core theme, to be appealing to the multiple publics who could benefit from that product or service. Similarly, the message that makes sense and is enticing for a specific population of the community may have limited value for a healthcare professional from that same specific population. Further, a message that plays well on television may have limited value on a web site. However, consistency of the core message and appearance is necessary to provide perceptual linkages to the basic service. Therefore, gaining familiarity with the organization's marketing endeavors and being sufficiently aware of community and professional needs to support or redirect marketing activities and foci are two challenges for chief nursing officers (CNOs).

MARKETING DEFINED

The term *marketing* refers to the process of defining and describing customers, relating their needs to the core mission of the organization, determining the organization's capacity to meet the needs, and assessing the competition's potential. The CNO's task is to be involved sufficiently with organizational marketing activities, to provide information about nursing that potentiates a marketing opportunity, and to provide insight about customers' needs based on community and healthcare directions. If marketing is a part of corporate culture, the view that "marketing is everyone's job" prevails.

Marketing is based on an exchange of need and supply. Need, or demand, refers to the desired quantity and type of services. Supply relates to the available quantity of services to meet the need or demand. Basically, marketing involves meeting the needs of the potential consumers by responding to those needs and conveying messages that help consumers make choices. Obviously, the intent of marketing strategies is to have potential consumers select the marketed products and services.

Marketing begins with the target population, the customers (consumers). Without appropriate market research, the nature of services and the intensity of those services' availability cannot be developed appropriately. In healthcare the key target is the community or some component of it. However, that target is not sufficient. Another key target is the healthcare professionals who are (or could be) attracted to work with a given organization. In many instances, what benefits one group benefits the other. For example, the healthcare organization with high qualifications such as Magnet or Baldrige designation can attract more patients, and more patients create the need to recruit more professionals. In addition, both designations include what is right about the workplace, which is also attractive to patients. The difference between marketing to the community and marketing to professionals is in how the message is crafted to portray the levels of relevance and quality that exist within an organization.

Understand your customers. It's the basis of
business success.
LARRY BOSSIDY

The goal of marketing is to create customer equity: "the sum of a customer's lifetime value across all of a company's customers" (Waite, 2002, p. 40). Waite described three kinds of equity that drive customer equity. The first driver is *value equity*, which healthcare organizations frequently reference as *value added*. In other words, what this new service or product does in the eyes of consumers is add value to remaining loyal to an organization. The second driver is *brand equity*. In other words, this driver would be viewed as another reason to remain connected to an organization because it carries the "trusted, known" brand. Clearly, one of the value-added benefits to Magnet designations (an example of brand equity) is the marketing potential (Woods & Cardin, 2002). The third driver is *relationship equity*. It might also be called *retention equity*. For example, many people choose not to switch primary healthcare providers simply because the current provider "knows my condition and my family." Therefore, rather than switching providers for financial reasons, a consumer may be driven by the relationship.

Customer Equity:
- Value
- Brand
- Relationships

Creating the image of quality is frequently nebulous. Person A may have had excellent experiences during a recent service encounter and person B may have had mediocre ones. If customer equity has not been established because the quality is consistently high and valued, the consumer is less likely to return to the prior place of service.

KEY CONCEPTS

The core mission is an important element in marketing considerations. When an organization is *mission* driven, every function has to be described in terms of the core. If a function does not relate and the organization pursues the function, the result is mission drift. The more frequently an organization drifts from its core mission, the less clarity exists about the organization. Therefore marketing efforts, like other efforts within the organization, have to relate to the core mission.

Even if some new function fits the core, *organizational capacity* must be considered. For example, a hospital may desire to expand its neurosurgical services, but insufficient staff, space, and support services may exist. How those insufficiencies can be corrected in a timely manner would need to be considered before any major marketing endeavor were undertaken. On the other hand, if no such insufficiencies are typical and additional consumers can be served, capacity drives marketing considerations in a different way.

In addition, the *competition's potential* to match or exceed an organization's services must be considered. An organization may choose to offer a service that has already saturated the market. This decision may be driven by a desire to describe the organization as having comprehensive services, or it may be driven by a new approach to a service that has been stagnant. Many organizations offer services comparable to every other organization and attempt to compete because of some different approach to meet consumer demands. The ability to differentiate among types of services helps consumers make choices about their care.

Porter and Teisberg (2004) suggested that the wrong competition has led to an inefficient, ineffective healthcare system. In comparing competition in healthcare to that of most other businesses, the authors drew the following conclusion regarding healthcare:

Costs are high and rising, despite efforts to reduce them, and these rising costs cannot be explained by improvements in quality. Quite the opposite: Medical services are restricted or rationed, many patients receive care that lags currently accepted procedures or standards, and high rates of preventable medical error persist. There are wide and inexplicable differences in costs and quality among providers and across geographic areas. Moreover, the differences in quality of care last for long periods because the diffusion of best practices

is extraordinarily slow. It takes, on average, 17 years for the results of clinical trials to become standard clinical practice. Important constituencies in health care view innovation as a problem rather than a crucial driver of success. Taken together, these outcomes are inconceivable in a well-functioning market. (pp. 65-66)

In light of this perspective, marketing to individuals is becoming more important because of the increasing research findings that suggest many diagnoses occur differently in different populations and that treatment also varies. Matching the consumer's needs with relevant services is a major function of marketing.

In *Blue Ocean Strategy,* Kim and Mauborgne (2005) suggest that rather than focusing on the typical "pool" of consumers, we expand our view to a larger "pool." The authors describe how Cirque du Soleil developed—not to compete with the circus or the theater, but rather to combine the best of those two formats to create a new approach. The unmatched success of Cirque du Soleil holds lessons for healthcare.

The Four Ps of Marketing

Probably the most basic and most frequent terms associated with marketing are the "four Ps": product, price, place, and promotion.

Because this concept was developed within manufacturing, the term *product* historically referred to an actual product. In the current perspective, that *P* refers to actual products and also to services. An argument also can be made that service is what product manufacturers sell too, but *services* more commonly describes what healthcare organizations offer. In manufacturing, customer loyalty often is related to the service behind the product. In healthcare, service is the face of customer loyalty.

The second *P*, price, refers to the costs to the consumer, or in the case of healthcare, the consumer and the consumer's insurance provider. Because this is such a complex system, price is a concept that may be the driver in healthcare decisions for the consumer, although it may be more so for the determiner of care, such as the employer or the insurance provider.

The third *P*, place, refers to such aspects as accessibility and comfort. Many inner-city hospitals have expanded sites to suburban areas to "be" where the consumers are. Additionally, the ambiance of hospitals can enhance one place over another. This concept explains why some newly built or renovated hospitals have rooms with convertible chairs, sofas, and Internet access (The Patient Room, 2004).

The final *P*, promotion, refers to the communication plans for conveying information about the product, price, and place. This stage involves advertising whether via the Internet, television, radio, brochures, and newsletters. Halm and Denker (2003) described an example of a diverse marketing program. In creating a primary prevention program for women at risk for heart disease, they dedicated a telephone line for direct access; they used internal marketing (word of mouth, signs, business cards, pamphlets, and newsletters); and they used external marketing (public service announcements, articles for community newsletters, television coverage, Internet access, speakers, and advertisements). They used a steering committee of influential women and they set the price of the service based on a survey of women who first used the services. This example shows that multiple

strategies are used in successful marketing plans and that the consumer is involved.

CONNECTING WITH TARGET POPULATIONS

To connect with specific groups of people for specific services requires defined marketing strategies. These strategies stem from the way in which the potential consumer base is described.

Segmentation, Targets, and Positions

These three activities are essential to successful marketing. Nursing often can assist in this aspect in indirect ways. Table 13-1 identifies examples of nursing's involvement with each of these essential activities.

Breaking groups into smaller, better defined subgroups (*segmentation*), whether patients or professionals, further enhances effective marketing. Typical segmentation has been focused around age, gender, language, and lifestyles. Although these continue, even more information is available about consumers so that the potential to relate to specific services, such as complementary therapies, is captured. One of the current market segment mapping activities in the business world has

Table 13-1 EXAMPLES OF NURSING'S CONTRIBUTION TO CONNECTING WITH TARGET POPULATIONS

Marketing Activities	Key Focus	Examples of Nursing Contributions
Segmentation	Distinct subgroups	Analysis of a clinic population to determine groups that could benefit from primary prevention strategies and groups that would benefit from tertiary care
Targets	Selection of a subgroup to provide services	Analysis of a cost-effective, but long-range, strategy to provide primary prevention services
Positions	Conceptualizing the value	Descriptions of how a service leads to quality care

resulted in fractional ownership of jets. It is a way to deal with the cost of fuel, fixed schedules, and travel to atypical places. The analogy for healthcare is a challenge CNOs can address (e.g., Can area hospitals provide a core educational program to prepare staff for specialty services?).

An emerging market segment that will continue to intensify is the technology-focused market. Whether the technology is high-tech equipment or web-based services to garner information or to schedule appointments, the key is that some people make decisions about a range of elements in their lives based on technologic advantages. As the population of "tech saavy" people grows, having the appropriate technologic supports will be important to marketing.

Targets are those segments selected as the focus of the marketing effort. Target segments are often niches that are attractive from a mission and/or financial perspective. Targets are often underserved populations from the perspective of the service to be provided. Creating a gastric bypass service, for example, is not a service associated with the traditional view of the underserved. *Underserved* in this context means few basic services are available. If no other organization is performing gastric bypass, if the procedure is a covered service, and if a segment of the community is obese, this may be a service to this previously underserved population.

Finally, *position* refers to the way in which the service is viewed, not necessarily the service itself. For example, if all hospitals offer a specially priced delivery service, it is difficult for parents-to-be to select one organization over another. If, however, one organization offers 24-hour call-in service for questions about the baby and a weekly cleaning service for 2 weeks, this organization may be seen as more desirable. Some current examples of positioning strategies are Internet connectivity in patient rooms and pager services for expectant fathers and families of surgical patients. Such services are designed to acknowledge consumers as busy people who need an organization that is sensitive to their needs.

CNOs have two primary populations about which to be concerned. The first, of course, is the prospective and actual patient population. Another source of influence associated with this population is family and friends (Roper, 2005). Thus connecting with family and friends of satisfied patients has great potential. In some cases, especially with family, these people decided where their significant other would receive care.

According to Keller and Berry (2003), "Roughly 1 in 10 of the adult population of the United States, the Influential Americans, are the people who make the society, culture and marketplace run" (p. 1). Although the influence of the individuals is widespread and diverse, some of their documented influence is in the healthcare marketplace. These Influentials also are likely to act on concerns that they have. In other words, if they have had an unsatisfactory experience, they are likely to provide feedback that indicates the problem and sometimes even offers solutions. When those sources of information are ignored, one source of information is limited and the potential for loss of an Influential is increased. Although Keller and Berry did not look specifically at healthcare, the idea of influential consumers creates different ways for thinking about the consumer population.

Depending on the type of healthcare organization, some connections are more likely than others. For example, rural hospitals are usually well integrated into the community. Public health departments frequently are seen as amorphous, and a school-based clinic tends to be connected with the grass roots at that school. Specialized services have a loyal following even though it may be a narrowly focused group. The concept of adjacency, which refers to finding a new market for what an organization offers or finding something new in the current market, is important here (Tecker, Frankel, & Bower, 2004). Connections to people and to key products and services and to the appropriate markets can enhance the way services are offered.

The second primary population with which CNOs are concerned is healthcare professionals.

By virtue of the quality of the workplace and the care provided, nurses, physicians, and others can be recruited. Marketing to these populations is different from marketing to the public, but both are about quality. Healthcare professionals want to work in safe, quality-oriented organizations in which patients are held in high regard. They want to have a "say" about care and they want to be supported when taking risks. Nurses in particular seek professional development support. Marketing to this group differs considerably from marketing to the public. Professionals obviously want to know about salaries and benefits, but they also want to know how the organization conveys the messages to the public and if those messages include key patient-centered issues.

A final and less frequently encountered group is the payers. Although the CNO is typically not the one negotiating with payers, the CNO needs to know best practices in the nursing services and how they fit in the community perspective so that internal messages are clear. What this means is that the negotiator for the healthcare organization must be convinced the organization can deliver the negotiated services. Furthermore, the key services to sell are those that can be received only within that facility; and nursing is a major factor.

MEETING THE MISSION

Because healthcare needs are constantly changing based on new strategies, technologies, and therapies, the demands for services also are evolving. With all of the current pressure on healthcare organizations, it is easy to become distracted from the mission and focus on the latest quality issue or the latest source of revenue. Thus the key strategy that every CNO must employ is a critical assessment of the services provided in terms of the organization's mission. Assuming that an organization is focused on high-value healthcare, managing for financial impact alone is no longer possible. Theoretically, in part, the mission of an organization is derived from an analysis of the target population, whether that is a community,

an age group, a clinical system, or a societal segment. In many organizations, the chief financial officer (CFO) represents the financial aspects of the organization's operation. The CNO typically represents the quality aspects of the organization's operations. It is the balance of the finances and the quality in terms of such issues as positive outcomes for patients and staff that make one organization more marketable than another.

Porter-O'Grady and Malloch (2002) devised an equation for value that has relevance to marketing.

Healthcare value = Resources + quality + service

Resources include funds, labor, and supplies; *quality* is the appropriateness of interventions; and *service* is the satisfaction and effective relationships. Together they equal healthcare value.

Therefore the mission must be to provide value to the population and to manage the finances and quality (or resources, quality, and services) to achieve the mission. Capitalizing on all three elements in marketing decisions can create stronger approaches.

Another major consideration is the nature of the expectations for services themselves. In other words, as healthcare has evolved, once a service or product became available, numerous demands were made to provide the service or product to all who were interested. One example is the availability of Viagra moving from a small self-pay population to major insurance coverage. The marketing created the desire for the product and the resultant demand changed funding practices. What then could happen if services were narrowed to focus more closely on quality in a given area? What if services were reorganized to emphasize prevention rather than treatment? For example, in January 2004 Blue Cross & Blue Shield of Rhode Island launched a broad-based prevention program based on an economic analysis of long-range costs savings (Harkey, 2004). Some "boutiques" offer such prevention services as part of their special practices (MacStravic, 2004). What if this approach became a trend? These are examples of how the mission must be thought of in the context of what the population needs and wants.

Another way to consider the total market potential is portrayed in Figure 13-1. Of any total market, an organization has some current base of service, called *market share*. A portion of the total market probably is unknown; for example, little may be known about the "members" of the subgroup. The *potential* growth is where additional success or failure awaits. The high potential areas are obviously the most desired, but they may not be readily identified. Filtering the evident community needs with the results of forecasting activities can set key targets.

So what must be done to meet the mission and current societal expectation about healthcare? Clearly cost is one element. At one time, that was the key driver. Since 2000, when the Institute of Medicine (IOM) report *To Err is Human* was released, the emphasis has focused increasingly on the beginning element of quality: safety. From the perspective of the providers and the public, statistics about failure to rescue, morbidity and mortality, and other relevant negative outcomes of care

are becoming more valued and more public. As a result, even though the idea of cost effectiveness has existed for decades, it will become increasingly easier to use the data of cost and quality to show which services and products, and thus which organizations, are effective and which are not.

A major difficulty exists, however, when the service is too costly or the quality is insufficient or when, despite poor finances or quality, the community expects the service will remain. Such is a common case for many rural hospitals. The quality they provide is excellent for the resources they have. However, the quality typically does not match that of a large teaching facility. Both organizations would have complaints about money, but because the scale of payment is so limited in rural settings, their finances are consistently critical. However, the citizens of those communities want "our hospital" to stay open and to provide the needed services. The dilemma of how to deliver care effectively in rural facilities remains a challenge. The potential is great for any redesigned approach that places rural hospitals in a more competitive stance.

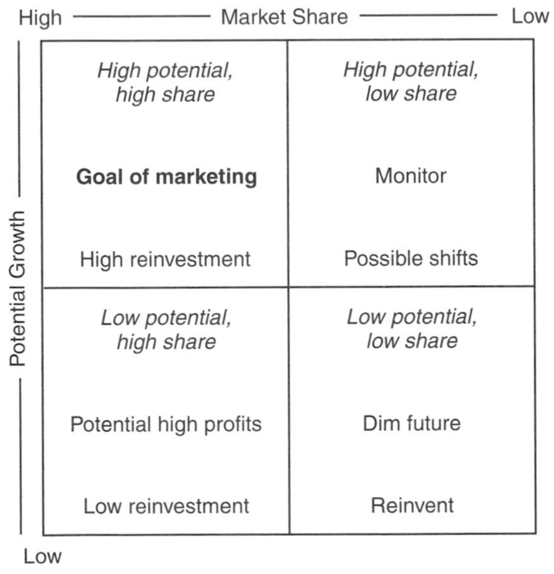

SPECIAL CONSIDERATION

Whatever strategy evolves from market analysis activities, the result is a business plan that, when well constructed, can distinguish one organization from another. If limited enthusiasm surrounds the plan for a new or revised service, caution dictates reconsideration of the analysis and conclusions. Committing to marketing decisions is important to the organization in meeting its mission.

External Influences

Several examples of marketing strategies relate to external forces. Baldrige and Magnet programs are marks of achievement in meeting performance criteria. Organizations with these designations use those achievements to market to customers and professionals. Leapfrog is another example of an attempt to improve the organization to subsequently

High ——————— Market Share ——————— Low	
High potential, high share	*High potential, low share*
Goal of marketing	Monitor
High reinvestment	Possible shifts
Low potential, high share	*Low potential, low share*
Potential high profits	Dim future
Low reinvestment	Reinvent

(Vertical axis label: Potential Growth — High at top, Low at bottom)

Figure 13-1 Market potential.

improve care. The Leapfrog Group is a national coalition of large healthcare purchasers attempting to wrestle with patient safety. The initial focus for Leapfrog was (1) computerized physician order entry systems; (2) staffing ICUs with on-site, skilled physicians (hospitalists); and (3) evidence-based hospital referrals for select high-risk procedures. Unfortunately, in 2003 (3 years after Leapfrog started), only 6% of the hospitals had fully implemented these expectations (Devers & Liu, 2004). Based on the fact that they targeted only the 12 communities in the Center for Studying Health Systems Changes 2002-2003 report, the goal of meeting this initial set of criteria most likely will take some time. However, connection with Leapfrog provides marketing potential to specific groups, especially health plans.

Patient Satisfaction

Patient and employee satisfaction reports also create important messages. For example, such surveys usually are thought to answer the question, "How have we done?" However, they also can indicate, "Why come here?" HealthGrades and Press Ganey Associates are examples of satisfaction surveys available to the general public. According to Press Ganey (2003), patient and employee satisfactions may be predicted from each other. A 60% likelihood exists of predicting patient satisfaction from employee satisfaction and vice versa. Satisfaction surveys also reveal sources of dissatisfaction. As these criticisms are addressed, to be open and verbal about the "new strategy" is important so that the public and employees know their concerns are not only heard but also addressed. The Literature box suggests decentralizing satisfaction data to increase the potential for improvements.

All of the recent IOM reports emphasize the need to work as a team. Breaking down the discipline silos becomes critical to ensuring an overall atmosphere of quality. Although each discipline must be discipline competent, the key is how the disciplines interact with each other on behalf of the patient. When a culture of focusing on excellence

exists, the entire workplace operates differently. Two growing factors that the public expects to hear about as they make healthcare decisions are staffing and interdisciplinary teamwork.

Staffing

Staffing has been documented increasingly in hospitals, especially in general acute care hospitals. It too can be used to sell one organization over another to a community and to professionals. The 2003 IOM report that focused on the workplace is an example of an external document that can provide internal movement to address an issue (staffing) that is of great concern to the public and to professionals. Issues such as staffing are critical for healthcare organizations to resolve.

Aiken, Clarke, Sloane, Sochalski, and Silber (2002) found that adding patients to a registered nurse's patient care load increased the potential for death after common surgical procedures. Additionally, Aiken, Clarke, Cheung, Sloane, and Silber (2003) found that a better-educated workforce also led to better patient outcomes. Both of these studies may indicate to some CNOs that they would want to demonstrate the best standards in their work setting. Therefore, if the CNO made this commitment, marketing would need to adjust its focus to help prospective employees understand the rationale behind lower patient ratios and an expectation of higher education. Then messages about how the ratio and education factors relate to quality would need to be crafted for the general public so that they understood the importance of these two factors.

Less attention has been paid to community organizations such as assisted living facilities. In a study conducted by Phillips, Munoz, and Sherman (2003), the researchers found that the presence of a full-time registered nurse was correlated with less chance of a resident moving into a nursing home. In other words, no registered nurse presence correlated with a higher chance that an assisted living facility resident moved into a nursing home. Although most assisted living facilities are not large enough to support a full organized nursing service, nurse administrators in other types of facilities can use this research finding to their advantage. By creating an information network that conveys this finding along with a list of relevant, local assisted living facilities for patient referral for nursing staff, the staff can help families make critical decisions about which assisted living facility to select when such is needed. Furthermore, if a major healthcare organization has related services connected with it, what a marketing advantage this information would be to assure people that their older family members would have less chance of being institutionalized.

Interdisciplinary Teamwork

Wherever healthcare occurs, some form of an interdisciplinary team is at work. Why, then, would research about interdisciplinary teamwork still occur? The answer is simple but alarming: because teamwork is not always effective. Without research to uncover specifically what is not working, attempts to alter practice are based on the experiences of others or are made with logical but random attempts to improve operations. One study of high-risk areas in acute care facilities reported about one third of the nurses surveyed believed disputes about patient care often were decided on who was right versus what was best for the patient. They also rated experiences with primary physicians, consulting physicians/surgeons, and anesthesiologists as low or very low; and the same held true for their experiences with nurse managers (Kaissi, Johnson, & Kirschbaum, 2003). Clearly, the task of the nurse administrators is to work with the nurse managers to develop their abilities to interact with staff so that experiences are seen more positively. Nurse administrators must also work with the physician staff to develop relationships that put the patient at the center and that limit the number of occasions when disputes seem to be based on *who* not *what* is right for the patient. The key is then to translate these outcomes into positive marketing messages.

Liability Issues

As Maar (2004) pointed out, issues of liability always must be considered. "Any sort of internal and external marketing activity can potentially subject your hospital to liability and needs to be undertaken with great care. What may seem like a harmless team-building newsletter or recruitment tool may cause unintended consequences. Communication or marketing material that a patient may have access to should be created with due diligence" (p. 522). This warning should not arrest the development of innovative communication. It should, however, alert nurse administrators to being certain that statements are truthful and, whenever possible, documentable. This concern for veracity also suggests that advertising materials would be better if dated and either have a global focus to use for an extended period or have targeted content that reflects current conditions; the latter is probably more cost effective. Working with other professionals has certain obligations; those increase in complexity and scope when working with the general public. Screening printed matter with a new view toward liability may be an example of an increased awareness of this concern for accuracy of marketing. Communicating clear, precise, and hopeful messages is the key to successful marketing with any potential audience.

SUMMARY

Each of the previous examples creates a different way of thinking about marketing. Marketing must focus on providing services that align with knowledge about the community and create messages that resonate for the community and healthcare providers alike. Looking at marketing merely as advertising is no longer possible. Assuming that marketing is someone else's job is also not possible. Being proactive to link the services frequently provided by the nurses within an organization with what the community needs is critical to the overall success of the healthcare organization.

Marketing is a complex element of organizational management. The CNO does not have final authority or accountability for marketing decisions in most organizations. A CNO can make two major contributions in this area: serving as a resource and marketing to professionals.

KEY POINTS TO LEAD

1. Analyze marketing activities of an organization from the perspective of equities.
2. Evaluate differences in marketing strategies between consumers and professionals.

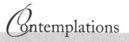

Literature Box

Typically organizations plan, implement, and analyze marketing activities at an organizational level. This has been true for some organizations for patient satisfaction also. Because patient satisfaction is so important to the success of an organization, it becomes more important to understand area-by-area results. Unit level systems often function as tightly woven, decentralized areas with standards and abilities that differ from the entire organization. Incremental opportunities to improve quality can be enhanced by patient satisfaction data. A drill down approach of the focal point (to the unit) and the content (the practitioners and services) yields potential data for improvement. In addition to the differences in patient population, the differences in the unit subcultures of an organization can produce variances among patient satisfaction data.

In addition to targeting problems with such data, the potential for new services and approaches can become apparent. Improved patient satisfaction also led to improved staff satisfaction in at least one service cited.

Scalise, D. (2005, January). Zeroing in. *Hospitals and Health Networks*, 48-51.

Contemplations

- What would happen if we applied new marketing approaches to healthcare?

- What healthcare issues exist that can be answered in a new way?

LEADER STORY ✒

GEORGIA FOJTASEK
PRESIDENT AND CEO
FOOTE HEALTH SYSTEM
JACKSON, MICHIGAN

Our Health System has nine vice presidents; one is the Vice President for Patient Care Continuum and another is the Vice President for Business Development and Marketing. We work as an integrated team, and at the end of the day, we all own responsibility for the success of the organization. We don't want marketing promising something we cannot deliver, and we all value the importance of how marketing helps us do our jobs and the effect on how both our staff and the public see us. Finance, Nursing, Marketing, Information Systems, etc., have equal say at the table, and this is key to our success.

Our Health System was referenced in a *Harvard Business Review* (HBR) article (January 2002), "Leading in Times of Trauma." The University of Michigan has a research project known as Compassion Labs. The researchers were actually here talking with our staff on September 11, 2001. They had been here about a day and a half collecting data on compassion in the workplace, and the trauma of that day ended their research at our organization because continuing it would have produced skewed results. That work, however, was part of the *HBR* article about the researchers' experiences with compassion within our organization.

As noted by the *HBR*, our staff wanted to do what they could for victims' families and friends in the aftermath of September 11. That led to significant staff donations of vacation time to the Red Cross. We discovered in this process that there had been a very quiet program whereby staff had been donating their vacation time to co-workers who needed it. I realized how, as leaders, we routinely reinforce values that drive the organization. No one had "asked permission" to implement this program. Staff suggested and Human Resources supported it, because it was the right thing to do.

Later, I discovered a different, but related, situation. We have a medication program for the uninsured, with certain limits on spending. It went way over budget at a time we couldn't afford it. I asked, "How could this happen? What are the controls?" Staff responded, "We understand our commitment to the poor, and we couldn't shut it off." Our internal "marketing," if you will, conveyed, both directly and indirectly, our organizational values. Staff is aware of whether the organization lives its values. When it does, it creates a high-performing organization in terms of patient care quality, patient safety, and long-term financial viability. Staff reflects these values in their actions. Our internal face must match external marketing or the organization's reputation will be negatively affected.

Employee satisfaction is related to internal marketing in other ways. Over the past 6 years, we've progressed on a nationally benchmarked tool from the 66th percentile to the 90th percentile on employee satisfaction, and this was while we were doing a major financial turnaround including some staff reductions. By engaging and involving our staff, we were able to do some pretty extraordinary things. That connection with the staff is internal marketing.

An internal marketing program that preceded external marketing involved a missed step in cleaning equipment used in patient care. Although we were certain that patient outcomes weren't affected, based on reviews by the Centers for Disease Control and Prevention and the state health department, we decided that, given the circumstances, our value of integrity required that we tell our patients. For our staff, the fact that we were totally transparent with all stakeholders and supportive of the staff in the area where this occurred was viewed very positively. We were clear that it was a system problem not a people problem. There was a great deal of organizational pride in how we handled a difficult situation. We had massive communication efforts directly involving patients, staff, volunteers, trustees, and media. We invited the media in. Internally, we talked about how our values led to our decision to inform our patients and how we could all learn from this issue. That had a marked effect on our organization. Our CNO was the executive leader for this matter, including the decision about "What are we going to do afterwards." We needed to be sure that our community knew that we took patient care quality and patient safety seriously and that our citizens could rely on us. Having the CNO active in this whole experience was very important to the organization. Our patients and the clinical issues were at the forefront. We put together a comprehensive response of testing and retesting patients and information hotlines staffed by nurses. Our CNO led that effort.

Another example of our CNO's involvement in marketing was when we created a joint venture with a small osteopathic hospital with a fairly busy Emergency Department (ED). The health system owners of the osteopathic hospital decided they were going to close inpatient and ED services, adding 20 patients daily to our inpatient volume, as well as moving all community emergency services here. We had been planning to expand our ED because it was 20 years old and not serving the volume needs that we already had, but we were just in the beginning stages of expansion planning. Our ED reports to the CNO, and she provided patient volume information and collaborated with marketing to mount a very vigorous public relations campaign to help patients choose the appropriate place for care and the service that met their needs: when to use our nurse call center for information, when to go to the primary care physician,

when to visit an urgent care center, and when to visit the ED. That campaign worked in part. We learned there are numerous intervening variables in deciding the right place for care, for example, insurance coverage requirements, families who can only access care after normal working hours, and, of course, the lack of access to primary care for Medicaid and uninsured patients. It is a constant struggle to direct patients to the right place and to balance demands on the hospital and our staff.

Meanwhile, we are building a new ED, a 2-year-long project. Because of the high visibility and high demand for ED services, it has been a constant effort for the CNO to keep everyone informed about the project. She is really focused on this being a community facility. Because the actual construction process is very disruptive to the neighborhood where we are located, she holds regular meetings with neighborhood groups to keep them well informed about progress and plans. She also makes regular presentations to city and county officials so that key leaders are well informed. We use ads and newspaper notices informing people about changes in parking and how best to access the facility during this construction period.

Being a nurse has significantly shaped what I do as a leader and has given me a different perspective. For example, I can relate to the demand that reduced length of stay has on nurses who must be sure that patients are ready for discharge, whereas nonclinical leaders may see only the business issue of length of stay. We are at a time in healthcare when our understanding and skills as nurses are more valued and more essential in top leadership roles.

It has been important to me to remain in close proximity to patient care areas. Several years ago, we purchased an old bank building about a mile from our main campus to use for nonclinical space needs. Most people assumed we would move our executive offices there to be away from the hectic pace of the hospital campus and in more executive-type space. I've elected to remain on campus with the key operations leaders. To be where our patients and staff are and to have daily reminders of the real business we are in helps balance my decisions.

Overall, we are beginning to witness much greater balance in leadership and acceptance of diverse thinking. Nurses are moving into chief operating, chief financial, and chief executive officer roles. They are bringing to the table strong collaborative and nurturing skills and a focus on the patient in decision making, along with solid business skills.

Dutton, J. E., Frost, P. J., Worline, M. C., Lilius, J. M., & Kanov, J. M. (2002, January). Leading in times of trauma. *Harvard Business Review,* 54-61.

Given where healthcare is today, this leadership balance is critical. We cannot survive without strong business acumen and ability to make hard decisions. But how hollow our work would be without a full understanding that our business is patient care and that our decisions affect this care.

For me, being a nurse and serving as a CEO during these very turbulent times is such a privilege. Creating an environment in which excellent patient care can be delivered, where staff and physicians believe they are in the best place to give care, and, at the same time, ensuring that the business enterprise not only survives but thrives is a challenge. Those times when it all comes together in excellent performance are enormously rewarding.

Chapter References

Aiken, L. H., Clarke, S. P., Cheung, R. B., Sloane, D. M., & Silber, J. H. (2003). Educational levels of hospital nurses and surgical patient mortality. *Journal of the American Medical Association, 290,* 1617-1623.

Aiken, L. H., Clarke, S. P., Sloane, D. M., Sochalski, J., & Silber, J. H. (2002). Hospital nurse staffing and patient mortality, nurse burnout, and job satisfaction. *Journal of the American Medical Association, 288,* 1987-1993.

Devers, K., & Liu, G. Y. (2004, February). Leapfrog patient-safety standards are a stretch for most hospitals. HSChange Issue Brief. Retrieved on February 25, 2004, from http://www.hschange.org/CONTENT/647/?words=.

Halm, M. A., & Denker, J. (2003). Primary prevention programs to reduce heart disease risk in women. *Clinical Nurse Specialist, 17*(2), 101-109.

Harkey, J. (2004, January 23). Health plans consider making the business case for prevention. Health Leaders. Retrieved January 29, 2004, from http://www.healthleaders.com/news/print.php?contentid=51793.

Institute of Medicine. (2000). *To err is human: Building a better health system.* Washington, DC: The National Academy of Sciences.

Institute of Medicine. (2003). *Keeping patients safe: Transforming the work environment of nurses.* Washington, DC: The National Academy of Sciences.

Kaissi, A., Johnson, T., & Kirschbaum, M. S. (2003). Measuring teamwork and patient safety attitudes of high-risk areas. *Nursing Economics, 21,* 211-218.

Keller, E., & Berry, J. (2003). *The influentials.* New York: The Free Press.

Kim, W. C., & Mauborgne, R. (2005). *Blue ocean strategy: How to create uncontested market space and make competition irrelevant.* Boston, MA: Harvard Business School Publishing.

Maar, S. P. (2004). Healthcare marketing liability: Avoiding possible pitfalls. *The Journal of Nursing Administration, 34,* 520-523.

MacStravic, S. (2004, February 9). Do boutiques deliver better care? *Health Leaders.* Retrieved February 9, 2004, from http://www.healthleaders.com/news/print.php?contentid=52125.

The patient room. (2004). *Hospitals & Health Networks, 78*(5), 34-51.

Phillips, C. D., Munoz, Y., & Sherman, M. (2003). Effects of facility characteristics on departures from assisted living: Results from a national study. *Gerontologist, 43,* 690-696.

Porter, M. E., & Teisberg, E. O. (2004, June). Redefining competition in healthcare. *Harvard Business Review*, 64-76.

Porter-O'Grady, T., & Malloch, K. (2002). *Quantum leadership: A textbook of new leadership*. Gaithersburg, MD: Aspen Publishers.

Press Ganey. (2003). Undeniable: Patient and employee satisfaction linked. Retrieved November 3, 2003, from http://www.pressganey.com/scripts/news.php?news_id=84.

Roper, A. S. W. (2005). Once in a generation: Critical. Retrieved May 25, 2005, from http://www.gsm.ucdavis.edu/innovator/winter2004/onceinageneration.pdf.

Scalise, D. (2005, January). Zeroing in. *Hospitals and Health Networks*, 48-51.

Tecker, G., Frankel, J., & Bower, C. (2004, August). Big myths. *Association Management*, 66-74.

Waite, T. J. (2002, February). Stick to the core—or go for more? *Harvard Business Review*, 31-41.

Woods, D. K., & Cardin, S. (2002). Realizing your marketing influence, Part 2. *Journal of Nursing Administration, 32*(6), 323-330.

Financial Leadership and the Chief Nursing Officer

Karen Kelly

A billion here, a billion there, and pretty soon you're talking about real money.
EVERETT MCKINLEY DIRKSEN

Today's chief nursing officer faces formidable challenges daily. Nursing leaders manage multimillion dollar budgets to ensure adequate resources to provide quality patient care. This chapter explores basic financial concepts that nursing leaders must master in today's healthcare environment. The chapter examines healthcare economics, reimbursement systems and issues, budgeting processes and plans, and nursing as a business within the context of the role of nursing leaders.

AS THE LARGEST DISCIPLINE OF PROVIDERS of healthcare services, nursing currently represents a cost center in a healthcare organization's operating budget and an essential source of revenue. However, nurse leaders are still relatively new players in the game of healthcare finance. Around 30 years ago even the chief nursing officer (CNO) had little or no control over the budget for nursing. CNOs were clinical leaders but not the financial leaders of their departments. That has changed dramatically. CNOs now oversee budgets that rival or exceed the budgets of many businesses within their communities. Competence with financial concepts is a basic skill in the toolbox of

today's nurse leaders to ensure nursing's place at the executive level. This chapter examines essential concepts for the financially savvy nurse leader.

HEALTHCARE ECONOMICS AND NURSING ADMINISTRATION LEADERSHIP

Nurses, for much of the profession's modern history, have not been engaged fully in the economics of healthcare. Before the introduction of prospective payment systems (PPSs—e.g., diagnosis-related groups [DRGs]) and managed care, nurses had little incentive to be cost effective in delivering care or to comprehend the basics of reimbursement of healthcare. Thirty years ago, physicians determined when patients would be admitted and discharged from the hospital. Most people had employer-paid healthcare insurance. Healthcare organizations billed for the costs of healthcare and were paid accordingly. Aspirins might be billed for $3.00, although they cost the hospital only pennies. Into the cost of the aspirin, as administered, charges were added for handling and storing the drug in the pharmacy, the time taken by the pharmacist to prepare the drug for distribution to the patient unit, the time of the nurse to prepare and administer the dose, and the time of the clerk in patient billing to post the charges to the patient account. In addition, some cost shifting of unpaid charges could have occurred for patients who had no insurance or resources to pay their bills. A small profit also was rolled into these charges. And these charges were paid as billed. So much has changed in the past 30 years that the need for nurses, from staff nurse to CNO, to be knowledgeable about healthcare economics has never been more acute.

The Sciences of Economics and Nursing

Economics is a science that focuses on the exchange of goods and services for money. Just as psychology, biology, and sociology have long been recognized as essential sciences for the foundation of professional nursing, so is economics. Economics focuses on the costs of healthcare and on the supply and demand for nursing services, a key underlying factor of the causes and effects of the current nursing shortage. Nurse leaders need to be competent in basic concepts of economics to compete in today's healthcare arena (Price, 2001).

Supply and demand is an economic force that nurse leaders must face routinely. Supply is reflected in the quantity of a product that a supplier can provide for a given cost in a specific period of time. Demand is reflected in the willingness of a user to purchase a product. When supply exceeds demand, the supplier may need to reduce production or reduce the cost of the product to stimulate demand. The demand for a certain piece of equipment that incorporates the latest technology may exceed the manufacturer's ability to supply the technology. This is likely to keep the cost high until production meets demand. At some point, the price may be reduced when supply exceeds demand, or the next generation of technology improves upon this piece of equipment (Chang, 2001; Cleland & Kibbin, 1990; Penner, 2004).

Likewise, the supply and demand for nursing services serves as a constant economic force for nurse leaders. During the 1970s, 1980s, and 1990s, cyclic nursing shortages and surpluses of nurses occurred. The introduction of Medicare's DRGs

in the 1980s created a brief surplus of nurses as hospitals reduced nursing positions in response to decreased reimbursement from Medicare. In the 1990s, the growth of managed care and the redesign of many healthcare organizations, especially acute care facilities, created an oversupply of nurses. Nursing positions in hospitals were reduced, and nurses began to move from acute care to community-based agencies and other employers. When a new shortage emerged in the late 1990s, competition for nurses began again as the demand for nurses became greater than the supply. In other decades, shortages often were addressed by an increase in the supply of students by schools of nursing. But changing demographics and other social and economic forces have made nursing a less desired career choice than in the past. New strategies for increasing the supply of nurses have been linked with changing nursing care delivery models, creating new incentives to recruit and retain nurses, and reshaping the nursing work environment. Among other efforts, these have brought nursing service and nursing education together to create new partnerships to address nursing supply and demand (Pfoutz & Price, 2001).

Utility reflects the satisfaction with a product that is sold. The satisfaction that defines utility is shaped by many factors, including the personal preferences, values, and culture of the consumer of a product (Penner, 2004). Healthcare consumers view their care as having positive utility when the care provides hope for renewed health or improved functioning. Negative utility is associated with care that offers risk or complications. Consumers seek products or services, such as healthcare, that offer a perceived positive utility, avoiding that which reflects a negative utility (Penner, 2004).

Nurse leaders have come to understand the economy of scale in recent years. Economy of scale is defined as "a situation in which the long-run average costs decline as output increases, thus enabling the producer to maximize profits" (Penner, 2004, p. 17). Two hospitals in a community may recognize the need to collaborate, rather than compete, to provide certain services to take advantage of the economy of scale. High-cost outpatient oncology services, for example, might be needed in the community. Because the two hospitals want to provide these services, but demand is not high enough to support two separate services, collaborating to provide a joint venture may offer the economies of scale that enable both facilities to retain their patient base in a cost-effective manner.

Nurse leaders must comprehend the economic principles that support the daily and long-term operations of healthcare organizations (Lemire, 2000). The *Scope and Standards for Nurse Administrators* (American Nurses Association, 2004) identifies the responsibility of the nurse administrator to evaluate and administer the resources of the nursing service department (p. 30). To manage multimillion-dollar budgets, nurse leaders must be able to understand the reimbursement systems that support the operation of their organizations; payment systems for nursing services; and the most cost-effective systems to ensure that the appropriate supplies needed for the delivery of nursing services are available. Nurses need to be prepared to explain to patients (i.e., their customers) forces such as reimbursement that influence length of stay. Quality care can be provided only when all nurses within an organization understand the economic underpinnings that support the healthcare organization.

NURSING LEADERSHIP IN FISCAL PLANNING

The cost of healthcare in the United States is an issue of continuing concern. Close to $2 trillion is spent annually for healthcare (Centers for Medicare and Medicaid Services, 2004), yet millions of individuals, indigent and employed, have no healthcare insurance and limited or no access to healthcare services. Despite the huge expenditures for healthcare in the United States, infant mortality in the United States is higher than in most other industrialized nations, life expectancy

is lower, and breast cancer rates are higher. As healthcare leaders, nurse leaders are involved in managing healthcare costs, healthcare budgets, and healthcare resources in an effort to support the community's health and well-being.

Nursing Fiscal Control: Past and Present

Nurse managers and administrators once had little control over the budget matters related to their units, departments, or divisions. Instead, they focused on managing patient care, with little or no control over the fiscal resources that supported patient care and the human resources that provided that patient care. The management of nursing resources was limited to scheduling and hiring/firing functions. Nurse administrators and managers, in some cases, had no voice in setting salaries and wages for nursing staff. Human resource personnel would determine pay rates with little or no input from the nurse leaders. This was rarely questioned and generally accepted as the way to run the healthcare organization.

Today's nurse leaders engage in short-term and long-term fiscal planning. Many organizations are on 3- to 5-year budget planning cycles, dealing with the current year's budget and planning for the next several years. These prospective budgets are subject to multiple reviews and revisions until the time they are submitted to governing boards and bodies for approval, based on trends and factors such as reimbursement rates; third-party payer contracts gained, lost, or renewed; market share gains or losses; changing patient demographics; changes in the number of admissions and the average length of stay; and the closure of some services and programs and the development of new service lines.

The Impact of External Forces on the Nursing Budget

In the current healthcare system, a wide range of social, political, and economic factors influences the role of nurse leaders in shaping healthcare budgets. Population and economic forces in a community can have a significant impact on healthcare organizations. Sometimes these forces can be predicted during budget planning; some occur without warning.

The sudden influx of migrant workers without healthcare insurance into a rural area may tax the resources of a community clinic. A change in the political party in power in the state legislature may alter drastically the way Medicaid reimburses for the care of children and indigent adults. The closure of a manufacturing plant that was the community's largest employer may result in a high unemployment rate, a loss of insurance coverage for some residents, and a loss of population, all of which change the community's pattern of usage of a healthcare organization's inpatient and outpatient services. A plant closure also may change dramatically the usage patterns of the hospital's emergency department (ED). The projections for the ED may have been built on the assumption of a steady 8% growth per year, based on historical trends. The sudden loss of insurance benefits may result in the increased use of the ED for primary care among the unemployed and their families, resulting in a sudden increase of 15% in the ED's patient population. This increase in the patient population has significant impact on the use of the ED's human and physical resources and consumable supplies.

Although the nursing shortage is an internal force, it is also an external force that shapes budget planning. The nursing shortage is an example of an external force that influences the budget planning and implementation. For example, a healthcare organization has depended on the local university and community college to meet its needs for new nursing staff for several decades. Over the past several years, the enrollment has decreased at both programs, which resulted in faculty cuts. Now both programs are seeing an increase in applicants but do not have enough faculty to meet the demands of additional students. In addition

to having cut the budgeted number of faculty positions, both educational institutions are unable to compete with local healthcare organizations for salaries to attract nurses with graduate and doctoral degrees. The CNO must consider this factor in all budget and program planning. More healthcare organizations are entering a variety of financial partnerships with educational institutions to ensure a supply of nurses to meet their institutional needs.

Nurse leaders must respond, sometimes on a daily basis, to the changes resulting from a range of social, political, and economic factors. Staffing patterns must be revised, selected clinical services may be reduced or eliminated while others are expanded, or purchasing practices must be altered. CNOs must not only plan for and implement these changes but also explain these changes to nursing staff and others, obtain their support in implementing these changes, and maintain the changes until the next wave of fiscal change hits. At the same time, they must deal with the ongoing forces of changing standards from accrediting bodies, an increased concern among the public and regulating bodies concerning patient safety issues, and new regulations concerning patient privacy related to healthcare services and reimbursement.

The Impact of Internal Forces on the Nursing Budget

The nursing shortage is also an internal force that affects the nursing budget. When nursing positions are vacant because of turnover and the creation of new positions, the budget is affected by the use of overtime pay and the use of agency nurses to fill shifts. When large numbers of graduates are hired each spring to fill new and vacant positions, the nursing budget is enlarged to cover the costs of orientation of a new cohort of nurses.

The expansion, reduction, and elimination of other services within a hospital may have an impact on the nursing budget. If the hospital's open-heart surgery program is eliminated because the surgeons have moved to another city, the nursing budget will be affected because the budgets for the surgical unit, intensive care unit, cardiac catheterization lab, and cardiac rehabilitation are all reduced to reflect the change in services. If an independent home health agency is acquired by a hospital to supplement its own home health service, the nursing budget may be expanded if home health service reports through the CNO. Interdepartmental competition for control and administrative reassignment of clinical services also may influence the nursing budget. If a hospital's home health service is moved from the control of the CNO to the vice president of outpatient services, or moved from the control of the vice president of outpatient services to the CNO, the nursing budget also will be affected.

CNOs: Changing Roles and Financial Responsibility

CNOs now control the largest portion of the budget in most hospitals and other healthcare organizations. Nursing resources account for a large portion of any operating budget. The role of the CNO has expanded to that of the chief executive of patient care services to include non-nursing and multidisciplinary departments, such as radiology, pharmacy, therapy services, social services, and outpatient services. As a result of this role expansion, the CNO has come to control an even larger part of an organization's budget. There is power in money, and CNOs are becoming more powerful as their roles evolve. Along with this change for the CNO comes change in the role of others in the hierarchy of nursing leadership in organizations. In large, complex healthcare organizations, midlevel executives (i.e., clinical, service-line, or department directors) may control multimillion-dollar budgets in conjunction with their front-line managers. Some directors, and even nurse managers, may control budgets larger

Box **14-1**	ADMINISTRATIVE ACCOUNTABILITY

Healthcare economics
Leadership in financial planning
Reimbursement issues
Budget process
Nursing as a business
Developing a business plan

than some local corporations, with multimillion-dollar operating budgets (Box 14-1).

The CNO must be able to work effectively with the full executive group to ensure that nursing's voice is heard in financial matters (Noonan, Weiss, Stichler, Looker, & Jones, 2002). One of the most common problems in the development of personnel budgets that support healthcare staffing is the lack of knowledge and cohesion among the full executive group. The leadership of the finance department, including the organization's chief financial officer (CFO), may not fully appreciate the intricacies of staffing a 24/7 service, such as nursing. Although the finance department runs on a typical business day schedule (e.g., Monday through Friday operations, open from 8:00 A.M. until 5:00 P.M.), nursing goes on 24 hours each day, 7 days a week. Although the finance department staff will work around the vacation days and sick time of workers, nursing must replace staff during vacation and sick time (Goddard, 2003). Gormley and Verdejo (2000) detail how the critical partnership of the CFO and the CNO enabled one healthcare system to manage a major budget shortfall that resulted, in part, from reductions in Medicare and managed care reimbursement and an increase in the uninsured and underinsured in the community's population resulting in more bad debt. This partnership allowed the organization to work through the shortfall without compromising the quality and quantity of healthcare delivered.

REIMBURSEMENT ISSUES

A Brief History of Healthcare Reimbursement

Healthcare insurance became an expected part of American life after World War II. Such coverage had existed to a limited degree before the war, but in the postwar years, employer-provided healthcare insurance became the norm. Fee-for-service programs were the typical form of coverage. Healthcare providers billed their fees, and the fees were paid by the insurers. There were deductibles and co-payments paid by the insured persons. However, providers rarely negotiated fees with insurers. In the 1960s, Medicare and Medicaid were initiated by the federal government to provide healthcare coverage for the elderly and the indigent, respectively. During the next 30 years, more changes in healthcare reimbursement would occur as managed care expanded and came to dominate healthcare benefits, changing the way healthcare organizations operated and were reimbursed for care. By the year 2000, all healthcare organizations, including acute care, home care, and community-based services, had experienced dramatic changes in how healthcare services were reimbursed.

Diagnosis-Related Groups and Prospective Payment Systems

In the early 1980s a major change in Medicare revolutionized healthcare financing. Until that time, Medicare and Medicaid were very profitable for healthcare organizations. Providers billed their charges and they were generally paid an amount that approximated what they billed. In 1983 Medicare introduced the PPS. DRGs were created, after much study, to create a system that paid for healthcare based on expected actual costs, by region of the country. Billing for healthcare became driven by coding that flowed from the documentation of physicians, as well as nurses, with DRGs assigned on the basis of the diagnosis and expected treatment plan. If a healthcare organization could provide care for a patient with a particular DRG code for less money than the

DRG paid, the organization got to keep the difference. If care in that organization cost more, the hospital provided care at a deficit.

An Introduction to Managed Care: A Driving Force

Although managed care has roots that precede World War II, managed care became a force in healthcare beginning in the 1970s. Health maintenance organizations (HMOs) began to appear throughout the country. By the 1990s, managed care was visible in most communities throughout the country. Numerous models of managed care exist, but all have common characteristics that deal with cost control. Case management, preauthorization, and gatekeepers became part of the healthcare vocabulary as managed care grew (Box 14-2).

Evolution of Healthcare Reimbursement

Healthcare reimbursement and the impact of third-party payers are driving forces in healthcare today. Healthcare organizations and individual providers live and die by the adequacy of reimbursement. Beginning with the debut of DRGs and PPSs for Medicare in the early 1980s, healthcare organizations and their delivery systems have been experiencing an ongoing evolution. The emergence of managed care has revolutionized the American healthcare system as cost-reduction efforts are driven by third-party payers. Reductions in Medicare rates to providers have resulted in more physicians declining to accept Medicare patients in their practices. The expansion of managed care plans, including preferred provider organizations (PPOs) and Medicare HMOs, has changed the way providers deliver care, organizational expectations of reimbursement for care, and consumers' access to care.

The Uninsured in America

Although different sources will report slightly different figures, strong evidence exists that 45 million

Box **14-2** Examples of Managed Care Plans

Staff model HMOs Physicians, nurses, and all other staff are employees of the HMO; offers highest level of cost and quality control **Closed panel HMOs** Network that includes staff models and group models (HMO contracts with physician specialty groups) **Open panel HMOs** Network that includes individual practice associations and group practices that contract with HMO **Point of service plans** Plan that allows HMO members to self-refer to providers outside the HMO network, with member incurring higher cost	**PPO** Member of PPO selects from list of preferred providers to obtain care at lower out-of-pocket cost but may self-refer out of network while incurring higher costs **Commercial insurance plans with managed care elements** Traditional fee-for-service plans evolved into plans with elements of managed care, including preauthorization for care, negotiated fees with preferred providers, and prescription services with restricted formularies; provides the lowest level of cost and quality control

Modified from Pulcini, J. A., Neary, S. R., & Mahoney, D. F. (2002). Healthcare financing. In D. J. Mason, J. K. Leavitt, & M. W. Chaffee (Eds.) *Policy & politics in nursing and healthcare* (4th ed., pp. 241-297). St. Louis: W. B. Saunders.

people were without healthcare benefits in the United States, up from 43.6 million, in 2002 (DeNavas-Walt, Proctor, & Mills, 2004; Kaiser Commission on Medicaid and the Uninsured, 2000; Rhoades & Cohen, 2004). Many of these are the working poor who exist on minimum-wage jobs. They fail to seek healthcare they cannot afford. When they are seriously ill, they often are absorbed into the healthcare system as charity or unreimbursed care. However, others without healthcare benefits include white-collar workers and professionals who work for small companies without healthcare benefits for employees. Many of these white-collar workers and professionals cannot afford private healthcare insurance. So they take their chances and hope they never experience a catastrophic health problem.

The United States spends more on healthcare per capita than any other industrialized Western nation. Unlike these other nations, the United States has disproportionately more people without access to appropriate healthcare. However, healthcare organizations are expected to care for those without third-party reimbursement. Often such people present for care late in their illnesses, when their lack of early access to preventive or primary care has resulted in significant morbidity or the high risk of mortality from an illness that was treatable but went untreated.

Comparing the Old and New of Healthcare Reimbursement

Before the introduction of Medicare DRGs and other PPSs and the emergence of managed care, providers (e.g., hospitals, physicians) submitted bills to insurance companies, Medicare, and Medicaid for services rendered at costs determined by the provider. Reimbursement was based on the amount billed. The payment might be a percentage of the billed amount, but the payment was still based on costs determined by the provider. The introduction of DRGs signaled a dramatic change in the way third-party payers reimbursed for healthcare services to hospitals, nursing homes, physicians, and other providers.

It was a revolutionary move from payment based on billed costs to a system that based payment on what care "should" cost. Diagnoses were clustered and categorized by a range of factors (e.g., alcohol detoxification without medical comorbidities vs. alcohol detoxification with medical comorbidities) and average payment rates. These payment rates adjusted for geographic differences in cost (e.g., higher for large coastal metropolitan areas than in rural Midwestern areas). If a hospital could provide care, for example, for an appendectomy case for less money than what the DRG paid, the organization got to keep the difference. However, if care cost more than what would be reimbursed, no additional payment would be forthcoming.

In the days before DRGs, when unreimbursed care was provided, the deficit could be passed on in the way of additional costs for care of those with insurance. PPS ultimately extended into other models of reimbursement and brought about the expansion of alternative models of reimbursement (e.g., HMOs, PPOs, contracts, capitation), nearly eliminating the traditional fee-for-service model. Rolling over unreimbursed costs no longer worked under the new system. Managed care has changed the way healthcare is reimbursed and delivered forever, including rural health (Box 14-3).

Medicare Managed Care

Medicare managed care has been offered for about a decade, and some states have adopted managed care programs for Medicaid. Many of these Medicare managed care plans have been withdrawn from the market after determining that they could not make sufficient profits on Medicare plans. Some of the original programs that opened in the mid-1990s soon reduced their geographic market or dropped out of the market. Although Medicare HMOs provide prescription drug coverage and other wellness benefits that Medicare does not provide, these HMOs may provide a lower level of coverage when severe illness occurs. For example, one hospital where this author worked contracted with four or five Medicare HMO plans when they first came into the marketplace.

Box 14-3 SETTING INFLUENCES

Rural hospitals may apply to the Centers for Medicare and Medicaid Services for status as a Critical Access Hospital. A CAH is eligible for cost-based Medicare reimbursement. CAH status ensures rural communities will have access to vital healthcare services. Participating hospitals must meet rigid criteria to be granted CAH status. The hospital can be for-profit or not-for-profit. The hospital must meet the following criteria:

- Have an average length of stay of 96 hours
- Have no more than 25 beds with swing beds (e.g., 15 acute beds maximum and 10 swing care beds [beds that can be used for acute or long-term care] maximum)

- Be rural and 35 or more miles to nearest hospital or another CAH (15 miles in mountains or if state certifies as "necessary provider")
- Provide emergency services available 24 hours daily; staffed with experienced, trained personnel; on-call staff must be available in 30 minutes
- Offer mandated services: inpatient care, laboratory, radiology, some ancillary, and support services may be offered part time off site
- Have at least one physician and may use mid-level practitioners
- Network with at least one other hospital to contract for referral and transfer and other selected services

From Busby, A., & Busby, A. (2001). Critical access hospitals. *Journal of Nursing Administration, 31*, 301-310.

This hospital had a well-respected, accredited comprehensive rehabilitation program for those who have had strokes, amputations, and other such disabling conditions. The Medicare HMOs would not approve treatment in this rehab unit, where patients received approximately 6 hours of active therapy each day. They would only pay for nursing home care with 6 to 8 hours of therapy per week. The 2003 Medicare reform (December, 2003), which gives senior citizens limited drug benefits, is fully effective in 2006 and encourages seniors to enroll in Medicare HMOs to get the highest level of drug benefits (Centers for Medicare & Medicaid Services, n.d.).

Incentives and Reimbursement

As the healthcare system was being reshaped by the forces of third-party reimbursement, a variety of new factors arose in an effort to maintain quality while containing cost. These incentives have implications for the CNO's budget work.

HMOs and PPOs offer incentives to physicians who work for them in clinic-like settings or who contract to provide services in their private practices. Primary care physicians who see patients every 15 to 20 minutes in private practice may be told by an HMO or PPO to see more patients, moving them through every 10 minutes or less to meet their daily quota of patient visits. Meeting the quota may bring a bonus, or a financial incentive reward, at the end of the fiscal year. Referring patients to specialists at a higher price can cost primary care physicians money by reducing their year-end bonuses by deducting an amount for each specialist referral.

Hospitals gain incentives for being cost effective. First of all, a greater margin (nonprofit organizations) or profit (for-profit organizations) exists for cost-effective organizations. They simply make more money for being cost effective. Cost-effective organizations may be more successful in gaining contracts from managed care organizations, which ensures that a body of patients will seek healthcare from their organizations, including the hospital, home health agency, and hospital-affiliated clinic.

Hospitals also gain when they can provide office space to physicians, at a profit, who also are affiliated with the healthcare plan and who will now use this hospital over a competitor, binding the physicians to their organizations.

Employees also may earn incentives for being cost effective in delivering healthcare. For example, some healthcare organizations offer employees incentives to propose cost-saving measures. Many times the cost-saving measures are tied to a bonus paid to the employee: for example, the employee gets 10% of the savings from the proposal submitted and implemented.

The CNO and Reimbursement Issues

With diminishing reimbursement for care, CNOs must take an active role in improving reimbursement. Cost-containment measures, such as lowering length-of-stay averages and eliminating expensive procedures that are not essential, are the main approaches to maximizing reimbursement. However, other efforts also may improve reimbursement. For example, improving documentation by physicians and nurses is another approach to improving reimbursement. Documentation directs the coding procedures that lead to billing for care. Although a small study by Bonace (2000), using a homogenous patient group in one hospital, did not demonstrate an impact on reimbursement, others have found that improving documentation can improve reimbursement. Adom et al. (2001) used clinical care coordinators (RNs) to conduct concurrent reviews of patient records to evaluate documentation. When deficiencies were noted, the clinical care coordinators coached the house staff and other physicians to enhance their documentation to reflect more accurately the severity of patient illness and to improve their assignment of diagnoses to support more appropriate coding for DRGs. This resulted in the development of a clinical documentation management program. The authors reported that millions of dollars were captured in reimbursement, although only 15% of the patient population were included in the review process. Nursing championed the issues of increasing reimbursement for the benefit of the whole health-care organization. CNOs need to explore a variety of ways to improve reimbursement.

THE BUDGETARY PROCESS

As Finkler and Kovner (2000) note, "A budget is a plan" (p. 239). In the current healthcare environment with low reimbursement and ever-tightening budgets, the cynical view of the budget process would indicate that the budget manager should plan to cut most accounts within last fiscal year's budget to create the next fiscal year's budget. New budgets for new programs and services often are created from the cuts taken from existing, less lucrative programs. However, the economic constraints of the current healthcare environment only emphasize the need for expert budget planning (Box 14-4).

Each budget cycle within a healthcare organization operates on a timetable or budget calendar. Many organizations operate on a 3-year planning/implementation cycle: current fiscal year, next fiscal year, and the second fiscal year ahead. Others operate on an annual budget cycle for most budget managers, with longer range budget planning (e.g., 1 or 2 years ahead), occurring only at the executive level, not with middle or front-line

managers. The steps in the budgetary process are not necessarily sequential. They tend to overlap and may repeat themselves during the planning processes.

The examples used in this narrative focus largely on the budget planning for a hospital, as a matter of convenience. However, the same processes apply to all healthcare organizations. This narrative also supposes a large enough division of nursing and patient care services to justify three levels of management: CNO, clinical/department directors (overseeing several departments or patient care units), and managers who report to the directors. Smaller organizations may have only two levels of management; very large organizations may have an assistant CNO. In the following discussion, *budget manager* is anyone from the CNO to a front-line manager who controls a budget.

Types of Budgets

Different budgets deal with different "pots" of money. Operating and capital budgets are two examples of these different "pots" and are a major focus of the CNO's budget work. The operating budget includes many components, including expenses and revenues; supply budgets; personnel budgets; and statistical budgets that delineate patient days, clinic visits, surgical procedures, and other discrete events. The operating budget may include fixed and flexible subaccounts. Service contracts on equipment, certain supplies, and salaries for management employees are examples of fixed budget items; flexible budget items rise and fall with volume and may include the wages of direct care staff and patient supplies.

The capital budget includes monies for equipment that costs over a set amount (often over $500 to $1000) and has a specific longevity (e.g., 3 to 5 years). This may include some kinds of furniture (e.g., patient beds) or large amounts of computers, televisions, and surgical equipment. Capital budgets also include expenses for remodeling or other construction projects. Repairs and minor improvements may be included in the

---

Box **14-4**   Steps in the Budget Process

- Setting the timetable: operating and capital budgets
- Assessing the environment
- Determining goals, objectives, and policies
- Identifying assumptions
- Specifying program priorities
- Setting the measurable operating objectives
- Budget preparation
- Negotiation and revision
- Control and feedback

operating budget rather than the capital budget, if the costs are lower than the threshold for capital expenditures.

Nurse leaders may encounter other kinds of budgets. Some examples of these are presented here.

- *Cash:* projects the cash flow in and out of the organization, enabling the organization to manage disbursements in timely manner. This kind of budgeting occurs at the organizational level, not usually at the departmental or unit level (Penner, 2004).
- *Program:* plans for revenues and expenditures for a single program, which may cut across departments (e.g., a cardiac care program that includes the critical care unit, the ED, medicine/cardiology, cardiac rehabilitation, marketing, and patient education/community services) (Finkler & Kovner, 2000).

- *Product line:* similar to an operating budget with a focus on a single clinical specialty or type of patient (e.g., maternal/child care) (Penner, 2004).

Budget Timetable

Setting the budget timetable is an executive function that includes the CEO, COO, CNO, and other top executives (Table 14-1). Usually the operating budget and the capital budget planning cycles differ by only days or a few weeks. For a fiscal year that runs July 1 through June 30, budget planning for the next fiscal year may begin at the top executive level with the July 1 initiation of the current fiscal year's budget. Forecasting for the next fiscal year's operating budget requires analysis of current budget trends. Capital budgets generally are due for submission shortly before or after the

Table **14-1** SAMPLE BUDGET TIMETABLE

Budget Timetable for County Hospital Operating and Capital Budgets FY 07-08	
Event	Date
Implementation of FY 06-07 budget	July 1
Executive team retreat and budget planning session, review of FY 06-07 budget	September 1
Executive team meeting on budget assumptions, goals, objectives, and policies	October 5
Budget packets to budget officers with budget training program	October 25
Budget officers meet with VPs and directors to set divisional, departmental, and unit goals and objectives	November 1 through 5
First draft of budget to VPs	December 5
Final budget to VPs	December 15
VPs' meeting with COO/CEO	December 16 through 18
Executive team review of budget	January 15 through 16
Budget review: VPs with budget managers: capital and operating budgets	January 20 through 25
Final budget review by executive team	January 28 through 29
Budget to hospital trustees for approval	February 2
Budget to executive team	March 1
Budget returned to budget officers	April 1
FY 07-08 budget implemented	July 1

operating budget, but much of the planning must be concurrent. Utilization of capital resources depends on the human resources included in the operating budget. A highly specialized piece of equipment for the surgical service, for example, may require a very expensive service contract that must be included in the operating budget.

For the July 1 fiscal year beginning, budget managers likely will receive the budget packet, often containing the operating and the planning budget packet (sometimes called "rollouts") by mid-November. This may occur after a management meeting or inservice session on this year's budget-planning process. Instructions are received in the inservice session and in a cover memo with the budget packet. The instructions may vary from very simple to very complex. Some years the forms change, which requires additional time for completion of the budget paperwork. Typically, the instructions indicate which budget subaccounts within the departmental account's operating budget may be increased with a cost of living allowance (COLA) or inflationary factor increase. Other budget subaccounts may be targeted for reduction, holding at last year's funding level, or increased at less than the rate of inflation. Some subaccounts may be targeted for elimination (e.g., training funds for outside educational programs).

Usually the budget manager has 2 to 4 weeks to review the current fiscal year's trends and to revise the budget. During this time a front-line manager typically reviews the budget with the department director, and the director reviews the operating budget with the CNO. These reviews may be repeated during the budget planning period. The CNO, in turn, takes the divisional budget to the executive bargaining table. In the budget timetable for operating and capital budgets, usually an extended period of weeks to several months lapses before the final budgets are issued to budget managers.

Capital budget planning is usually concurrent and sequential with the operating budget. Plans for new equipment may require the inclusion of special staffing needs, service contracts, staff education, or rental fees for temporary replacement of malfunctioning equipment. Plans for remodeling or renovating an area may require additional operating costs to maintain the current level of service during construction; the service may, alternatively, need to be reduced or suspended during renovations. Staffing and other costs also have to be adjusted for this time period.

Assessing the Environment

This step of the budget process is actually ongoing throughout the budget year but is intensified during the budget preparation period. Many data about the internal and external environment are available to the budget manager from the organization's strategic planning process. Other data sources include staff and patient satisfaction surveys, public (and grapevine) information about the plans of competitors, trends in reimbursement, historic data related to patient census and service utilization, and community expectations for services and programs—all critical to a well-organized budget planning process. The need to adjust a budget (up or down) can be justified effectively only through the use of such data. If the competing hospital is going to close its behavioral health program or pediatric unit, the shift in patient population may justify an increase or at least maintenance of a budget previously slated for reduction. Using historic census data can enable the CNO and other nursing leaders to identify low census units that can be consolidated to create fewer units where higher occupancy (e.g., 85%) can be ensured (Kirkby, 2003).

Patient satisfaction data, for example, may indicate gaps in services, dissatisfiers (e.g., slow nurse response to call lights), or other issues that may need to be addressed in program and new service planning, as goals, objectives, and policies are set. If patients consistently are dissatisfied with nurse response in one area of a nursing unit, perhaps the problem lies in an antiquated call light system that needs to be replaced. The costs for the new system may be captured before the actual budget planning period if this assessment process is ongoing during the budget year.

Determining Goals, Objectives, and Policies

Goals, objectives, and policies related to the programmatic planning aspects of the budget process flow from the strategic plan and interrelate to the environmental assessment noted in the previous section. They are critical to supporting organizational assumptions. Budget goals must be realistic and consistent with the organization's availability of appropriate physicians, nurses and other human resources, the corporate culture, the healthcare market environment, economic climate of the community, and the organization's payer mix. Objectives must be measurable and must flow from the goals. Policies must be realistic and must fit with goals and objectives. If the budget policy is to cut all staffing budgets by 10% in the next fiscal year, setting goals to increase patient volume in selected services by 15% is not realistic. There must be goodness of fit among goals, objectives, and policies.

Identifying Assumptions

Some of these organizational assumptions are the product of educated guessing. Others flow from the strategic plan and the current assessment of the internal and external environment. Some assumptions are derived from the organizational and community grapevine through informal communication channels. If the organization assumes that Medicare reimbursement will be cut because of legislative plans and 55% of the hospital's inpatient population is covered by Medicare, such assumptions have significant impact on the budgetary process. If an aggressive for-profit outpatient physical rehabilitation corporation announces plans to break ground for a new facility three blocks away from the hospital, budget planners would have to carefully consider prior ideas about extensive expansion of the hospital's existing rehab program. Another example might be a new

department director hired from the competitor across town brings information about plans for expanding cardiac surgery services. This information must be treated as a potential assumption until it is validated or proven incorrect. These assumptions may reshape the goals, objectives, and policies as the budget planning process continues.

Specifying Program Priorities

These priorities start at the top levels of administration. Many influences shape these program priorities. Customer expectations for services can be a strong influence. If other organizations in the area offer mother-baby rooms and the hospital wants to expand its maternal/child market share, renovations to offer this kind of service must be considered a priority. The hospital's emphasis may be building market share for cardiology services as a result of vigorous physician recruitment for cardiologists, cardiac surgeons, and interventional cardiologists. These physicians expect new equipment, additional space, and the expansion of professional and support staff to support the growing program. This may translate to a budget emphasis for operating budgets in the critical care unit (CCU), telemetry, cardiac surgery services, cardiac cath lab, and cardiac rehab services, including home health. Capital and operating budgets also would be affected by these priorities. Budgets in other program areas may be reduced to help support these institutional priorities.

Priorities such as the clinical priorities noted above influence the budget-planning process for nursing. Expansion or change in any service that involves inpatients and most outpatient services often affects nursing budgets, both operating and capital. However, other priorities, consistent with the organization's strategic plan, also may surface in the budget-planning process. For example, in the last budget cycle, staffing (hours per patient day, or HPPD) was reduced for the general medical unit of one hospital. In the year since those cuts were implemented, patient satisfaction survey scores have fallen by 25% to below 70%, nursing turnover has risen from 8% to 22%, and family and patients are critical during their hospital stays about the failure of nursing staff to respond to their calls for help in a timely manner. However, the hospital's strategic plan calls for patient satisfaction scores above 85% and for nursing turnover of less than 12%. This may significantly affect budget planning for the division of nursing/patient care services. The CNO must mediate this planning process to meet both sets of priorities within the limits of the projected budget.

CAPITAL BUDGETS

Capital budgets often are considered "wish lists" that reflect organizational priorities. As noted earlier in this chapter, capital budgets focus on expenditures for equipment and projects that have a set minimum cost and lifespan. These budgets can include desirable, but not essential, capital items that can be deleted from the budget during negotiations. For example, the clinical director for a behavioral healthcare unit directed the nurse manager to include in each year's capital budget extra items that were desirable but not essential. The director knew, based on history, that behavioral healthcare was a low priority service in the organization's strategic plan, and most or all the capital budget items would be denied, even when less than $2500 was requested. Cardiovascular and surgical services topped the organizational priority list and garnered most of the capital budget each year. Therefore each year the manager added an $8000 blanket warmer (for the geropsychiatric patients) and one or two stretchers for the electroconvulsive therapy (ECT) rooms, in addition to miscellaneous items and replacement items, such as new pieces of furniture for the lounges and conference rooms. When the director had to negotiate the capital budget with the CNO, $10,000 to $15,000 in requests always had to be to cut from the budget when cuts had to be made. The director always developed a well-considered justification for these items that could be dropped readily. Most years the department actually managed to obtain one or two

smaller items that were new acquisitions instead of just essential replacement items.

Setting Measurable Operating Objectives

These can be set at several different levels. Top administration may set an objective to increase inpatient admissions by 5% to 10% by each clinical service. This directly affects inpatient nursing departments and involves the CNO, department directors, and unit managers. Flexible staffing must address this increased patient load, with increases for total HPPD translating into more nursing hours to be paid. Consumable supplies, housekeeping, and other subaccounts that support the provision of inpatient care also may need to be adjusted. This is, of course, based on the premise of increased reimbursement for these additional patient admissions.

Within the nursing/patient care services division, the leadership team may set a goal to provide more support to staff through internal continuing education and inservice education programs in order to maintain clinical competency and to improve nursing retention. This may be expressed through an objective to provide 10 additional hours of staff development programs each month. If some of this programming is to be contracted out to paid consultants, this must be calculated for the budget. If the educational programs are to be provided without additional personnel costs, using internal experts or by faculty of nursing programs that use the hospital as a clinical facility, budgets may need to be adjusted for increased materials, such as handouts and workbooks, and even food to provide a learner-friendly environment.

Budget Preparation

This is a two-phase process: First, after the initial planning is completed by top administration, the finance department issues the necessary budget information to all budget managers, as noted earlier (see Table 14-1). This may be preceded or followed by a meeting with all budget officers to outline this year's budget preparation forms, procedures, and deadlines. Second, each budget manager spends hours gathering information and then calculating the numbers to fill in the blanks on the budget forms. Additional meetings with directors or the CNO follow. These meetings become part of the process of negotiation and revision.

Negotiation and Revision

This is a process of moving up the organizational hierarchy. The manager may review the budget(s), operating and capital, with selected staff and then with the department director. The director and manager meet with the vice president to review the budget(s). At each stage, figures are checked and recalculated and challenged. The process may be reiterated. Even if the bottom line of the budget is on target, some reductions still may be taken in subaccounts to provide a pool of monies to transfer to another budget. The CNO then takes the divisional budget to the COO/CEO. Further revisions are likely to occur at this level and when the budget goes to the board of trustees for final approval.

Control and Feedback

Budget managers receive monthly reports that go by many names, including responsibility reports, variance reports, monthlies, rollouts, and budget reports. These monthly reports provide feedback as to how well the plan (budget) is working. The most important data these reports provide are the variance data: how much over or under each subaccount is, as well as the overall department budget. The budget manager must justify or explain the variances. The budget manager uses this feedback to evaluate how effectively the budget is controlled. Each budget manager's supervisor also receives the monthly report to provide data for budget oversight.

In some institutions addressing variance reports is a very formal process. Managers must meet with the CNO and painstakingly explain all variances, whether justified by patient day or procedure volume increases or decreases. In other institutions, a memo by each manager may serve as the feedback mechanism for variance reports. Budget officers are accountable for variances and should expect to report on the causes of such variances.

Favorable or positive variance results, for example, when volumes are high and actual revenues exceed budgeted revenues. Unfavorable or negative variance can occur when nursing wages exceed the amount budgeted because of higher-than-budgeted HPPD (from the statistical budget). If the higher-than-budgeted HPPD are the result of increased patient acuity or longer length of stay, increased revenue is unlikely to offset this variance. However, if increased patient days with increased revenues result in increased HPPD, the manager can easily justify the variance in staffing costs.

Institutional policies on variance investigation and reporting always drive this control and feedback process. Other reasons for investigating budget variance include the following:

- Data entry errors related to statistics, revenue, or expenses
- Expenses that exceed revenues
- Unbudgeted expenses
- Unusual variances (e.g., variances in office supply costs)
- Continued variances within a subaccount over several months
- Concerns about impact on budget if variance continues through the fiscal year
- Experience with and personal knowledge of budget (Penner, 2004)

The "Budget Game"

The efforts of the behavioral healthcare director related to the capital budget, as cited on p. 284, are part of the "budget game." This budget game is a reality of administrative practice and is played well by successful CNOs and other nurse leaders. This is not a game of chance but actually the use of strategies to negotiate desired outcomes.

Negotiation of budget issues focuses on program priorities but can be shaped by other influences, such as institutional politics and staff or physician demands. The CNO who understands how to be effective at the negotiation table will know how to use the strategies of the budget game successfully. The CNO understands the gaming strategies, whether seated at the negotiating table with directors bringing the CNO their departmental budgets or with the CEO with the nursing or patient care services budget. This strategizing process is used to ensure that one's department, division, or service gets a fair share of the organization's resources, human, fiscal, and physical. In addition to the formal negotiation strategies built into any budget process, informal negotiations among and between managers, department directors, and executives may occur to ensure the adequacy of resources as part of the "budget game."

In addition to the "game" strategy identified in the example of the behavioral healthcare director, many other strategies may be used. For example, moving funds from one budget category to another is another budget game. For the next budget, a nurse manager may seek to increase the hours of paid time for continuing education for the department's nursing staff, in response to the organization's goal to improve nurse retention. The nursing staff has experienced a change in the patient population for whom they care and need to expand their skills to provide effective care. However, the manager's department director firmly believes that the unit's nurses should be able to care for the new patient population without additional education (i.e., "a nurse is a nurse is a nurse" thinking) and refuses to expand the budgeted hours for education. The nurse manager may need to move funds from underused subaccounts for seldom-used supplies or contracted services to the education subaccount.

NURSING AS A BUSINESS

Typically, nursing services are considered a "cost center" in a healthcare organization's budget, often without consideration that nursing services generate revenues from both inpatient and outpatient services. Not long ago people were inpatients when they came to hospitals for routine examinations now performed as outpatient services. Hospitals often served as hotels for relatively healthy persons requiring diagnostic services or screening for potential health problems. Patients requiring inpatient care today are inpatients because they require sufficiently intensive nursing assessment and care throughout a 24-hour day. In any hospital, nursing services often represent the largest group of employees, consuming the largest portion of wage and salary dollars. However, no inpatient services could be delivered without the presence of the nursing staff; many outpatient services would likewise be undeliverable without nursing care. Nurse leaders need to recognize that they are running revenue-generating businesses on their units and in the departments they manage. Nursing is an art and a science, but it is also a business. Many nurse managers and administrators are responsible for multimillion-dollar budgets, not unlike those who run corporations.

Intrapreneurial nurses identify opportunities to develop new nursing services within the healthcare organization (e.g., developing a wide-ranging community health education program covering all age groups that ties participants to the hospital's healthcare services). They also seek to make the business of nursing core to the effectiveness of the healthcare organization by promoting, developing, and monitoring the quality and scope of nursing services within the organization. These nurses can see unmet patient or community needs within their organizations and develop a nursing service response to these needs.

Intrapreneurs can be characterized as nurses who fit the following criteria:

- Enjoy exercising professional autonomy while having access to organizational resources
- Demonstrate a strong goal orientation and a high level of self-motivation
- Respond to organizational rewards and recognition

- Can work effectively and efficiently within self-imposed and organizational timelines
- Can manage a range of tasks and still delegate effectively
- Demonstrate a high level of self-confidence and courage
- Are moderate risk-takers

Entrepreneurs, like intrapreneurs, have a can-do attitude. They demonstrate the same characteristics as intrapreneurs but may tolerate a higher level of risk-taking. Entrepreneurial nurses create new nursing business opportunities outside of existing healthcare organizations (e.g., independent nurse psychotherapists, consulting services, speaker services, home care agencies, staffing agencies). New businesses must fill a market niche, meeting a need that no one else meets, no one else already in the business can meet fully, or no one else is meeting satisfactorily. The proliferation of home health agencies in the 1980s and 1990s is an example of meeting a market niche. Healthcare reimbursement was forcing the early discharge of patients to home, yet these patients still needed nursing care because the patients or their families could not yet provide full self-care. New home healthcare agencies, some founded by nurses, were developed to meet this need. During times of nursing shortages, staffing agencies and travel nurse agencies flourish to meet the ever-fluctuating needs of healthcare organizations; many of these are owned by nurses.

Entrepreneurs may establish their business ventures in a variety of ways. They may start new companies, as sole proprietors or within the framework of a corporate partnership; buy an existing business; buy into a franchise arrangement; or take on other roles, such as working part time in a healthcare organization and doing freelance consulting work on a part-time basis.

Strategic planning is essential to any new business venture, whether entrepreneurial or intrapreneurial. This strategic planning process is essential to the development of a business plan. The business plan, which is outlined in the following section, is the road map for the new venture. A business plan is essential as the intrapreneur seeks approval of a new venture, including funding,

within the healthcare organization. For the entrepreneur, the business plan is also critical for the creation, direction, and evaluation of the new venture and is essential for external funding, whether funds are sought through a grant (e.g., start-up monies for a not-for-profit nurse managed healthcare clinic) or other sources (e.g., a Small Business Administration loan for start-up funds for a home health agency).

THE BUSINESS PLAN

A business plan includes basic information by which others can evaluate the merit of the plan for a new venture (Box 14-5). Various formats can be found in reference books (Finkler & Kovner, 2000; Storfjell & Smith, 2000). Most healthcare organizations will have their own format for the submission of a business plan. However, the key elements tend to be the same in all formats.

The business plan outlines the following:

- What the new business seeks to accomplish: the goals and objectives
- How the need for the new business was determined and validated: the market analysis
- How the new business will be marketed: the marketing plan
- What resources the new business will use: the projected operating and capital budgets
- How the new business will be managed and staffed: the personnel plan
- How the business will be implemented: timelines and potential for third-party reimbursement if a clinical program
- How the success of the new business will be evaluated: both short-term and long-term plans

For the intrapreneurial nurse leader, the business plan communicates the proposed venture to the administrative team of the healthcare organization, the board of trustees, and the entire nurse leadership team. For the entrepreneurial nurse, the business plan is the communication tool used for securing funding through grants and loans. It is the critical tool for initiating a new business venture.

Box 14-5   Business Plan Format

COVER PAGE
- Business name
- Name of principal(s)
- Date

EXECUTIVE SUMMARY OF THE PLAN
  (not to exceed one or two pages)

DESCRIPTION OF THE SERVICE/BUSINESS
- Background, rationale, goals
- Discussion of the services/products to be provided and by whom

MARKET ANALYSIS
- Target market
- Need for service
- Existing or similar services/businesses in the market area

RESOURCES REQUIRED
- Human
- Fiscal
- Physical

MARKETING PLAN
- Strategies/targets
- Initial

- First year
- Second and third years

FINANCIAL PLAN (first 3 years)
- Operating budget
- Capital budget (start-up needs in first year budget)
- Potential for third-party reimbursement/ payer mix

ORGANIZATION AND MANAGEMENT
- Corporate structure/management structure

IMPLEMENTATION PLAN WITH TIMELINES
- Initiation of business/service
- Operating plan for first 3 years

EVALUATION PLAN
- 1 month
- 3 months
- 6 months
- Annual

SUMMARY

The CNO is in a unique position to use financial savvy to promote nursing services within a healthcare organization. Nursing services represent the largest portion of the personnel budget of most healthcare organizations, especially hospitals. Although nursing traditionally has been viewed as a cost center, CNOs and other nursing leaders need to view nursing as a revenue source, because nursing is a unique business within the healthcare system. Nurse leaders must have the financial savvy to recognize the unique role of nursing in generating revenue in a healthcare organization, not just serving as a cost center. Comprehending the complexities of reimbursement, mastering budget development and management, and assessing the multiple forces that influence the nursing budget are key skills for the nurse leader in any type of healthcare organization.

Key Points to Lead

1. Explore concepts of healthcare economics related to the role of the nurse administrator.
2. Examine the role of the nurse administrator in fiscal planning.
3. Explore reimbursement issues.
4. Value the role of the nurse administrator in the budget process.
5. Analyze the concept of nursing services as a business.
6. Develop a business plan for a nursing service.

Literature Box

The changing role of the nurse administrator requires financial savvy and skills that enable the nurse leader to integrate clinical and business skills. A survey of nurse executives and CEOs from different medical centers in all 50 states demonstrated strong agreement on a list of nine financial management skills/knowledge that CNOs needed. However, the CNOs and the CEOs were less likely to agree that current nurse leaders held those skills and knowledge. The CNOs and CEOs were asked to rate the financial management knowledge of nurse leaders in a series of questions. The grand mean of the CNOs' responses was 2.95 (on a 4-point scale). The CEOs' grand mean for the same items was only 2.34.

Findings of this survey resulted in the development of a financial management course for the graduate program in the researcher's school of nursing. Many nursing administration faculty, like nurse leaders, have learned their financial skills on the job without a solid academic background in finance and are not well prepared to teach the complex financial skills and knowledge that CNOs need today. Nine course objectives that focus on financial skills critical for nurse executives are presented with plans for practicum experiences in financial management.

Lemire, J. A. (2000). Redesigning financial management education for the nursing administration graduate student. *Journal of Nursing Administration Quarterly, 30*, 199-205.

Contemplations

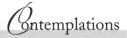

- Explore an example of how the practice of a nurse leader is influenced by economic forces and an example of how the practice of a staff nurse is shaped by these same economic forces. Compare these two nursing experiences.
- What impact do managed care, Medicare rate reductions, and problems with Medicaid reimbursement have on your organization? Give one or two examples.
- How does the current reimbursement system differ from the system in place 20 or more years ago, before the introduction of PPSs? Identify at least three differences.

- Examine your thoughts about the implications of caring for the uninsured in an overburdened, under-reimbursed healthcare system.
- What new service line could be developed in your organization? How would you conduct the market research for a business plan? If you have ever considered a nursing business, how would you begin the market research for this business? How would you develop the data needed to construct a solid business plan?

LEADER STORY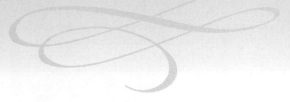

Maxine Johnson
Administrator, Outpatient Services,
Edwardsville Health Center, Gateway
Regional Health Services
Former Chief Nursing Officer for Gateway
Regional Medical Center
Granite City, IL

I have been with the hospital for 29 years in a variety of management and administrative roles. I became the CNO when the hospital changed ownership in 2002. After more than 75 years as a community hospital owned by an order of Catholic nuns, the organization became Gateway Regional Medical Center when the medical center was purchased by Community Health Systems of Brentwood, TN.

I have seen the growth of the hospital in the 1970s and 1980s and have witnessed the dramatic change in both the hospital and the community over the past decade. Once a bustling steel town, many of the community's industries have downsized, closed, or been taken over in mergers, significantly changing the economy and the population of the community.

This is a changing healthcare organization in a changing community marked by several external forces:

- An aging population with a shifting middle class, marked by the flight of the educated middle class to other nearby communities
- An increasing population of the young and the poor, with an increase in section 8 (subsidized) housing
- A single-parent population that is increasing as middle-class, two-parent families move to nearby communities
- Changes in employers among those who live in the community, with less commercial insurance that was once the standard in the manufacturing plants in the community

These changes have had a significant impact on the financial status of the community, the healthcare organization, and many of the residents who live in the surrounding community. For example, because the hospital serves a community with a rising rate of poverty, it receives a disproportionate share of Medicaid reimbursement from the state of Illinois—$1 million per annum.

The religious order that previously owned the healthcare organization created clinics to serve the poor of the community. With the change in ownership and a change in program priorities, these clinics were divested to another organization that focuses on primary care for the poor through its foundation-funded clinics. Those clinics continue to operate within the community, including one that operates within the hospital building.

As the new CNO, I was actively involved in the organization's transition from nonprofit to for-profit status. During the transition, 100 FTEs (full-time equivalents), out of about 1000, were cut. Some of these reductions in FTEs were accomplished through attrition. A few employees left because of change in the organization's status. Some attrition was related to the strict productivity standards that were implemented in the first 6 months after the change of ownership.

I am the only senior manager from the prior administration who remains with the healthcare organization. All other administrators are new to the organization. I hold an MBA, a corporate preference of the new ownership. As part of the top administrative team, I meet with the rest of the team and review the prior 24 hours each business day.

This reflects the corporate culture of the new ownership related to financial accountability.

The new CEO had turnaround experience with other organizations. In the first year of operation as a for-profit under his leadership, the hospital went from a $2 million loss in 2001 to an $8 million profit in 2002. This was a $10 million turnaround in the first year, marking a dramatic financial change for the healthcare organization.

One of the significant changes for nursing was a switch to a daily monitoring system that looks at staffing on a 4-hour basis for nursing in order to stay on target for budgeted nursing HPPD. Because of the 4-hour reviews of staffing needs, nurses know that they may be sent home halfway during a shift or added mid-shift. This is a dramatic change in nursing operations, where the norm is 8- or 12-hour reviews.

Another change for nurse managers, related to the financial operations of their departments, are monthly financial meetings with the CFO. In these monthly financial meetings with the CFO and the CNO, the managers review and explain variances in their budgets. These meetings represent the organization's changing expectations for higher levels of accountability for these variances. I also meet individually with managers weekly to discuss progress toward financial goals that have been set for their departments.

To improve the effectiveness of case management, nurses are now the case managers on the acute units. They handle utilization as well as discharge planning. A social worker is the case manager for the skilled nursing and acute rehabilitation units. Using a model of case management from the corporate ownership, the case managers are making progress in managing cost-effective care. Under the previous ownership, social workers served as the acute care case managers. The new model has resulted in more cost-efficient care.

For Gateway Regional Medical Center, the ED accounts for 53% of all hospital admissions. All ED cases that meet criteria for admission but are not admitted are reviewed and evaluated.

Because the ED is so critical to the hospital's success, $4.5 million has been earmarked for a new ED, along with money for other capital improvements. This ED has already undergone major renovation twice in the past 25 to 30 years.

The hospital has offered a comprehensive behavioral health program for more than 30 years. This service accounts for 35% of admissions. A new behavioral healthcare administrator came on board in the transition to support and grow the service, noting that behavioral healthcare is a program priority for the organization. Behavioral healthcare includes two adult units, both adolescent and child units, and a geropsychiatric unit. The units include 70 beds, take involuntary admissions (unlike some other programs in the area), and include two hospital psychiatrists who help cover patients admitted.

The medical center is located in a two-county region (Madison and St. Clair Counties in Southwestern Illinois) that has lost almost 200 physicians in the past few years because of dramatic increases in liability insurance rates. The region is viewed as a haven for personal injury and malpractice lawsuits. Gateway Regional is the only hospital in Madison County that helps physicians pay their liability insurance. The affiliated foundation pays up to 50% of any increase in fees if physicians are active staff with an office in the hospital's community.

Some other significant changes were introduced during the transition to a for-profit organization, in an effort to support the financial health of the organization.

Billing changes were introduced by new ownership. Patients pay their co-pays at the time of service for ED and outpatient services. The billing department is working more aggressively to collect bad debt. Charges are entered and monitored daily, another change in procedure for the organization.

There is a marketing department that regularly visits physicians and other referral sources to support inpatient admissions and outpatient services.

Statistics on physician admissions are monitored for decreased admissions, with follow-up with the physicians to determine the cause.

Corporate headquarters set the budget target (revenue) annually. The hospital's administrative team then determines how this target will be met, setting goals for patient days, outpatient visits, procedures, and other revenue sources and then determining what resources will be expended to achieve these goals. This is known as EBITDA (Earnings Before Interest, Taxes, Depreciation, and Amoritization).

Nursing is viewed as a revenue center, not just a cost center, by the corporation.

I offer these pieces of advice for CNOs dealing with a healthcare organization's change from nonprofit to for-profit status:

- Master the concepts of finances.
- Comprehend the financial concepts and accountability that are unique to a for-profit, publicly traded corporation.
- Recognize that you and your budget managers will be held fully accountable for the budget, customer/patient satisfaction, and quality of care, much more accountable than in a nonprofit healthcare organization.

Chapter References

Adom, N. K., Adom, D. F., Cole, J., Davilman, C., Dennis, R., Forbes, M., Motta, A., Rebuquiro, P., Roeth, N., Scott, M., & Zyloney, P. (2001). An expanded professional nursing role: Increasing hospital reimbursement. *Journal of Nursing Administration, 31*, 7-8.

American Nurses Association. (2004). *Scope and standards for nurse administrators* (2nd ed.). Washington, DC: Author.

Bonace, A. L. (2000). Documentation's effect on reimbursement for rapid treatment status patients. *Journal of Nursing Administration, 30*, 295-297.

Busby, A., & Busby, A. (2001). Critical access hospitals. *Journal of Nursing Administration, 31*, 301-310.

Centers for Medicare and Medicaid Services. (n.d.). *Medicare Modernization Act*. Retrieved August 21, 2004, from http://www.cms.hhs.gov/medicarereform/.

Centers for Medicare and Medicaid Services. (2004, January 8). Press release: Health care spending reaches $1.6 trillion in 2002. Retrieved January 22, 2004, from http://www.cms.hhs.gov/media/press/release.asp?Counter=935.

Chang, C. F. (2001). Market, demand, and supply. In C. F. Chang, S. A. Price, & S. K. Pfoutz (Eds.), *Economics and nursing: Critical professional issues* (pp. 37-57). Philadelphia: F.A. Davis.

Cleland, V. S., & Kibbin, R. C. (1990). *Economics of nursing*. Norwalk, CT: Appleton-Lange.

DeNavas-Walt, C., Proctor, B. D., & Mills, R. J. (2004). Income, poverty, and health insurance coverage in the United States: 2003. (Current population reports, pp. 60-226). Retrieved September 8, 2005, from http://www.census.gov/prod/2004pubs/p60-226.pdf.

Finkler, S. A., & Kovner, C. T. (2000). *Financial management for nurse managers and executives* (2nd ed.). Philadelphia: W. B. Saunders.

Goddard, N. L. (2003). The five most common flaws in healthcare staffing and personnel budgets. *Nurse Leader, 1*(5), 44-48.

Gormley, K. K., & Verdejo, T. (2000). A systems approach—budgeting for the 21st century: Turning challenges into triumphs. *Nursing Administration Quarterly, 24*(4), 51-59.

Kaiser Commission on Medicaid and the Uninsured. (2000, March). *Uninsured in America: Key facts*. Retrieved August 24, 2004, from http://www.pbs.org/newshour/health/uninsured/.

Kirkby, M. P. (2003). Number crunching with variable budgets. *Nursing Management, 34*(3), 28-34.

Lemire, J. A. (2000). Redesigning financial management education for the nursing administration graduate student. *Journal of Nursing Administration, 30*, 199-205.

Noonan, M. D., Weiss, K., Stichler, J. F., Looker, P., & Jones, M. L. (2002). Learning to speak the language of finance. *AWHONN Lifelines, 6,* 124-133.

Penner, S. J. (2004). *Introduction to healthcare economics & financial management.* Philadelphia: Lippincott.

Pfoutz, S. K., & Price, S. A. (2001). Application of economic principles to nursing. In C. F. Chang, S. A. Price, & S. K. Pfoutz (Eds.), *Economics and nursing: Critical professional issues* (pp. 120-140). Philadelphia: F.A. Davis.

Price, S. A. (2001). The economics of nursing and healthcare. In C. F. Chang, S. A. Price, & S. K. Pfoutz (Eds.), *Economics and nursing: Critical professional issues* (pp. 3-36). Philadelphia: F.A. Davis.

Pulcini, J. A., Neary, S. R., & Mahoney, D. F. (2002). Healthcare financing. In D. J. Mason, J. K. Leavitt, & M. W. Chaffee (Eds.), *Policy & politics in nursing and healthcare* (4th ed., pp. 241-297). St. Louis: W. B. Saunders.

Rhoades, J. A., & Cohen, J. W. (2004, June). *Statistical brief #24: The uninsured in America—1996-2002. Estimates for the civilian noninstitutionalized population under age 65.* Retrieved August 24, 2004, from http://www.meps.ahrq.gov/papers/st24/stat24.htm.

Storfjell, J. L., & Smith, C. M. (2000). Nursing as a business. In L. M. Simms, S. A. Price, & N. E. Ervin (Eds.), *The professional practice of nursing administration* (3rd ed., pp. 179-194). Stamford, CT: Delmar.

15 Creating a Culture for Promoting Nursing Research and Clinical Scholarship

Patricia Messmer

Jacqueline L. Gonzalez

The test of a leader is taking the vision from me to we. JOHN C. MAXWELL

This chapter focuses on an element of growing importance in nursing administration: research in the clinical setting. With the advent of evidence-based practice foci, the nursing organization must make decisions based on research that defines practices appropriate to the organization. Approaches for developing a research program and examples of research are included.

EMBRACING A PRACTICE CULTURE THAT encompasses inquiry and evidence-based practice is critical to the success of achieving high standards. Nurse researchers and chief nursing officers (CNOs) must encourage staff, foster collaboration, and provide support for the dissemination of research findings. Through their vision and implementation of a culture of support for research and scholarship, CNOs guide research and its application to evidence-based practice. This chapter is designed to show how research can be implemented within the clinical setting and how the results can be shared widely so that all may benefit.

Various nursing research studies are integrated throughout this discussion and may stimulate interest in replication at other clinical sites.

NURSING RESEARCH IN HEALTHCARE ORGANIZATIONS

Traditionally, nursing research has been associated with college and university programs in nursing. Early research focused primarily on students in nursing schools and not on registered nurses, their practices, or patient outcomes. Over the past several years, many nursing service organizations have made a commitment to using nursing research to advance practice. Many also have committed to conducting research studies so that they would know firsthand what best practices are appropriate for their patient populations, what produces positive outcomes with nursing care, and what administrative strategies produce the best results.

Many nurse executives have instituted a program of nursing research. The impetus for some of these programs is the desire to base decisions on substantive data. In addition, the American Nurses Credentialing Center's (ANCC) Magnet Recognition Program has spurred the intensity and adoption of programs of research. For example,

Messmer, Jones, and Rosillo (2002) proved how one medical center successfully used nursing research projects to highlight how the institution met Magnet standards. Messmer and Gonzalez (2003) stressed the importance of providing evidence of clinical scholarship and evidence-based practice to attain the (then) Magnet Standard XIII, Research. Nursing research in healthcare organizations creates the opportunity for nurses to be the best for patients and for the practices that support nurses in their provision of care. That is the ultimate goal of research.

THE VISION

A successful nursing research program begins with the CNO's vision for nursing research. This vision should relate to the overall vision for nursing services. It must be relevant for patients and nurses. Thus research may relate to clinical studies that focus on nursing interventions in the care of patients and to role studies that focus on various aspects about the nurses' interactions in the workplace. An example of the former may be control of postoperative pain; an example of the latter may be determining if using electronic games maintains or enhances surgical nurses' dexterity.

Kerfoot (2002) stated that the most strategic asset a leader has to work with is the competency of the staff to perform at a level of excellence, which should include research skills. In addition, the CNO must be supportive and have an understanding of the research process from development to implementation to dissemination through publications and presentations. The CNO also must have an awareness of the time and resources necessary to accomplish and sustain this challenging task. A nursing research program can be beneficial for patient care and instrumental for the effectiveness and success of a nursing service.

The ANCC Magnet Recognition Program and the Malcolm Baldrige National Quality Award (MBQA) expect that research is ongoing. Neither dictates how a vision is created or used, but both are based on data relevant to a particular organization.

Therefore, without a vision for research, an organization may not be achieving its best results.

PROCESS

If a CNO inherits an established research program, the focus may be on enriching activities that occur within that program. On the other hand, if no program exists, the CNO may need to begin with a campaign to convince staff of the value of such a resource. The CNO must provide research resources in such aspects as funding statistical analysis software packages and release time for staff members to collect, code, analyze, and interpret data. The process may include selection or authorization of consultants for components of the statistical analysis.

The CNO must support financial resources for nursing leadership, including providing advanced practice nurses and the nursing staff support to disseminate their results. In other words, whether dissemination occurs only within the organization or if it includes external presentations and publications, the findings and implications must be shared with others in some deliberate manner. This may include authorizing a section of the organization's web page, or it may require a publications budget for internal dissemination and a plan for external dissemination. In addition, staff members need to be recognized for their efforts to present papers and posters at local, regional, state, national, and international conferences. Beyond the direct expenses of preparing slides and posters and travel to support the individual(s) at conferences, the CNO also may wish to create a type of award or incentive to encourage participation in such activities.

The nurse researcher can drive these initiatives. For example, a program of nursing research is a vital component within the expectations of the Magnet Recognition Program (Messmer, Jones, & Rosillo, 2002). The role expectations of nurse researchers within an organization bring life and meaning to the vision for research by creating the processes that produce results.

APPROACHES FOR DEVELOPING A PROGRAM OF RESEARCH

Several different approaches can be taken to implement a program of research. The most common ways are the following:

- Employ a full-time nurse researcher
- Develop collaborative relationships with a college or university to secure consultation from or part-time availability of a nurse researcher
- Contract for services from an independent nurse researcher
- Encourage innovative ways to meet the demands for research

Hiring a full-time nurse researcher provides the most intense approach to developing and implementing research. This approach is found commonly in larger organizations and in academic health centers. It is frequently the result of years of other efforts that eventually culminate in one or more full-time positions. It also can be used when an organization decides to "fast track" involvement in research. Because so much emphasis is placed on evidence-based decisions, it is possible that this "fast track" approach will be prominent for a few years until most major healthcare organizations consider adopting this approach. In some cases it is not until redesignation that hospitals are able to provide the funding for a full-time nurse researcher. For example, Wake Forest University Baptist Medical Center employed a doctorally prepared researcher and placed that person in charge of the shared governance model. By creating a nursing research council within the shared governance model, nursing staff members were able to engage in various research endeavors and evidence-based practice, such as "Choosing a Wound Cleanser in Tracheostomy Care for Patients" (Hudson-Barr & King, 2004; King, 2004a, 2004b). One challenge to this methodology is the current and impending shortage of doctorally prepared nurses.

Developing a collaborative relationship to secure consultation from or employment of a part-time nurse researcher is also a common strategy. In fact, it is probably the most common approach in current practice. Most commonly, as indicated above, this strategy involves a school of nursing where research has been a part of the mission for a period of time. Commitment to improvement of clinical practices should be evident in the work of the collaborating school. One approach may be to have a part-time contract with the organization for one of the faculty to lead or advise on projects important to the organization. Another may be to form a committee with major involvement of faculty researchers as a way to guide research efforts. The key, however, is that research activity is increased in clinical areas. Doctorally prepared nurse researchers can mentor staff in designing research studies, refining skills in collecting and analyzing data, and presenting at various conferences. Supporting staff through presentation activities not only disseminates results of the studies, but also creates networking opportunities with other nurse researchers to discuss future research projects.

Contracting for services with an independent nurse researcher is also possible. Currently the number of individuals engaged in such services is limited. However, as qualified nurse faculty retire from full employment in schools of nursing, it is possible that some will turn to contracting as a way to continue contributions to the profession. Based on the various predictions about the number of retirements before 2010, some growth may occur in this format for services. The key in using this approach is to be clear about expectations. Research may consume a great deal of time and produce results that were not anticipated. Although this outcome is seen as disappointing for some, it further contributes to nursing's overall body of knowledge.

Whether the CNO is conducting research personally, the knowledge of how to conduct research is critical to role implementation success. Most nursing administration graduate programs include nursing research content, and many specifically address the needs for successful nursing administrators (Frank, Aroian, & Tashea, 2003).

Baker, Bingle, Hajewski, Radant, and Urden (2004) advocate a service-learning project designed to assist master's degree students in nursing administration to submit a Magnet application in conjunction with a local hospital. Students use the ANA (2004) *Scope and Standards for Nurse Administrators,* ANCC (2003) *Health Care Organization Instructions and Application Process Manual,* and the ANCC web site http://www.nursecredentialing.org. As of January 2005, Research and Evidence-Based Practice became a component of Force 6 Quality of Care of the 14 Forces of Magnetism (ANCC, 2005, pp. 47-49). However, the component remains a critical and integral part of documenting and substantiating the value of conducting nursing research studies in this Force and throughout the application and site visit.

Each of the above approaches uses a more established, traditional way to develop a program of research. Several institutions, however, have used innovative approaches, including creation of a hospital-based nursing research fellowship for staff nurses (Hinds, Gattuso, & Morrell, 2000). Hinds et al. described a primary focus on clinical research that included clinical trials and research methods from behavioral sciences and clinical strategies. They conducted qualitative and quantitative research on hope in adolescents with cancer. In addition to providing fellowships for staff nurses, their approach included a multidisciplinary team of direct care providers to have a broader range of impact. Hinds et al. (2003) also demonstrated how a hospital-based interdisciplinary team successfully translated psychosocial research findings into evidence-based practice guidelines.

In another example, the CNO of a university hospital and an associate dean of a school of nursing worked together to position doctorally prepared nurses in clinical practice settings so that research flourished at the unit level (Berger, Eilers, Heermann, Warren, Franco, & Triolo, 1999).

Although a case can be made for all organizations to engage in an organized approach to research, not all are necessarily ready. To determine the readiness of an organization for implementing

a nursing research program, Snyder-Halpern (1998) developed an instrument, the Innovation Readiness Scale (IRS). The IRS was developed from research-based contextual cues identified by nurse researchers as supportive of successful hospital-based nursing research programs. The IRS provides decision makers with a measure by which to judge an institution's readiness to implement a nursing research program. The following cues were validated for the IRS instrument (Snyder-Halpern, 1998, p. 231):

- There is a commitment to providing ongoing funding for a formal researcher position.
- A variety of research consultation services are readily available.
- Administration is committed to providing ongoing funding to support a formal research program.
- A researcher can network readily with external and internal resources to facilitate research.
- Data-based decisions are valued.
- The culture values the contribution that research can make to patient care.
- Administration supports the creativity and independent thought necessary for research.
- A spirit of investigation and curiosity exists.
- The mission is compatible with research.
- There is support for development of a climate that fosters professional practice.
- There is encouragement of faculty and student research.
- Leaders view research as an integral component of professional practice.
- Administration displays a flexible attitude toward practice to accommodate the research process.
- There is commitment to recognizing and rewarding those who participate in research.
- Administrators facilitate staff participation in research activities.
- Staff are committed to using research findings in their practice.

RESEARCH PROGRAM

A research program is shaped by a cadre of clinical scholars dedicated to advancing the knowledge base for nursing education and practice.

Most importantly, however, it has an impact on patient outcomes. The research program is integral to the philosophy of the nursing services and the overall organizational mission. The design derives from the research questions that serve as the basis for methodology. For example, if a nursing organization believes in family-centered care, one example may be determining approaches to having family present during codes and rounds. Such a study may compare care for those who have designated others as active participants in care with those who have not made such designations. Such a study could include qualitative aspects, such as focus groups of patients and their families to determine their views about family presence. A quantitative aspect could be achieved by using a valid and reliable instrument with physicians and nurses regarding their views of family presence. Results of such a study could drive education programs and policy decisions.

A program of research can be implemented using either qualitative or quantitative methods or a combination of both (as discussed previously). Combining both approaches, called *triangulation*, provides a rich approach to clinical research. Quantitative and qualitative research approaches complement each other because they generate different kinds of knowledge that can be useful to CNOs and nurse researchers as they validate programs of research.

Quantitative research often is viewed as "hard" science because it involves numerical quantification of an outcome, employs the use of valid and reliable instruments, and depends on statistical techniques to determine significance. An example of quantitative methods is using survey research to measure satisfaction (e.g., with nurses, physicians, and/or patients) or attitudes toward some aspect of practice or care (e.g., staffing patterns, communications between professions, pain control). Measuring outcomes can determine the effect of an intervention or provide insight into the feelings and experiences of patients and their families.

Qualitative research, often referred to as "soft" science, depends on demanding systematic processes to describe life experiences and give meaning to those descriptions (Burns & Grove, 2003). An example of qualitative research may be for the nurse researcher to conduct a one-to-one interview with selected nurses, physicians, or patients to determine their views on a subject. Unlike a quantitative approach, in which words or phrases are preselected and the respondent is asked to select a specific choice or rate or rank items, the qualitative approach begins with asking questions and provides a framework for the nature of responses generated by the respondents.

INVOLVEMENT OF NURSE MANAGERS AND STAFF

Nurse managers and staff most commonly are not experts in conducting research. In addition to having skills at reading and interpreting research to determine relevance for clinical practice, these two groups have distinctive knowledge about the realities of practice and thus are invaluable in shaping research. Nurse managers and staff raise the questions that require research because the literature may lack clarity about best practices, yet they practice in a specific way, almost intuitively. Their desire is to validate or report their current practice so that they do the best for patients. When the research process documents best practices inherent in intuition, it helps to validate the expertise that nurses contribute to an organization. Knowing how patients actually respond and what staff members say are legitimate concerns that can shape the way a study is designed and implemented. Therefore determining common complications associated with nursing interventions, the effectiveness of various nurse-patient ratios or educational preparation of the staff, the use of technology in the clinical setting, or the correlation of salaries with nurse demographics and satisfaction contribute to the quality of an organized nursing service.

OUTCOMES

The key outcomes of a nursing research program in a clinical setting are (1) decisions made at a more informed level and (2) practices based more firmly on evidence. As a result, clinical policies and procedures in addition to clinical practice guidelines or pathways are developed according to current literature. Nurses no longer practice in the context of "how we have always done it." Rather, they create the policies and procedures based on scientific evidence.

Journal clubs and research roundtables are outgrowths of findings within the literature and within the organization's research efforts. Research roundtables are an interactive means for providing novice nurse researchers and nursing students with the skill sets required to drive applications of existing evidence into nursing practices and to conduct further studies to derive new evidence (Maljanian, Caramanica, Taylor, MacRae, & Beland, 2002).

When the culture for research and scholarship is nurtured, the outcomes can be dramatic. As Table 15-1 shows, the intensity of research at Miami Children's Hospital reflects the

Table 15-1 RESEARCH PRODUCTIVITY AT MIAMI CHILDREN'S HOSPITAL

Study	Key Findings	Knowledge Dissemination
Nurse Job, Work Satisfaction, Stress and Recognition in a Pediatric Setting	Older nurses with more years of experience and more years at the hospital had less job stress and were less concerned about pay and task requirements than their younger counterparts.	Poster session presented at Florida First Magnet Nursing Research Conference, Tampa, FL, February 2004. Poster session presented at STTI Biennial Convention Toronto, Canada, November 1-5, 2003. Paper presentation at SNRS Conference Orlando, FL, 2003. Publication: Ernst, M., Franco, M., Messmer, P. R., & Gonzalez, J. (2004). Nurses' job satisfaction, stress and recognition in a pediatric setting. *Pediatric Nursing, 30*(3), 219-227.
Walking a Tightrope: Living with Your Child's Congenital Heart Disease	The study indicated a need for nurses to identify themselves to the patients and their family because the parents knew the nurse by name only with a long stay but knew the physician's name only in a short stay. The findings from this study served as the impetus for revising the Informed Consent because the families expressed that they could be more fully informed.	STTI Research Congress in St. Thomas, Virgin Islands, July 2003. Paper presentation at First Florida Magnet Nursing Research Conference in Tampa, FL, February 2004. MCH Nursing Research Committee South Florida chapter meeting of the Society of Pediatric Nurses (SPN) held at MCH.

Table **15-1** Research Productivity at Miami Children's Hospital—cont'd

Study	Key Findings	Knowledge Dissemination
Perceptions of Nursing Toward Bar-Coding Technology (BCT) for Medication Administration Satisfaction and Program, Difficulty with the BCT System	The quantitative data indicated that perceptions of the effect of the BCT on medication errors, timeliness of medication administration, and patient satisfaction were significant in the areas of less difficulty learning the system and an increase in patient satisfaction. The qualitative data demonstrated that although the nurses perceived that it took more time to bar-code the medication, they believed that the system saved children's lives, which became the most important focus. There was a noted increase in the awareness and self-reporting of "near misses."	Paper presentation at STTI International Research Congress Dublin, Ireland, July 22-24, 2004. Paper presented at Florida International University (FIU) School of Nursing Annual Research Improving Health Care Quality through Research, October 14, 2004. Poster session presented at First Florida Magnet Nursing Research Conference in Tampa, FL, February 2004. Poster session presented at SNRS Conference in Louisville, KY, February 2004. Poster session presented at Eighth Annual Magnet Conference in Sacramento, CA, October 15-17, 2004. Publication: Topps, C., Lopez, L., Messmer, P., & Franco, M. (2005). Perceptions of pediatric nurses toward bar-code point of care medication administration. *Nursing Administration Quarterly 29*(1), 102-107.
Use of Nitrous Oxide as Sedation for Short Minor Procedures	Results indicated that nitrous oxide was a cost-effective and efficacious alternative to conscious sedation or general anesthesia for children undergoing minor procedures.	Paper presented at STTI Research Congress in St. Thomas, Virgin Islands, July 2003. American Pediatric Surgical Nurses Association Annual Conference in Ponte Verde, FL, April 2004. American Pediatric Surgical Association Meeting, 2003. Publication: Burnweit, C., Diana-Zerpa, J., Nahmad, M., Lankau, C., Weinberger, M., Malveszzi, L., Smith, L., Shapiro, T., & Thayer, K. (2004). Nitrous oxide analgesia for minor pediatric surgical procedures: An effective alternative to conscious sedation. *Journal of Pediatric Surgery 39*(3), 495-499.

Continued

Table 15-1 RESEARCH PRODUCTIVITY AT MIAMI CHILDREN'S HOSPITAL—CONT'D

Study	Key Findings	Knowledge Dissemination
Testing Three Pain Management Modalities in the Postoperative Pediatric Appendectomy Patient	The study findings demonstrated that patients demanded more patient-controlled administration (PCA) of medications when receiving only Toradol. This finding resulted in the hospital's pain intervention treatment plan including Morphine PCA with or without Toradol.	Poster session presented at Mosby Pediatric Nursing Conference, Las Vegas, NV, October 10, 2002. Poster session presented at World of the Hospitalized Child, Miami, FL, November 2003.
Use of the Sport Bed in Status Post Rod Placement Patients for Non-Pharmacological Pain Management	Results indicated that the pediatric patients had reduction of pain and better sleep patterns with less utilization of narcotic analgesia to control pain. Nurse perceived less physical strain and injury, resulting in improved satisfaction.	Patient Safety Conference in Orlando, FL, March 2003. American Pediatric Surgical Nurses Association Annual Conference in Ponte Verde, FL, April 2004. Poster session presented at Florida International University (FIU) School of Nursing Annual Research Program, Improving Health Care Quality through Research, October 14, 2004.
Effect of Inappropriate Size of Endotrachial Tubes in a Neonatal Transport	A review of 100 charts was conducted to determine whether the inappropriate endotrachial tube size results in an adverse event. Researchers found an identified need for improved documentation on the specifics of the endotrachial tube size during the transport.	Poster session presented at Florida International University (FIU) School of Nursing Annual Improving Health Care Quality through Research Conference, October 21, 2005.
Skin Prevalence Study	Results indicated that the rate at this site was 5.9% lower than the national rate at 15.5%. Replication is occurring March 2005.	Poster session presented at Florida International University (FIU) School of Nursing Annual Improving Health Care Quality through Research, Program Conference, October 21, 2005.
Staff Attitudes Toward Family Presence During Invasive Procedures, Cardiopulmonary Resuscitation and Rounds to Promote Family-Centered Care	More than 325 nurses, physicians, respiratory therapists, social workers, and child life specialists were surveyed on their attitudes toward family members allowed to stay during rounds, CPR, or invasive procedures.	Paper presented at the Florida International University (FIU) School of Nursing Annual Research Program, Improving Health Care Quality through Research, October 14, 2004. Poster session presented at the Second Annual Magnet Nursing Research Conference, Tampa, FL, February 3-4, 2005.

Table 15-1 Research Productivity at Miami Children's Hospital—cont'd

Study	Key Findings	Knowledge Dissemination
		Paper presented at the Second International Family Centered Care Conference, San Francisco, CA, February 21-23, 2005.
Use of the Human Patient (Pediatric) Simulator (HPS) to Enhance Critical Thinking Skills in New Graduates	Interviews conducted with the new graduates revealed that taking the Critical Thinking test and completing several scenarios on the HPS improved their chances of passing NLCLEX.	Poster session presented at the Second Annual Magnet Nursing Research Conference, Tampa, FL, February 3-4, 2005.
Enhancing Nurse-Physician Collaboration Using a Human Patient (Pediatric) Simulator	50 nurses and 55 medical residents, divided into code teams of six, participated in the study. Each team was evaluated on three code scenarios. In the first scenario, nurses talked only to nurses, while the medical residents communicated only with the other residents. In the second scenario, both disciplines began to work together as a team with greatly improved results. By the third scenario, each team worked together cohesively and collaboratively with optimal patient results.	Paper presented at the Florida International University (FIU) School of Nursing Annual Research Program, Improving Health Care Quality through Research, October 14, 2004. Poster session presented at the American Academy of Nursing (AAN) Conference in Washington, DC, November 2004. Poster session presented at the Nineteenth Annual SNRS Conference Atlanta, GA, February 4, 2005.
Effect of a Support Group for New Graduate's Retention	The findings except for 2 out of 32 participants were satisfied with their job and indicated no intention of leaving their position. The one who was not satisfied with the job indicated no intention of leaving the job.	Paper presented at the Florida International University (FIU) School of Nursing Annual Research Program, Improving Health Care Quality through Research, October 14, 2004. Poster session presented at the NLN Annual Summit in Orlando, FL, September 30-October 2, 2004. Poster session presented at the First Florida Magnet Nursing Research Conference in Tampa, FL, February 2004. Poster session presented at the Second Annual Magnet Nursing Research Conference, Tampa, FL, February 3-4, 2005.

commitment of the nursing organization to using research to shape practices.

Clearly, having an extensive program of research provides ongoing products to be disseminated. Although many organizations cannot produce the level of work described here, the key is that researchers have engaged staff members in active roles and have used numerous strategies to create studies and disseminate findings.

INTERDISCIPLINARY RESEARCH

Nursing research programs frequently include studies that reflect more than the nursing profession. Although an interdisciplinary approach may present challenges, other disciplines must be included to bring breadth and depth to projects. In addition, most practices within an organization include multiple disciplines in the daily implementation of care. Although different disciplines may see the problem to be addressed from a different perspective, agreement about the type of answer sought typically creates a more focused project. Unless other institutions are involved in the research endeavors, only one Institutional Review Board (IRB) process is used. Determining who is "in charge" of a particular study and how findings will be disseminated are necessary preliminary decisions before the research is designed or implemented. Also making certain who is collecting data is an example of role clarification activities that must be decided before work is begun.

Because multiple disciplines provide various perspectives, application of findings may have implications for numerous policies and practices. The key would be that the policies and practices are comparable or compatible so that care is improved from multiple perspectives.

Processes for achieving ANCC Magnet Recognition and the MBQA rely on research as the way in which practices within the organization are improved. The research efforts are the driving force in determining that desired outcomes are achieved and, where possible, that improvements are made. Evidence-based practice indicates that staff members are using current findings to support their practice. Examples of outcomes using a retrospective approach are found in the Literature box. The role of research and its impact on nursing practice is an important element in advancing the quality of care within healthcare organizations. The CNO sets the expectation and provides the support needed to achieve goals.

SUMMARY

More important than the way in which a nursing research program is implemented is the fact that one exists and that it drives practice. Although the CNO need not be the researcher, the CNO, however, does create the culture for the value placed on research within the facility and its utilization in practice. CNOs need to consider how to facilitate a milieu for research to happen. In doing so, they need to instill value within the setting for the quality of research conducted and for the avenues for disseminating the research findings within the organization and the profession. By creating an atmosphere of scholarly inquiry that fosters staff involvement, the CNO establishes a practice environment of professional development and clinical excellence.

KEY POINTS TO LEAD

1. Value the key research mission of nursing service organizations.
2. Discuss the role of the CNO in promoting research and scholarship.
3. Define the research standard established for Magnet programs.

Literature Box

Aiken's primary interest was to understand how the structure, culture, and organization of hospitals affected nurse and patient outcomes. When Aiken and colleagues started their research, they found that measurement of organizational traits of hospitals was relatively underdeveloped. Most studies focused on nurse staffing. Although Aiken felt staffing was very important, it had to be viewed in the context of organizational climate and whether it enhanced or detracted from the effects of nurse staffing on patient and nurse outcomes. Aiken indicated that until the nurse work environment could be measured, it would be difficult to understand why some hospitals were more successful than others in attracting and retaining nurses and producing good patient outcomes. Registered nurses were selected as informants about the organizational traits of hospitals because they tended to be at the nexus of interactions of the key groups within hospitals, including physicians, support services, management, patients, and their families. The instrument used to collect the data was the Nursing Work Index (NWI), developed by Kramer and Hafner (1989), based upon their research on (reputational) Magnet hospitals. It was revised and became the NWI-R.

The evidence base in support of superior outcomes for Magnet hospitals is extensive. Magnet hospitals have been shown to achieve substantially more favorable outcomes for patients when compared with non-Magnet hospitals. Research documents that the ANCC Magnet Recognition Program is successful in identifying hospitals with professional nursing practice environments. Magnet designation provides valuable information to consumers, which enables them to select the best hospitals. Magnet status also serves as a guide to nurses seeking employment and to nursing students who desire the optimal work environment. Attracting and keeping nurses addresses this nursing shortage. The ANCC Magnet Recognition program promotes the excellence in nurses' work environments that is vital to successful recruitment and retention of nurses worldwide.

Aiken, L. (2002). Superior outcomes for Magnet hospitals: The evidence base. In M. McClure & A. S. Hinshaw (Eds.), *Magnet hospital revisited: Attraction and retention of professional nurses.* Washington, D. C.: American Academy of Nursing.

Contemplations

- What process could be used in your healthcare organization to construct a program of research?
- What are the top issues to be researched within your organization?

LEADER STORY ∽

JACQUELYN L. GONZALEZ
SENIOR VICE PRESIDENT/CHIEF NURSING OFFICER
MIAMI CHILDREN'S HOSPITAL
MIAMI, FL

Miami Children's Hospital (MCH) in Miami, Florida, was an early pioneer to have a full-time equivalent, doctorally prepared nurse researcher with teaching responsibilities at an area university. At this pediatric hospital, the nurse researcher was responsible for developing and coordinating the nursing research program. The hospital-based nursing research program enabled pediatric nurses and graduate nursing students to identify and develop nursing research projects that evaluated the best methods of providing quality patient care. In the early 1990s, when the nurse researcher resigned to take a full-time faculty position, the researcher position was not filled with a full-time researcher because of financial constraints. One of the strategies used to engage in nursing research and scholarship was to contract with a local university for half-time consultative services for nursing research. This approach yielded limited outcomes because of competing priorities and did not achieve the desired results of creating an atmosphere of scholarly inquiry and staff involvement and interest in research.

In 2002, after evaluation of the previous model, the position was again fully funded and a full-time nurse researcher was employed. The application and process for the Magnet program served as the impetus for redirection and funding support, because one of the challenges of "Going for Magnet" included increasing and integrating nursing research into the practice culture.

A housewide nursing research project was studied to identify the level of nurses' job satisfaction, stress, and recognition in the hopes of generating interest and participation in nursing research. Out of 534 pediatric nurses, 249 (46%) participated in the study, "Nurse Job Satisfaction, Stress and Recognition in a Pediatric Setting." The Nursing Department launched its research program!

Nursing research was facilitated by addressing patient safety with the "Bar-Coding Technology (BCT) for Medication Administration" study, with the result that the hospital became a national leader for this technology in children. Before implementation of the technology, a survey was administered to the nursing staff eliciting their perceptions of the effect of the BCT on medication errors, timeliness of medication administration with BCT, effect of the BCT on patient/family satisfaction, and difficulty with the BCT system. About 6 to 8 weeks post implementation, another survey was administered that measured staff perceptions of BCT. This study involved the collaboration of nursing with pharmacy, respiratory, and the medical staff. The qualitative data demonstrated that although the nurses perceived that it took more time to barcode the medication, they felt that the system saved children's lives, which became the most important focus.

The Nursing Department is fortunate to have an endowment fund, the Frida Hill Beck for Nursing Innovation and Excellence Fund, to support research endeavors. In turn, the nurse researcher seeks additional funds from philanthropic foundations, pharmaceutical companies, professional organizations, and governmental agencies to support nursing research studies and innovative educational projects. The Nursing Research Council is part of the Governance Council and is chaired by the nurse researcher and co-chaired by a clinical nurse specialist (CNS). Staff nurses are members of the Nursing Research Council and are paid to attend these meetings in addition to unit-based clinical practice committees if the meetings occur on their day off. At these unit-based clinical practice committees, staff nurses share the information presented at the Nursing Research Council and make recommendations for changes in policies and procedures based on findings from the studies.

A commitment to quality of nurse retention was a focus of the board of trustees and the executive level of administration in addressing the nursing shortage crisis. With a continuous focus on improvement by promoting a positive practice environment, the vacancy rate went from 20.1% in 1998 before the Magnet application to 2.65% in 2003 at the time of the ANCC Magnet site visit and the Magnet celebration. This is well below both the national and state levels. All the nursing projects are listed on the hospital web access site (http://www.mch.com).

Studies have been initiated by the nurse administrators, directors, clinical nurse specialists, and staff nurses in addition to the nurse researcher. Nursing staff must first clarify and share their findings by presenting their work either as a poster or paper and then by publishing the article for scientific dissemination. The nurse researcher attends conferences with the staff nurses. It is important to identify performance improvement projects that are suitable for nursing research studies. For example, in preparing for a prevalence of pressure ulcer study, a Skin Protocol based on the Modified Braden Q scale was created on the computer for documentation to provide further analysis.

Faculty from the area universities in addition to faculty from across the country have expressed an interest in conducting their studies at MCH. For example, several faculty members from an area university are conducting a study, "Death in the PICU/NICU: Parent and Family Functioning" in collaboration with MCH nurses

and physicians. It is important that facilities support faculty and doctoral students' research and assist them through the IRB process. One of the staff nurses in the Cardiac Intensive Care conducted a study in fulfillment of her doctorate in nursing on "Walking a Tightrope: Living with Your Child's Congenital Heart Disease." This was a qualitative study dealing with parents experiencing their child's critical illness. The results of this study served as the impetus to revise the IRB Consent form to be more "parent friendly."

The nurses in the pediatric intensive care unit (PICU) are testing the "Use of Chlorhexidine as a Mouthwash for At-Risk Pediatric Patients to Reduce Noscomial Infection Rates." The PICU nurses also developed a protocol based on research, "Prevalence of Deep Venous Thrombosis in the Lower Extremities of Children in the Intensive Care Unit." Finally, another nursing research interest focusing on "Pediatric Palliative Care Across All Units" was expressed by the Medical-Surgical as well as the PICU, Cardiac Care ICU, and NICU nursing staff. These are three examples of how staff nurses have learned to critique nursing research studies and integrate evidence-based outcomes into their practice. In most cases a staff member from the facility is on the protocol to ensure that the reports are submitted in a timely manner.

At this facility, the nurse researcher serves on the IRB with the me as an alternate. The minutes are available through a controlled web site and on a CD for staff nurses who may be interested in any of the protocols, including the pharmaceutical protocols. The nursing leadership and staff are offered the opportunity to participate in and take advantage of the hospital-wide educational programs on Protection of Rights of Human Subjects. Before approval to conduct any nursing research study, they must present proof that they have obtained the CITI course in the Protection of Human Subjects certification on-line. The nurse researcher was appointed to the Board of Trustees Research

Committee and is involved in strategic planning for research initiatives.

INTERDISCIPLINARY RESEARCH

Although it may present challenges, it is vital to include other departments to bring breadth and depth to the projects. For example, the nurse researcher is conducting studies using patient simulation. One study, "Use of the Human Patient (Pediatric) Simulator to Enhance Critical Thinking Skills in New Graduates," was funded by the Hugoton Foundation. Another study, funded by the hospital foundation, determined the nurse-physician collaboration developed over time as one of the outcomes of using clinical simulation, "Enhancing Nurse-Physician Collaboration Using a Human Patient (Pediatric) Simulator." Nursing collaborated with Education and Medical Education to implement this study. Clinical nurse researchers have opportunities to conduct research studies in conjunction with other departments.

Frequently the nursing leadership team and staff are enrolled in graduate programs and conduct their projects or studies at the clinical institution where they are employed. One of the staff nurses conducted a study in the emergency room to fulfill her academic class assignment, "Evaluation of Three Tier vs. Five Tier Triage Acuity Rating in Emergency Department." This is beneficial to all nurses who come in contact with the study, because it stimulates interest and discussion about research. Nurses in other areas of the hospital are involved in research, especially the neuroscience area. A program of research had

been conducted by the advanced nurse practitioner and includes the most recent study, "Outcome of Epilepsy Surgery in Patients under 3 Years of Age."

A study conducted by a director, nurse researcher, clinical nurse specialist, and educator is the "Effect of a Support Group for New Graduate's Retention." The study was funded by Florida Nurses Foundation (FNF) and Sigma Theta Tau International (STTI), Beta Tau chapter. The findings of this study in improving retention among this vulnerable population were essential to sustain financial support for its continuation of the program. The program includes the use of a "clown care unit" for humor, therapeutic relaxation, and meditation and the psychiatric staff to facilitate dialogue in the support groups. Except for one, all the other 31 participants were satisfied with their job and indicated no intention of leaving their position. The one who was not satisfied with the job also indicated no intention of leaving the job.

Involvement in clinical scholarship activities such as STTI and other nursing professional organizations, including the American Nurses Association (ANA), is strongly encouraged. The nurses at this pediatric facility are very fortunate to live in an area with four university STTI chapters that sponsor annual nursing research conferences: MCH nursing leaders and staff are involved and hold offices in these chapters and present papers and posters at the conferences. In addition, staff also present their research at the Florida Nurses Association (FNA) biennial convention, Florida League for Nursing (FLN) annual conferences, and the annual Florida Magnet Nursing Research Conference. These opportunities are very successful in highlighting the nursing research projects to the community.

Chapter References

Aiken, L. (2002). Superior outcomes for Magnet hospitals: The evidence base. In M. McClure & A. S. Hinshaw (Eds.), *Magnet hospital revisited: Attraction and retention of professional nurses.* Washington, D. C.: American Academy of Nursing.

American Nurses Association. (2004). *Scope and standards for nurse administrators* (2nd ed.). Washington, DC: Author.

American Nurses Credentialing Center. (2003). *Health care organization instructions and application process manual 2003-2004.* Washington, DC: Author.

American Nurses Credentialing Center. (2005). *Magnet Recognition Program application manual 2005.* Washington, DC: Author.

Baker, C. M., Bingle, J. M., Hajewski, C. J., Radant, K. L., & Urden, L. D. (2004). Advancing the magnet recognition in master's education through service-learning. *Nursing Outlook, 52*(3), 134-141.

Berger, A. M., Eilers, J. G., Heermann, J. A., Warren, J. J., Franco, T., & Triolo, P. (1999). State-of-the-art patient care: The impact of doctorally prepared clinical nurses. *Clinical Nurse Specialist 13*(5), 259-266.

Burns, N., & Grove, S. (2003). *The practice of nursing research: Conduct, critique & utilization* (4th ed.). Philadelphia: W. B. Saunders.

Frank, B., Aroian J., & Tashea, P. (2003). Nursing administration graduate programs. *Journal of Nursing Administration, 33*(5), 300-306.

Hinds, P. S., Gattuso, J. S., Barnewell, E., Cofer, M., Kellum, L.K., Mattox, S., Norman, G., Powell, B., Randall, E., & Sanders, C. (2003). Translating psychosocial research into practice guidelines. *Journal of Nursing Administration, 33*(7/8), 397-403.

Hinds, P. S., Gattuso, J., & Morrell, A. (2000). Creating a hospital-based nursing research fellowship program for staff nurses. *Journal of Nursing Administration, 30*(6), 317-321.

Hudson-Barr, D., & King, C. R. (2004). From nursing research committee to nursing research council. *Journal for Specialties in Pediatric Nursing, 9*(4), 139-141.

Kerfoot, K. (2002). On leadership. The leader as chief knowledge officer. *Nursing Economics, 20*(1), 40-41.

King, C. R. (2004a, November 11-13). *An innovative nursing research council within shared governance.* Poster session presented at the American Academy of Nursing Annual Meeting and Conference, Washington, DC.

King, C. R. (2004b, November 11-13). Choosing a wound cleanser in tracheostomy care for patients. Poster session presented at the American Academy of Nursing Annual Meeting and Conference, Washington, DC.

Maljanian, R., Caramanica, L., Taylor, S. K., MacRae, J. B., & Beland, D. K. (2002). Evidence-based nursing practice Part 2. *Journal of Nursing Administration 32*(2), 85-90.

Messmer, P. R., & Gonzalez, J. L. (2003). March to Magnet. *Reflections on Nursing Leadership* 4th quarter 2003, 14-15.

Messmer, P. R., Jones, S. G., & Rosillo, C. (2002). Using nursing research projects to meet magnet recognition program standards. *Journal of Nursing Administration 32*(10), 538-543.

Snyder-Halpern, R. (1998). Measuring organizational readiness for nursing research programs. *Western Journal of Nursing Research 20*(2), 223-237.

16 Working with Human Resources to Develop a Strategic Partnership

Carol Haun

Eleanor T. Lawrence

Human Resources should be defined not by what it does, but what it delivers. D. ULRICH

This chapter focuses on the cooperative relationship between the chief nursing officer (CNO) and the human resources (HR) department. The many responsibilities of HR in large facilities are examined in view of the supporting role HR has toward other departments in the facility. HR is a valued resource that eases the many personnel questions and issues faced by nurse leaders. The American Organization of Nurse Executives (AONE, 2005) included in the *Nurse Executive Competencies*, developed in 2004 and 2005, a major subsection on the importance of HR. The work to be done by the CNO as it relates to HR builds on a collaborative relationship with the HR department.

THROUGHOUT THIS CHAPTER AN EMPHASIS is placed on the importance of people and their contributions to the competitive success of an organization. Human resource management (HRM) deals with the design of formal systems in an organization to ensure the effective and efficient use of human talent to accomplish organizational goals. In a hospital (e.g., for-profit, not-for-profit, community, or tertiary) the management of HR involves the design and delivery of recruitment, compensation, training, and development services. The relationship and interface between the CNO and HR and the relationship and critical interaction of HR and staff nurses with their managers are integral to ensure the effective and efficient use of human talent to accomplish organizational goals. The CNO has a significant impact on strategy formulation, HR planning, strategy implementation, and key HR functions such as hiring, performance management, training and development, and employee relations.

HUMAN RESOURCES AND NURSING: A STRATEGIC PARTNERSHIP

Knowing what HR can provide to ensure the success of the organization through the contribution of each employee is critical for CNOs. The best nursing and HR leaders collaborate. They work together as strategic players to make the best things happen for the internal and external customers. The CNO and the chief human resources officer (CHRO) and other members of the executive team form a partnership to align the business strategy of the organization with a culture that supports the contribution of each employee. They focus on the congruency of strategy and the initiatives of work design, productivity, selection, development, rewards, and communication (Ulrich, Losey, & Lake, 1997). Each of these elements in the HR system is designed to maximize the overall quality of human capital as an asset to the organization (Becker, Huselid, & Ulrich, 2001).

HR has to structure each element of the HR system to support and reinforce a high-performance culture. To build and sustain a talented, high-performance workforce requires linking selection and promotion decisions to the skills and competencies and to develop compensation and performance management and development policies that attract, retain, and motivate employees (Becker et al., 2001). The HR practices, polices, and procedures must maximize the contribution of the employee to implement the organization's strategies. The HR system is the linchpin that influences employee behavior and performance. The most potent action that the CNO and the CHRO can take is to ensure the alignment of the HR infrastructure and its components to cultivate talented, recognized, and rewarded employees that deliver superior performance.

Understanding and using an investment perspective is required before nursing and HR executives can have an influential role in the management in any organization. "I am constantly amazed at the contrast between the concern that organizations show for potential capital costs and the casual indifference they tend to display toward the potential human resource costs until, of course, the latter have gotten completely out of hand" (Dyer, 1983, p. 263). The conceptual framework for the nursing/HR partnership is based upon an investment orientation toward people, as presented in Figure 16-1. It comprises a mission

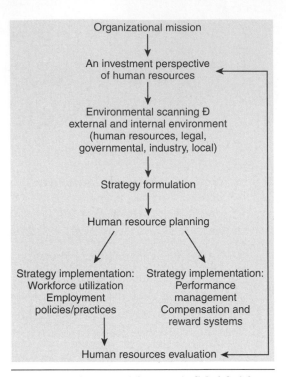

Figure 16-1 Conceptual framework. (Modified from Greer, C. R. (© 2001). *Strategic human resource management: A general managerial approach.* (2nd ed) p. xiv. Reprinted by permission of Pearson Education, Inc., Upper Saddle River, NJ)

statement and the functions that draw from the principles of human capital theory, strategic management/planning/implementation, hiring, compensation reward systems, performance evaluation, and development/training.

THE SCOPE OF PRACTICE IN HUMAN RESOURCES

The people that comprise an organization are its key assets. Successful organizations understand that behind every single business issue lies a human issue. Where effective HRM is an integral part of management, where HR is included in the executive team, people issues are integrated with business issues and optimum outcomes are achieved (Ulrich et al., 1997).

Human Resource Systems

Organizing and managing people will continue to be the quintessential business challenge well into the twenty-first century. The HR system provides the infrastructure to recruit, train, nurture, develop, recognize, reward, and ultimately retain employees. A connection exists between the service and the value the organization generates and the people it employs. By hiring the right people; matching them to the right position; and managing, orienting, training, supporting, and recognizing and rewarding them, healthcare organizations will be able to deliver exceptional patient care and retain their most valued resource.

The CNO must possess a solid understanding of the HR processes and operations that affect the care of the patient. It is equally important for HR to comprehend how excellent patient care is delivered and exactly how that care is provided. With a shared understanding of how excellent patient care is linked to the people, operations, goals, strategies, and HR systems, an organization can design a model that specifies the employee competencies and skills needed (Becker et al., 2001). The CNO, as a partner to HR, plays an important role in identification of the desired employee behavior and performance. The current role of the CNO is to be involved with HR to translate the organization's strategy and operational goals to influence employee behavior and performance in the desired direction.

The relationship between HR and the CNO and his or her executive team becomes one of collaboration and support. Communication between the CNO and HR is a critical component to developing a high-performance healthcare organization. Working with HR is a partnership toward a shared vision, congruent personal and professional values, and fulfilling the organization's staffing needs, whereas communicating and resolving issues are essential to providing excellent outcomes. HR personnel must work with nurse leaders on a regular basis. As partners, they build a nursing culture that nurtures, supports, and actualizes the potential of those who care for patients.

Responsibilities of Human Resources

The major activities and typical responsibilities that the CNO can expect from HR professionals are determined by the scope, size, and complexity of the hospital. The expectation is that HR will be a partner helping the organization to build a high-performance workforce that emphasizes and recognizes the importance of the contribution of each employee to deliver excellent patient care.

1. *Advice and counsel.* HR serves as in-house consultant to the supervisors, managers, and executives. HR possesses knowledge of internal employment policies, labor agreements, and past practices. HR professionals understand the needs of employees in addition to external trends in legal issues and employment data. HR is concerned with supporting the operating and productivity goals of the managers and supervisors.
2. *Service.* HR designs and delivers multiple technical services and functions such as recruiting, selecting, testing, planning, conducting training and development programs, and listening to and responding to employee concerns and complaints.
3. *Policy formulation and implementation.* HR proposes, drafts, revises, and interprets employee-related policies and procedures for the executives, managers, and staff.
4 *Employee advocacy.* HR serves as the employee advocate and listens to employees' concerns, issues, and needs and represents their views to management.

Human Resource Planning

HR planning is fully integrated and linked with organizational strategy formulation and implementation. HR personnel and nurse executives need to be able to forecast and plan for the future availability of employees to carry out the strategies of the organization. The literature often indicates that HR planning is an evolving source of potential competitive advantage (Greer, 1995). Organizations are concerned about providing an adequate supply of competent and skilled employees.

HR planning (Greer, 1995) encompasses the following factors: (1) interfacing with strategic planning and scanning the environment, (2) taking an inventory of the organization's current human resources (workforce), (3) forecasting the demand for human resources (labor demand), (4) forecasting the supply of human resources from within the organization and the external labor market, (5) comparing forecasts of supply and demand, (6) planning the actions and tactics needed to manage the anticipated needs—both shortages or overages, and (7) feeding back the information into the strategic planning process.

In the healthcare industry, shifting labor demographics, the increasing proportion of total costs accounted for by labor costs, competitive pressures, governmental and legal oversight, and reimbursement constraints are just some of the primary reasons cited for engaging in effective HR planning. Evidence demonstrates that the greater the involvement of all executives in HR planning, the greater the strategic impact (Greer, 1995). With the recognition that a skilled and competent workforce is a source of competitive advantage for the organization, involvement in HR planning is an important role for the CNO.

Staffing

The hospital's strategic plan provides the framework for the staffing plan. A sufficient number of staff members is based on the determination of the appropriate skill mix and patient acuity to safely meet the care, treatment, and service needs of the patients. Allocating employees as needed to meet patient and unit needs often is done in conjunction with the nursing supervisor.

Long-term staffing is the process of planning the number and type of employees who will be needed to fill a unit's complement of positions. It typically is based on projected patient volume and a specified or desired nurse-to-patient ratio.

Daily staffing is the process of making the daily adjustments to staffing and usually is coordinated through a "staffing office" supported by the nursing division.

Scheduling is the process of planning when staff members are assigned to work their shifts. Several computerized staffing programs exist to help with this complex and sometimes emotionally charged task. Schedules usually are completed several weeks in advance so that employees may anticipate their upcoming work schedule. Scheduling takes into account vacation requests and other days off. When staff are accountable for self-staffing, they make determinations within a framework of criteria such as employment policies and staffing ratios. HR may need to validate the framework to determine compliance with laws and policies whenever the criteria are revised.

Staffing Effectiveness

Staffing effectiveness is a complex issue that is a major concern for nursing. The hospital may select data on clinical/service screening indicators in combination with HR screening indicators to assess staffing effectiveness. A minimum of four screening indicators (two clinical and two HR indicators) are selected for data compilation and trending. The focus is on the relationship between the clinical/service and HR screening indicators to determine staffing effectiveness.

Defining direct and indirect caregivers in the HR screening indicators is critical to determine any impact that may be related to patient outcomes. Data must be collected and analyzed in combination and in collaboration with other disciplines or areas of the hospital. The hospital provides evidence of any actions taken and reports at least annually to the leaders of the organization in regard to staffing effectiveness data and any actions taken to improve staffing.

HUMAN RESOURCES AND NEW EMPLOYEES

HR has many responsibilities in the process of hiring new employees, including working with the CNO in recruiting new staff, initial screening, and other basic requirements. In addition, HR and the CNO must collaborate on work-life balance programs to attract and retain the younger generation of nurses.

Recruiting and Hiring the Right Talent

Recruiting and hiring the right person for each position is mission-critical in healthcare organizations. In most organizations, the workforce represents the largest expense. Successful organizations treat this not as an expense but as an investment. They view their employees as assets, talented individuals who need to be involved, developed, supported, and fully engaged. It starts with the hiring process. HR and administration share the responsibility to ensure that the best people and the best processes are in place to make that happen (Meisinger, 2004). The recruiting process is designed to increase the number of applicants whose qualifications meet job requirements and the needs of the organization.

Hiring Process: Selection

Selection is the process of choosing those individuals who have the relevant qualifications to fill existing or projected vacancies (Bohlander, Snell, & Sherman, 2001). Selection of applicants for hiring is determined by the applicant's ability to perform job functions, his or her education, experience, aptitude, and ability to be trained in specified programs. Decisions regarding the recruitment and selection of employees are made on the basis of job-related criteria and in accordance with state and federal laws. HR works with managers on updating existing job descriptions and developing new ones, based on the competencies and criteria needed to fill the desired position.

Positions are "posted" for a period of time to allow applicants to apply for an open position. All positions must have a written job description.

The design and delivery of the selection program is the formal responsibility of the HR department. The line managers make the final decision about hiring people into their unit. Therefore nurse executives and nurse managers must understand the objectives, policies, and practices used for selection. In broadest terms the goal of the CNO and the nurse manager is to maximize "matches" and avoid the "misses" in their selection decisions (Bohlander et al., 2001).

Position Descriptions

A position description or job description is developed for each position to include functions of the job in addition to known physical and environmental demands of the position. The description is a mechanism for sharing job expectations and standards and competencies for the position. Position descriptions are developed to provide applicants and employees with specific standards and expectations and to comply with regulatory agencies.

Screening

Once a candidate is selected for interviewing, HR performs an initial screening and forwards qualified candidates to a manager for an interview. HR is responsible for checking references, completing background checks, and verifying licensure and past employment. After a conditional offer is made to the best-qualified applicant, employment-related medical examinations and disability-related inquiries are permissible, as long as they are required of all new employees in the same job category. If, based on such post-offer examinations, a manager chooses not to hire an individual, he or she must be able to show that the applicant cannot perform the essential functions of the position, even with reasonable accommodation.

Consistency in handling applicants is a key to supporting hiring decisions. Nurse managers must use a standardized format for recording the responses of each applicant during interviews and ask the same questions of each applicant for a specific position.

In reviewing a resumé, the nurse manager should look for information that indicates the candidate's competence for the position based on the description and standards for the particular position (Box 16-1). Education, experience,

---

Box 16-1   CHECKLIST FOR REVIEWING RESUMÉS OR APPLICATION FORMS

- Review the position description(s) for the position(s) to fill. Note requirements from the description needed and refer to them often during the review of resumés/applications.
- Ignore the applicant's name, address, or personal information to limit subconscious biases.
- Attempt to ignore superficial issues such as writing style and typographic errors in favor of content, unless such issues are directly related to the position for which the person is applying. Such scrutiny may unintentionally rule out members of protected classes.
- Check work experience for applicability to the position for which the applicant is applying, length of time in each position, promotions or awards received, and reason for leaving each position.
- Note gaps in employment but do not assume they were caused by negative reasons.
- Check educational background for qualifications necessary to successful performance based on the position description.
- Note special skills (e.g., computer software, office equipment) as stated on the position description.
- Note on a separate piece of paper any pertinent questions that arise when reviewing the resumés/application and ask those during a telephone screen.

---

accomplishments, employment changes, and reasons for leaving positions are indicators of a candidate's qualifications. Gaps in employment, frequent employment changes, degrees/certifications, salary requirements, and specific skills should be noted before scheduling an interview. The resumé should be searched for "red flags"—areas of concern that merit additional review or focus during an interview. Some tips for nurse leaders to use in screening a resumé or application and how to address these concerns in an interview are presented in Table 16-1 (Society for Human Resource Management, 2003).

Interviewing

HR will screen applications for minimum qualifications based on the position description before referring candidates to nurse leaders for consideration. Conducting an interview is an opportunity to access candidates' qualifications and "fit" or "match" for the position. In addition, it is an opportunity for nurse leaders to provide a great impression of nursing and of the organization. Nurse leaders may not choose to hire the person being interviewed; however, they will want to formulate their perceptions during the interview process. Hiring decisions are based on selecting the most qualified person for the position. "Qualified" includes skills, competencies, work experience, motivation, and position fit. Persons are entitled to equal employment opportunity regardless of race, color, religion, sex, sexual orientation, national origin, age, disability, or any other non–job-related characteristic as required by local, state, and federal law. Every effort must be made to employ the best-qualified candidate for the position. The CNO must be aware of interview protocols. The Society for Human Resource Management prepared the information in Table 16-1 as a guide.

Behavioral Interviews

Conducting an interview using a series of behavioral interview questions provides a more accurate assessment of how successfully a candidate will

Table **16-1** INTERVIEWING QUESTIONS TO ASK/NOT ASK

Category	May Ask	May Discriminate By Asking
Sex and family arrangements	If applicant has relatives already employed by the organization	Sex of applicant Number of children Marital status Spouse's occupation Childcare arrangements Healthcare coverage through spouse
Race		Applicant's race or color of skin Photo to be affixed to application form
National origin or ancestry	Whether applicant has a legal right to be employed in the U.S. Ability to speak/write English fluently (if job related) Other languages spoken (if job-related)	Ethnic association of a surname Birthplace of applicant or applicant's parents Nationality, lineage, national origin Nationality of applicant's spouse Whether applicant is citizen of another country Applicant's native tongue/English proficiency Maiden name (of married woman)
Religion		Religious affiliation/availability for weekend work Religious holidays observed
Age	If applicant is over age 18 If applicant is over age 21 if job-related (e.g., bartender)	Date of birth Date of high school graduation Age
Disability	Whether applicant can perform the essential job-related functions	If applicant has a disability Nature or severity of a disability Whether applicant has ever filed a workers' compensation claim Recent or past surgeries and dates Past medical problems
Other	Convictions, if job-related Academic, vocational, or professional schooling Training received in the military Membership in any trade or professional association Job references	Number and kinds of arrests Height or weight, except if a bona fide occupational qualification Veteran status, discharge status, branch of service Contact in case of an emergency (at application or interview stage)

From Development Dimensions International, Inc. (2003). *Legal considerations in selection; U.S. version.* Bridgeville, PA: Author.

perform in the job. The premise behind behavioral interviewing techniques is that "past behavior predicts future behavior" (Development Dimensions International, 2003). Conducting an interview using behavioral questions is designed to elicit as much information as possible about how a prospective employee views a situation and then acts on it. Seeking details about an actual situation, the action that the employee took, and the outcome adds to the richness of understanding how a person performs in real-world situations. These components provide insight into how future employees may react in changing situations based on their past behaviors and experiences. A variety of behavioral

interviewing techniques is available, and some examples are contained in Box 16-2. Box 16-3 provides a summary of important guidelines for the interview/hiring process.

Employment Testing

In many industries tests play an important role in the hiring process as a method to measure or predict skills and abilities. Employers commonly ask applicants to undergo other procedures, such as testing, as part of their selection process. Although a detailed discussion is beyond the scope of this chapter, following are some of the more important

---

Box 16-2   BEHAVIORAL INTERVIEW QUESTIONS/COMMENTS

- Tell me about a time when you found it challenging to be a member on a team. What did you do, and what was the outcome?
- Sometimes decisions are made that we don't agree with. Tell me about a time when you did not agree with a decision or a change that was made by a supervisor or administration. How did you respond, and what happened as a result?
- Sometimes it is necessary to work in unsettled or rapidly changing circumstances. When have you found yourself in this position? Tell me what you did. What was the outcome?
- Describe a time when you chose to be honest, even though being quiet or agreeable might have been easier. What happened?
- Tell me about a time when you made a decision that was not in line with a policy. What were the circumstances? What was the result?*
- Describe a time when you took action to provide a quick response to a problem with a manager or direct report.
- What actions have you taken when you've been asked to significantly change

- a policy or process and how you communicated that change to your nurse leaders?
- Tell me about a time when something that you were doing was ineffective. What did you do? How did the change affect you?
- Describe how you improved productivity in your department. How did you identify these opportunities for improvement?
- Tell me about a time when you had many opportunities to coach others in your department or area of responsibility.
- Describe a situation in which you had to approach a physician in regard to a sensitive issue. What was your approach and what was the outcome?
- Tell me about your experience in developing quality indicators and patient care initiatives.
- How would the nursing staff describe your management style? Physicians? Top management?
- Describe your experience with documentation and regulatory compliance as it relates to this position.

*Modified from Development Dimensions International, Inc. (2003). *Legal considerations in selection; U.S. version.* Bridgeville, PA: Author.

Box 16-3   IMPORTANT GUIDELINES FOR
           THE INTERVIEW PROCESS

- Prepare questions in advance on an interview guide.
- Take accurate and complete notes, without writing on the resumé or application.
- Save interview notes of all the candidates interviewed, in case of potential legal challenges.
- Use behavioral interviewing techniques in addition to skills assessments. When feasible, include an additional person in the interview process.
- Confirm that HR will conduct thorough reference and background checking.
- Collaborate with HR before extending an offer, promising compensation, and scheduling orientation planning.
- HR will prepare an offer letter of employment for the CNO's signature.

issues to consider before implementation of testing procedures. An employment test is "an objective and standardized measurement of a sample of behavior that is used to gauge a person's knowledge, skills, abilities and other characteristics (KSAOs) in relation to other individuals" (Bohlander et al., 2001, p. 195).

The same tests should be administered under the same conditions to all applicants for the same position. If using preemployment, job, or skill-based testing, the nurse manager should be certain that tests are validated relative to the position. Other considerations are cost, time, ease of administration and scoring, and the relevance of the test being used to the individuals being tested (validity). Tests can be used as a supplement to the interview. Tests should not be the sole basis for decisions about candidates; they are one component of the overall selection procedure.

Employment tests are classified as measuring either aptitude or achievement. Aptitude tests measure a person's capacity to learn or acquire skills. Achievement tests measure what a person knows

or can do now. Employment tests may measure (1) cognitive ability, such as mental capacity, general intelligence, verbal fluency, and numeric and reasoning ability; (2) personality and interest inventories, including disposition and temperament; (3) physical ability; (4) knowledge related to an understanding about a particular role/position; and (5) work samples, which require performance of tasks that are actually part of the work required (Bohlander et al., 2001).

Other types of tests frequently used during the selection process are drug tests. State and federal laws (especially federal contractors and employers governed by Department of Transportation or other federal agency regulations) should be consulted before using drug tests as part of the selection process. Applicant consent must be obtained before testing. Confidentiality and standard procedures for confirmation tests should be established, if they are not already specifically regulated for the industry (Society for Human Resource Management, 2004).

If an organization is considering the use of tests, the managers should have a basic understanding of the technical aspects of testing and the contribution that tests can make to the selection process. Professional test consultants are recommended to improve testing programs and to meet legal guidelines. More information on employee testing is available at the web site for the Society for Industrial and Organizational Psychology at http://www.siop.org/workplace.

Categories Most Commonly Tested

Numerous standard tests are available, and most organizations do not have an interest in developing their own. The focus for testing may incorporate four common categories:

1. Cognitive tests measure learning and thinking ability.
2. Personality tests look at the habitual ways that people act.
3. Interest tests measure work interests.
4. Specialized tests measure specific skills.

The American Psychological Association has standards for test development and use. Industrial test developers are available to assist an organization in the design and development of tests or the selection and validation of appropriate standardized tests (Society for Human Resource Management, 2005).

How Personality Assessments Work

The exempt population and/or executive management receive personality and interest tests. Often the personality and interest results are used for succession and career planning. Personality assessments shed light on a person's needs, attitudes, motivations, and behavioral tendencies. More than a century of research has led some experts to focus on a small number of personality factors that seem to relate to performance in the workplace (Society for Human Resource Management, 2005).

Consensus is building in the research community that five factors shape one's overall personality, and researchers and testing firms are trying to use all five to measure job fit. The five dimensions are (1) the need for stability, (2) solitary or social, (3) striving for more innovation or efficiency, (4) sticking to positions or accepting others' ideas, and (5) linear or flexible in approaching goals. Personality tests consist of series of questions that assess a person's natural comfort level within these categories. Personality tests have no wrong answers—only results that suggest one individual is better suited to one type of work than another type of work (Society for Human Resource Management, 2005). Personality test scores should be used in tandem with other factors believed to be essential to the job—such as skills and experience—to create a comprehensive evaluation of the merits of each candidate. Those criteria then are applied identically to each applicant (Society for Human Resource Management, 2005).

However, the most ardent advocates of personality tests note their limitations. Employers also should be careful that their use of personality

tests does not violate Title VII of the Civil Rights Act, the Americans with Disabilities Act, and the guidelines of the U.S. Equal Employment Opportunity Commission in addition to various state laws aimed at discrimination prevention and other unfair practices (Society for Human Resource Management, 2005). Related resources for specific tests are The Society for Industrial and Organizational Psychology, The Association of Test Publishers, and The Personality Project (Society for Human Resource Management, 2005).

Drug Testing

Other types of tests that are used frequently during the selection process are drug tests. State and federal laws should be consulted (especially federal contractors and employers governed by the Department of Transportation or other federal agency regulations) before drug tests are used as part of the selection process. Applicant consent should be obtained before testing. Although drug tests themselves may be administered pre-offer, employers who conduct post-offer medical exams typically combine the two to save money and time. Confidentiality must be maintained and procedures established for confirmation tests, if they are not already specifically regulated for the particular industry (Society for Human Resource Management, 2004). If an organization is considering the use of tests, the managers should have a basic understanding of the technical aspects of testing and the contribution that tests can make to the selection process. Professional test consultants are recommended to improve testing programs and to meet legal guidelines. More information on employee testing is available at the web site for the Society for Industrial and Organizational Psychology at http://www.siop.org/workplace.

References and Background Checks

Verification of references, licensure, and background information is critical to the interview and selection process. Healthcare organizations conduct a thorough background check, including previous employment, criminal history check, license verification, personal and professional reference checks, and education verification. Drug screening is conducted after a job offer in a healthcare environment because of the easy access that healthcare workers have to medications and because most healthcare institutions are drug-free work environments. Background checks include a criminal history, verification of employment, and verification of education and personal and professional references. HR will confirm references and background checks.

In smaller facilities the HR function may not be delineated in the same way that it would be in a larger or tertiary facility. In small or rural facilities, the CNO may need to be more personally involved in handling reference and background checks. The CNO should ask the candidate for the name of an executive in the organization for which the candidate last worked so that the CNO can talk to that executive regarding the candidate. Executive-level references are invaluable in addition to those obtained through HR. The CNO would gain important knowledge regarding the candidate by asking the following questions: "Would you hire this manager again?" "What can I do to ensure the success of the manager being considered for employment?"

Cost of Poor Selection

Hiring the wrong person for the job can be costly. Costs are incurred in time and expense associated with interviewing candidates, training new managers, advertising, recruitment fees, contract labor for interim nurse managers, travel, relocation, severance pay, and administrative processes. In addition, hidden costs include disrupted patient care, manager orientation, incomplete projects, patient and employee satisfaction, and more. The challenge with the nursing shortage is to continue to select the right manager in spite of limited

resources and desperate times. The amount of time and energy required to mentor or counsel a manager that was a poor hiring decision far outweighs any amount of time spent on the selection process. A marginal nurse manager can incur complications such as costly employee relations issues, high staff turnover, disgruntled staff and physicians, decreased patient volumes, administrative complaints, and legal repercussions. The CNO must choose a manager who will be operational yet administrative, confident yet humble, and inspiring yet rational and grounded.

HUMAN RESOURCES AND EDUCATIONAL SUPPORT FOR NURSING

Performance Management

Evaluations

Performance reviews or evaluations are conducted periodically (at a minimum, annually) to provide a mechanism for employee feedback and to comply with the Joint Commission on Accreditation of Healthcare Organizations (JCAHO) and other regulatory agencies. Performance competencies and standards for evaluation should be objective, measurable, and obtainable. Periodic review of performance evaluation tools is necessary to maintain the integrity of the evaluation tool and to respond to changes in the environment. Merit increases often are tied to performance evaluations. Individual performance improvement plans may be created at the time of evaluation for those individuals identified as needing to improve their performance in specific areas. Peer evaluations may provide additional feedback to employees beyond a management evaluation. For feedback from multidisciplinary teams and at all levels, 360-degree evaluations may be used. Employee self-evaluations may be used in conjunction with any of the previously discussed evaluation methods as an approach to getting employees to acknowledge their own success and opportunities for development. The CNO may become involved directly in an employee evaluation when an employee and manager disagree. The CNO would serve as a mediator in reviewing the concerns with both parties.

Staff Development, Training, and Education

Staff development, training, and education are necessary to engage and retain nurses and to remain compliant with regulations. Although the nursing department may have its own staff development related to ensuring that the nurses and their support members are able to practice within the best practice available, HR typically remains accountable for generic training and development, such as safety, employment standards (e.g., nondiscrimination and zero tolerance for abuse), and new institution-wide protocols. HR also may be accountable for general leadership development strategies. Further, it is typical that the HR department is accountable for succession planning although leaders of various departments also have a plan in place.

We don't work for each other.
We work with each other.
STANLEY C. GAULT

HUMAN RESOURCES AND EMPLOYEE ISSUES

Significant issues in the course of work affect the nursing division. Several of these are related to enhancement of the workplace, whereas others are of a more sensitive nature.

The CNO works closely with nurse managers and HR in dealing with sensitive personnel issues and potential risk/liability factors that arise in daily operations. The key to dealing with employee relations issues is to educate nurse managers on preventive approaches. Corrective counseling is to

inform an employee that his or her conduct or performance is not meeting expectations or standards. The counseling is to encourage understanding of what is expected and to provide the employee an opportunity to respond and improve his or her performance. Coaching may be appropriate before use of any formal corrective counseling. Coaching begins when the nurse manager identifies a performance problem and meets informally with the employee in an attempt to bring performance up to standard.

Managing Staff Requests

Employees may request to be excused from participating in an aspect of a patient's care or treatment in situations in which the prescribed care or treatment presents a conflict with the employee's cultural values, religious beliefs, or sense of ethics. For example, assisting with terminating a pregnancy, assisting with discontinuing life support, or administering blood may conflict with certain employee values or beliefs. Employers generally encourage staff to request reassignment or to notify employers in advance for special considerations. Nurse managers and HR could handle staff requests at an operational level. The CNO needs to be informed of any unique situations or patient safety issues as they relate to managing staff requests and needs to ensure that the requisite care is available.

Grievances

Facilities or organizations often use a grievance procedure as a mechanism for employees to resolve issues related to interpretation or application of policies or in response to a termination. Grievance policies and procedures are designed to be an internal process. They do not include outside participants or attorneys and are not recorded. Grievances are not generally a process that managers can use. Managers who have disagreements or conflicts should deal directly with the CNO. In cases in which the issues are not resolved effectively, an outside mediator or coach may be retained to assist in resolving the issue.

Counseling and Disciplinary Issues

On occasion, an employee's performance may be affected by absenteeism, a single incident (such as reported sexual harassment), or poor interpersonal relationships on the job. Corrective actions may range from simply counseling the employee to formal disciplinary procedures.

Most organizations have specific, detailed processes for managing situations that could be punitive to an employee. The best first strategy is to determine as much information as possible and then seek the view of the person whose performance is in question. In a blame-free environment, some issues may result in new policies or strategies. However, some behaviors, such as persistent absence or abusing patients, require formal action. The situation and resultant disciplinary action must be documented in as much detail as possible. Further, HR should be notified so that the nurse leader is supported in subsequent action. The current intervention and subsequent consequences also must be clear. The disciplinary action should be presented in a slow, calm manner. Critical listening and note taking are important. After the discussion is concluded, any subsequent employee performance and progress must be monitored.

The nature of discipline is progressive and includes employee counseling in the form of verbal warnings, written warnings, suspension, or final written warnings and termination as appropriate. The CNO must be certain that all managers understand the process and involve HR in each step. Depending on the circumstances, employees may progress through one or more of these steps before termination. The CNO will want to be involved in final decisions regarding employment and disciplinary action to support nurse managers and to avert potential litigation or other negative outcomes.

When efforts to improve employee performance fail, or when significant occurrences warrant immediate termination, managers should consult with the CNO and with HR before finalizing a termination. In many circumstances, an investigation may be warranted before termination. Suspending an employee, pending investigation into an incident or complaint, is a recommended step before termination. On rare occasions an employee's overall performance or a single major violation of conduct may justify involuntary termination for cause.

HUMAN RESOURCES AND THE FINANCIAL ASPECTS OF THE NURSING DIVISION

CNOs must support the nursing division's administrative structure in their understanding of the specific issues that affect nurses. Particularly the nurse manager group must understand compensation packages, productivity, and benefits. An overview of classifications of hours appears in Box 16-4 and base pay systems appears in Table 16-2.

Compensation

Base pay is the rate or salary assigned to employees in the position for which they were hired. Base pay does not include any shift differentials or on-call or overtime pay. Guidelines for overtime pay to nonexempt employees are in accordance with the federal Fair Labor Standards Act and the current state law.

Nursing compensation historically has been an issue of debate and challenge. Nurses make life-and-death decisions. Traditionally, nurses have not been paid at the level they feel they deserve. Compensation has been blamed as a reason for high turnover. Recent trends are to place more emphasis on "total compensation" or "total rewards" as a philosophy for managing compensation. The total compensation model includes compensation, benefits, and the overall work-life experience.

Box 16-4   Classifications for Hours Worked

Regular full-time: A regular full-time employee is scheduled to work on a regularly scheduled basis, usually for 32 to 40 hours per week.

Regular part-time: A regular part-time employee is scheduled to work less than full time (e.g., scheduled to work 20 to 32 hours per week). Part-time employees working less than a certain number of hours per week are not generally eligible for health and welfare benefits.

Temporary: A temporary employee is an individual whose work assignment is expected to be of limited duration. Temporary employees are not eligible for health and other benefit programs. It is prudent to evaluate a position that is temporary every 90 to 180 days to determine the business necessity.

PRN, per diem, or supplemental: An employee who is classified as PRN, per diem, or supplemental is one whose employment is for no definite term and who works on an "as needed" basis. Work hours are not guaranteed; rather they are determined and scheduled according to business needs. These positions are not normally eligible for health and other benefit programs.

The concept of total compensation includes the following:

- Attract and retain talented employees
- Be competitive with the market in terms of overall wages and benefits
- Recognize employee education, skill, and experience through hiring and promotion guidelines
- Recognize and reward individual and organizational performance
- Provide increases or rewards based on merit

- Reflect market and business strategy
- Facilitate formal and on-the-spot recognition programs in the workplace
- Seek new ways to improve the work experience for employees

The total compensation model includes pay structures. Positions generally are assigned to grades, based on market data. A pay structure normally is designed with a minimum, midpoint, and maximum range for base pay, based on years of experience and market average. Nursing compensation is assessed continually to maintain the integrity of the compensation structure and to be competitive enough to recruit and retain nurses. The structure is adjusted in accordance with market changes. Healthcare organizations use multiple survey sources and conduct market surveys using geographic area and skill sets in addition to looking at the industry on a national basis. Certain jobs (e.g., nursing) are benchmarked using market data. Although nursing salaries have increased gradually over recent years, talk continues about special pay in addition to base pay or hourly wage.

Some examples of special pay plans would be additional pay for certification, for nursing specialties (e.g., OR, ICU, ED), or pay for academic degrees. Nurses tend to promote special pay; however, some argue that a medical/surgical nurse works just as hard as an ICU nurse and therefore should have equal compensation. For example, many CNOs tend to be reluctant to pay a premium for BSNs, in part because of the nursing shortage. Yet, many CNOs also declare a preference for hiring bachelor and higher degree prepared nurses.

Productivity

Productivity management is a concept that nurse leaders and HR professionals must embrace in the current world of healthcare management. Most productivity measures are based on either paid or productive hours. Productive hours are hours worked. Nonproductive hours include any hours paid but not worked. Nonproductive hours include sick time, vacation time, holidays, extended illness

Table 16-2 Comparison of Base Pay Systems

System	Advantages	Disadvantages
Flat-rate system	Best for routine, simple jobs that offer little opportunity to vary performance; simple to implement and administer; preferred by unions	Does not reflect individual performance or skills
Time-based system	Best for routine jobs in which competency level increases with time; provides opportunity to reward long-term employment	Does not reflect varying proficiency rates or performance differences; may raise average pay levels over time even if performance is below average
Performance-based pay	Best used when individual performance is valued and accurately measured; rewards superior performance	Requires good performance appraisal system; can be manipulated by supervisors; may discriminate against protected groups
Productivity-based pay	Best when quantity of work is accurately measured; encourages high level of productivity	Quality of work may be sacrificed without careful supervision
Competency- or skill-based pay	Best where skill/knowledge levels are well-defined and employee development is valued; encourages flexibility and training; supports work teams; emphasizes cooperation and teamwork	Administration and training may be costly; requires flexibility in making job assignments

Modified from http://www.shrm.org (member only access).

benefits, jury duty, or funeral leave. Educational hours generally are considered nonproductive as well. Total paid hours are the sum of productive hours and nonproductive hours (The Healthcare Company, 2001). Budgeting processes most often focus on paid hours. A paid full-time equivalent (FTE) is an employed or contracted group of people or an individual paid for doing a job. It is not a job or position. Paid FTEs typically are used in budgeting because they incorporate all hours that an employee must be paid for, whether productive or nonproductive. FTE calculations typically include contract labor in addition to employed and agency labor.

The CNO needs to have a broad perspective on overall hospital budgeted FTEs while relying on nurse managers to handle productivity on an operational basis. Nurse managers are responsible for the process of making the daily schedule and for adjustments to staffing. The CNO needs nurse leaders who can stay attuned to constantly changing staffing needs and who are adept at increasing or decreasing staffing in response to patient needs and acuity.

Productivity can be measured at the individual employee level, at the departmental level, and at the facility level. The CNO will be most concerned with the facility productivity and staffing. The CNO will want to work with nurse leaders on negative trends or overall productivity concerns and budget variances. Often a facility adopts a standard set of workload volume statistics so that the measurement of work output or productivity is objective and consistent. Sometimes workload measures are defined as units of service. Units of service may range from counting numbers of procedures, treatments, or patient days to more complex methods of evaluating a weighted count of procedures, treatments, or patient days. Monitoring the pure count of workload measures is less complex and is used as a basic measure to indicate volume of work produced by a department or business unit.

Some examples of unit of service measures would be the following:

DEPARTMENT OR SERVICE AREA:	UNIT OF SERVICE MEASURE:
Surgery or outpatient day surgery	Operating room minutes
Clinics	Number of procedures performed
Physical therapy	$1/4$-hour increments of therapy treatments
Nutrition services	Equivalent meals
Registration or admissions	Number of registrations

(The Healthcare Company, 2001)

Adjusted Patient Days

The term *adjusted* indicates that volume numbers are being adjusted to reflect overall workload of a facility. This may include multiplying inpatient volumes by an outpatient volume factor. Productivity is not always easily definable. In some cases, a department measure would be more useful if it included an adjustment for overall workload (The Healthcare Company, 2001).

Average daily census (ADC) is the measure of inpatient volume. It is calculated by dividing the total inpatient days for a given time period by the number of days in that time period. Average daily census in a hospital generally is calculated by counting the number of inpatients at midnight.

$$\text{ADC} = \frac{\text{Inpatient days (Total)}}{\text{Number of days in a period}}$$

Adjusted average daily census can be calculated once the average daily census is known. The adjusted average daily census gives an overall volume of work for a facility by multiplying the average daily census by an outpatient factor. Adjusted average daily census may be calculated by taking the outpatient factor and multiplying it by the average daily census. It takes into account additional components beyond inpatients (The Healthcare Company, 2001). Equivalent employees per occupied bed (EEOB) is a term used to calculate the number of paid or productive FTEs divided by the adjusted average daily census. This unit of measure is useful to the CNO and nurse managers in evaluation of efficiency and productivity as they relate to actual patients.

Manager Effectiveness

Manager effectiveness is one of the most important drivers of staff nurse retention. Higher turnover occurs among new nurses than among existing or more seasoned nurses. This might be logical because many new graduates "test" an employment site before making career decisions or they are gaining experience before returning to school for other education. A poor manager can also contribute to short-term employment. Turnover is related directly to support received as a new employee and to support from management. The best nurse leaders are those who exhibit a sense of knowledge and confidence balanced with humility. They serve as a role model and advocate for all nurses. The best leaders demonstrate a voice for nursing and are "nurses' nurses" (Strachota, Normandin, O'Brien, Clary, & Krukow, 2003). Effective strategies must be created continually to better train, reward, satisfy, motivate, and inspire employees. The CNO needs to model behaviors that in turn inspire and reward nurse managers. Providing support to managers during challenging and changing times is critical to retaining the most talented leaders.

To support managers, hospitals are developing and instituting a wide range of strategies. To respond to the reality that employees leave *managers*, organizations are providing more leadership training and development. Flexible scheduling and more weekend options are being used. Special positions such as an admission and discharge nurse to assist with patient turnover and "Give Me a Break" nurses (whose sole job is to relieve staff for breaks or educational sessions) are developing. HR can support each of these efforts.

Satisfaction Surveys

HR is often the department to conduct or facilitate employee surveys. Satisfied and engaged employees result in more satisfied patients and increased patient safety. Employees who are satisfied with their managers are likely to be more satisfied overall and to stay with the organization longer. Further, a supportive culture contributes to the development and enhancement of self-esteem, affiliation, achievement, and autonomy (Strachota et al., 2003). Because higher performing organizations have employees who respond more positively about their workplace, it is important to have ongoing data about nurse and other employee satisfaction collected.

Increasingly, organizations are turning to their HR and organizational development departments to assist with change efforts. Climate surveys and employee satisfaction surveys can be valuable tools to assess where the organization is and to look toward opportunities for improvement. Unfortunately, many hospitals do not conduct employee satisfaction surveys.

Employee satisfaction surveys can be invaluable in assessment of a variety of workplace issues. Some of these include turnover, productivity, manager effectiveness, overall job satisfaction, communication, and quality. When employees take the time to complete a satisfaction survey, they must receive some feedback and communication in regard to findings, and they must be included in an action plan to make improvements. Many reputable companies can be used for the purpose of conducting an employee satisfaction survey. Many organizations have a relationship with a particular employee satisfaction vendor or tool. Some advantage exists to following up with the same survey tool year after year in terms of trending results and assessing progress on action plans.

The purpose of a climate survey is to evaluate the general work environment in terms of teamwork, opinion of management, and potential challenges that an organization may encounter as it approaches future changes. Climate surveys generally are used to help leaders strategize for upcoming changes and reorganizations. They do not require development of an action plan that is communicated back to respondents. Climate surveys are used more often to benchmark an organization's progress toward a goal.

Benefits and Work-Life Enhancement

The cost of attrition is higher than providing people with benefits that will keep them working. A summary of benefits away from work is found in Box 16-5.

Work-life enhancement has become a priority in high-performing organizations. In healthcare especially, the challenge has been to create new and innovative approaches that help employees balance work life with home and community life. Companies outside of healthcare began to offer work/life programs in the 1980s and 1990s, often to support women and children. Current programs are not gender-specific and are much broader than providing childcare options. Employees want flexibility and control over their work and personal life (Lockwood, 2003).

In healthcare, nurses juggle their work obligations of caring for acutely ill patients with low staffing, high stress, and long hours along with managing personal responsibilities, financial considerations, families, and stress at home. The estimated cost for replacing a medical/surgical nurse is $42,000 and a specialty nurse is $64,000 (Strachota et al., 2003). The cost of lost productivity alone is nearly 80% of the total turnover cost. More and more emphasis is being placed on taking care and consideration for the "whole person" in the workplace to attract and retain the best talent.

Box 16-5   TIME AWAY FROM WORK BENEFITS DEFINITIONS

Type of Leave*	Mandated by Federal Law	Mandated by Some State Laws	Not Mandated
Vacation			X
Holidays			X
Sick leave			X
Family and medical leave	X	X	
Short-term disability leave		X*	X
Long-term disability leave			X
Military/reserve duty	X	X	
Jury duty	X	X	
Bereavement leave			X

Modified from http://www.shrm.org (member only access).
*Currently mandated by only six states.

Terms Used in Table:

Vacation: Leave for vacation time is granted by most employers and is considered a benefit that accrues as the employee works. Many states consider accrued vacation leave a benefit that is payable upon termination of employment.

Holidays: Individual company policy governs which holidays are taken by employees for private companies (they are mandated in the public sector). Most companies use the federal holidays as a guideline and offer many of the same holidays to their employees. Customary holidays include New Year's Day, Memorial Day, Independence Day, Labor Day, Thanksgiving, and Christmas.

Sick leave: The amount of paid sick leave an employee earns, if any, is governed by the policy of each employer. Many employers provide between 5 and 12 days per year as a standard, often allowing employees to accrue more as length of service increases. Most companies do not allow carryover of unused sick leave from year to year beyond a reasonable amount.

Family and medical leave: Family and medical leave is governed by federal law. The basics: Employers with 50 or more employees must grant up to 12 weeks of unpaid family and medical leave to their employees for the serious illness of the employee or immediate family members, or the birth or adoption of a child; healthcare benefits must be continued during family and medical leave, and the employee must be reinstated to his or her former position or an equivalent position at the end of the leave. Employees are eligible for family and medical leave if they have worked for the employer for the past year, have worked 1250 hours or more in that year, and are at a work site where there are at least 50 employees within a 75-mile radius. Leave may be taken in increments as short as what the employer's payroll system will allow (e.g., 8 minutes), or as long as 12 weeks.

Short-term disability leave: Many employers provide full or partial income replacement to employees who are unable to work because of illnesses or injuries whose duration exceeds that of regular sick leave benefits. It is common for employers to provide 50% or more in income replacement for periods of up to 26 weeks after a short waiting period (usually 1 to 2 weeks). Some employers include provisions for benefit continuation and job security in their policies, and most employers self-fund their plans,

Box 16-5   Time Away from Work Benefits Definitions—cont'd

rather than insure them. Additionally, six states mandate temporary disability benefits: California, Hawaii, New Jersey, New York, Puerto Rico, and Rhode Island.

Long-term disability leave: Long-term disability benefits are most commonly provided through insured plans and are designed to pick up where short-term disability benefits end. Employees who receive long-term disability benefits are generally not expected to be able to return to work in the foreseeable future. Benefits usually range from 50% to 70% of the employee's salary (including any Social Security benefits, if applicable) and are customarily payable after a waiting period of 3 to 6 months.

Military/reserve duty: Employers must grant leave to employees who are drafted or voluntarily enlist in the U.S. Armed Forces, or who volunteer for the National Guard and Military Reserves. Employees returning from those duties are entitled to full reinstatement to their former jobs after discharge from the military, or to positions of like seniority, status, and pay. Reservists must be granted time off for fulfillment of their duties, plus travel time, in addition to any vacation leave they may have accrued. Federal law does not mandate that reservists be paid by their employer for their time away from work but does specify requirements for vesting in pension plans. In practice, many companies pay full wages or the difference between their employees' reserve wages and regular pay for short periods such as the annual 2-week training that reservists must perform.

Jury duty: Employers are required to grant leave to employees who are called to serve on juries in federal and state courts. Several states have also passed laws requiring employers to grant leave when an employee is subpoenaed to testify as a witness. Discharge, discrimination, and retaliation against employees called to jury duty are strictly prohibited. Some state laws govern payment of wages to employees on jury duty leave, but most leave this policy decision to the employer. Many employers continue to provide full pay to employees on jury duty (partially offset by remuneration paid by the court).

Bereavement leave: Although not mandated by state or federal law, it is common practice to grant leave to employees who experience a death in their immediate family. Most policies specify and define immediate family, and most offer paid leave for several days.

In healthcare, and within nursing in particular, attention is increasingly being paid to "soft benefits"—benefits beyond the traditional medical, dental, and vacation time offered to employees. Soft benefits include things that go beyond meeting basic needs and expectations. They include such things as on-site dry cleaning drop off and delivery services, grocery shopping, on-campus childcare services, options for sick child care, elderly care, adoption benefits, concierge services, on-site oil changes and tire rotations, grocery shopping, and much more. Several dozen hospitals in the United States have instituted a paid concierge service for employees. The concierge plans vacations, makes travel arrangements, provides pet care, delivers food to the units, takes cars in for service, and runs errands for staff during the day or for night staff while they sleep.

Currently, no research quantifies the value of soft benefits or the return on investment; however, feedback from employees is tremendously positive in those organizations that offer the services. Some organizations have started a "meals to go" service through their nutrition department for staff who are working late or are too busy to prepare a well-balanced meal after working a 12-hour shift. Nurses who work can enjoy the benefits of having other business taken care of through the employer so that they can relax or spend time with family when they are not at work.

Additional ideas to consider for promoting work-life enhancement include the following:

- Family-friendly benefits such as wellness plans, discounted events and vacation packages, domestic partner benefits, tutoring, partner support, scholarships for children of employees
- Employee assistance programs and financial assistance or peer assistance
- Total life planning: encouraging employees to look at their lives as a whole and assess relationships, emotional and physical well-being, careers, spirituality, and their personal financial situation
- Critical incident and daily operations stress debriefing programs

Types of Alternative Work Schedules

Although the nurse leadership team establishes work schedules, HR is frequently involved to fit innovative ideas within labor requirements and benefit plans. Flextime permits employees to work the same number of hours as is customary each day, but they arrive and depart either earlier or later than usual. Most policies specify core hours (i.e., 10 AM to 3 PM) when all employees must be at work. This schedule is best for employees who have commuting, childcare, or educational issues that can be better managed by a regular adjustment to their schedule. A compressed work week allows employees to work the same number of hours in a week, but they compress the hours over fewer days (e.g., four 10-hour days). This works best for employees who want to maximize their work and their personal time. Job sharing is when two employees share the responsibilities and benefits of one full-time job. One employee may work mornings and the other afternoons. The two

employees communicate through notes or as they cross paths during the day. This schedule is best for employees who want to work part-time but need some benefits and are willing to partner with another employee with similar needs to share one job. Telecommuting capitalizes on employees' skills that can be used from home. Telecommuters receive the same compensation and benefits and should be communicated with on a regular basis regarding work assignments and performance. This arrangement is best for jobs that require little face-to-face contact, which can be performed individually and without daily access to office resources (Society for Human Resource Management, 2004).

REGULATORY COMPLIANCE AND LEGAL ASPECTS

Regulatory compliance related to nursing and human resources varies, depending on the venue where nurse leaders work. Hospitals are required to meet certain conditions of participation to comply with federal, state, and local laws. All hospitals must be in compliance with all applicable federal labor laws, which are summarized in Box 16-6. The state health department oversees a number of regulatory compliance issues, specific to the state. The state health department regulates building plans, licensure, quality management, access to patient medical records, patient grievance procedures, facility obligations to the patient, single-use disposable medical devices, patient rights, occurrence reporting, and involuntary restraint. Periodic on-site surveys are conducted to ensure compliance.

The JCAHO is the primary regulatory agency for purposes of hospital accreditation. The mission of the JCAHO is to improve the safety and quality of care provided to the public through the provision of accreditation and related services the support performance improvement in healthcare organizations (Joint Commission on Accreditation of Healthcare Organizations, 2004). The 2004 Hospital Accreditation Standards (HAS) were designed to facilitate a hospital's continuous

Box 16-6 Federal Labor Laws by Number of Employees

FOR 1 TO 14 EMPLOYEES:

- Civil Rights Act of 1964, Title VII, and Civil Rights Act of 1991, (for employment agencies and labor organizations). (See the list for 15 to 19 employees for other employers.)
- Consumer Credit Protection Act of 1968
- Employee Polygraph Protection Act of 1988
- Employee Retirement Income Security Act of 1974 (ERISA) (if company offers benefits)
- Equal Pay Act of 1963
- Fair Credit Reporting Act of 1970
- Fair Labor Standards Act of 1938 (FLSA)
- Federal Insurance Contributions Act of 1935 (FICA) (Social Security)
- Health Insurance Portability and Accountability Act of 1996 (HIPAA) (if company offers benefits)
- Immigration Reform and Control Act of 1986 (IRCA)
- Labor-Management Relations Act of 1947 (Taft-Hartley Act)
- National Labor Relations Act of 1935 (NLRA)
- Uniform Guidelines on Employee Selection Procedures (1978)
- Uniformed Services Employment and Reemployment Rights Act of 1994

FOR 11 TO 14 EMPLOYEES, ADD THE FOLLOWING:

- Occupational Safety and Health Act of 1970 (maintain record of job-related injuries and illnesses)

FOR 15 TO 19 EMPLOYEES, ADD THE FOLLOWING:

- Civil Rights Act of 1964, Title VII, and Civil Rights Act of 1991

- Americans with Disabilities Act of 1990 (ADA), Title I

FOR 20 TO 49 EMPLOYEES, ADD THE FOLLOWING:

- Age Discrimination in Employment Act of 1967 (ADEA)
- Consolidated Omnibus Budget Reconciliation Act of 1985 (COBRA)

FOR 50 OR MORE EMPLOYEES, ADD THE FOLLOWING:

- Family and Medical Leave Act of 1993 (FMLA)
- EEO-1 Report filed annually with the Equal Employment Opportunity Commission (EEOC) if organization is a federal contractor

FOR 100 OR MORE EMPLOYEES, ADD THE FOLLOWING:

- Worker Adjustment and Retraining Notification Act of 1988 (WARN)
- EEO-1 Report filed annually with the EEOC if organization is not a federal contractor

FOR FEDERAL CONTRACTORS, ADD THE FOLLOWING:

- Executive Orders 11246 (1965), 11375 (1967), and 11478 (1969)
- Vocational Rehabilitation Act of 1973
- Drug-Free Workplace Act of 1988
- Vietnam Era Veterans' Readjustment Assistance Act of 1974
- Davis-Bacon Act of 1931
- Copeland Act of 1934
- Walsh-Healy Act of 1936
- Service Contract Act of 1965

operational improvement in addition to the self-assessment of its performance against the standards. Beginning in January 2004, the JCAHO began implementing a new initiative to focus the survey on the actual delivery of care, treatment, and services. A shift was made to focus the survey on operational improvement as opposed to survey preparation. The primary standards that apply to nursing and HR are the following:

- Assessment of patients
- Care of patients
- Education and competencies
- Medication management
- Improving organizational performance
- Leadership
- Management of human resources
- Nursing

Nursing and HR standards require collaboration to provide the adequate number of staff members to meet the needs of patient populations served. The staff must be competent and have the appropriate experience, education, and abilities required to perform their roles. HR must ensure adequate orientation, training, and ongoing education.

OSHA

HR is the department for ensuring compliance with Occupational Safety and Health Administration (OSHA) standards. The Department of Labor oversees the Occupational Safety and Health Act of 1970 (29 USC 657) to ensure compliance with safety regulations in the work environment. Specific requirements exist for building safety, emergency action plans, fire prevention, equipment, ventilation, noise exposure, radiation exposure, flammables and combustibles, hazardous materials, and other toxic substances. Employers must maintain records of all work-related injuries and illnesses on an OSHA log (Form 300). Documentation of any care given to employees as a result of a workplace injury or illness and records must be provided to appropriate government representatives (http://www.osha.gov).

Safe Medical Practices

HR may be accountable for or coordinate the requirements about safe medical practices. The Federal Food, Drug, and Cosmetic Act (21 USC 321h) defines certain criteria for compliance in identification of medical device–related incidents as soon as possible after an occurrence to ensure corrective action and to prevent or minimize the occurrence of similar incidents. Facility-specific records and written reports must be maintained to comply with federal law, Food and Drug Administration regulations, and the Department of Health, in addition to JCAHO. The Needlestick Safety and Prevention Act (HR 5178) was signed into law in November 2000. This act requires that healthcare facilities use "safe medical devices" that have built-in safety features to prevent blood exposures caused by needlesticks (Nelson & Spitzer, 2003).

Major Legal Considerations in Employment

HR is accountable for compliance with employment laws. The goal of employment law and legislation is to provide fair employment opportunities to all citizens and to prevent the hiring of illegal aliens. Federal, state, and municipal laws dealing with employment discrimination have been in effect since the 1940s. The Civil Rights Act was passed in 1964 and prohibits discrimination based on race, color, religion, sex, or national origin in all employment practices. This includes hiring, firing, internal transfers, promotion, compensation, and other terms or conditions of employment.

The EEOC was created to administer Title VII and to ensure equal treatment for all in the workplace. In 1967 presidential executive orders mandated equal employment standards for federal contractors. In the same year, Congress passed the Age Discrimination in Employment Act (ADEA), prohibiting employment discrimination against individuals age 40 and over. In 1973 the

Rehabilitation Act was passed, providing equal protection for individuals with disabilities (Development Dimensions International, 2003.)

In July 1990 Congress passed the Americans with Disabilities Act (ADA). In 1991 Congress passed the Civil Rights Act of 1991 that strengthened previous federal civil rights legislation (Development Dimensions International, 2003).

Section 504 and ADA

The American with Disabilities Act of 1990 prohibits discrimination on the basis of disability in the delivery of healthcare services and in employment (Development Dimensions International, 2003). The regulation requires that sensory-impaired persons, including the blind and hearing impaired, be provided with auxiliary aids at no cost to allow them an equal opportunity to participate in and benefit from healthcare services. Failure to properly assess and subsequently provide adequate accommodations or services is punishable by fine to the provider or employer.

Classifications of Personnel

Most employers are covered by the Fair Labor Standards Act (FLSA). It covers public agencies and businesses engaged in interstate commerce or providing goods and services for commerce. The FLSA provides guidelines on employment status, child labor, minimum wage, overtime pay, and record-keeping requirements. It determines which employees are exempt from the Act (not covered by it) and which are nonexempt (covered). It establishes wage and time requirements when minors can work. It sets the minimum wage that must be paid and mandates when overtime must be paid.

Additional information, as well as the full text of the regulations, is available on the Department of Labor's FairPay web site at http://www.dol.gov/fairpay.

SUMMARY

Executives and managers throughout the organization are accountable for the effective use of all resources available to them. Therefore effective management of human resources is an integral component to any executive's role, whether as the CNO or nurse director/manager. Perhaps even more importantly, cooperation and collaboration with the people that specialize in HR and the other leaders are critical to organizational success. Economic and technologic change, workforce availability and quality concerns, and demographic and diversity issues have become prevalent challenges in the healthcare industry (Mathis & Jackson, 2000). HR must be built to maximize the capabilities of all the diverse human resources. HR must ensure the talents of all the people inside the organization are used and attract the best of the diverse external population. More effective management of the human resource is seen increasingly as positively affecting organizational performance. CNOs and the HR officer who work as partners contribute to organizational success through the development of strategies that ensure that HR dimensions are considered.

KEY POINTS TO LEAD

1. Evaluate personnel practices that require HR involvement.
2. Ponder the complexities of personnel issues.
3. Value the need for nursing and HR to work together.

Literature Box

Dynamic change in the healthcare environment has created a demand from healthcare organizations, health management professional associations, and educational institutions to identify what it means to be a fully competent healthcare executive. The article describes five sets of entry-level behavioral competencies required to address clusters of critical issues facing healthcare. This study uses a sample of the American College of Healthcare Executives (ACHE) affiliates from different geographic regions and health industry segments to construct the framework of competencies and healthcare issue clusters.

The article identifies competencies or SKAs (skills, knowledge, and abilities) required for early-career executives to manage effectively within the framework of key issues in the healthcare environment. The study combines qualitative and quantitative data sources and uses a set of quantitative analytic procedures to develop a comprehensive array of critical issues in the healthcare environment and specific competencies for addressing them.

COMPETENCIES TO ADDRESS HEALTHCARE ISSUE GROUPS

Five clusters of perceived critical healthcare issues are used as a framework to guide healthcare executives in identification of the specific behavioral competencies, or SKAs, required by those entering the field. Specific behavioral competencies are designated for each competency area. They are (1) healthcare operations management; (2) patient or consumer focus; (3) political, legal, and ethical concerns; (4) financial and economic issues; and (5) medical and physician relationships. Each of those areas, or clusters, as they are called, has specific competencies. The competencies or SKAs were generated and prioritized by a panel of ACHE affiliates.

The identified items were generated in response to each cluster of critical healthcare issues in the framework.

Competencies associated with healthcare operations management include communications (the key item), team building, credibility, listening skills, analytic skills, and the ability to adjust to constant change.

Competencies associated with patient or consumer focus include understanding the healthcare continuum (the most important item in this cluster), public or community knowledge, regulatory knowledge, knowledge of community healthcare needs, and political savvy.

The third cluster of competencies relates to political, legal, and ethical concerns. They include management ethics training (the most important item in this cluster), knowledge of demographics, doing what is right for the patient, knowledge of patient rights, cultural competency, organizational structure and philosophy, and general legal skills.

The fourth cluster relates to financial and economic issues. These include competencies related to knowledge of healthcare public policy (viewed as the most important element in this cluster), stewardship, analytic and data management skills, quality drivers, and negotiation skills.

The final cluster, medical and physician relationships, has seven defined competencies. These competencies include understanding the legal and malpractice process, conflict-management skills, problem-solving skills, research/organizational/bioethics (the ethics trinity), knowledge of error and risk reduction strategies and techniques, consensus building, and knowledge of the physician education process.

The most highly rated item overall is communication skills. This is no surprise to any employee

Literature Box—cont'd

in healthcare because it is so critical to patient safety. Public policy and management ethics are also viewed as important, as are legal and malpractice process and the healthcare continuum.

Each of these areas is likely to be viewed as important due to the influence each has on healthcare and how it is delivered.

The article augments the developing body of knowledge of required competencies for health care executive. Entry-level healthcare executives may benefit from reviewing the competencies, assessing their abilities related to each, and creating and implementing a plan to develop these competences

Garmen, A. L., Tyler, L., & Darnell, J. S. (2004, September/October). Development and validity of 360-degree feedback instruments for healthcare administrators. *Journal of Healthcare Management, 49*(5), 307-322.

Contemplations

- How many people are needed for organizations to meet their objectives?
- Which knowledge, skills, and abilities do staff members and new hires need?
- Can new positions be filled from within the organization, or would the company benefit by bringing in new workers?
- What training is required?

- What is the best compensation strategy?
- How does the organization's overall direction affect employees' career plans?
- What will you do as the nurse leader to contribute to the building blocks of performance? Are you prepared to create a workplace where people have the ability, motivation, and opportunity to succeed?

We have a very active and productive HR department at our institution. I work extremely well with the VP for HR. In addition, there is a specific HR consultant assigned to the nursing division. This person is well versed in nursing issues and is our primary resource person. Whenever there are difficult personnel issues in nursing management, there is a specific person who assists the managers. The manager works with the HR person to develop a plan regarding how they will proceed.

Considerable time and effort are being exerted toward leadership development, and several organizational development people in HR work with training and education both in leadership development and in succession planning. Senior leadership establishes retreats and identifies both the strengths and areas for growth of all members of the team. 360s are done on all managers under the supervisor of the patient care services clinical directors, who establish action plans for each person. There is a discussion of any positions that will turn over and the "stars" and possible replacements for each of these positions. Several staff members are being developed for manager roles, and several managers are being developed for director roles. The university has 3000 employees, including 1453 in nursing, pharmacy, rehabilitation, and cardiology. The HR department has 35 people, including the education group.

I highly recommend that CNOs actively work at creating a relationship with the VP for HR. I served on the interview team when this VP was hired. We look at strategic goals as the senior executive team. This includes serious, meaningful discussions about recruitment and retention because HR is so important to the clinical divisions.

The right complement of people is essential, as is sustaining the workforce. We work closely together, and offices are in close proximity, and we talk frequently. By working together, leaders can outline strengths; develop a report card for employee satisfaction, turnover, etc.; and learn a great deal from exit interviews. This information can be related to overall staff and physician satisfaction. Quality scores for the organization as a whole are important and can then be related to the employees and the overall growth of services by HR. In addition, we have long-term employees who serve as coaches and advisors to preserve the quality of patient care.

I worked closely with HR to support the initiation of an Associate Degree nursing program. We actually fund some of the faculty positions. We support LPNs going back to school. We actively support new graduates with additional orientation, training, and precepting. We also support these new graduates in pursuing their BSN with tuition reimbursement. We do provide differential pay to staff who have completed their BSN.

In addition, we are building a new facility, which adds 100 beds. HR has helped in building teams for the new area. We've done many team-building activities, including Ropes Courses. This has been a major effort to build teams and establish a clear vision of where we are going in the new facility.

I have worked on many special projects with HR. They have been very supportive of our shared governance model and have helped with the resource councils. The HR representatives keep asking the councils, "What would work better?" They have helped with solving employee issues such as by creating "Instant Pay" when a staff member works an extra shift; they are paid the next morning. There are also "high volume" dollars that were created so that staff wouldn't feel a need to go someplace else and work additional shifts. HR created a hotline for staff to call with recommendations or questions. This is one way to stay current on issues that arise within the staff and to identify them early. Leadership works closely with HR to stay on top of these suggestions. For example, when the organization does well financially, the entire staff receives a bonus. We gave $200 to every employee last December for the exceptional year we had financially. There was great celebration. At the same time, if the year is not good, the focus is then on action plans for staff and areas in which problem solving is operationalized for whatever issues are identified as not working well.

We have a Spirit of Caring program, in which employees go off site for 2 days and also have follow-up classes. They are encouraged to look one more time at why they are in healthcare. These 2 days provide an opportunity to refocus on what is important and why. They review the importance of communicating with patients. They role-play being an elderly patient: being cold, thirsty, and alone with the sense that no one cares. They have learned that even 2 to 3 minutes of time with a patient can make such a difference.

If graduate students came to me to ask for advice, I would encourage them to volunteer for activities and classes associated with succession planning. I would encourage involvement in the many succession-planning projects.

We've had many special projects. University Hospital was an original Magnet Hospital in 1983. The Magnet characteristics have been in place here for quite some time. This has supported the maintenance of a satisfying environment for staff. We have had the Shared Governance Model with identified councils. The council has looked at both resources and benefit practices. We have a fairly low turnover rate. We have also looked at the issue of wellness. The VP for HR and I were involved in asking the questions about supporting higher

levels of wellness in the community and in an organizational healthy environment. We have several nurse practitioner clinics, for example, one focused on congestive heart failure that looked at creating healthier life styles.

HR did an analysis of what was increasing health premiums. It was the employees with chronic conditions that were increasing the costs. If the hospital goal is to increase health in the community, it would be good to start with our organization. The senior administrative team put everything on the line. All employees do a health risk profile. As a result of the profile assessment, they can choose to lower the co-pay on the healthcare benefit by committing to improve on one wellness factor from the profile each year. HR worked on all of the reward programs and put together all the programs including smoking cessation, weight management, diabetes wellness, and the employee assistance program (EAP).

The employees receive wellness dollars for enrolling in the program and for reaching their goals. They can participate in smoking cessation with wellness coaches to help them. If they are overweight, they can volunteer for a weight reduction program, and if they achieve a 5% improvement toward their optimal weight, they maintain their 10% co-pay. If they are not successful, they go to 30% co-pay. There are many programs to support employees such as stair steppers, yoga classes, etc. The cafeteria is set up with the South Beach diet. There is a walk at lunch program with distances marked off around the campus. The thinking is that it is unfair to the total population of employees if a few who are not healthy increase the premiums for the remainder of the employees. The VP for HR is responsible for the development of the Sporting Club.

An example of working closely with HR occurred when two trains crashed into each other and there was a serious chlorine gas spill just outside of Graniteville, across the state line in South Carolina. I was called at 2 AM and told about the disaster, and there were already 10 firefighters down. Within 30 minutes, there were 20 victims and they were still on the outside of the spill area. The hospital in Aiken, Georgia, was shut down because of the emergency and needed to evacuate patients. All my staff are licensed in Georgia. HR rose to the occasion and got temporary licenses in South Carolina so that our staff could help transfer all the patients. Our VP for HR, just as he has risen to the occasion so many times, facilitated the problem solving for licensees. This relationship is so important to me and to nursing.

Chapter References

American Organization of Nurse Executives. (2005). AONE Nurse Executive Competencies. *Nurse Leader, 3*(2), 15-21.

Becker, B. E., Huselid, M. A., & Ulrich, D. (2001). *The HR scorecard: linking people, strategy, and performance.* Boston, MA: Harvard Business School Press.

Bohlander, G., Snell, S., & Sherman, A. (2001). *Managing human resources.* Australia: South-Western College Publishing.

Development Dimensions International, Inc. (2003). *Legal considerations in selection; U.S. version.* Bridgeville, PA: Author.

Dyer, L. (1983). Bringing human resources into the strategy formulation process. *Human Resource Management, 22*(3), 263.

Greer, C. R. (1995). *Strategy and human resources: a general managerial perspective.* Englewood Cliffs, NJ: Prentice Hall.

HCA The Healthcare Company. (2001). *Plus—a productivity management tool: The basic language of productivity.* Nashville, TN: HCA.

Joint Commission on Accreditation of Healthcare Organizations. (2004). *Hospital accreditation standards.* Chicago: The commission.

Lockwood, N. R. (2003). Work life balance: Challenges and solutions. *HR Magazine, 48*(6), S1.

Mathis, R. L., & Jackson, J. H. (2000). *Human resource management* (9th ed.). Australia: South-Western College Publishing.

Meisinger, S. (2004). Thank God it's Monday. *HRMagazine, 49*(7), 10.

Nelson, B., & Spitzer, D. (2003). *The 1001 rewards & recognition fieldbook.* New York: Workman Publishing.

Society for Human Resource Management. (2004). *HR functions.* Retrieved July 17, 2004, from http://www.shrm.org.

Society for Human Resource Management. (2005). *Personality tests: More than meets the eye.* Retrieved September 17, 2005, from http://www.shrm.org.

Strachota, E., Normandin, P., O'Brien, N., Clary, M., & Krukow, B. (2003, February). *Journal of Nursing Administration,* 111-117.

Ulrich, D., Losey, M., & Lake, G. (1997). *Tomorrow's HR Management: 48 thought leaders call for change.* (Eds). NY: John Wiley & Sons.

U.S. Department of Labor. *OSHA Regulations (Standards 29CFR): Workplace safety and health.* Retrieved March 2005, from http://www.osha.gov and http://www.dol.gov.

17 Governing and Being Governed

One person seeking glory doesn't accomplish much. Success is the result of people pulling together to meet common goals. John C. Maxwell

W hether the chief nursing officer (CNO) is in the administrative role and being governed by an organizational board or is a member of the organizational board (or another one) and governing others, key concepts apply to being effective. This chapter describes these key concepts.

GOVERNING AND BEING GOVERNED

For many years, CNOs were highly accountable regarding patient care and had great internal organizational dialogues. They did not, however, have dialogues with the board that governed the organization. The board heard the fiscal components of healthcare in detail, but they did not hear about the quality or effectiveness of healthcare in detail. However, now boards increasingly expect to hear about the effectiveness component as well. This interest has created new opportunities for CNOs to be involved directly with the board and, in some instances, to serve on the board as a corporate representative.

What Governing Means

A board comprises a group of individuals with the authority to create policies and plans to achieve a mission and to hold the staff accountable for the implementation of the resultant work. The ultimate authority of any healthcare organization is its board. Not all decisions require board action, but when the board acts, it is the final authority.

All boards are controlled by a set of ethics about board governance and obligations to be accountable. Boards also are controlled by various laws and regulations that apply to the nature of the business they govern. The real value of a board derives from the questions the board poses (Chait, 2004). These questions can maintain a board at its current level of functioning or take the board to new levels. If the board asks the right questions, the board leads the organization to renewal, new goals, or really meaningful advancement of the mission. For example, asking what matters and how to reexamine problems and opportunities (Chait, 2004) are probably more dynamic questions than where the organization is with meeting budget or what progress has been made on the building endeavors.

Ryan (2004) suggests that boards govern in three modes: fiduciary, strategic, and generative. Fiduciary, discussed later, is the board's stewardship role. The strategic mode is what is thought of as strategic planning. Most boards exercise both of these activities and accountabilities on a regular basis. What often is missing is the third element, the generative mode. This element is the one in which the board frames and reframes problems and makes sense of the whole. It is also the element that takes boards to new levels of leading the organization.

CNOs may be included as a regular executive staff attendee, or the CNO may become a member of the board (Matisoff-Li, 2004). The CNO obviously needs to value the concept of governance and how it influences the ongoing operation of the organization.

Policies

One of the key governance strategies is policy development. Policies typically are developed to prevent or intervene in a problem or issue. Public policy involves some level of governmental decision; health policy may not necessarily involve any governmental agency, but its focus is on some aspect of health. Policies work best when they are based on some form of evidence. According to Rutledge and Grant (2002), three sources of such evidence exist. The first, and most reliable, sources are research-based evidence policies. These result from organizational, or broader, research that provides direction for a policy. The research must be constructed in well-designed approaches and often involves complex statistical analyses. The second are theoretic evidence policies. These are based on theories and constructs that have not necessarily been tested. However, they reflect sound thinking. The third are nonresearch evidence policies. This type of policy involves case studies, legal opinions, cost analyses, and standards of care.

The board is accountable for developing/approving policies and for evaluating their implementation. Staff of an organization may suggest policy and even develop it. They may provide the evidence about policy effectiveness, but the board is accountable for the overall policy direction and has the final authority in matters of dispute.

Plans to Achieve the Mission

The other major strategy that boards use to accomplish their work is the creation of plans and strategies to achieve the mission of the organization. Often staff members make suggestions for the board's consideration. In such cases, the board often needs to weigh one option against another. Because the board's commitment is to the long term, the level of the plans is broad; the staff members create the details once the board sets the direction. Once again, the mission is critical to the development of this work. Thus the work associated with considering the mission and its relevance for the future must precede any work about the plans.

Boundaries

The separation of roles is an important factor to consider so that neither the board nor the staff is trying to do the other group's job. Hirschhorn and Gilmore (1992) provide a way of thinking about the boundaries that matter. They suggest four boundaries to consider. First is the authority boundary. The key question to consider is, "Who is in charge of what?" (p. 7). Answering this question often prevents a blurring of roles of the board and the staff. Second is task boundary. It is designed to answer the question, "Who does what?" (p. 7). The answers to this question help to promote clarity about how the work will actually get done. The third boundary is one of politics. The political boundary is focused on, "What is in it for me?" (WIFM). For a board or a staff to take risk, some benefits must be evident. Answering this boundary helps to see those benefits and alert board members when a conflict of interest might occur. The final boundary is that of identity, and it is designed to answer the question, "Who is and isn't us?" (p. 7). The answers to this question help build pride in the teamwork that must occur between board and staff and create clarity about what the enterprise's work comprises.

Duties of Care, Loyalty, and Obedience

All board members have the duties of care, loyalty, and obedience (Figure 17-1). Although elaborate definitions exist of each of these elements, an individual must be committed to an organization, have only declared conflicts of interest, make decisions based on what is best for the organization, and abide by laws and regulations associated with the organization.

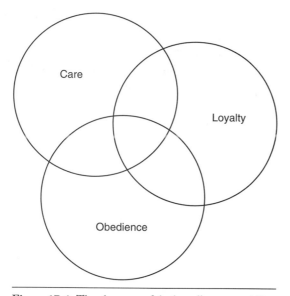

Figure 17-1 The elements of the board's accountability.

Care means that board members commit to being informed and to participating in decisions. In other words, if serving on a board sounds like a good "resumé builder," it is not. Key work is involved. Care also requires that people act in good faith. That means that board members should ask what a prudent person would do in such a situation and then act accordingly.

Loyalty involves such aspects as keeping confidential those decisions and discussions that should be kept confidential. It also involves speaking in positive ways in the larger community. It is based always on the premise of acting in the interest of the organizations and disclosing conflicts of interest. Few, if any, board members are without some form of conflict of interest. For example, a board member may own stock in a business that provides (or could provide) services to the organization. In another example, a board member could determine that if a particular decision were made, it might affect another organization with which the board member is associated. In such cases, the board member could ask to be recused from the discussion, the decision, or both, or, at a minimum, declare a conflict of interest so that others are aware of the conditions that exist as a topic is discussed. For the CNO serving on the board, this same kind of conflict might exist if the CNO is especially concerned with the nursing service in preference over other units within the organization. This is what Banaji, Bazerman, and Chugh (2003) suggest is in-group favoritism. It happens almost unconsciously and is a bias that favors "your" group.

Obedience requires that board members not only know about the laws, regulations, and standards affecting the organization but also act in accordance with them. On a higher level, it means always protecting the mission of the organization. As an example, the Joint Commission on Accreditation of Healthcare Organizations (JCAHO) considered the complexity of information board members needed to track as they reduced the number of standards and criteria with which the board needed to be concerned. JCAHO expects that communication and collaboration is a two-way process so that the board is well informed about performance reports (Thompson, 2004). This example illustrates that boards need to be apprised and that appraisal needs to be clear and concise.

Fiduciary Responsibilities

Boards also have fiduciary responsibilities. This means that the board must act prudently and in accordance with the stated mission. Thus the non-financial documents take on new importance because they form the yardstick against which the financial decisions are measured. The budget is simply the financial tool to achieve the organizational goals. The board typically does not know the details of a given budget, but they should know the general costs of a service, what it provides for that cost, and what the anticipated outcomes are.

There are no problems we cannot solve together,
and very few that we can solve by ourselves.
LYNDON B. JOHNSON

Clarity of Board and Administrative Staff Roles

Effective governance of any organization occurs through the collaborative work of board members and the administrative staff. Each has a distinct role in meeting the overall work of the organization and those distinct roles need to be complementary. When administrative staff members are members of the board, they have a dual accountability, one to the ultimate governance of the organization and the other to the ongoing implementation of policy to ensure that the intent of the governing body is accomplished.

Board Roles

Boards are accountable for setting the strategic direction of the organization. They must align goals and objectives with the vision and mission of the organization. Thus they are also accountable for monitoring the implementation and for evaluating the results. Boards determine direction through such activities as trends analyses and strategic planning and approving implementation plans and the budget. They set policy for the organization. They conduct oversight through the duty of care, loyalty, and obedience (see previous discussion), and they evaluate the results (receive reports). In addition, boards are accountable for selecting and evaluating the CEO. This involves supporting the CEO in performing the duties and expectations of that role or providing feedback so such expectations can be met.

How the board sets integrity as an expectation is critical to the filtration throughout the organization. Creating a climate of honesty, trustworthiness, and truthfulness must be as evident in the boardroom as in the patient room. The board always should be "thinking ahead" so that effective organizational planning is always timely. The board is accountable for bringing insight from various perspectives to the table as strategic planning occurs.

Boards of nonprofit organizations have several areas of accountability that require distinctive input of the administrative staff. Perhaps the most critical element is determining the mission and purpose of the organization. The board by specific action can redirect an organization totally and what it is designed to do by redefining the mission and purpose of an organization. Moving from an organization that provides care to all populations to addressing only an age group or diagnosis is an example of how a board might redirect its work and that of the organization. Although the administrative staff must convey information about the organization's effectiveness of mission, the board has the right and authority to alter the direction.

Kocourek, Burger, and Birchard (2003) proposed seven principles for what the authors call soft governance, or the ability to work together and with management (Box 17-1). Each principle requires time. Together, however, the principles create a high-functioning, competent board. Whether the chair of the board assumes these duties or designates one or more board members to achieve this work, each element is critical. Even with the right people in place, keeping them well versed in the best and latest business practices and clinical issues is important. The CNO can play a critical role in this ongoing development. Especially as the public becomes more concerned with honesty, trustworthiness, and transparency in their healthcare organization, knowing what is happening clinically and the major changes that are designed to produce better outcomes are the

---

Box 17-1   Governing Well

Select the right people
Train, train, train
Inform and communicate
Balance the CEO's power
Establish new behaviors
Devote the time
Evaluate and improve

Based on work by Kocourek, P. F., Burger, C., & Birchard, B. (2003, Spring). Corporate governance: Hard facts about soft behaviors. *Strategy+Business, 30*, 1-12.

sorts of information that board members must understand. The Literature box relates to how governance is linked to clinical outcomes. If the board uses these strategies, the CNO also must be prepared for the potential that an open agenda would allow for unplanned topics. Thus having overall knowledge of the organization and specific knowledge about nursing will be important.

To implement their roles, board members need to know 12 things, according to Kocourek et al. (2003). Table 17-1 identifies the 12 areas. This information forms the basis for the enrichment of

Table 17-1 WHAT BOARD MEMBERS NEED TO KNOW AND QUESTIONS TO CONSIDER*

Need to Know	Questions to Consider
Strategic direction	Where are we headed? Is it what is needed for the future?
Resource allocation	Are all of the resources in place (personnel, plant, financial) to achieve the desired goals? Are the resources appropriated to meet the needs?
Management organization	How does the executive level work together? What happens if the CEO leaves?
Financial accountability	Are the systems and controls sufficient to provide some degree of comfort in dealing with a complex organization? What do the auditors say?
Operational controls	Are we benchmarking? How do we rate?
Constituency protection	Are we functioning as needed based on laws, regulations, and standards? Are we doing the best for patients and their families? Are we aware of employee needs?
Litigation and disputation	What are the big legal issues? What actions are being disputed? Are we changing practices to be responsive and proactive?
Crises and contingencies	What risk-management strategies are in place? How do we deal with data that indicate a need for change in practices?
Management priorities	What needs to happen when? Are immediate priorities being acted on without excluding progress in longer-term goals?
Past and present performance	How have we performed as an organization before? Are we better now?
Underlying causes	What does a SWOT (strengths, weaknesses, opportunities, and threads) analysis indicate to us? What do root cause analyses show?
Performance potential	Are we growing appropriately? Are there strategies that need to be more competitive?

*Based on work by Kocourek, P. F., Burger, C., & Birchard, B. (2003, Spring). Corporate governance: Hard facts about soft behaviors. *Strategy+Business, 30,* 1-12.

board members' individual and collective abilities to grapple with the numerous issues facing the governing board of a healthcare organization.

Table 17-2 provides some key abilities to which a board member needs to commit to be effective. These key abilities are as applicable to the CNO in a board role as to the CNO in an executive role. "What distinguishes exemplary boards is that they are robust, effective social systems" (Sonnenfeld, 2002, p. 109). This means that part of every executive team member's role is to facilitate the development of trust, respect, honesty, and trustworthiness to produce the best possible boards.

One final aspect important to consider is the politics of governance (Table 17-3). As if the work of the board and its interrelationship with the staff is not complex enough, politics may influence an otherwise solid process. Each of the common issues cited in Table 17-3 can be further complicated by an overlap/interaction with staff. Clear communication, trust and respect, and clarity about role differences help delimit the politics of governance.

Staff Roles

The key function of staff in governance is to provide the necessary support for the board to make substantive decisions. This support almost always is provided through the executive level staff, even though other members may be called into specific discussions to ensure that the most comprehensive knowledge is available for any discussion. Realistically most organizational reports are developed and implemented at other levels of the organization, so many other administrative personnel have a vested interest in what the board does.

In many organizations, it is difficult for the staff members not to think that they know best. After all, they are there full time. However, that is one of the dangers of the relationship between board and staff. The staff members are accountable for the quality of information provided to the board so that the board can make the best decision possible. The staff members also are accountable for implementing the policies and directions

the board establishes and for providing them with the necessary support for them to be effective representatives of the organization. Thus staff must be timely in their reports, which must be brief enough to be useful to board members. The staff members are the technical and professional support for the implementation of the mission. Therefore, after the board sets the mission and the strategic direction of the organization, the staff is accountable for preparing plans to implement the mission and the work plans to accomplish the goals.

Staff members provide the details of planning and budgeting so that the board can create the global plans and accept budgets. The staff members monitor and counsel and assure the board that the work that the board does is translated throughout the organization on a daily basis. Further, staff members frequently draft policies for the board's consideration. DePalma (2002) suggests six elements to include in policy proposals (Box 17-2). Each is important. Without a clear statement of an issue, confusion will reign. Evidence drives much in current society, and it is no less important here. Also, knowing what stakeholders think adds another dimension. A plan with specific objectives and a view of feasibility helps the board do their best for the organization.

Emerging Issues

Numerous issues are always evolving, but one of the clear issues in recent years has been the Sarbanes-Oxley legislation (DiConsiglio, 2003). Although this legislation was designed to focus on for-profit organizations and thus has direct implications for some healthcare organizations, the results have evolved into best practices for organizations regardless of their IRS designation. In short, Sarbanes-Oxley was designed to provide greater transparency between executive staff and boards and between that group and the employees. Focusing mostly on accounting practices to prevent irresponsibility, Sarbanes-Oxley laid out certain expectations about accounting rules and auditing

Table 17-2 ABILITIES OF EFFECTIVE BOARD MEMBERS

Key Abilities	Examples
Show up.	Attend board and social events.
Speak up.	Be sure that dissenting views are heard as well as support for popular ideas.
Ensure no surprises.	Alert the board chair and/or the CEO of good as well as bad news.
Criticize in private, praise in public.	Respect the need to share information appropriately. (Note: if cause for concern exists, praising in public can be seen as insincere. If the criticism is by a board member with the CEO, the board chair should be informed appropriately.)
Role model membership.	Pay attention, follow through with commitments, recruit other strong board members, champion diversity, cultivate other members and nonmembers.
Be timely.	Respond to mail, e-mail, and phone messages as soon as possible.
Expect follow through.	Request that unanswered issues be carried forward so that closure is achieved.
Keep the mission statement visible.	Know why you are there and where you are headed.
Schedule all events.	Be accountable for showing up.
Ensure that ongoing development occurs.	Expect, and hold accountable for, board development activities so that the board is better at being a board.
Expect compliance with organizational policies.	Hold the CEO to the organizational policies, including those about evaluation and vacations.
Plan for transitions.	Determine in advance who is a likely successor so that board leadership and executive functions continue without a crisis.
Stay out of the management functions.	Remember the separation of board and staff roles.
Ask questions.	Get to the root of issues and strategies to ensure understanding of complexities.
Seek legal guidance.	Use the corporate attorney or seek additional expert information about legal issues.
Be informed.	Read materials submitted, listen actively, sense the board's compatibility.
Ensure quality governance.	Review board policies and procedures on an ongoing basis and maintain current policies for effective operations; expect to assess board performance.
Create the practice of accountability.	Be accountable and open.
Plan for the future.	Be flexible and willing to embrace change.
Insist on clarity of terms and actions.	Use accurate terms, clarify acronyms, be clear about actions intended and timelines.
Create the climate.	Encourage openness, honesty, and frankness.

Table 17-3 THE POLITICS OF GOVERNANCE

Common Issues	Politial Implications
Use of power	Although some members of a governing group may have more credentials or greater prestige or more connections than other members, using those factors to gain a vote or influence others' thinking is a short-term strategy at best.
Persistence	Sometimes a decision appears to have been reached easily. The case often is, however, that the topic has been discussed before. Sometimes this discussion has been in a closed (less public) session or so long ago that others have forgotten that the issue was previously discussed. True commitment to an issue may require addressing the same issue multiple times in multiple formats to gain support.
Cultural differences	Cultural differences that relate to gender, age, economics, ethnicity, or religion are typically viewed as cases for nondiscrimination. However, a board needs to make considerations related to those factors. How to provide for services that are unique to one gender or a service devoted to an age group and how to support consumers without sufficient financial means to pay for services are examples of how cultural differences must be addressed. Framing the issues so they can be discussed without becoming discriminatory is the challenge for leaders.
Getting to the truth	When a discussion occurs that appears to be one sided or to expose accurate but insufficient information, a leader may need to redirect conversations to expose the greater picture. One strategy is to pose questions that require explanatory responses so that others may hear additional information.
Resiliency/flexibility	The ability to "bounce back" is critical. If it seems as if a leader has taken something personally, he or she may lose effectiveness. Rather, the ability to put forth one's best effort on an issue and then "move on" conveys that the individual does see the effort as one of team rather than one of "me." That does not mean that a leader might not return to the topic again.
Penny wise and pound foolish	The old saying is important to remember because some issues aren't worth fighting over. Knowing how to balance issues in the scheme of the big picture is what leaders are expected to do. Being able to make decisions about huge expenditures is as important as making decisions about smaller issues.
Being in the "in group"	Avoiding cliques altogether is a lofty goal and one that is not readily accomplished. Always siding with a particular person or set of people is limiting. In addition to conveying a lack of independence of thought, individual influence is diminished. In the worse case scenario, those not part of the group may feel compelled to create their own clique.
Avoid surprises as much as possible	No one likes to appear uninformed or inadequately prepared. This means that there is a need for additional work between formal meetings, especially if new information or omitted information needs to be shared. Keeping colleagues apprised

Table **17-3** The Politics of Governance—cont'd

Common Issues	Political Implications
	of what is known on a topic can be seen as valuable if for no other reason than they are not surprised in public.
Avoid public arguments	It is possible that leaders may disagree on a topic; but it serves no good purpose for arguments or disagreements to turn public. "Egging" someone on has no place in a leadership position. Creating "power plays" to force someone to appear as a loser or to retaliate to comments only lowers the esteem of the total group. If these have occurred, create new expectations for behavior, even if the potential is to influence only a few people. Once a decision is reached, it is one to be supported publicly by all members.
Keep confidential what is	If a discussion occurs in a closed or confidential setting, an obligation exists to keep the conversation confidential. If an individual knows that he or she must share some portion of the confidential information, it is useful to identify this at the time so that all are clear what will be said and who has the authority to share more. Further, it is critical to protect confidential papers/email/faxes.
Avoid favoritism	Whether only people who are supportive or a member of the "in group" are reappointed to a group or always chair subgroups, an appearance of favoritism is raised. Once that happens, a team becomes divided and thus less effective. Deliberately seeking input from and offering leadership roles to those who aren't part of the normal leadership group creates a greater openness and provides for new insights. The person making those broader decisions about leadership is subsequently viewed as being fairer and more goal oriented.
Elevate the discourse	Many groups become comfortable with the status quo. They know how to move the agenda quickly. They know there will be no tough conversations that could lead to any embarrassment. Elevating the discourse creates discomfort for such groups and it simultaneously creates greater relevance for the organization. Using the group first to discuss the change in the content and level of discussions can help the group move to a more relevant involvement. Although there may be a temptation to delay such discourse, effectively leaving it to a subsequent group, facing issues head on provides for a timely and often less dramatic response to an issue.
Represent the care component	Boards historically focused on the finances of the organization. Increasing public awareness of safety issues has also increased the need to discuss care at a level equivalent to the financial aspects. The CNO is often the one with the greatest perspective about care issues and has the moral obligation to share insights into patient care issues within the organization so that better governance results.
Respect and trust	To be most effective, any group has to respect its individual members and trust that they will do what they say they will and that they are being honest when they speak. Respect and trust are integral to sound board/organizational governance and have to be promoted consistently.

Box 17-2   KEY FACTORS IN POLICY
            PROPOSALS

Clear statement of issue
Evidence to delimit scope of issue
Stakeholders' views
Proposed action plan
Objectives that lead to outcomes
Feasibility of proposed action

DePalma, J. A. (2002). Proposing an evidence-based policy process. *Nursing Administration Quarterly, 26*(4), 55-61.

requirements. Detailed information is available at http://www.sarbanes-oxley.com.

One of the key requirements is that organizations form an independent audit committee (separate from the management team and uncompensated for their work) and that that group includes a person with a strong financial background. In addition, the CEO is expected to sign a document that validates the veracity of financial reports from the organization's perspective. The law also requires a records retention policy. That along with retaliation against informants are the two criminal provisions, and they are viewed as covering all organizations. Nonprofit organizations are not *required* to examine their practices; for-profit organizations are.

Despite the benefits, the costs of complying with the new law have been extensive (Hamel, 2003). Part of the expense comes from the more elaborate accounting activities. Another part that is slow to emerge is compensation for board members. According to Gilbert (2003), approximately 12% of nonprofit healthcare organizations compensate their directors. In part, this low percentage is due to the ability of nonprofits to attract qualified board members who can give sufficient time and abilities to meet the expectations of the legislation.

Kocourek et al. (2003) also suggest that the board engage in self-evaluation activities to improve their own performance. Although the CEO is the key staff accountable for this activity, the CNO can be invaluable by virtue of the number of people who report directly and the extensiveness of evaluation in which the CNO and nursing are engaged. Sonnenfeld (2002, p. 113) puts it a different way: "People and organizations cannot learn without feedback." Assessment of the board's effectiveness can be simple or complex. Partridge (2000) advocates for asking a series of simple questions, such as if the goals are clear, if board roles are clear, if the board is effective in problem solving, and if it handles conflict effectively. If no assessment has occurred before, this would be a less threatening way to determine how the board is functioning.

SUMMARY

The balance between board and staff and the clarity of understanding each other's role are critical to the effective functioning of the organization. Regardless of whether the CNO is a member of the board, certain support and expectations are inherent in the role. Key obligations of the CNO for effective board operations include making certain that the board understands the nature of the business they are governing—patient care—and assisting the board in understanding the complexities of quality and patient safety.

KEY POINTS TO LEAD

1. Evaluate the CNO role for differences when being governed and when governing.
2. Analyze the strengths needed to interact in a successful manner with governing boards.
3. Assess the CNO's involvement in governance within the organization and how it could be enhanced.

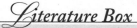
Literature Box

Although the concept of governance is evolving, the authors believe that it will support a broader community level that will reflect six roles:

1. Be comprehensive in structure
2. Be comprehensive in ongoing evaluation (including social and justice systems as need measures)
3. Provide outcomes for consumers so they can select services
4. Conduct studies that include care and social issues
5. Identify areas of need
6. Facilitate transitions to meet areas of need

During the board orientation process, the CNO should provide information about nursing and performance improvement areas of the organization. The CNO also can help board members understand the language of healthcare and the significance of issues, such as medication errors and nosocomial infections. In addition, the CNO needs to be aware of how the CEO interacts with the board, because sometimes the CEO sees the board as his or hers and thinks about how to manage the board. If the CEO suddenly left, the CNO may be a logical replacement.

Because governance is not a key focus in graduate healthcare education, the CNO may need to study this topic and make keen observations about how it is lived. In addition, that knowledge can be useful to achieving goals for the nursing organization.

Genovich-Richards, J., Gorenberg, B., & Deremo, D. E. (2000). The role of governance in improving clinical outcomes: Opportunities for nurses. *Nursing administration Quarterly, 24*(2), 62-71.

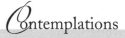
Contemplations

- What gains or losses does the CNO experience when serving as a member of the governing board?
- What influence does the CNO have with the board that other executives are missing?

- Which clinical areas would serve as showcases if you were trying to expose a board member to the richness of intensity and complexity of nursing care? Why?

LEADER STORY

THOMAS SMITH
SENIOR VICE PRESIDENT, NURSING AND PATIENT CARE SERVICES
THE MOUNT SINAI HOSPITAL
NEW YORK CITY, NEW YORK

Chief nurse executives are first clinicians, so we've learned how to balance many simultaneous activities. That's one of the reasons we make such great leaders. We also are based in relationships with others; they're the foundation of our practice. We are good at juggling work and competing interests and how people approach their work. I don't think about relationships with the people I am "governing" or the people who are "governing" me as causing me to be "in the middle." To me, it is more that we are all focused on the same mission and in the hospital setting it is about providing the best possible patient care. On the other hand, I am directly in the middle of everything! I am in the middle of dialogue and discussions and decisions about patient care delivery. I am in the middle between the board and nurses. I am in the middle of issues that affect nursing. Every one of those "in the middle of" situations allows me to be present so that nurses are represented. I just don't think about relationships in a hierarchic manner.

As the leader of a clinical discipline, my work is about creating voice. As nurses, our work is often about creating voice. It works for us at all levels. Frontline nurses have voices of agency or advocacy for their patients. One of the primary parts of my job is to give voice to patients and nursing practice. When I meet with nurses in their orientation, I really emphasize this important role of professional nursing. Suzanne Gordon described this in the book, *From Silence to Voice.*[*]

I don't see myself as being in the middle of a hierarchy, with people at the bottom or the top. I see myself, as the CNO, in the middle of a great mission. And, nurses are at the forefront of that work. I am absolutely passionate about nursing and cannot imagine myself doing anything else. I am proud to give voice to this work, whether to the board or to a clinical nurse or to a nurse colleague, whether patient care is being discussed or actually being performed in front of our eyes. I think of it as a web of connection.

Dan Pesut describes what I am thinking of in the work on clinical reasoning; he talks about clinical reasoning webs: spinning and weaving them in multiple directions.[†]

Being in the middle of the web with linkages to the nurse at the bedside and also to the CEO or board chair creates distinctive opportunities. First of all it is about creating relationships. And, as I said, nurses are great at this, because creating relationships is at the center of everything we do. This allows us to create the venue and the opportunities to tell our stories. And that is the second big opportunity. Our stories are our strength in connecting people who aren't in healthcare with the impact and poignancy of our care. The third big opportunity is our ability to influence decisions. More of my influence potential is not at the board level *per se*. Rather it is at the individual board member or committee level. That is where many decisions are made, at least in my organization. It is the opportunity to talk with a board member

---

*Gordon, S., & Buresh, B. (2000). *From silence to voice: What nurses know and must communicate to the public.* New York: Cornell University Press.

†Pesut, D., & Herman, J. (1999). *Clinical reasoning: The art and science of critical and creative thinking.* Albany, NY: Delmar.

on a one-to-one basis or to discuss important information in a specific committee that eventually shapes a decision at the board level.

There is only one nurse who goes into that board room, so that makes me *the* voice for nursing there. Being a CNO is a lonely spot. Often a CNO is the only nurse involved in any decision and sometimes that nurse is the only clinician. So, it is very important that I be articulate and passionate. I cannot be silent. I must speak for those in the web. I must address the core issues of the members of that web. I am the spokesperson, the translator, and the interpreter and that works both ways. I function in a constellation of forces, voices, agendas, people, and issues. My job is to touch all. There isn't an area of the hospital that nursing doesn't touch. So I have to be an integrator.

Nurses are the largest group of providers, so I have to be at the board meetings to represent our practice and our discipline. We are what brings people to the hospital. We are the 24/7 group.

I think there are some real keys to employ in working with a board. First, never go to the board and be silent. Always participate in the meeting. Even if you are new, speak up so that at least the board can recall that the new CNO spoke up. Never be seen as a wallflower…never, never, never.

Second, study who is on the board. Get a list of their names and figure out who they are, where they work, their backgrounds. This personal information is often the basis for being comfortable in interacting with the board. You can do that with ease, if you have a personal connection.

Third, get on board committees. That is often where important decisions are made and you can be most influential there. You may need to push in that regard.

Fourth, cultivate individual relationships with board members in situations beyond the board too. They need to know you as a person and you need to know them that way too. I also invite board members to nursing events and write them letters about issues and nursing activities.

Fifth, go early to meetings and stick around afterwards and do business. Those are the times when you can interact with individuals about some important item. Even though you have to be prepared during the board meeting, it is often those other times that make a difference.

Sixth, take board members on rounds. Most will love it and I make a big deal of it. Some people are on boards because they want to be around important people; but most people are on boards because they have some connection to the mission and purpose of the organization. In our case patient care is the mission and board members like to see what is happening. They like to know why our hospital is special. It's a really great opportunity to showcase nurses and nursing excellence. Board members remember these experiences.

I happened to be working late one night and the chairman of the board came in with his mother-in-law. The emergency department (ED) couldn't have been busier or more crowded. This is an ED you would expect to see in the middle of an inner-city community in a large metropolitan area. He was there with his wife and mother-in-law for about 4 hours. I can assure you I didn't leave their sides! What an opportunity to interpret the care! They had the opportunity to watch nurses execute great care and to watch me as the leader of nursing as I interacted with others. I was concerned with the outcome of care, of course, but more concerned with the information he could take away about the difference a nurse could make in the care of a loved one and to see that I could interact with staff so that my stories were later valued. When he saw I was comfortable in the clinical area, he could walk away with a great sense of my connection to caregiving and nursing practice. He could see me as a leader of nursing and be transported back to that experience. He could see me as credible, comfortable, and able to manage and influence the environment. He knew I was not a stranger to patient care and that that is where I was rooted. I wanted him to feel my presence. That made all of my subsequent clinical stories more believable. The chairman of the board hasn't stopped talking about it. In fact, he referred to that when we had our Magnet site visit in such a meaningful, personal way. He described my leadership and presence and the excellent care his mother-in-law received.

Whenever I am having a bad moment, all I have to do is go find a patient and a nurse. Then, everything is okay.

Chapter References

Banaji, M. R., Bazerman, M. H., & Chugh, D. (2003, December). How (un)ethical are you? *Harvard Business Review*, 56-62.

Chait, R. P. (2004). The problem with governance. *Board Member, 13*(4), 6-7.

DePalma, J. A. (2002). Proposing an evidence-based policy process. *Nursing Administration Quarterly, 26*(4), 55-61.

DiConsiglio, J. (2003). Keeping up with Sarbanes-Oxley. *Board Member, 12*(6), 6-8.

Gilbert, P. (2003, April 26). Compensating nonprofit directors: A consequence of Sarbanes-Oxley? *Health Leaders News*. Retrieved April 30, 2004, from http://www.healthleaders.com/news.

Hamel, W. W. (2003). Keeping up with Sarbanes-Oxley. *Board Member, 12*(6), 6-8.

Hirschhorn, L., & Gilmore, T. (1992, May-June). The new boundaries of the "boundaryless" company. *Harvard Business Review*, 1-16.

Kocourek, P. F., Burger, C., & Birchard, B. (2003, Spring). Corporate governance: Hard facts about soft behaviors. *Strategy+Business, 30*, 1-12.

Matisoff-Li, A. (2004, April). Chief nursing officers: A seat at the table. *HealthLeaders*, 36-44.

Partridge, W. G. R. (2000, January). Getting the board to measure up. *Association Management*, 59-63.

Rutledge, D. N., & Grant, M. (2002). Introduction to evidence-based practice in cancer nursing. *Seminars in Oncology Nursing, 18*(1), 1-2.

Ryan, W. P. (2004). Governance as leadership. *Board Member, 13*(4), 8-9.

Sonnenfeld, J. A. (2002, September). What makes great boards great. *Harvard Business Review*, 106-113.

Thompson, R. E. (2004). The Joint Commission in 2004: What the board needs to know. *Hospitals and Health Networks*. Retrieved January 14, 2004, from http://www.hospitalconnect.com.

18 Creating Relationships and Working with Physicians and Service Leaders

Leadership is influence, nothing more, nothing less. That means it is by nature relational.
JOHN MAXWELL

Relationships are critical to effective leadership. In this chapter, these relationships are examined, beginning with factors that serve as the basis of relationships and progressing through to the strategies for building relationships. The American Organization of Nurse Executives (AONE) Competencies concerning the importance of relationship building are incorporated (2005).

IN THE EARLY 1990S, MARGARET WHEATLEY led the effort to look at organizations from a new perspective, applying what she had learned from quantum physics and chaos theory. She was particularly interested in leadership and complex organizations. Furthermore, organizational study had subsets, such as followership, empowerment, and leader accessibility that particularly intrigued her in view of such thought processes as chaos theory. She identified ethical and moral questions as key elements in the relationships that leaders have with staff, suppliers, and stakeholders. "If the physics of our universe is revealing the primacy of relationships, is it any wonder that we are beginning

to reconfigure our ideas about management in relational terms?" (Wheatley, 1992, p. 12). Wheatley believed that relationships were at the core of organizations and their accomplishments. Consequently, this chapter focuses on establishing relationships and how the nurse leader relates to staff, to the administrative team, to peers, to superiors, and to major stakeholders such as physicians.

RELATIONSHIPS: DEFINITION AND BASIS

Being in relationship with another human being implies a connection with that person. These connections are critical in complex organizations. Relationships are the glue that holds the people, teams, and organizations together. To have a cohesive team, the relationships must be solid. In the Nurse Executive Competencies developed by AONE, (2005), relationships are emphasized in the first competency on Communication and Relationship-Building. This competency identifies relationship management as building trusting collaborative relationships with staff members, peers, other disciplines, ancillary services, physicians, vendors, community leaders, legislators, and nursing educational programs. This competency identifies relationship management, in part, as the ability to deliver "bad news" in such a way as to maintain credibility. The leader must follow through on promises and explore concerns or issues expressed by anyone associated with the facility. The leader must be able to manage difficult situations with unhappy or dissatisfied patients and their families. The leader must be able to care about people as individuals and demonstrate empathy and concern. However, this caring cannot usurp or undermine organizational goals and objectives. The focus must be on accomplishing goals through persuasion and facilitating celebrations of success and accomplishments. A part of building relationships enables the leader to assert his or her views in a nonthreatening and nonjudgmental way.

The Basis of Relationships

In an attempt to build relationships that meet the competencies as described in the previous section, the reader must understand the basis of solid relationships, which includes common background, common interests, common beliefs and values, and common vision and goals. *Common background* begins with family and implies being from a similar socioeconomic group. For example, people who grow up together in a rural area, those who grow up together on the streets of Brooklyn, or even those who grow up in the country club set have shared economic backgrounds and come from similar social groups. People tend to form relationships in groups with which they have many things in common. Thus people often stay together in ethnic groups (e.g., the ethnic neighborhoods of large metropolitan areas such as the Polish and the Italian neighborhoods or the African-American and Hispanic neighborhoods). Religious groups also cluster, such as in the Jewish neighborhoods or in the Muslim neighborhoods in metropolitan areas. Many of these groups began as immigrant groups that spoke the same language and shared the same customs.

In addition, people also tend to form groups and networks based on their educational background. They attended the same schools or the same sororities and fraternities and lived together. Many nurses' friendship circles comprise primarily nurses, just as is true among physicians or academics. In addition, people can form friendships based on athletic activities (e.g., runners develop friendships with other people who run). These relationships often remain connected because of the closeness during the formative years growing up or attending college.

Common interests may include sports participation or attendance, crafts, reading, and like activities. Because of these interests, people in these various groups form relationships. Activities and topics of conversation emerge around these interests.

Within schools, fraternities, and professions, friendships and relationships frequently develop based on *common beliefs and values*. People share a commitment to integrity, honesty, and hard work. They may make a concerted effort to have humor in their lives and to make each other laugh. They may have a belief in quality patient care or the principle that "the patient comes first." They may have a strong focus on religious values and living these values in everyday life. With these common values, people may spend time together outside of the workplace. Kanter's classic work (1977) found that these factors were the most powerful in explaining the men at the top of America's corporations. They all went to school together, were in the same clubs together, and ultimately ran a company together.

Vision or *goals* may be shared, such as a focus on learning and growing as an adult, or being on a "journey" through life. The goal could be creation of a positive work environment, in which all team members treat one another with respect. The vision could be attaining Magnet status for the hospital. A concerted effort is possible to create a learning environment that focuses on research or a scientific process to discover solutions to patient care and staff problems. Another possibility is an intense focus on education to support staff members in personal growth and professional advancement, or in best clinical practices, which support the best possible outcomes for patients. Because of these goals or visions, people work together toward higher-level accomplishments.

Differences

Differences between people create problems in relating to one another. Problems begin with different backgrounds: socioeconomic, education, ethnicity, or religion. Rarely is this more obvious than in medicine and nursing. Physicians have an average of 12 to 14 years of post-secondary education as compared with nurses who have as little as 2 years to qualify for the licensure examination. These two individuals who have such disparate educational backgrounds and knowledge bases are supposed to be in relationship with one another! They have very few interests in common. Clearly bridges between these two professions have to be built based on issues other than a common background in such areas as education. However, they may build a bridge based on quality patient care.

Unfortunately, differences may breed *fear*. Fear stimulates judgments, gossip, bickering, and blaming. At the risk of stereotyping a particular group, an example of one difference could be expression of feelings. Female nurses may be more prone to displaying emotions and feelings with patients and peers in extremely stressful or sad situations. Physicians traditionally have resisted sharing or demonstrating feelings openly. It is not perceived as professional behavior. Some nurses make negative judgments about the physician who refrains from expressing feelings, and some physicians make negative judgments about the nurse who displays emotions.

Differences in beliefs may stem from such issues as the belief on the part of some physicians that nurses ought to be more deferential to them because they are the captain of the ship and responsible medico-legally for the patient. This can create defensiveness in nurses, who are prepared to think for themselves and function more independently. Nurses and physicians may differ in beliefs regarding how to relate to patients or families or about communication, respect, and the elements of an effective team. It is easy to see how relationships can break down or never even begin because of such differences.

LEVELS OF RELATIONSHIPS

Three basic levels of relationships exist (Figure 18-1). The first level of relationships is the one that forms around activities. In this level, the activity is more important than the relationship. Other people may be present or needed for the activity, but the people are interchangeable. For example, in performing emergency surgery, the most important thing is the patient and the procedure. The people involved are whoever happens to be "on call" for the operating room: the anesthesia person, the scrub and circulating nurses, the assistants to the surgeon, and the support staff. Level 1 relationships are by far the largest group of relationships in the work setting.

On the other hand, level 2 relationships consist of activities in which being with the person is more important than the actual activity.

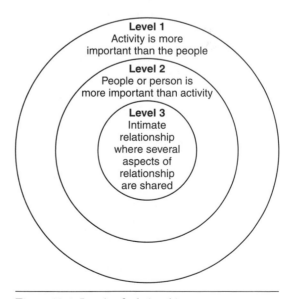

Figure 18-1 Levels of relationships.

For example, the activity is probably unimportant when a person has the opportunity to spend the day with an old nursing school classmate. Shopping or walking in the mall, having lunch together, or going camping in the mountains may be acceptable. The most important thing is the time together, talking, catching up, and sharing, reciprocally, various life events. The number of level 2 relationships for one person may be a couple of dozen throughout a lifetime, significantly fewer than for level 1. In the workplace, most relationships would be level 1 and sometimes level 2 relationships.

The third level of relationships is an intimate relationship in which several aspects of the relationship are shared between two people. The list of shared life areas is found in Box 18-1. Whitfield (1993) estimated that at least three of these areas must be involved for the relationship to qualify as intimate, or level 3. For example, a couple may be involved in an emotional life area, which means they share feelings and emotions. They also may share the affectional area, characterized by touching, tenderness, and a sense of being special to each other. This could be accompanied by the sexual life area, in which physical intimacy occurs. The number of level 3 relationships per person could be counted on one hand.

STEPS IN BUILDING RELATIONSHIPS

According to Acuff (2004), building relationships consists of three essential steps, beginning with the right positive mindset, collecting information by asking the right questions, and demonstrating professionalism through thoughtful, unexpected acts of kindness that demonstrate the importance of the relationship (Figure 18-2).

Creating the right positive mindset begins with thinking the relationship is important. The most important aspect of this mindset is believing that you are someone whom other people would like to know better and with whom they would value time spent. The leader must feel positive and believe that he or she has experiences, skills, abilities,

Box 18-1	AREAS OF LIFE THAT MAY BE SHARED IN CLOSE RELATIONSHIPS
Social:	An area that consists of a group experience
Intellectual:	The sharing of thoughts and ideas; a discussion of these
Emotional:	Feelings and emotions shared between two people; often in conjunction with life stories
Physical:	Working together; often physical labor
Recreational:	Sharing a recreational activity such as hiking or biking together
Aesthetic:	Sharing what is beautiful or artistic such as art, music, or natural beauty
Affectional:	Sharing affection through touching, tenderness, or special caring
Sexual:	Having a significant relationship; deep closeness is possible
Spiritual:	Sharing a spiritual experience, not only religious

Modified from Whitfield, C. L. (1993). *Boundaries and relationships: Knowing, protecting and enjoying the self.* Deerfield Beach, FL: Health Communications.

and knowledge that others value. A positive self-concept is essential. In addition, the leader must think positively about other people and attempt to see and understand the other person's perspective. This means thinking positively and respectfully about individuals whose behavior may be inappropriate or disrespectful. Judging such people as "jerks" or worse does not support building a relationship or create effective problem solving.

Collecting information about the person by asking questions in a meaningful way for the right

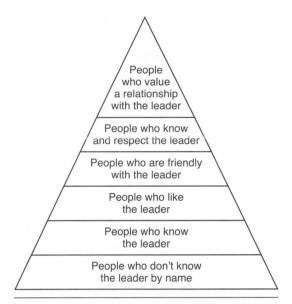

Figure 18-2 The relationship pyramid. (Modified from Acuff, J. (2004). *The relationship edge in business: Connecting with customers and colleagues when it counts.* Hoboken, NJ: John Wiley & Sons.

reasons is a key in building relationships. The purpose of the questions is to discover common ground, interests, values, goals, or mutual friends. If few commonalities exist, the leader may be able to *learn* about something that the other person cares for passionately.

The third step is for the leader to *demonstrate professionalism, integrity, caring, and knowledge* toward the other person, perhaps a physician. When it is appropriate, the leader can do unexpected, inexpensive, or thoughtful acts based on what has been discovered about the person. These unselfish, thoughtful acts can create respect, credibility, and trust because such acts demonstrate caring. The leader does this not in expectation of "payback" but as a thoughtful gesture one person would do for another. For example, perhaps a physician loves sailing and has a sailboat. The leader may see a book or article that would be of interest and may send it to the physician. Thoughtfulness and helpfulness create meaningful relationships.

KEY COMPONENTS OF RELATIONSHIPS

In examination of relationships from a different perspective, particularly as they apply to leadership, six behaviors and the value of integrity provide additional insight into advancing relationships with stakeholders of the facility.

Behaviors

Active Listening

Active listening is a significant part of entering into a relationship and meeting each other's needs. Listening is such an integral part of building a relationship that without it, no relationship exists. If the leader does all the talking, staff members, physicians, and peers begin to practice avoidance. People do not like to be with someone who never asks questions or listens to other people's thoughts and ideas. Leaders should not be afraid to ask people about their needs and desires: "What could make things easier for you?" Then the leader listens carefully.

The content and the intended meaning may be verified by repeating what was heard. At social events, a leader ought to ask more questions than he or she answers by at least 5:1.

Asking Questions

Asking questions is the most powerful tool leaders have. Certainly to ask questions is important when information is sought from staff. (For an additional discussion on questions, see Chapter 9.) As previously mentioned, in social situations, the beginnings of relationships are created by asking questions. A key aspect of this process begins by remembering someone's name. If remembering names is a problem, leaders can insist that staff members wear nametags. Even using a deck of 3 × 5 cards or a Personal Digital Assistant to organize personal information can be helpful. The cards can serve as a desk reference. Seemingly inconsequential helps such as this assist the leader in building self-confidence in this basic skill.

Frequency of Interaction

Interacting frequently over time with people creates greater possibilities of relationship building. Remembering staff or physician names occurs more readily when frequency of interaction occurs over time. For relationships to develop, it is helpful to see a person happy, upset, sad, exhausted, highly motivated, or deep into a project, and this is more likely to happen with ongoing contact. By seeing the person in a variety of settings and circumstances, more and more can be learned about the person. Relationships develop from frequent interaction.

Follow-Through

One of the more important behaviors is following through with commitments, responsibilities, and promises. Unfortunately promises are frequently made "in the heat of the moment" that are difficult to follow through with after the excitement and passion of the moment have passed. Following through with the commitment often means doing tasks that may not be favorites. These tasks should be performed anyway. When anyone fails to follow through, a "nagging little voice" may send negative messages, which creates negative self-talk. The little voice can create sleeplessness or wakefulness in the middle of the night. Follow-through means a great deal to physicians and staff. If the leader does it consistently, relationships will grow, and he or she will be perceived as competent.

Demonstrating Competence

The nurse leader must demonstrate competence. This is not necessarily current clinical competence, yet it is valuable to have been clinically knowledgeable and competent at some point in a career. Frequently, competencies of leaders lie in such areas as administrative skills, including visioning, problem solving, communication, administrative knowledge base, financial issues, and knowledge of current healthcare issues.

CNOs must be perceived as competent in creating positive relationships with staff and nurse leadership groups. This could include such possibilities as creating a learning environment in the nursing division, focusing on succession planning at each administrative level within nursing, providing mentoring, and having frequency of interaction with directors, nurse managers, and charge nurses. Competence in holding directors and nurse managers accountable for skills, behaviors, and outcomes is an essential part of leadership and relationships. It also supports development of this next level of leaders within the organization. Concurrently, the CNO can demonstrate building relationships with physicians and other stakeholders, including key people in the community.

Competence most likely extends to such areas as the healthcare environment, including knowledge about various delivery models and work design. This could include an understanding of health policy, particularly state and federal laws and regulations, in addition to national accreditation regulations. It also could include a thorough and complete knowledge of all aspects of nursing care that affect patient safety, including facilitating design and monitoring of safe clinical systems, processes, policies, and practices.

Reciprocity

Reciprocity is a cornerstone of relationships. First a desire must exist, regardless of the motivation, to meet each other's needs. If only one person has his or her needs met, soon the other person will become disillusioned and cease making an effort to meet the needs of the first person. Usually a period of "testing" the relationship occurs; a period of trial and error in which both people find out what works and what does not. An example of this testing occurs between physicians and the "new" CNO. It includes an assessment of knowledge base, clinical judgment, critical thinking, levels of cooperation, and the ability and willingness to solve problems. If the nurse appears competent after this trial, reciprocity is a clear possibility and the relationship can progress.

INTEGRITY AND BUILDING RELATIONSHIPS

Integrity is not determined by circumstances; integrity is a choice. The problem for many is that they look outside themselves for explanations and justifications of any shortcomings with regard to integrity. However, as Maxwell (2003) states so clearly, integrity is an "inside job." It is tied to the choices made throughout life. Leaders can choose the positive, which enhances character and integrity, or they can choose the negative, which detracts from character and integrity.

A leader can become deluded into believing that value is based on status, credentials, or job descriptions, particularly as the leader advances in the organization. However, character and integrity are different from credentials. Credentials add value to only one person, whereas character adds value to many people. Likewise, credentials focus on the rights of the person holding the position or the titles, whereas character focuses much more on the responsibilities of specific roles or titles. Credentials are built on past accomplishments (e.g., the entitlement that comes with academic tenure) versus the drive to build a legacy for the future. Credentials can evoke jealousy in others, where outstanding character and integrity generate respect. Credentials can open the door for the CNO, but strong character and integrity keep him or her in the position. No degrees, titles, or awards can substitute for basic integrity and character.

Sometimes people confuse integrity and reputation. A good reputation exists because it is a reflection of a leader's integrity and character. It is helpful to focus less on what people think and focus instead on developing and maintaining integrity. The questions in Box 18-2 allow evaluation of integrity. Integrity is highly valuable. When others criticize, integrity allows the leader to hold his or her head high and to refrain from striking back or from saying things that damage relationships. When others have identified accurately a problem or issue with the leader's behavior, integrity helps a person accept feedback and

Box 18-2   QUESTIONS TO HELP YOU MEASURE YOUR INTEGRITY

1. How well do I treat people if I gain nothing?
2. Am I transparent with others?
3. Do I role-play based on the person(s) I'm with?
4. Am I the same person in the spotlight as I am when I'm alone?
5. Do I quickly admit wrongdoing without being pressed to do so?
6. Do I put people ahead of my personal agenda?
7. Do I have an unchanging standard for moral decisions, or do circumstances determine my choices?
8. Do I make difficult decisions, even when they have a personal cost attached to them?
9. When I have something to say about people, do I talk *to* them or *about* them?
10. Am I accountable to at least one other person for what I think, say, and do?

From Maxwell, J. (2003). *Relationships 101: What every leader needs to know*, p. 61. Nashville, TN: Thomas Nelson.

continue to learn and grow. When a leader with integrity attempts to influence staff or co-workers, these people know that he or she acts because of the opportunity to support them and add value to their lives rather than attempting to manipulate them.

Becoming a person of integrity involves a commitment to honesty, reliability, and the ability to keep confidences. This is not necessarily an easy road, particularly because everyone loves a good story. Sharing information without the permission of the person about whom the story is being told is an easy habit to assume. This information is sometimes shared in a somewhat demeaning way, if it is funny. The rule of thumb should be this: Can you tell the story in the same way using the same tonality if the person who is the subject of the story were present? If not, the story should not be told, regardless of how funny it is.

Leaders must decide that they *cannot* be bought or used. For leaders unable to commit to integrity, the purchase price could include money, power, status, pride, or revenge. Bending principles or relinquishing integrity for any of these "rewards" puts relationships at risk. Attitudes and skills that expand integrity should be practiced every day. Such practice lays the foundation for building strong relationships in careers and in families. It opens the door to success. Without holding to the principles of integrity, the leader will surely not be successful.

RECOMMENDED AREAS OF NURSE AND PHYSICIAN COLLABORATION

The relationship between the nurse leadership group and the corresponding physicians is so important that AONE (2005) devoted an entire section of the Nurse Executive Competencies on Communication and Relationship-Building to medical staff relationships. The nurse leader must first build *credibility* with physicians as a champion for patient care, quality, and nursing professionalism. He or she also represents nursing at the medical executive committee and other medical committees. If another member of the nursing leadership team is appointed in place of the CNO, the nurse leader must be assured that the appointee represents the nursing division in the way the CNO would choose. This could be a coaching or role modeling opportunity for the CNO to work with the nurses who represent nursing leadership. Likewise, the CNO or the designee serves as the representative to work with medical staff in determining and evaluating needed patient care services, the equipment associated with these services, and developing the corresponding patient care policies, protocols, and procedures.

Positive working relationships support outstanding performance within the organization. Many lessons can be learned through development of such relationships. Several of these are identified in Box 18-3. Focusing on methodologies to improve relationships is quite productive.

NURSE-PHYSICIAN RELATIONSHIP BREAKDOWNS

Clinical Performance Issues

When the problem is substandard clinical practice on the part of the physician, substantiating data and immediate interventions are necessary. Failure to act puts patients and the facility at risk. Data consist of chart review and any documentation (e.g., an incident report) in conjunction with the specific situation, which is initiated by another professional. The first level review is by medical peers, and if the problems are not resolved, administration becomes involved and then outside entities such as another professional who can participate in peer review and provide an unbiased approach can be involved. The last level of intervention comes from the state medical board.

Inappropriate Physician Behavior Toward Staff Members or Patients

Confronting the inappropriate behavior of a physician is never an easy situation. Thompson (2004) provides some suggestions for coping with such behavior. He suggests that determination of a cause for disruptive behavior can begin with exploring the existence of a medical condition such as diabetes, depression, or dementia. A brain tumor has even been documented to explain outbursts of uncontrollable anger. Strategies should be designed to deal with the cause of the adverse behavior.

Box 18-3   RELATIONSHIP LESSONS

Ways to improve organizational performance:

1. The essence of positive working relationships is the strength of the connections between physicians, nurses, ancillary staff, support staff, and patients and their families.
2. Strengthening relationships in the workplace relies on developing people.
3. Developing stronger relationships is accomplished by the following:
   - Understanding mutual interests and needs
   - Linking these interests and needs to quality patient care and positive outcomes
   - Constructing a meaningful plan for how to achieve these strong relationships
   - Implementing the plan in an effective, efficient manner
4. Workers' skills need to be developed in ways that are consistent with the organization's espoused mission.
5. Experiential learning or simulation to gain this learning helps the organization, especially when learnings are applied to a real-time, mission-focused project.
6. New relationship behaviors must be recognized, rewarded, and measured repeatedly.
7. A focus on improving and changing behavior in ways that strengthen the connections between various levels and members of the staff, physicians, and other departments within the organization is productive.

From Cohen, S. L. (2004, July). Performance improvement through relationship building. *T & D Magazine*, pp. 41-47. Copyright © July 2004, Reprinted with permission of American Society for Training and Development.

Because "hope is not a plan," to simply hope the problem will resolve itself without intervention is unacceptable. If the physician clearly is being disruptive and no medical explanation exists, immediate action is necessary. One of the first steps is to document the behavior in time, place, and specific actions. Groups who can assist in such situations include a medical quality committee or another group of physicians within the facility who can undertake the responsibility. Programs to help physicians are usually available through employee assistance or the state medical board.

Disruptive and acting out behaviors are not acceptable in employees and therefore are unacceptable in physicians. Most of these situations can be resolved by productive, nonjudgmental confrontation. However, if behaviors are not confronted, physicians have no opportunity to change, and damage can be done to patients, employees, colleagues, and to organizational integrity. The number of patients admitted by the offending physician cannot influence the necessary action. If initial interventions by the senior administrative team are unsuccessful, it may be possible to find a consultant who can help devise a plan or even work with the physician. If the situation ends in suspension, it also must be clear what circumstances would allow for reinstatement. The less judgment and upset from the staff and administration, the better the chance for constructive resolution.

Dispute Facilitation

Physicians commonly approach the CNO with complaints about a specific nurse. It would be easy and ineffective to assume that a physician's interpretation of the situation is completely accurate. The CNO must know how to collect appropriate information from staff members in such situations and then bring both parties to the table while serving as mediator for resolution of the issue or problem.

PHYSICIAN-NURSE COMMUNICATION

Interprofessional Communication

Improving the communication between nurses and physicians is a first step in improving relationships and improving care to patients. Poor communication, in which individuals argue, blame, and are generally disrespectful to one another, makes for a difficult work environment and can endanger the patient. Clear, direct communication between physicians and nurses can eliminate much of the relationship damaging problems. Guidelines for effective communication can be found in Box 18-4.

A study done by the Institute for Safe Medication Practices indicates that physicians who intimidate or berate caregivers such as nurses, pharmacists, and other health professionals contribute to the incidence of medication errors by reducing the likelihood that nurses, for instance, will ask questions or express concerns about medication orders (Morrissey, 2004). Physicians were found to use condescending language or were impatient with questions from nurses twice as often as anyone else. About 69% of respondents reported they had been told (in the past 12 months), "Just give what I ordered." About 43% of respondents said they had been recipients of verbal abuse or threatening body language at least once in the past year. Around 7% reported being involved in a medication error in which intimidation clearly played a role. On the other hand, Braggs, Schmitt, and Mushlin (1999) found a positive association between increased nurse-physician collaboration and a lower risk of negative patient outcomes and readmission to the ICU and risk of adjusted mortality. In a study by Boyle and Kochinda (2004), a focused intervention with physician and nurse leaders, including collaborative communication-building skills, had a significant improvement in communication with physicians. In addition, lower stress levels for physicians and nurses were reported and the nurse turnover rate decreased. Also, an increase in the ability to meet patient and family needs and an increase in the quality of care were reported.

Box 18-4   COMMUNICATION WITH PHYSICIANS: SUPPORT AND ROLE MODELING FOR STAFF

1. Determine the need for contacting the physician. Be sure to assess the patient thoroughly and check the chart thoroughly, especially the orders.
2. Be completely prepared before making the call. Have the chart with you when placing the call. Have pertinent information at your fingertips, including such things as recent laboratory results. Be clear about your assessment of the patient.
3. Identify yourself and the patient you are calling about. If speaking with someone in the physician's office, determine the person's name. Follow all the policies regarding telephone orders, particularly reading the order back and indicating the name of the person who provided you with the order.
4. Think carefully about whether the call can wait until morning when calling at night. Follow all of the above directives carefully. If any uncertainty exists, consult with other nurses on the unit.
5. Be sure the other nurses know you are calling in case they need the same physician for something.
6. Let another nurse know you called the physician if you leave the unit for any reason.
7. State your request briefly and completely when speaking to the physician. Clearly ask for what you want.
8. Document all attempts to reach the physician.
9. Speak to a rude or abusive physician calmly and request he or she do the same. Ask for clarification if you receive criticism.

Remember, the patient comes first.

Blickensderfer (1996) identified strategies that can be used to enhance collaboration:

1. Establish nurse-physician liaison committees. These can be an effective first step. In these committees, mutual concerns and problems can be addressed.
2. Create opportunities to learn about each other's roles. A better understanding of each other's roles has been shown to improve collaboration. Some type of program in which shadowing occurs between the professions often works.
3. Schedule meetings to ensure collaboration. Routine joint meetings can be scheduled during which case examples of communication and collaboration breakdown can be presented and then discussed by the whole group.
4. Capitalize on interprofessional education. Curriculum changes in nursing and medical schools, including joint nurse/physician classes, professor exchanges, and frank discussion of the problems between nurses and physicians can be very helpful. Joint classes can occur in such content areas as communication and nutrition.
5. Use joint quality assurance committees in which policies and procedures are reviewed and discussed and patient problems or serious errors are discussed. These committees also can serve as an appropriate reference group for complaints concerning inappropriate physician behavior. This group could suspend the physician, revoke privileges, or report the physician to the state licensing board (Trossman, 2003).

No doubt other areas could be considered in creating an improved culture of collaboration. Evaluation would be particularly helpful on an individual level, including the nurse's responsibilities in the collaboration and the breakdown. Blickensderfer (1996) and Trossman (2003) have identified important aspects of productive communication, which the nurse leader can teach, role model, and support in the nurse manager and the staff nurses.

1. Demonstrate respectful behavior in all communication with physicians even when there is upset with the involved parties. For example, the nurse could say, "I feel distressed and confused. I cannot continue this conversation unless the manner in which it is conducted changes."
2. Demonstrate support for other nurses, both in communication with each other and communication with physicians. Support for one another means refusing to participate in or listen to gossip, blame, or judgment of others. Support in communication with a difficult or out-of-control physician could mean instituting a "Code Pink" exercise, in which other nurses simply come to the aid of their co-worker by surrounding the physician who is out of control and saying nothing.
3. Be assertive, direct, open, and honest in communication that indicates respect for self *and* the other person. Ask directly for what is wanted. Refrain from acting in an indecisive or uncertain way, which can be a "set up" for a lack of respect. Confront, respectfully, any inappropriate behavior.
4. Be a lifelong learner, which includes staying current in clinical skills and knowledge base or administrative skills and knowledge base. Take responsibility for continuing education. Reflect upon and acknowledge strengths rather than focusing on errors. Work to be an expert in the field of practice.
5. Enhance self-esteem through relinquishing perfectionist thinking. Rather strive for continuously improving skills. Focus on what is good and right about a co-worker or a physician rather than what is negative or wrong.
6. Take personal care by managing stress. Nurses who are healthy and relaxed are much better able to deal with conflict and effectively confront situations. Always maintain a sense of humor and play.

Learn what is nurturing and make time for such activities on a regular basis.

7. Commit to working collaboratively with the team of physicians and nurses. This might include an agreement among team members to establish trust, act respectfully, accept one another, and forgive any past problems.

8. Remember always that the primary purpose remains care of the patient. The team is committed to the best possible care to this human being and his or her family. *The patient comes first.*

ASSESSMENT OF RELATIONSHIPS

Building solid relationships relies on the following characteristics: respect, shared experiences, and trust (Maxwell, 2003).

Respect is defined as the desire to place value on other people, to hold them in special regard, or to hold them in high esteem. Obviously, if the leader holds a person in high esteem, the person is important. It is not possible to make the other person feel important if secretly the leader feels he or she is a "nobody" or an unworthy human being, or if the leader simply does not like the person. Often this describes the interaction between nurses and some physicians. A few physicians (and nurses) are not very likable. The key is to treat every other person with respect before they have done anything to "earn" it. Conversely, leaders must expect to earn respect from others.

Shared experiences are critical to building relationships. It would be extremely difficult to be in a relationship with someone you do not know. Being in relationships requires shared experiences over time. If most of the leader's interactions are in groups, such as meetings, he or she could plan thoughtfully for what those interactions would be like and how they would be created to make them as meaningful as possible.

Trust, the faithful reliance on the character, strength, or truth of another, is an integral part of building relationships. Without trust, relationships cannot be sustained (Galford, 2003). Trust also is discussed in Chapter 7. Maxwell (2003) says, "When your words and actions match, people know they can trust you." Covey (1989, 2004) connects this to integrity or an adherence to a code of values that are incorruptible. With integrity, a leader commits to character development over personal gain; to people rather than things; and to service over power, to principles over convenience, and to long-term goals over the expediency of the moment. These behaviors create trust.

Furthermore, Wall (1999) believes that relationships break down when assumptions are made about the other person's intentions, character, or personality. Of course, when anything is negative in these assumptions, the relationship begins to unravel. If issues are somewhat ambiguous, disagreement exists regarding goals, or these goals diverge, estrangement can occur. If, even because of confusion or lack of clarity, agreements are not kept, relationships can begin to unravel. Like the majority of the previous discussion in this chapter, these issues can occur in the CNO's relationships with physicians just as they can with the nursing leadership group or with staff. Regardless of the people involved in the relationship, the opportunities and the risks are the same.

RELATIONSHIPS WITH ACADEMIC INSTITUTIONS

Because of the severe nursing shortage, CNOs must be concerned about nurse preparation and education. A collaborative relationship should be developed with nursing educational programs to provide required clinical practice sites for future nurses. Developing collaborations requires determination of the current and future supply and demand for nursing care and assistance in planning for how the demand will be met.

Rather than identification of all the shortcomings of the graduating nurses, collaboration with the nursing programs in evaluation of the quality of the graduates and development of mechanisms to enhance their abilities would be helpful. In consideration of the faculty shortage, examination of possible options would be helpful to support clinical teaching of students through the development of models that use the clinical experts in the facility. Often students like experiencing clinical rotations with instructors who work in the setting and who know all the special emphases, rules, and informal structures of facilities and ways to complete work expediently. When students have very positive clinical experiences, they are more apt to select that facility as a work setting after graduation.

Further, the CNO can serve on academic advisory councils and collaborate with nursing faculty in nursing research in addition to participating in evidence-based studies and implementing nursing research into practice (AONE, 2005). The CNO also is responsible for the identification of educational needs of the existing staff. Mutual benefit and mutual dependency exist between nursing service and nursing education, and it behooves the CNO to develop the relationships with education that support all of these common interests.

SUMMARY

No doubt, a decade ago, a suggestion that a chapter dedicated to relationships appear in a textbook on nursing administration and leadership would have resulted in considerable scoffing. However, today it is clear from the AONE Nurse Executives Competencies; papers from the Institute of Medicine (IOM); and from such organizations as the American Association of Critical Care Nurses (AACN), which has established the AACN Standards for Establishing and Sustaining Healthy Work Environments, that each of these documents addresses the importance of relationships in the work setting. Consequently, relationships have been defined, the basis of them has been explored, and key components of relationships have been examined. Correlations between these aspects and the factors related to building relationships with physicians, peers, and nurses have been explored. Many nurse leaders have come to understandings about relationships intuitively. In the next decade, it is time for creating relationships consciously and systematically and for increasing the understanding and importance of how this task is accomplished.

KEY POINTS TO LEAD

1. Analyze three important relationships, identifying the basis of each relationship.
2. Analyze these same relationships for the specific components used to build the relationships.
3. Evaluate three strategies you currently use or would like to implement to increase positive nurse-physician relations in your facility.
4. Develop a plan to support staff members in resolving difficult physician situations.

Literature Box

This small pocket book is a typical Maxwell book; however, it is very clear and succinct about the importance and the need for relationships at work and at home. He uses stories, poems, and sayings to keep the reader interested. However, the CNO will find helpful information regarding the important aspects of relationships. He begins with why relationships are important, including what keeps relationships solid. He identifies the important things to know about others and what stumbling blocks exist when attempting to formulate relationships.

He is specific about the building blocks that form relationships, including encouraging others, becoming a believer in people, and supporting them to be successful. Maxwell shares specific skills and tools about how to connect with people and the results of connecting with people in the workplace. He has specific ideas about the importance of listening to others and ways to become a better listener.

Maxwell also has ideas about growing relationships and the trust and integrity required to do so. He highlights the importance of following through and the self-discipline to do the things you should do before the things you want to do every day. He emphasizes the importance of family relationships and how to work on these. This small book is an easy read and can stimulate some very important self-reflection.

Maxwell, J. (2003). *Relationships 101: What every leader needs to know*. Nashville, TN: Thomas Nelson.

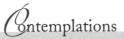

Contemplations

- Reflect on the key physician relationships you currently have.
- Reflect on the physician relationships that are important to cultivate.
- Determine what prevents a relationship with these physicians.
- Consider what additional steps you could take to improve the relationships.
- Reflect on which directors or nurse managers with whom you have limited relationships.
- Consider what prevents you having a more meaningful relationship with these nurses.
- Decide what you could do this week to significantly improve the relationships.
- Reflect on the senior administrative team.
- Think about a team member whom you dislike, consistently disagree with, or have considerable judgment about.
- Work on a plan (at least three steps) that you could implement to improve the relationship.
- Perform a self-assessment, using what was identified in this chapter to discover what the similarities and differences are with all of these relationships.

LEADER STORY

Lois Sonstegard
President
Friends of CHT, Pakistan (a 501(c)(3) organization)
Minneapolis, MN

Working with physicians and others doesn't just happen. This work takes deliberate focus to build and enhance relationships that have real meaning for the effectiveness of our work on behalf of people needing healthcare. This is true whether you are in a paid employment position or whether you are in an unpaid voluntary position.

Leadership in the nonprofit sector and within volunteerism requires an attitude of servant leadership. Servant leadership requires that you show up fully as yourself and without judgment. Your job is not about fixing people or organizations; that drives people away, because people do not want to be fixed. Rather people want to be in a relationship that focuses on support, caring, and concern for their welfare and the work they do. So, leadership is all about relationships.

Most people who volunteer are fully engaged in busy careers or businesses. They don't have time for inefficiencies. Many are somewhat skeptical as they have seen ideas dwindle to nothing. This disillusionment results from lack of being meaningfully engaged. Increasingly, in a world of scarce resources where time may be more scarce than money, those who volunteer want to know how much value a project can have long term.

Currently, I am working to create a "virtual hospital" and teaching network for a remote hospital on the border between Afghanistan and Pakistan. It is a stronghold of the Taliban. Conditions are primitive and the United Nations has declared the area to be "the sickest of the sick and the poorest of the poor." And, in this region a mission hospital has faithfully served people for 150 years! It has provided badly needed medical care and hope to the community. The hospital operates 77 beds, 3 operating suites, 15 outreach clinics, and a school

of nursing. They do this with four physicians and nurses who are taught by two of the mission nurses. They all work incredibly long hours every day of the year. The care is good, the facilities adequate, and the needs unending.

One day, I received a desperate call for help. The mission physicians and nurses were exhausted. They needed equipment and specialist help. After numerous conversations with the hospital and the involved mission organizations, we decided to form a 501(c)(3) organization to provide assistance. We are determined to secure the medical, nursing, and rehabilitative services and equipment needed. Supplies are being gathered and will fill a 40-foot shipping container. We are identifying, recruiting, and sending medical, nursing, administrative, and other teams to help meet specialized medical and healthcare needs of the area. In particular, there is need for surgical teams, gynecologists, ophthalmologists, rehabilitation specialists (of all kinds, including vision loss rehabilitation), orthopedic surgeons, cleft lip and cleft palate specialists, and family physicians. Nurse educators are needed to help with the school of nursing, which operates on site and is the major nursing resource for the hospital. This is a huge undertaking; it requires the involvement of physicians, nurses, hospital administrators, accountants, pharmacists, and the business community.

Leadership in such a venture requires a track record. Business leaders who may put themselves on the line to help raise money want to know, "Can I do the job?" They want to know what my track record is for organizing people to get done what is seemingly impossible. Business leaders evaluate projects very critically. They know money is hard to come by. They have earned each penny. They know the sweat and the tears that went into creating their own success. They also know how easily sales, business, and money can disappear. So if they invest, they want to know the investment will produce a net value. It is the leader's track record that helps them answer their key question.

Leadership requires partnerships with unusual groups. It means I have to be able to talk many languages. I need to be able to go from finance to university faculty to hospital management and understand each of their value systems and concerns. Partnership also means I don't need to take credit. It's all too easy to get caught in the fame game. Recognition is not important in servant leadership. It is the end-result and the process that's used in getting there that's the most important. That is all about relationships!

Establishing partnerships requires careful relationship building. This is especially true when working with women. Faith Popcorn has done some fascinating research on marketing to women in which she found that women are loyal customers when they find that the service or product that they purchase creates a context through which they can experience relationships. So soccer moms like going to soccer games not only to watch their children play soccer, but also to find out how other mothers are managing their lives. There's a sharing that takes place. Women choose healthcare providers in the same way. Recently I went to see my OB-GYN. Each year she has a questionnaire focused on a specific issue that I have to fill out. This year the questions were all about safety. Do I wear a helmet? What sports do I play? We had a wonderful discussion about safety issues that had nothing to do with obstetrics or gynecology per se. I left feeling connected and very cared for. We need to take these ideas of marketing to women and "going beyond" to create new relationships that will have real meaning for patients and their safety.

If a novice nursing leader came to me for advice regarding creating relationships with peers, with organizational leadership, with physicians, or with other healthcare providers, I would say that genuine concern for people is the key. I can't say that often enough! If I don't have an interest or commitment to people, I have no business in leadership. In developing leadership skills and relationships I examine my interactions with others each day and ask these questions:

- Is it the truth? When I talk about something, is it absolutely the truth? To what extent have I added hyperbole? In creating a relationship, integrity is key. Without it nothing else will happen.

- Will all people benefit from the relationship? I can't be the only one benefiting. It can take a lot of time and effort to sort through how others will benefit, but that's what keeps the relationship working. No one wants to be used or participate in a one-sided relationship. That is true of our work and volunteer efforts as well. Thinking this way takes more time and effort and sometimes money. It is the only way a long-term project can be accomplished.

- Is it fair to all I will work with? The process is critical. The end result is important but never more important than the process. Be fair. If you can't be—don't get involved. It will take too many years to undo any damage that you created. Years after a project is completed, people may forget the project and remember the feeling. That's the process. They don't remember specifics, so never underestimate the importance of the process you used. A worthwhile litmus test for this is: "When someone sees me again, do they smile and seem excited or do they look for the first possible exit?" If they are looking for an exit—you did something that was not perceived as fair or desirable.

- Have I burned a bridge today? In the heat of the moment and upset, it is easy, although thoughtless, to say or do something hurtful and damaging to another person. Be careful and thoughtful. Never burn a bridge. You never know when you might need the bridge or the relationship months or years into the future. It simply isn't worth the moment of pleasure in making another person wrong or less than.

I think novice leaders need to focus on making a difference. People want to buy into ideas and concepts that are strategic, that solve problems, and that are workable. They want to work with something that will make a difference in this world, something that has meaning. I advise new leaders to learn and participate in an effort or a project that gets them excited and desirous of getting up in the morning. It doesn't matter who the others are with whom you work. Whether others are physicians, other nurses, business leaders, or the patient, relationships are important. All of these efforts require a genuine commitment to creating, building, and maintaining relationships.

Chapter References

Acuff, J. (2004). *The relationship edge in business: Connecting with customers and colleagues when it counts.* Hoboken, NJ: John Wiley & Sons.

AONE. (2005, February). AONE Nurse Executive Competencies. *Nurse Leader,* pp. 15-21.

Blickensderfer, L. (1996). Nurses and physicians: Creating a collaborative environment. *Intravenous Nurses Society,* 19(3), 127-131.

Braggs, J., Schmitt, H., & Mushlin, A. (1999). Association between nurse-physician collaboration and patient outcomes in three intensive care units. *Critical Care Medicine,* 27(9), 1991-1998.

Boyle, D., & Kochinda, C. (2004). Enhancing collaborative communication of nurse and physician leadership in two intensive care units. *Journal of Nursing Administration,* 34(2), 60-70.

Cohen, S. L. (2004, July). Performance improvement through relationship building. *Training and Development,* pp. 41-47.

Covey, S. (1989). *The seven habits of highly effective people: Restoring the character ethic.* New York: Simon and Schuster.

Covey, S. (2004). *The eighth habit: From effectiveness to greatness.* New York: Simon and Schuster.

Galford, R. (2003). The enemies of trust. *Harvard Business Review,* 81(2), 88-96.

Kanter, R. (1977). *Men and women of the corporation.* New York: Basic Books.

Maxwell, J. (2003). *Relationships 101: What every leader needs to know.* Nashville, TN: Thomas Nelson.

Morrissey, J. (2004). *Survey on workplace intimidation.* Institute for Safe Medication Practices. Retrieved March 31, 2004, from http://www.ismp.org/survey0311.asp.

Thompson, R. E. (2005). Common mistakes in managing problem physicians. Retrieved December 3, 2005, from http://www.hhnmag.com/hhnmag/hospitalconnect/search/articlesjsp?dcrpath=HHNMAG/PubsNewsArticle/data/05030IHHN_Online_Thompson&domain=HHNMAG.

Trossman, S. (2003). Professional respect: The CWPA and Magnet facilities work to improve nurse-physician relationships. *American Journal of Nursing,* 103(3), 65-67.

Wall, B. (1999). *Working relationships: The simple truth about getting along with friends and foes at work.* Palo Alto, CA: Davies-Black.

Wheatley, M. (1992). *Leadership and the new science: Learning about organization from an orderly universe.* San Francisco: Berrett-Koehler.

Whitfield, C. L. (1993). *Boundaries and relationships: Knowing, protecting and enjoying the self.* Deerfield Beach, FL: Health Communications.

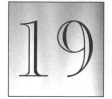

Working with Regulatory and Accrediting Bodies

Mary Beth Mancini

Coming together is a beginning. Keeping together is progress.
Working together is success. HENRY FORD

This chapter describes the major regulatory and accrediting bodies that affect the functioning of current highly controlled healthcare organizations. As major areas of concern for nurse leaders, this chapter covers the Centers for Medicare and Medicaid Services (CMS) and its Conditions of Participation (CoP) in addition to the Joint Commission on Accreditation of Healthcare Organization (JCAHO) and its accreditation process. A brief overview of the Health Insurance Portability and Accountability Act of 1996 (HIPAA) and the Emergency Medical Treatment and Active Labor Act of 1986 (EMTALA) is provided, which reflects the significant impact of these acts on healthcare organizations in general and the nurse leader in particular. The unique role of the nurse leader in maintaining continual readiness for review is summarized. From setting the expectation for compliance to coordinating site visits, this chapter highlights key factors nurse leaders must consider for their organizations to maintain required certification and accreditation.

To PROTECT THE HEALTH AND SAFETY OF the communities and patients they serve, healthcare organizations are licensed, regulated, and accredited by a variety of governmental and nongovernmental agencies. By virtue of their position and education, nurse leaders often are involved actively in the regulatory and accreditation processes regardless of the type of organization in which they work. From setting the expectation for compliance to representing the organization during site surveys, nurse administrators and nurse managers are key to obtaining and maintaining licensure, certification, and accreditation. As such, all nurses must have a thorough understanding of the regulations and accreditation standards that affect their organization's ability to function and be prepared to take a leadership role during interactions with regulatory and accrediting agencies.

REGULATION

In the current environment, government is involved inextricably in the American healthcare system. At various levels, government serves as provider, payer, and regulator of healthcare services (Mason, Leavitt, & Chaffee, 2002). At the local level, cities and counties actually own or operate public clinics, health departments, hospitals, and health systems. In addition, municipalities commonly promulgate fire, safety, sanitation, and public use ordinances that healthcare organizations must follow. At the state level, government serves as a regulator of healthcare by licensing healthcare providers in addition to healthcare facilities. State government serves as a payer of healthcare by virtue of administering Medicaid programs. Some states also serve as direct providers of healthcare services by virtue of their ownership of hospitals and/or long-term care facilities.

Through the Medicare program, the federal government is the principal payer of healthcare costs in the United States. Since its creation in 1965, Medicare has become the country's largest health insurance program. It currently provides healthcare funding for more than 40 million individuals. These individuals are not just persons over the age of 65. Regardless of age, Medicare provides coverage to individuals who have certain permanent disabilities, such as end-stage renal disease. Because of the scope of Medicare penetration into the healthcare market, the federal government serves as the foremost regulator of healthcare services. It does so through the requirements it establishes for healthcare practitioners and organizations that wish to participate in the Medicare program (Kovner and Jonas, 2002).

Medicare policies and procedures are administered by CMS. Medicare participation is regulated by a complex set of rules outlined in a lengthy set of guidelines, the CoP. The CoP outlines the specific requirements that healthcare organizations must meet to be eligible to receive Medicare and Medicaid reimbursement. The requirements set forth in the CoP are used by CMS to improve quality and protect the health and safety of Medicare and Medicaid beneficiaries. The CoP specifically addresses the responsibility of healthcare organizations to protect patient rights and ensure systems are in place for measuring patient outcomes and resource utilization. In addition, the CoP outlines specific business and billing practices that organizations must implement to maintain program integrity and prevent fraud and abuse.

Beyond administration of the Medicare program, as its name implies, CMS works in partnership with the states to administer Medicaid and the Children's Health Insurance Program (CHIP). Although CMS has its headquarters in Baltimore, Maryland, it has 10 regional offices that work with states to administer the programs under its purview. In this partnership, the state and federal governments work together with the intent of creating an efficient mechanism for monitoring compliance with a comprehensive and consistent set of regulations that healthcare organizations and providers must meet to participate in the Medicare, Medicaid, and CHIP programs. This partnership draws upon the proximity of state agents to survey sites and evaluate complaints in a timely manner. Unfortunately, because of the significant differences among state programs, the goal of efficient implementation and monitoring of consistent state and federal regulations is not always met. On occasion, a change in a regulation at either the state or federal level creates a challenge to complying with regulations at the other level. This situation highlights the need for nurse leaders to develop specific strategies for monitoring federal and state regulations to be able to respond rapidly to changes in either set of regulations. The use of a consistent cadre of state personnel to monitor compliance with the Medicare, Medicaid, and CHIP programs has the benefit of allowing nurse leaders to build relationships with these surveyors.

Building a positive working relationship with local surveyors helps the nurse leader ensure an efficient and collegial survey when it occurs. Nurse leaders can follow certain strategies for creating effective working relationships with surveyors. These include immediately meeting the surveyor when he or she arrives for an announced or unannounced survey, establishing a common set of expectations with regard to how the survey will be run, and anticipating resources the surveyor will need, such as a convenient space for confidential interviews and review of records. Being proactive and responsive to surveyors is, in the long run, the most successful approach to dealing with a survey. However, nurse leaders must be well versed in what constitutes an appropriate scope of review for a survey and when it is necessary to refer a surveyor's request to the facility's legal counsel for review and guidance.

Beyond involvement in the Medicare and Medicaid programs, CMS has administrative responsibility for sections of HIPAA and EMTALA. Because of the scope and impact of both of these acts, nurse leaders must be well versed in their regulations and implications also.

As the title of the Act indicates, HIPAA was designed to protect health insurance coverage for workers and their families when they change or lose their jobs. For that reason, the Department of Health and Human Services, the Department of Labor, and the Department of the Treasury each has a role in implementing HIPAA's insurance reform provisions. Included in the Act, however, are "administrative simplification" rules that have had a profound impact on basic healthcare processes; this is where CMS becomes involved with nurse leaders in relation to HIPAA. Along with requiring creation of unique identifiers for healthcare providers and use of specific transaction and code set standards for electronic health transactions, HIPAA specifically mandates that organizations will ensure the privacy and security of all patient information (Glass, Rebstock, & Handberg, 2004).

HIPAA privacy and security rules fundamentally changed how healthcare practitioners interacted with each other and their patients in regard to obtaining and sharing patient-specific information (LePar, 2004). The Act specifically outlines policies and procedures that must be implemented to protect patient information. Further, it establishes penalties for failing to do so. Thus nurse leaders must not only be familiar with the key elements of HIPAA privacy and security regulations but also ensure that the appropriate policies and procedures to safeguard patient information are in place throughout the organization. The nurse leader must take an active role in helping the organization meet the challenges associated with HIPAA compliance. Foremost among these challenges is the need for a significant culture change in how physicians and nurses communicate with patients, family members, and each other about personal health information. The key elements of HIPAA's privacy and security rules are outlined in Box 19-1.

Another Act that has had a major impact on healthcare organizations is EMTALA. EMTALA requires that all patients who present themselves for evaluation and care to an emergency department in a hospital that receives Medicare or Medicaid funding would be seen, receive a medical screening exam (MSE), and be treated or stabilized before discharge or transfer regardless of their ability to pay. The provisions of the Act are not limited to Medicare beneficiaries. They apply to all individuals who attempt to access emergency care.

This law is considered by many to be one of the most difficult to understand and the easiest to inadvertently violate (Glass, Rebstock, & Handberg, 2004). Enforcement of EMTALA is a complaint-driven process; that is, the investigation of an organization's policies, procedures, and processes are initiated by a complaint from an individual or a facility that alleges "patient dumping." Such an allegation of inappropriate care or transfer of a patient regardless of the ability to pay most often will result in a site survey. It is therefore necessary for nurse leaders to have an understanding of EMTALA and its mandates and interpretive guidelines to develop specific strategies to reduce risk of an inadvertent violation. Specific EMTALA requirements are outlined in Box 19-2.

In addition to paying for healthcare, CMS has a direct responsibility for the quality of healthcare

Box 19-1   Key Elements of HIPAA Privacy and Security Rules

PRIVACY RULE

The Privacy Rule protects all individually identifiable health information. This information is called "protected health information" (PHI). In addition to common demographic data such as name, address, social security number, and birthdate, PHI includes information related to the following:

- The individual's past, present, or future physical or mental health or conditions
- The provision of healthcare to the individual
- The past, present, or future payment for the provision of healthcare that identifies the individual or for which there is a reasonable basis to identify the individual

The purpose of the Privacy Rule is to define and limit the circumstances in which an individual's PHI may be used or disclosed. Most common situations in which PHI can be used or disclosed are the following:

- As the individual authorizes in writing
- For treatment, payment, and healthcare operations
- For public interest and benefit activities, specific law-enforcement purposes, and required reporting such as abuse, neglect, or domestic violence
- As a limited data set for the purposes of research, public health, or healthcare operations

There are several areas of the HIPAA Privacy Rule that are of particular interest to nurse leaders:

- Providing auditory and visual privacy in patient rooms, registration areas, prescription pick-up windows, clinic or procedure waiting rooms, and any other areas in which communication occurs between hospital staff and patients or their families

- Limiting the placement of patient names on unit boards or in clinics where individuals other than healthcare providers have access to them
- Limiting discussions about specific patients and/or patient care situations between physicians, nurses, and other staff in public areas
- Limiting discussions between medical staff and patient's family and friends without specific patient approval
- Controlling medical records and limiting visibility of PHI on computer screens and other devices accessible to other patients or visitors

SECURITY RULE

The Security Rule addresses the technical and physical safeguards required to protect electronic patient information. Covered facilities are required to develop and implement specific policies and procedures. Areas of particular interest to nurse leaders include the following:

- Establishing a Security Officer responsible for implementing and monitoring security-related policies and procedures
- Certifying that data transmission, storage, back-up, and access control are secure
- Obtaining Chain of Trust Agreements with partners who have access to PHI
- Creating contingency plans for computer systems and auditing that the plans have been tested and function as planned
- Devising specific plans to secure records and process them in an appropriate manner
- Ensuring security clearance processes for all personnel who deal with confidential information
- Training all personnel on HIPAA requirements

Box 19-2   EMTALA: Key Components

An individual presenting to a hospital offering emergency medical services will receive an MSE without regard to the individual's ability to pay.

An MSE is an examination provided by qualified medical personnel (QMP) within the capability of the emergency department. The examination includes ancillary services routinely available to QMP to determine whether an emergency condition exists.

QMP are individuals, such as physicians or nurses, who have been declared qualified by the organized medical staff to provide an MSE.

An emergency medical condition is a condition manifesting itself by acute symptoms of sufficient severity, including pain, psychiatric disturbances, and/or symptoms of substance abuse, such that the absence of immediate medical treatment could reasonably be expected to result in placing the individual in jeopardy of serious impairment or death. If the patient is a pregnant woman in labor, she automatically is considered to have an emergency medical condition.

If an emergency condition is present, the hospital must provide stabilization and treatment within its capacity and capability to do so.

The terms *capacity* and *capability* address the ability of the facility to provide care and treatment of a patient. Capacity includes consideration of an adequate number of beds, appropriately qualified staff, and equipment.

If the facility does not have the capacity or capability to provide care or if the patient requests transfer to another facility, the transferring hospital must contact the receiving hospital and the receiving hospital must formally accept the patient before the transferring hospital can transfer the patient.

A hospital with capacity and capability to provide the care required to stabilize and treat a patient cannot refuse to accept the transfer of such patient from a facility that does not have the capacity or capability to provide the care required.

To be compliant with the Act, organizations must do the following:

- Post signs in the emergency department that outline the rights of patients with emergency conditions to receive an MSE in addition to treatment and stabilization regardless of their ability to pay
- Maintain logs of individuals who seek care at the emergency department in addition to their disposition and lists of physicians who are on call to evaluate and treat patients with emergency medical conditions
- Maintain records of all patients who transferred to and from the hospital for a period of 5 years

provided through what it calls *quality-focused activities*. These activities include CMS's Quality Improvement Organization (QIO) program (formally called *Peer Review*), providing a financial incentive for hospitals to report quality data that will be used by patients to help them make decisions about hospital care and establishment of minimum quality standards for healthcare facilities.

The QIO program uses specially trained physician reviewers to determine if healthcare paid for by CMS is reasonable and medically necessary, meets the recognized standards for that care, and is provided in the most appropriate and efficient setting. Although this may appear to be a physician-dominated activity, nurse leaders are involved frequently in the process. Nurse leaders may be involved via their participation in facility-based utilization management activities or by virtue of their direct responsibility for nurse case managers. Nurse case managers often serve as the organization's interface with the physician-of-record. These case managers routinely monitor for appropriate physician documentation of medical necessity. They work with physician advisors to ensure that care follows the recognized standards and facilitates patient flow to the appropriate setting for care, either in the ambulatory or acute care setting.

In accordance with the belief that providing data on the quality of care provided is a vital first step in improving patient care, the Medicare Prescription Drug, Improvement, and Modernization Act of 2003 (MMA) created an incentive for hospitals, nursing homes, and home healthcare agencies to submit quality information to CMS. Those facilities that report the required data elements are eligible to receive the full Medicare payment for healthcare services provided in 2005. Those who do not voluntarily submit these data received a 0.4% reduction in their Medicare fee schedule for 2005. As of 2005, facility-specific data are available for consumers to access and use for reviewing and comparing selected performance and outcome indicators. Interested individuals are able to obtain this information on the CMS web site or by calling a toll-free CMS number.*

The data elements for the hospital quality initiative are drawn from the core measures CMS and JCAHO require hospitals to collect. These core measures are integral to efforts by CMS and JCAHO to improve the quality of care by collecting and reporting the actual results of care provided. The data elements collected include information on hospital performance related to three common medical conditions: acute myocardial infarction, heart failure, and pneumonia. The 10 specific indicators for these core measures are outlined in Box 19-3. These indicators have been reviewed and endorsed as reliable and valid indicators of healthcare quality by JCAHO and the National Quality Forum (NQF), a voluntary standard-setting organization representing consumers, providers, researchers, and purchasers. As individuals often directly responsible for quality

*http://www.cms.hhs.gov; 1-877-267-2323.

Box 19-3   HOSPITAL QUALITY INITIATIVE: CORE MEASURES

The Hospital Quality Initiative is designed to improve healthcare quality by providing consumers information about three serious medical conditions: acute myocardial infarction, heart failure, and pneumonia. These measures of appropriate care for each condition were selected after extensive testing of reliability and validity.

ACUTE MYOCARDIAL INFARCTION

Aspirin given upon arrival at the hospital
Aspirin prescribed at discharge
Beta-blocker given upon arrival at the hospital
Beta-blocker prescribed at discharge
An ACE inhibitor given if heart failure present

HEART FAILURE

Assessment of heart function performed
ACE inhibitor prescribed

PNEUMONIA

Antibiotic given in a timely way
Pneumococcal vaccination given
Oxygen level assessed

---

and performance improvement activities in addition to their commitment to the use of the data in formulating evidence-based nursing practice associated with these three conditions, nurse leaders need to be involved actively in the collection and dissemination of these data.

Nurse leaders also must be familiar with the Department of Health and Human Services' Quality Assessment and Performance Improvement (QAPI) program (Cady, 2003). To be in compliance with the CoP, hospitals must meet the requirements of the QAPI program. The program is designed to ensure that hospitals systematically examine the quality of care provided and that they use the data obtained to develop and implement projects that improve quality, enhance patient safety, and reduce medical errors. Six activities are outlined in the QAPI program:

1. Identify critical patient care and service elements
2. Apply performance measures predictive of quality outcomes
3. Collect and evaluate data on a continuous basis to identify opportunities for improvement
4. Identify and verify quality-related problems and underlying causes
5. Design and implement corrective action plan
6. Follow up to determine degree of success of interventions and detect new opportunities for improvement

The requirement that the hospital's governing body be involved in the institution's QAPI should be of particular interest to the nurse leader. The governing body must prioritize explicitly which processes will be monitored and analyze the effect of the program. Governing bodies, however, often comprise nonhealthcare providers. Based on background and experience, nurse leaders are commonly the hospital executive who interacts with the governing body on regulatory, accreditation, and quality-related activities. Responsibilities in this regard may include initial orientation of new board members to regulatory and accreditation standards, routine discussions related to quality activities, and annual review of quality plans including prioritization and evaluation. In this role, nurse leaders help translate technical aspects of care and operational systems into language and context that is usable by the governing body. It is especially important to assist the governing body in understanding the current state of the literature related to patient safety, medical error, and patient rights. With guidance from the nurse leader, the governing body needs to set the tone and establish the expectation for the organization's continuous focus on patient rights and patient safety.

With a focus on patient safety and the quality of patient care provided, CMS is responsible for the enforcement of its standards through its certification activities. For a healthcare organization to participate in and receive payment from Medicare and Medicaid, the organization must be certified as complying with the CoP. Healthcare organizations can obtain certification of their compliance with the CoP through two routes. One way is through a survey process conducted by a state agency on behalf of CMS. Alternatively, an organization can elect to be surveyed and accredited by a national accrediting body holding "deeming" authority for CMS.

"Deeming" is a process that CMS uses to ensure that the standards of an accrediting organization meet CMS standards. If CMS agrees that an accrediting body has and enforces standards that meet the federal CoP, CMS can grant "deeming" authority to that accrediting body. Healthcare organizations accredited by a body with such authority are therefore "deemed" as meeting Medicare and Medicaid certification requirements. Although healthcare organizations accredited by agencies with deeming authority are subject to random validation surveys and complaint investigations, they would not routinely be subject to certain additional CMS survey and certification processes. Exceptions in acute care hospitals are those state or CMS surveys associated with specific programs such as end-stage renal disease and dialysis, psychiatric care, and dedicated rehabilitation units. These targeted surveys usually are not covered by deemed status accreditation. Many states also accept voluntary accreditation by a national accrediting agency in lieu of other types of regulatory activity. For these reasons, healthcare organizations often prefer to seek CMS certification via accreditation by an accrediting body with deeming authority rather than through a survey process conducted by a state agency on behalf of CMS. They do so believing that this mechanism for meeting CoP requirements lessens the financial and bureaucratic burdens imposed by state and federal surveys.

ACCREDITATION

Accreditation refers to the approval of an organization by an official review board having met specific standards. Healthcare organizations can seek accreditation by organizations such as the American Osteopathic Association (AOA) and JCAHO. Both of these organizations have been granted "deeming" authority by CMS. The AOA is a professional association for osteopathic healthcare organizations that offers accreditation to acute care hospitals, mental health facilities, substance abuse centers, and physical rehabilitation centers. JCAHO accredits approximately 80% of acute care hospitals in the United States. JCAHO provides accreditation with deemed status options for ambulatory surgery centers, clinical laboratories, critical access hospitals, health maintenance organizations, preferred provider organizations, home healthcare agencies, hospices, and acute care hospitals.

JCAHO is an independent, not-for-profit organization governed by a 29-member board that includes physicians, nurses, and consumers (Longest, Rakich, & Darr, 2000). JCAHO evaluates the quality and safety of care provided at more than 15,000 healthcare organizations in the United States and internationally. Organizations accredited by JCAHO include ambulatory care organizations, assisted living facilities, behavioral healthcare organizations, critical access hospitals, clinical laboratories, healthcare networks, home care organizations, hospitals, long-term care facilities, and office-based surgery practices.

The explicit mission of JCAHO is to "continuously improve the safety and quality of care provided to the public through the provision of health care accreditation and related services that support performance improvement in health care organizations" (JCAHO, 2005, p. 11). To earn and maintain JCAHO accreditation, organizations must comply with an extensive set of standards and at least once every 3 years undergo an intensive on-site review by a team of JCAHO professionals.

The purpose of the review is to identify the organization's strength and weaknesses and evaluate its overall performance in areas that JCAHO believes affect quality patient care. In general, the accreditation process helps to inform and protect consumers, educate providers, and enhance organizational performance in ways that improve the quality of care provided. Box 19-4 enumerates a number of reasons healthcare organizations may seek accreditation.

In 1999 the Office of the Inspector General (OIG) completed a 2-year investigation into concerns that JCAHO was failing to protect the public from potentially inadequate or incompetent care in hospitals it accredits. In their report, "The External Review of Hospital Quality," the OIG claimed that traditional hospital accreditation

---

Box **19-4**   Reasons Healthcare
                Organizations Seek JCAHO
                Accreditation

Beyond complying with CMS's CoP, healthcare organizations seek JCAHO accreditation for a variety of reasons:
- Enhance community confidence
- Provide a report card for the public
- Offer an objective evaluation of the organization's performance
- Stimulate the organization's quality improvement efforts
- Aid in professional staff recruitment
- Meet requirements for having post-graduate medical education programs
- Provide a staff education tool
- Expedite third-party payment
- Fulfill state licensure requirements (may vary by state)
- Influence liability insurance premiums (may vary by insurer)
- Influence managed care contract decisions favorably

processes are too focused on teaching hospitals about quality improvement and that the triennial-announced survey process lacked adequate scrutiny to detect substandard patterns of care or individual practitioners with questionable skills. Responding to increasing concerns about its processes in addition to an expanding public interest in patient safety, JCAHO undertook a major review and redesign of its processes. In 2002 JCAHO announced significant changes to its accreditation processes. The new accreditation processes are designed to move the focus of organizations away from survey preparation and reposition their concentration onto the continuous improvement of operational systems critical to patient care and safety (JCAHO, 2004). JCAHO calls this new initiative "Shared Visions—New Pathways." The new processes were implemented with accreditation visits beginning in 2004. The six

innovations, or "pathways," through the JCAHO accreditation process are listed in Box 19-5.

Despite the significant changes that JCAHO has instituted in its accreditation process, the nurse leader must stay abreast of the continuing challenges being made to the reliability and validity of the JCAHO accreditation process. The Literature box describes a 2004 study by the Government Accountability Office (GAO), the former General Accounting Office, which once again examined the effectiveness of JCAHO's accreditation process. Based on a review of accreditation surveys during the period 2000 to 2002, the report called for giving CMS more oversight authority over JCAHO accreditation. This report may result in a fundamental realignment of the deeming authority that JCAHO now enjoys with CMS. Being aware of the state of the controversy will help the nurse leader prepare for any potential

---

Box 19-5   JCAHO's Shared Visions—New Pathways

Shared Visions—New Pathways includes the following changes in the accreditation process:

- A substantial consolidation of the standards was undertaken to reduce the paperwork and documentation burden associated with the accreditation process. The intent of this change is to increase the organization's focus on patient safety and healthcare quality by improving the clarity and relevance of the remaining standards.
- A midcycle, periodic performance review (PPR) is now required, during which the organization must evaluate its compliance with JCAHO standards. If noncompliance is noted, a plan of action must be developed and reported. Validation of PPR findings and corrections will be reviewed by JCAHO during the organization's next on-site survey.

- A priority focus process (PFP) is used to design each organization's on-site survey. The PFP uses the organization's core measures data, previous recommendations, demographic data related to clinical service groups, complaints, sentinel event information, and MedPar data to design a survey that is relevant to that organization's patient safety and healthcare quality issues.
- On-site evaluation is now focused on compliance to the standards in relation to the care experiences of actual patients in the facility. This process is known as the tracer methodology.
- Individual organizational performance reports have been revised to provide "Quality Reports," which include specific organizational performance information.
- Surveyors actively seek the engagement of physicians and other direct caregivers during the accreditation process.

changes in the processes and respond to questions from staff, governing board members, physicians, and members of the general public.

The *Shared Visions—New Pathways* initiative is a fundamental shift in JCAHO's survey process and requires the nurse leader to develop a new approach to the accreditation process. It is no longer possible for an organization to prepare once every 3 years for its anticipated and prescheduled accreditation survey. Now organizations must practice what is called "continual readiness." Continual readiness requires organizations to monitor important aspects of care continuously and ensure that they are in compliance with regulatory and accreditation standards on a daily basis. Organizations must demonstrate commitment to continuous improvement and be prepared to provide documentation of their ongoing efforts to that effect to the public, JCAHO during accreditation surveys, and CMS during site visits.

THE ROLE OF THE NURSE LEADER IN MAINTAINING CONTINUAL READINESS

As regulators, accreditors, and the public focus on patient safety issues, healthcare organizations are positioning themselves to stand the scrutiny of an outside surveyor at any time. Organizations are moving from a generation of accreditation and survey processes that were built upon a predictable cycle of scheduled reviews toward a future that includes continual compliance with standards. This requires organizations to create infrastructure and processes that are committed to ongoing performance improvement. The nurse leader is key to the organization's cultural transformation in this regard. By virtue of their position in the organization and their knowledge of the regulatory and accreditation processes, nurse leaders are situated uniquely to focus the organization on making this critical transition that directly affects the quality of patient care and enhances patient safety.

Change is not the same as transition. Transition is the psychological process people go through to come to terms with the new situation.
WILLIAM BRIDGES

The nurse leader can facilitate the transition through a variety of actions. For example, the nurse leader may give formal presentations on the topic of JCAHO's *Shared Visions—New Pathways* initiative, discuss the concept of continual readiness at all management meetings, and conduct walk-rounds on a routine basis to monitor compliance and assist staff to integrate the standards into their daily practice. Key staff members from all departments should be involved in performance improvement activities. Performance improvement targets for key clinical or service indicators can be posted for staff to review and the results of monitoring activities routinely reported so that progress can be seen by all.

SUMMARY

The nurse leader is commonly the face of the organization when dealing with regulatory and accreditation issues. The nurse leader is often the individual who articulates the organization's expectation for continual compliance with regulatory and accreditation standards. Setting that expectation starts with a commitment to providing high-quality patient care in a manner that is patient-centered, evidence-based, efficient, and effective. The challenge this places on the nurse leader is significant. Although this chapter dealt with the two major regulatory and accreditation entities—CMS and JCAHO—they are not the only entities with which the nurse leader must be familiar. Depending on the size and complexity of the organization in which the nurse leader works, more than a dozen agencies may monitor and evaluate operational processes or the quality of patient care services. Other regulatory agencies that monitor essential hospital functions include the Food and Drug Administration (FDA), the Occupational Safety and Health Administration (OSHA), the Equal Employment Opportunity Commission (EEOC), and state licensing boards for various health professions. Nurse leaders also must interact with non-JCAHO accreditation agencies, such as those associated with cancer and trauma programs, medical residency education, and nursing education. Clearly it takes a significant and concerted effort by the nurse leader to remain knowledgeable in the area of regulation and accreditation.

KEY POINTS TO LEAD

1. Discuss the involvement of various levels of government in the healthcare system in the United States.

2. Describe the role of CMS and its CoP in enhancing the quality of care provided in healthcare facilities.

3. Describe key elements the nurse leader must know in regard to EMTALA and the privacy and security sections of HIPAA.

4. Value the role of accreditation in improving healthcare quality.

5. Ponder the role and responsibilities of the nurse leader in ensuring compliance with regulatory requirements in addition to obtaining and maintaining JCAHO accreditation.

Literature Box

PROBLEM/PURPOSE

Hospitals accredited by JCAHO are deemed to be in compliance with CMS's CoP. The purpose of this GAO study was to examine the effectiveness of JCAHO's hospital accreditation process to detect noncompliance with CMS's CoP and validate the appropriateness of granting JCAHO deeming authority.

METHODOLOGY

Drawing from fiscal years 2000-2002 data, the GAO compared findings from state agency reviews or CMS validation surveys of 500 JCAHO-accredited hospitals with the findings from each hospital's most recent JCAHO survey.

RESULTS

Of the 500 JCAHO-accredited hospitals that received a follow-up visit by a state agency or a CMS validation survey, the study found "serious deficiencies" in 157 (31%). Serious deficiencies were defined as a situation that violates at least one of Medicare's conditions of participation. Of these 157 hospitals, JCAHO had failed to identify 123 (78%) as having Medicare deficiencies. More than half of the deficiencies missed by JCAHO were violations related to fire safety and other physical environment requirements.

CONCLUSIONS AND IMPLICATIONS

Failing to identify noncompliance with CMS CoP is of concern to the GAO and members of Congress. To oversee patient safety in hospitals adequately, the GAO believes that Congress should consider giving CMS more authority over JCAHO's accreditation process. Officials from JCAHO responded that although inspectors do occasionally miss problems during their accreditation surveys, they believe that the GAO's study was "based on a flawed study methodology and erroneous, alarming statistics that seriously mislead the public." They point to the fact that JCAHO has announced plans to move to an unannounced survey process in 2006. This move, they believe, will make it more difficult for hospitals to come into compliance just during the time of the accreditation visit. These findings are important to nurse leaders as they may portend even more significant changes in hospital regulatory and accrediting processes. 🖉

Tieman, J. (2004). Critical fallout. Lawmakers call for more oversight of JCAHO. *Modern Healthcare, 34*(30), 8-10.
United States Government Accountability Office. (2004). *CMS needs additional authority to adequately oversee patient safety in hospitals.* GAO-04-850, a report to congressional requesters. Retrieved July 2004, from http://www.gao.gov/cgi-bin/getrpt?GAO-04-850.

Contemplations

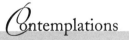

- What is the value of accreditation of your healthcare organization?
- What improvements related to accreditation standards is your organization achieving?

- How does your organization "stay ready"?

LEADER STORY

SHEILA EVERLY
VICE PRESIDENT & CHIEF NURSE EXECUTIVE
MEDICAL CITY DALLAS HOSPITAL
DALLAS, TEXAS

Medical City underwent its JCAHO accreditation visit in June 2004 using the new tracer methodology. My experience made me a fan of the new system and the overall change in the way the survey is conducted.

The reason? The tracer methodology of surveying is much more reflective of the true clinical processes that take place across the hospital. It is a more accurate reflection of the interdependence among hospital staff as patient handoffs occur from department to department. In the past, one could predict the format of the JCAHO visit and make sure that the best communicators represented the hospital. That is no longer possible. Because of the way the tracer methodology is employed, you don't know exactly where a surveyor is going to go, so there is no "up front" preparation. In the new system, you find out which patient the JCAHO surveyor has selected on the way to the unit where the patient is.

I think that's a good thing! It's a much more accurate reflection of the patient care across the continuum. It requires that *all* staff members know *all* the processes and that they *all* know what the JCAHO standards are. And that is why I'm such of fan of the tracer methodology. Innate knowledge about patient care and patient care standards must be a part of the culture for *every* staff member.

At Medical City, the new way of doing the survey gave various members of our staff the opportunity to speak to what they do every day. I saw firsthand the great pride members of our nursing staff took in exhibiting their knowledge and their expertise and in showing how they provide the highest quality of patient care. We were very fortunate with our nurse surveyor, who was the most skilled surveyor I have encountered in the 10 surveys I have been associated with. The way the nurse surveyor conducted the process helped keep the staff members who were called upon more at ease. In the past, the whole interdisciplinary team would be in the room during the interview process, which put more pressure on the individual staff member. This time the surveyor went individually to team members. I'm sure the people participating in the events felt nervous to some degree because they were the ones going through the interviews. That being said, I saw a whole different side to some people who are not our most articulate or outspoken staff members. It was very positive seeing how they handled themselves in the spotlight. One example I remember most vividly was a critical care nurse who was so natural throughout the interview process. She knew everything about that patient and could speak to all aspects of the interdisciplinary process. That is why I believe the survey is much more reflective of what happens every day in patient care.

The key is in how the tracer methodology works. The surveyor picks a patient from a whole list of patients. That patient is tracked or "traced" from entry into the system throughout their stay. In this way, the surveyor really examines what the patient process is like, which is a much more meaningful way to examine the continuum of care than the prior method. The old process was much more fragmented; the new method focuses wholly on communication and the clinical processes. This ensures that national patient safety goals are part of the day-to-day process in the care of the patient.

You might wonder how one prepares for the tracer methodology. A key to our preparation was that we already had a lot of structures in place that we continued to utilize for the survey. Our Quality Management Department carried us through the process with flying colors! We had a team focus on all of the survey—from staff preparation to administration. We are very fortunate that we have a director of Quality Management who provides regular updates to leadership and unit representatives at our monthly Performance Improvement Update meeting. Her goal is to ensure that all of us are survey-ready every day by giving us information on a regular basis over time instead of all at once. These continuous updates throughout the year and a monthly performance improvement newsletter, "The Que," help our staff remain "at the ready." That is essential, especially going forward with the unannounced surveys.

Another one of the ways in which we prepared for the JCAHO visit was to hold practice sessions in various departments to help the staff become comfortable with the new system. Any member of the staff should be able to state what it is they do on a regular basis and how the patient safety goals are achieved. Even though that individual may not have been caring for that particular patient, they know how to articulate the processes. For example, site verification for surgeries is a key process. You will do that for any patient who comes through the OR.

Being survey-ready at all times means you have a structure in place that will facilitate every staff member's education and understanding of the JCAHO survey process. From previous surveys, our staff was already familiar with presenting patients and pulling in the interdisciplinary team in that process. We built on those experiences to prepare for this survey. The structures Medical City has had in place remain in place today and will remain in place on a continuing basis.

By the way, I support the unannounced surveys 100%. It has always been my personal philosophy that in patient care, we do not do things because of any regulatory body. Instead, we think of systems and processes that improve outcomes for the patient because that is the right thing to do. I really don't have much tolerance for the attitude that "we are doing this because JCAHO says we have to."

The chief nursing officer (CNO) must play a key role in all of these processes, leading by example. I would advise my colleagues to embrace the process and to get the leadership team on board with the same enthusiasm. The CNO must model the behavior and approach they want to see in their staff. As CNOs, we must be supportive, set expectations, hold staff accountable, and set staff up to be successful.

If we have done our job in preparing the staff, then we allow them to be successful in the survey. We are doing what we do to improve patient care. Leaders need to be very consistent in that message. That is critical from the leadership perspective.

With proper preparation and a "can do" attitude from leadership and staff, you can look forward to a successful JCAHO survey that showcases the quality of care your patients experience every day.

Chapter References

Cady, R. F. (2003, June). DHHS's final rule on the quality assessment and performance improvement program. *JONA's Healthcare Law, Ethics, and Regulation, 5*(2), 29-31.

Glass, D., Rebstock, J., & Handberg, E. (2004, April-June). Emergency Treatment and Labor Act (EMTALA)—Avoiding the pitfalls. *Journal of Perinatal and Neonatal Nursing, 18*(2), 103-114.

Joint Commission on Accreditation of Healthcare Organizations. (2004). *Facts about shared visions – new pathways.* Retrieved November 30, 2005, from http://JCAHO.org.

Joint Commission on Accreditation of Healthcare Organizations. (2005). *Our mission.* Retrieved Sptember 22, 2005, from http://www.jcaho.org.

Kovner, A. R., & Jonas, S. (Eds.) (2002). *Jonas and Kovner's health care delivery in the United States* (7th ed.). New York: Springer.

LePar, K. (2004, April/June). Quality consciousness... Auditing for HIPAA Privacy Compliance. *Journal of Nursing Care Quality, 19*(2), 105-113.

Longest, Jr. B. B., Rakich, J. S., & Darr, K. (2000). *Managing health services organizations and systems.* (4th ed.) Baltimore, MD: Health Professions Press.

Mason, D. J., Leavitt, J. K., & Chaffee, M. W. (2002). *Policy and politics in nursing and health care.* (4th ed.) St. Louis, MO: Saunders.

Tieman, J. (2004). Critical fallout. Lawmakers call for more oversight of JCAHO. *Modern Healthcare, 34*(30), 8-10.

United States Government Accountability Office. (2004). *CMS needs additional authority to adequately oversee patient safety in hospitals.* GAO-04-850, a report to congressional requesters. Retrieved July 2004, from http://www.gao.gov/cgi-bin/getrpt?GAO-04-850.

20 The Chief Nursing Officer as the Chief Operating Officer

Sharon Pappas

The more removed individuals are from these front-line activities (and, incidentally, from direct hazards), the greater is their potential danger to the system. JAMES REASON

This chapter explores the combined role of chief nursing officer (CNO) and chief operating officer (COO) for a facility. The positive aspects of a combined role and the issues involved with such roles are identified and discussed. How such a role might influence the future of healthcare facilities is also investigated.

DURING THE PAST DECADE, MANY CHANGES have influenced healthcare settings, care providers, and reimbursement. Reduced reimbursement placed physicians in a competitive juxtaposition with hospitals for the healthcare dollar. Ambulatory, investor-owned centers are a common setting for providing less complex care, which leaves hospitals with the most acute, costly patients and significantly reduced profit margins. These changes have culminated in a hospital environment in which reduced margins create a culture struggling to balance productivity and quality. Such cultures design organizational structures around excellent patient care, which requires leaders to focus on clinical and financial processes and outcomes of patient care. The number of departments and whether the hospital is in a start-up or growth phase also influence the organizational structure. When hospital size, scope of services, philosophies, and needs allow, the CNO also may serve as the COO.

THE ROLE OF HOSPITAL OPERATIONS

Operational Responsibilities

The ultimate accountability of hospital operations is delivery of patient care. The daily activities necessary to deliver this product include active involvement in the process and the clinical and financial outcomes of care. A balanced perspective of ensuring effective operations including productivity and quality through the collaboration of multiple disciplines is the role of operations. In addition to operations, these administrators are responsible for vision and strategy. They also must be focused on creating value for patients, staff associates, and physicians by understanding daily operations and the role hospital culture plays in continued success. Healthcare leaders must be able to understand the clinical and financial accountabilities of the operational role. They must possess the leadership qualities to create the culture that delivers on the organizational commitments, and to have strategies for remaining knowledgeable and nimble in this environment of healthcare complexity and continuous change. To accomplish this within the executive team means roles have to be well defined and matched to the talents of the executives.

Historical Perspective

The history of organizational structures in hospitals has been hierarchic and bureaucratic; the hospital operated through policies, rules, and authority. Managers made decisions and employees implemented the decisions. Hospital organizational charts resembled organizational charts found in manufacturing. The charts were linear and defined the chain of command. Over time, as hospitals evolved into nonlinear structures, hospital operations were redefined entirely. Hospital leaders realized that the complex and multidimensional nature of patient care was best achieved through horizontal interactions (clinician to clinician) rather than the vertical (through the chain of command). The fact that many individuals had to interact simultaneously to achieve the best in patient care redefined traditional hierarchic operations of hospitals. This discovery led to the collapse of the traditional organizational structure and to an increased emphasis on the relationships involved in the process of care as opposed to hierarchic relationships. In many institutions, the previous roles of manager and employee have evolved to the point at which workers in the hospital, from the housekeeper to the CEO, have become associates, or "partners," in the business of patient care.

Reinventing hospitals resulted in an overhaul of the corporate, bureaucratic culture, a shift in the control-oriented management philosophy, and a commitment to seeking continuous improvement of operations at all levels (Sherman, 1993). This change required rethinking executive roles and a reinvented model ensured the decision makers had an extensive knowledge of patient care.

CNO as COO: The Balance

In the mid-1980s, a nurse in a large hospital might have been expected to choose between being a clinician and being an administrator. In that era, healthcare could afford a differentiation and segregation of duties. The evolution of healthcare has created a new set of accountabilities for its leaders, which build on clinical preparation and knowledge of the patient care process. Success requires creation of a culture and environment in which those who know most about patient care are the influencers of hospital operations. The leadership roles currently include balancing excellent patient care and fiscal accountability with the ability to engage employees as partners. This is a shift from the single focus on the bottom line. Leaders with strong clinical knowledge have a great advantage in creating this balance. Placing nursing leaders in operational roles can address the complexities of the operational leadership role successfully.

The importance of creating balance between excellent patient care, fiscal accountability, and positive work environment identifies one of the greatest benefits of the dual role of CNO as COO. The dual role is not the only structure that can lead to this balance; however, the dual role does contribute naturally to a balanced perspective (Figure 20-1), because many nurse leaders already think and behave in a manner that balances these three key factors. To operate a hospital solely in a financial model when the core business is quality patient care seems limiting. Meleis and Jennings (1989) related that the practice of nursing administration solely in a business model is analogous to practicing nursing in a medical model. The dual role of CNO as COO is one strategy that can restore a clinical focus to healthcare operations, and it is logical to consider a nurse in such a role. The balance of excellent patient care, fiscal accountability, and a positive work environment best summarizes the requirements of the dual CNO-COO role.

Excellent Patient Care

An understanding of excellent patient care must begin with evidence and the clinical research. Evidence-based clinical practice involves use of knowledge resulting from a synthesis of many sources of information. The sources include

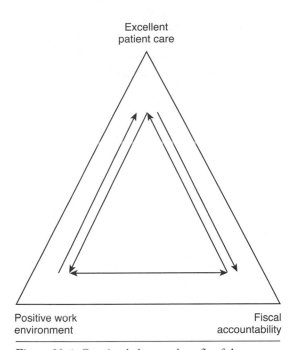

Excellent
patient care

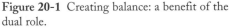

Positive work
environment

Fiscal
accountability

Figure 20-1 Creating balance: a benefit of the dual role.

research, retrospective or concurrent chart review, established standards, data from many sources (quality improvement, risk, infection control, costs, benchmarking), patient expectations, and clinical expertise developed from clinical practice (Goode & Piedalue, 1999). Evidence also emerges from current practice in any setting where the intent is to observe and learn from the daily work. Evidence is the basis of quality patient care.

Those who regulate healthcare and are guided by evidence have established outcomes they believe define excellent patient care. The Joint Commission on Accreditation of Healthcare Organizations (JCAHO) requires public reporting of outcomes for congestive heart failure, acute myocardial infarction, coronary artery bypass grafts, community-acquired pneumonia, lower joint replacement, and pregnancy. The Centers for Medicare and Medicaid Services (CMS) have created incentives for hospitals to report outcomes of these same patient conditions publicly (excluding

pregnancy outcomes). Eventually payment will be based on the results of patient care in these diagnoses, and hospitals perceived this "incentive" as the equivalent of pay for performance. JCAHO and CMS take an outcomes focus to evaluating quality. As healthcare enters a pay for performance era, leaders need to do the following:

- Embrace quality improvement as an essential business strategy
- Be relentless in the pursuit of performance improvement goals
- Give priority to quality improvement infrastructure needs when setting priorities and allocating resources
- Ensure that governing boards and nonclinical management have a working familiarity with clinical quality improvement principles, practices, and performance indicators
- Oversee clinical quality as closely as financial matters, construction projects, and service satisfaction
- Promote adoption of evidence-based care by medicine, nursing, and other disciplines

A business collaborative called Leapfrog set out to identify low-cost, high-quality centers to which businesses could send their employees for needed healthcare. They identified process elements that evidence says will influence quality of care for patients. These elements include computerized provider order entry (CPOE), medical coverage in the intensive care unit by physicians specially trained to care for critically ill patients (hospitalists or intensivists), and evidence-based hospital referrals, including threshold volumes for high-risk procedures (The Leapfrog Group, 2004). As part of the contracting process, many payers request patient care outcome data to make sure their subscribers are channeled to hospitals that provide high quality. In many cases when quality is the priority, the care is subsequently low cost. Although CMS, JCAHO, and other agencies are well-intentioned institutions establishing what the outcomes focus should be, the basis of how to accomplish this work is grounded in the relationships of the caregivers and the environment in which they practice. A JCAHO surveyor identified good communication among caregivers as the most important factor in the prevention of sentinel events (L. E. Kirven, personal communication, August 20, 2004).

The relationships among members of the clinical team play a significant role in patient care. The environment of care including the structures and accountabilities of teamwork are basic to how good relationships are established and maintained. Authorities on Magnet hospitals have identified the significance of nursing and physician relationships and established it as a tenet for nursing engagement and excellent patient outcomes (McClure & Hinshaw, 2002; Ritter-Teitel, 2002). The ability of a hospital operational leader to influence the design of these structures while emphasizing the clinical process is valuable. Many hospitals have succeeded in implementing a triad structure consisting of a business leader, nursing leader, and physician leader with authority and accountability for the success of key hospital services (Weber, 1990). This allows a blending of each perspective in the operation of the service.

Such a balanced operational structure also allows an equalizing focus on performance reporting, which includes service outcomes, clinical effectiveness outcomes, and financial outcomes. Measurement of operational results of care traditionally has been evaluated from a financial perspective at one table and from a quality perspective at another. A balanced organizational structure allows for a balanced evaluation of operational results that analyzes the financial results as they relate to clinical outcomes, caregiver engagement, and patient satisfaction. The CNO as COO is one way to ensure the balance.

Fiscal Accountability

The foundation of fiscal accountability is to evaluate the profitability margin for the hospital and the operating units. Some services operate at considerable profit to provide a significant margin that can balance services in which profits are nonexistent or deficient. Some of these low-margin services often are viewed as community services because they exist to provide needed services to the community where the hospital resides. Simplistically, margins also can be viewed as surplus once operational costs are deducted from what the hospital was paid for the services. This margin is essential to allow for the purchase of high-cost patient care equipment, employee pay increases, improvement of the physical plant, and overall capital growth of services. In the current environment, as reimbursement has declined, most of the excess costs have been eliminated from operations through programs of benchmarking, cost controls, and reengineering. Many of these methods have resulted in immediate gains but have not been sustained because the process of care was not changed. These methods of cost reduction have been approached largely as a financial project with limited focus on the impact on the quality of services.

A financial approach to improving margins often targets productivity by seeking to reduce the costs required to care for each unit of service provided to a patient. Most of the cost comprises labor costs but also includes cost of supplies and other non–labor-related costs. In the inpatient-nursing world, labor costs commonly are expressed as hours per patient day (HPPD), which reflects the nursing hours required for caring for each patient each day of hospitalization. In nursing homes these are hours per resident day (HPRD). An easy target in a financial approach to cost reduction is to focus on labor costs. With the current legislated staffing expectations in some states (Seago, Spetz, & Mitchell, 2004) and the growing evidence relating staffing to patient outcomes (Doran, 2003), a balanced approach to fiscal accountability is more likely to be encouraged by a dual CNO-COO role. The focus of the dual role goes beyond fiscal accountability and includes a focus on value. Value is defined as organizational accomplishments related to the costs of doing the work that achieves those accomplishments. Cost management does not only mean reduction of labor costs. Evaluating the processes of patient care for waste, in time and energy and for redundancy of these processes, adds value to patient care activities and manages costs. The CNO as COO can provide this focus on value.

Positive Work Environment

The dual role of CNO as COO provides a natural affinity for creating quality patient care because the CNO is first a nurse. The nursing background establishes the thought process for decisions about the application of resources, purchases of patient care equipment and supplies, and responses to changes in outcome trends, all with the patient in the forefront. The following question is a natural framework: "What is best for patient care?" When patient care outcomes are trended, the CNO as COO asks the appropriate questions and has a wealth of experience in searching for appropriate answers. The process of routinely asking for problem identification and possible solutions from clinical nurses helps create relationships of trust and engagement between staff members and the formal hospital leadership. One example in which a positive work environment was actualized occurred when clinical nurses were involved in the design of the renovation of their unit. The core support area of the unit was designed to combine the clean supplies and medications into one large room supported by multiple computer terminals. No architectural rendering had identified the need to design services in this manner, and the clinicians were met with strong resistance from the architectural team. However, the clinicians succeeded in obtaining the design, in part because of the clinical focus and understanding of the CNO-COO who influenced the remainder of the executive team. The subsequent change in the architectural design and improvement of the work flow enabled the clinical nurses to spend more time with patients without increasing HPPD. Often architectural designs of hospitals are created without caregiver input and are presented for their approval once plans are complete. In the traditional decision-making model, the work gets done; however, the opportunity is missed for creating a clinical design

that facilitates improved patient care while creating a positive physical work environment. This supports all members of the staff and provides for clinical nurse engagement. The input of the CNO as COO becomes significant in providing the clinical expertise needed for the best possible work space for the team.

The organizational structure also can contribute to associate engagement. A structural process can be created in which nurses and other staff associates feel so supported in their work and in their teams that their job satisfaction is high and they are greatly invested in their patients and their professional roles. In an organization in which the CNO has responsibility for clinical departments in which the main responsibility is not nursing care, a natural horizontal integration occurs. One option for the common scope of responsibilities for the CNO as COO includes nursing departments and other clinical departments such as laboratory, radiology, nutrition, and pharmacy. In the traditional view of separation of nursing departments from other clinical departments, adversarial relationships often were created. In an extreme example, one facility had a hypothetical group that comprised traditional "non-nursing" departments called *SPONGE* (the Society for the Prevention Of Nursing Getting Everything)! The goal was obvious. In the current environment in which mutual respect and support are essential, these values are facilitated by a balanced focus on outcomes with an inclusive team of excellent caregivers. Figure 20-2 provides a comparison of the two models.

THE OPERATING SYSTEM THAT MAKES THE CNO AS COO ROLE WORK

Structural Elements

Several structural elements allow the balanced focus on cost and quality to occur. One element is driven by the belief that those who provide patient care are in the best position to improve the care.

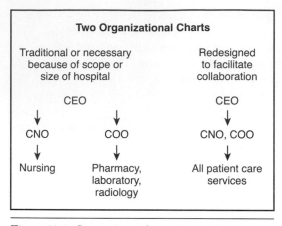

Figure 20-2 Comparison of organizational structures.

This belief is actualized through a flat organizational structure with a minimum of management layers between those providing direct patient care and the executive team. This enables a care environment in which decision making is close to the patient. A focus on what clinical nurses do for patient care and the value of this work overshadows the quantitative aspects of how many hours are required for direct care. Committees and teams work more effectively when they are comprised of individuals who care for patients. These individuals are in the best position to resolve issues and problems that are obvious to the public but invisible to management (Johnson, K., 2004).

A second influential structural element is the time allotted to managerial involvement in patient care. The ability of a manager to participate in unit-level operations at least 50% of the time makes a significant difference in daily operations. The manager's time on the unit facilitates business and clinical assessment and problem solving. It promotes working with clinical nurses, coaching them, and encouraging their personal and professional growth. This style of unit leadership is actually the microcosm of the dual CNO as COO role as the manager balances clinical operations, fiscal operations, and employee engagement.

A third significant structural element is the medical staff structure. Traditionally, the operating structure for physicians included clinical departments such as medicine and surgery; the subdivisions such as cardiology, oncology, and psychiatry; and the hospital-based departments such as radiology, anesthesia, pathology, and emergency medicine. Decision making and problem solving occurred in these departments without involvement from other disciplines. Although each section has a need for confidential medical peer review, this function can be transferred into another forum, and a new model can emerge. The establishment of a clinical excellence committee, including all relevant patient care disciplines, emphasizes patient outcomes, improves teamwork, and results in all participants who provide care becoming involved in the review and improvement of patient care. Some of the results of this collaboration have been the improvement in the care of patients with congestive heart failure because the team of clinicians evaluated the entire continuum of care and all caregivers became accountable for the patient outcomes. The time for a patient with an acute myocardial infarction to transition from the emergency department to the cardiovascular lab was reduced by half because the team focused on the time outcomes, not solely their individual roles in the care.

The Culture: The Individual, the Hospital, and the System

The previous section established three structural elements foundational to the balanced environment. Cultural characteristics also support balanced relationships. The cultural characteristics of the individual, the hospital, and the system play a significant role in whether a balance of excellent patient care, fiscal accountability, and engaged staff can be achieved. It may seem foreign to consider the individual as a component of the culture because the common concept of culture is the milieu consisting of all components operating simultaneously. When the evolution of hospitals is considered, it becomes clear that hospitals must change to sustain themselves as sources of excellent patient care. Therefore the organizational structure had to change, and the activities and processes performed by individuals, leaders, and caregivers had to change.

The Individual

First, the characteristics of each individual within the culture are foundational to the culture. Certain preparation is essential for the individual who occupies a dual CNO-COO role. The American Nurses Association (ANA) established qualifications and standards of professional performance for nurse executives. The qualifications include current state licensure, education, and experience. The nurse executive should hold a minimum of a baccalaureate degree in nursing and a graduate degree in nursing or a program that includes organizational science and management concepts. The nurse executive also should hold certification in nursing administration. Experience should include clinical and administrative practice that has allowed the CNO to draw from many areas of knowledge and research (Box 20-1).

The same ANA standards describe specific responsibilities for the nurse executive that include the following:

- Partnering with other disciplines and leaders for success in meeting patient and organizational outcomes through systems thinking and behaviors
- Acquiring resources essential for safe function and process of patient care in an environment in which priorities must be consistent with organizational strategy and safe patient care
- Ensuring development of policies, programs, and evidence-based practice consistent with standards of the professionals participating in patient care; this requires collaboration and communication among professionals so that the result is excellent patient care
- Being a visionary, strategic planner, change agent, and practice innovator who is always

Box 20-1 EXAMPLES OF KNOWLEDGE BASE OF NURSE ADMINISTRATOR PRACTICE

Care management systems, including measurement of patient needs, outcomes, nursing workload
Consumer healthcare issues
Evidence-based nursing administration
Fiscal management and financial outcome
Health and public policy
Healthcare evaluation and outcome measures
Management systems, processes, and analysis
Nursing research and other scholarly activities
Patient and employee safety
Performance improvement
Professional nursing practice and environment
Standards of clinical nursing practice and best practices
Systems for patient safety
Technologies, including data management
Trends in business practices

Modified from American Nurses Association. (2004). *Scope and standards for nurse administrators* (2nd ed.). Washington, DC: American Nurses Association, p. 10. Reprinted with permission from American Nurses Association. (2004). *Scope and standards for nursing administrators*. Silver Spring, MD: nursebooks.org.

scanning the environment for opportunity to improve patient care and nursing practice
- Being accountable for continuous quality improvement for the entire nursing system and the complex organization where nursing is practiced
- Ensuring nursing participation in decision making related to the culture of patient care and to the practice of nursing

These responsibilities are addressed by collaborating with individuals necessary to perform activities within the structure of the standards of professional performance.

The 2004 Institute of Medicine (IOM) report identifies five essential management practices, which also could be considered leadership talents and practices. These are balancing the tension between efficiency and reliability, creating and sustaining trust, managing the process of change, involving workers in work design and work flow decision making, and creating a learning organization. These practices consistently have been associated with the achievement of a culture that ensures safe patient care (Page, 2004). These practices require a broad range of leadership talents essential to effectively execute the CNO-COO role.

The most recent study of the responsibilities of nurse administrators with the accompanying educational recommendations describes how these are currently being addressed (Krejci, 1999). A convenience sample of 1000 nurse executives belonging to the American Organization of Nurse Executives (AONE) was surveyed. Krejci's study (1999) confirmed that administrator roles for nurses were prevalent, many with accountability for departments that did not provide direct nursing care. Most held master's degrees, some dual master's degrees, and more than 10% held a Ph.D. Those who completed the survey believed a master's in business administration (MBA) was not highly recommended when compared with the master's of science in nursing (MSN). These results indicated the continued need for healthcare leaders and administrators to possess a clinical background to be successful in the current healthcare era. Others believe this background is essential to understand the entirety of what the patient needs and to see hospital services through the eyes of direct caregivers (Matisoff, 2004).

Typical job functions for CNO-COOs follow.

- Provide leadership and inspiration for individuals working to achieve the goals of the organization
- Ensure effective operations and capital utilization to achieve opportunity and fiscal viability
- Ensure excellent patient care

- Develop mechanisms to ensure collaboration among hospital, physicians, and the community board
- Maintain conducive environment for staff
- Lead strategic planning activities to achieve community service and market share

The COO role has been defined in as many ways as there are COOs in the current healthcare world. Largely the COO role is one of ensuring effective daily operations, monitoring volumes, and identifying trends and opportunities for business growth. Individuals with financial backgrounds occupy many COO roles. When this occurs, the natural affinity of the COO is to focus more on the financial aspects rather than on the clinical aspects of operations. When a chief financial officer (CFO) is present on the executive team, the team could become unbalanced, which leaves the clinical operations solely to the CNO, and in some cases the chief medical officer (CMO). The ultimate role of a COO is to maintain the balance of operations between the quality process and outcomes and the financial outcomes.

The relationships and leadership beliefs within the executive team are critical to the culture of the hospital. In addition to the dual role of CNO-COO, organizations have a chief executive officer (CEO) and a chief financial officer (CFO). Leadership styles of these individuals can be enabling if agreement exists in the practices of decentralized decision making. If the style of the CEO is one of command and control and top-down decision making, the ability to create an environment that promotes risk taking, experimentation, and front-line focus is inhibited.

An example of one hospital's lack of alignment of decision-making philosophy occurred in a setting in which the CNO-COO working with one CEO had established environments in which clinicians had autonomy and accountability to make decisions and solve problems about patient care. This CEO transitioned to another position in the company and was replaced with a CEO who made all the decisions himself. The chaos that resulted and the loss of relationships between team members and the executive team were devastating. The executive team was not aligned in their leadership beliefs. The executive team's accountability is to establish the philosophic frameworks related to decision making and leadership among the members to ensure alignment and consistency in execution.

The Hospital

The hospital culture is also key to fulfilling the unwritten contract between hospitals and the communities they serve. The importance of the issue of patient safety has drawn attention from consumers and hospitals. The essential tenet of a culture of patient care excellence is grounded in the organization's ability to nurture healthy relationships among those providing direct patient care. These relationships are foundational to good communication that allows for questions to be asked, errors to be reported, and problems to be solved without intimidation or embarrassment (Page, 2004; Johnson, K., 2004).

In any executive role, CNO, COO, or CEO, the strategic priorities for administrative accountability are clear. In a healthcare system, hospital, or patient care department, the foundation for accountability rests on superior service, clinical excellence, and operational effectiveness accomplished through engaged associates (Centura Health, 2004). The administrative team has accountability for providing an environment that consists of "places with no needless deaths, pain, waits, helplessness, and waste" (Reinertsen, 2004, p. 1; Berwick, 2004).

The System

When the CNO is accountable for nursing or the CNO-COO is accountable for all clinical operations, the leadership characteristics are similar. When the leadership role exists within a single institution versus a healthcare system, different issues are present. Some hospitals are not part of larger systems; they are stand-alone facilities. In these single institutions, most of the work is simplified by the vertical organization with direct connection between components of the care. When a hospital is part of a larger system of hospitals or part of an integrated delivery system of hospitals, home care, long-term care, or physician practices, the complexity increases exponentially. Certain people and departments exist outside the hospital walls that the CNO-COO relies on to be successful in meeting the hospital goals. Excellent relationships and influence among a much larger and diverse group of individuals is necessary for the CNO-COO to operate the hospital. A healthcare system often exists because of the financial benefits and market leverage that result from centralization of services such as purchasing, patient business office, information technology (IT), managed care contracting, and human resources. To be effective in the role at the hospital, the CNO-COO must interact with related hospitals and the centralized, corporate providers to influence decisions that ultimately affect operations at the hospital. Some of the differences between operating within a single hospital and within a hospital that is part of a system are listed in Table 20-1.

THE IMPORTANCE OF THE CNO-COO ROLE TO THE FUTURE OF HEALTHCARE

Monitoring the Pulse of the Industry

The future of healthcare leadership relies on the integration of the business and clinical activities, not simply operating a business, which is the basis of much economic theory. The delivery of healthcare is largely private in the United States and subject to competition. Healthy competition in private systems usually results in improvements in service and quality, and subsequently prices fall. Healthcare competition is different from these traditional economic theories. Those who are not prepared to compete are subject to extensive restructuring or total business failure (Porter & Teisberg, 2004). Improvements in service and

Table 20-1 COMPARISON OF OPERATIONAL CHARACTERISTICS

Single Hospital	Hospital within a System
Simplified relationships among those individuals in the hospital	Multiple and multidirectional relationships among those in the hospital and system
Vertically integrated	Vertically and horizontally integrated
Responsible only for relationships with hospital departments (nursing, lab, radiology, nutrition, pharmacy of one hospital)	Responsible for relationships with hospital departments *and* for common departments horizontally across hospitals (ICU of one hospital to ICU of other hospitals)
Institutional leverage for contracting for supplies and with payers	System leverage for contracting for supplies and with payers
Limited need for standardization because the hospital scale is small	Value in standardization to achieve economies of scale because the system is large
Institutional interests and goals	Institutional and system interests and goals

quality do not guarantee a decrease in the price of healthcare; these improvements could increase costs and thus price. Healthcare in this new model of competition requires that hospitals compete on clinical value. A balance of clinical quality and cost by hospital leaders is essential or the price will escalate, which results in the hospital losing its competitive edge. Clinical knowledge is essential at the executive level, either in the form of a dual role of clinician (CNO-COO or CMO-COO) or in a team with clinical integration, in which each member of the team has direct knowledge of the patient care process.

Nursing

Nurses, including nurse leaders, are fixers. Nurses often practice first-order problem solving, or quick fixes, which provides only instant, short-term remedies. Second-order problem solving is more desirable because it takes action to address underlying causes, thus preventing problems from reoccurring. Often nurses do not participate in second-order problem solving because of inadequate time or sometimes because of lack of ability and awareness (Tucker & Edmondson, 2003) or because the organization does not value

their involvement. Nurses also work from a motivational perspective. Nurses are motivated to fix things patient by patient because they see immediate results and gratification. Motivation, from Herzberg's perspective (1968), says employees tend to be motivated by external factors that act as incentives for one to complete the work. Often employees are driven to accomplish work out of fear of failure or perhaps in the case of nurses, fear of negative patient consequences, those external factors described by Herzberg. When leaders consider the soulful connection of nurses to our work, would it not be more consistent to inspire nurses *rather than* motivate them?

Inspiration is based on love and comes from the soul, an internal factor. If nurses were inspired and equipped to solve patient care problems so that problems were permanently solved, would that get at the soul of the profession and recreate fulfillment for nurses in their daily practice? Nurses are motivated to fix problems on the first order, which results in temporary improvement. This may feed their ego and the problem occurs with the next shift or next patient. Second-order problem solving results from inspiration of a better work environment and help to their team. "What if we could inspire others by appealing to something within them that is far greater that the personality or the ego?" (Secretan, 2004, p. xxviii)

The successful future of hospitals depends on quality patient care and fulfilled nursing professionals. The importance of nursing cannot be ignored and could be at risk if walking the budgetary tightrope is the only focus of hospital leaders. A limited focus on nursing beyond the operational role of direct patient care results in diminished attention to advancing the practice of nursing. Advancing the practice of nursing deserves strategic attention in terms of developing environments in which nurses like to practice, establishing means for nurses to continue their education, and providing adequate staffing in numbers and in competency. In addition the view of nursing as an operational necessity, with attention to the practice of nursing as a strategy to hospital success because of who nurses are and what they do, guarantees the patient focus and caring patient interactions.

Frequently nursing care has been identified as the most significant predictor of patient satisfaction (Otani & Kurz, 2004). Clinical outcomes, financial results, and the satisfaction of those who receive care and services measure the quality of a healthcare organization. The demand for these outcomes is high, and an organization that takes a balanced approach to leadership will be most successful by balancing the clinical and financial talents of its leaders and viewing nursing as an essential component of the business and the strategy. The CNO as COO has a broad organizational perspective and the influence to create this environment that promotes nursing and the fulfillment of the individuals who comprise the nursing culture. The imperative to improve patient care calls on professionals providing care and inspires an organization to seek excellence to see results of settling for nothing short of the results of improved care.

> *Creating the opportunity for your soul*
> *to become an equal life-partner with*
> *your personality.*
> SECRETAN

Healthcare

The changes facing healthcare are unprecedented. Methods and relationships that traditionally have served healthcare leaders well are failing largely because adaptation cannot occur quickly enough for the rapidly changing environment. Those technical solutions that once served leaders well no longer are solutions for complex, adaptive problems. An example of this shift is the notion that increasing pay (a technical solution) would be the solution to nursing retention (a complex, adaptive problem). This shift forces leaders to search for new methods of problem solving that provide adaptive solutions. Dr. John Kenagy, an expert in healthcare process improvement, describes one solution to the future, which allows organizations to be nimble in navigating change. He proposes an Adaptive Design, which offers five essential links that improve the value in the process of providing patient care. Identification of the links creates a positive feedback loop that results in increased operational returns (Box 20-2) (Kenagy, Sundahl, and Udall, 2004). Adaptive Design is further illustrated in a case study of solving a complex problem, one that involved people, systems, and equipment (Box 20-3).

The Challenges of CNO as COO

Challenges of the dual role exist as the CNO-COO works to meet the expectations of the organizational strategy and professional accountabilities. Challenges evolve from the basic notion that the CNO as COO must maintain the delicate balance between support of nurses and support of all disciplines. For example, a challenge exists when individuals such as nurses, pharmacists, and technicians exist who continuously compete for what they perceive as scarce resources for various areas or departments within the facility. It is difficult for them to relinquish the perspective of care provided by individual departments and focus on the system as a whole, as well as patient care outcomes. In the current environment of staffing shortages and intense competition for the limited number of nurses, significant market-related salary increases have occurred for nurses. This has led to internal

Box 20-2   ADAPTIVE DESIGN

- *A new value proposition* is identified close to the work involving known science or evidence.
- *Relevance* creates obvious routine work and practices requiring improvement.
- These two links inform the organization how to *redirect resources* to do what is needed to realize the value of improvement that was identified from being close to the work. The organization employs *problem-solving methods,* which allow experimentation. This results in the realization by the organization of the *new value* from the work.

Modified from Kenagy, J. W., Sundahl, D. L., & Udall, J. (2004). *Delivering on the promise: An adaptive approach to information technology in healthcare.* Retrieved June 1, 2004, from http://www.microsoft.com/Resources/Healthcare/adaptivedesign.aspx.

competition between nurses and other professional groups whose salaries are not increasing at the same rate. The CNO-COO must manage this competition or relationships are destroyed and patient care is affected.

Conversely, when the CNO-COO addresses specific issues outside of nursing as dictated by the operational component of the role, nurses can view this attention to such issues as "abandonment of nurses and nursing issues." The CNO-COO must focus on excellent communication with all aspects of operations and the people who work in these departments to balance these aspects. One strategy for resolving this daunting task is to avoid the tightrope and the balancing efforts and to focus instead on excellent patient care. This is the common ground of all those who practice in hospitals.

One of the key issues regarding a combined position is, "Aren't you doing two full-time jobs? Are you working 120 hours per week?" Clearly considerable overlap exists in the two positions.

In addition, the important emphasis is on how this leader recruits and coaches the people who report directly to the leader, from nursing and the other operational areas. The key is supporting this next level of administration to be wonderful leaders for their specific groups. Some of the more successful CNO-COOs have identified a strong director of nursing who effectively leads the nursing division while working closely with the CNO-COO. Another key intervention is clear communication with all groups in addition to ongoing meetings, which create interaction between the nursing and non-nursing groups. When time conflicts arise, those problem areas that do not contribute to improving patient care can be made secondary to those that do. The ability of the CNO as COO to create a leadership culture that focuses on excellent patient care will support this approach to decision making.

SUMMARY

The combined role of CNO as COO is one way to hardwire excellence in hospitals. The executive desire to ask the Quint Studer question, "We want to make this a better place for you to work. What do I need to do?" (Studer, 2003, p. 13) of all clinicians, including physicians, becomes organizationally innate when effective clinical influence resides at the executive level.

Concerns are warranted with broadening the CNO role to include COO accountabilities. Where the CNO position was transformed from nurse executive (responsible only for nursing) into patient care executive (covering hospital departments in addition to nursing), support to direct care staff declined (Sovie & Jawad, 2001), and a diminished influence of nursing in institutional prioritization and weakened ties between clinicians and administrators occurred (Aiken, Clarke, & Sloane, 2000). These problems are real and can be managed through expert selection of the individual occupying the role and grooming the culture to accept this broadened role. Strong executive mentoring is also essential to allow a CNO to develop the knowledge and relationships essential

Box 20-3   Application of Adaptive Design

CASE STUDY

An inpatient cardiology unit in an urban, acute care hospital was perceived by hospital leaders as one of the best units in the hospital in terms of clinical outcomes and patient satisfaction. Because of the low turnover of staff, this unit was designated as a pilot unit for engaging the clinicians in problem solving and decision making to further improve unit operations. Members of the executive team engaged in the unit clinical operations. The leaders of this unit included a clinical leader who was the nurse manager, the CNO-COO, and physicians who cared for patients on this unit. Observations of the work on this unit were initiated. From the observations, problems were identified (relevance created) and experiments were conducted (resources redirected). Some experiments were successful and some were not. The successful experiments (problem-solving methods) resulted in various improvements, such as improved patient satisfaction with the discharge process, cost savings resulting from the process of medication administration, and improved rescue of patients when complications occurred (new value). These were all results seen immediately when changes were made. The clinical nurses on the unit learned how to effect informed change through collaboration within the unit team. By going to the source of problems they were able to create permanent resolution.

Some of the latent improvements observed on this unit came in the form of their engagement as measured by the biannual staff satisfaction survey. This unit also exhibited better than average retention of nurses. The feedback loop enabled continuous problem identification and experimentation because of the new value created.

The team on this unit deserved all the credit for improving patient safety and care. The involvement of executives, who either held clinical experience and focus or placed themselves in a position to gain clinical focus from observations and learning, enabled change to occur at a faster pace. The trust that resulted from building relationships between hospital executives and those who provided the care guaranteed this pilot would continue and expand and that the changes would be permanent. This unit, perceived to be one of the best, became even better. When the CNO-COO attended one of their unit team meetings to update the group of hospital changes, she witnessed clear nursing engagement. This occurred because the executives developed relationships with the staff and had been involved in the daily operation of this unit. No update was necessary because executives and staff interacted regularly, exchanging information. Instead, the teams spent the meeting time with the CNO-COO, presenting their plan on what they were working on next to improve care.

to the COO role. Internal leadership development programs, including those described by Kowalski (2004), establish the value of leaders spending time with those who report to them. The time includes time with aspiring leaders in groups in addition to one-on-one interaction, which leads to an environment that supports truth, vulnerability, and caring. This development is essential and well suited to nurse executive growth and role expansion.

Many nursing leaders have assumed executive roles. They all came to these positions in various ways. These leaders report mentoring, education, and seizing opportunity as key to their success (Gaskill, 2004). They also report the impact their actions have on patient care as paramount in their decision making. These executive nursing leaders covet their understanding of the work of clinical nurses, because they have lived it and view it as their inspiration.

KEY POINTS TO LEAD

1. Evaluate the role of CNO and COO.
2. Identify the three accountabilities of a clinical leader.
3. Identify key elements of preparation for this combined role.
4. Value the characteristics of a complexity-tolerant culture.
5. Describe features of the future healthcare industry this role will encounter.

Literature Box

Many individuals have succeeded in articulating new ideas about leadership. New ideas frame our current practices in a new way that organizes our greatest strengths to achieve broader influence and effectiveness. Refreshing traditional practices into new paradigms better suited to our changing healthcare and nursing cultures is essential to growth and improvement. One example of bringing forth such a new paradigm is the list of the principles that follow. Leaders who can use these principles as a measure of their own current practices can adjust and improve their effectiveness.

Leaders can become consumed by the daily work to the extent that they lose sight of the organizational potential. The role of the COO focusing on the daily work (including the nursing daily work) and the related complexity could cloud the vision of the future. Given the complexity of healthcare, these 10 principles can assist the leader in maintaining focus separating out those activities that best match the new world of work.

Principle 1: Wholes are made up of parts. Leaders live in the space between connections and they need to be focused on how integration of the parts facilitates the work of the organization.

Principle 2: All healthcare is local. If a healthcare provider is not directly providing care to a patient, the associate is serving someone who is. Patient care is the core business.

Principle 3: Adding value to a part adds value to the whole. Everyone has accountability to add value to the system.

Principle 4: Simple systems make up complex systems. A leader's commitment to the system gives the leader focus and a framework for the work.

Principle 5: Diversity is a necessity of life. If everyone says the same thing and thinks the same way, the truth will not emerge.

Principle 6: Error is essential to creation. Error indicates where someone is on the journey and the only unacceptable error is the error that is repeated.

Principle 7: Systems thrive when all of their functions intersect and interact. The primary job of a leader is to manage relationships and interactions.

Principle 8: Equilibrium and disequilibrium are in constant tension. Absolute stability is the absence of life. Leaders walk the tightrope between stability and chaos and tend to favor chaos.

Principle 9: Change is generated from the center outward. A system will thrive only if those at the point of service own their decisions that are made where they work. Unnecessary structure (including management) can draw resources away from the accomplishment of the objectives and interferes with its ability to achieve success.

Principle 10: Revolution results from the aggregation of local changes. Leaders, as the agents of change, bring the vision and context of change so that the caregivers can develop the content of change.

Porter-O'Grady, T., & Malloch, K. (2002). *Quantum leadership.* Gaithersburg, MD: Aspen, pp. 46-75.

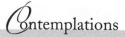

Contemplations

- What is adequate business knowledge for one to be successful in the combined role?
- What is the requisite knowledge of the hospital financial system, budgeting, and decision support needed in this joint position?
- What should the relationship be between this joint position and the CFO?
- What structural elements aid in keeping nursing visible in an organization without a CNO with only nursing responsibilities?
- What mechanisms can be employed to ensure the application of nursing belief system related to decision making and professional standards in patient care areas and the professional environment?

- How is patient safety influenced by a combined role?
- What strategies ensure collaboration among professionals and demand standards of effective communication so essential to patient safety?
- What strategies can be used to incorporate the smooth interaction between nursing, allied health departments, and support departments?
- What role does communication play in the successful implementation of this joint position?
- How is a culture of value and appreciation for every employee created?

LEADER STORY

JOYCE JOHNSON
SENIOR VICE PRESIDENT OPERATIONS AND CHIEF
NURSING OFFICER
GEORGETOWN UNIVERSITY HOSPITAL
WASHINGTON, DC

My vision of leadership is the capacity to deliver a service through others with *passion*. A passion for helping others is the reason that most healthcare workers—nurses, doctors, and therapists—entered their professions. It is my job to see that this passion, compassion, and energy are not siphoned off in coping with logistic issues. The leader must be certain that the staff, at the point of service, have what they need to do their job. This includes resources, policies, a clear and dependable decision-making process, and support. I feel an awesome responsibility to the staff. It is entirely the responsibility of leadership to create the environment in which caregivers (and those who support caregivers) are engaged and nourished in their desire to help our patients. It is such an environment that fosters employees who articulate that they "love being here at Georgetown." Staff and physicians, in addition to our patients, know that Georgetown is where 5000 individuals are energized to pull together to make the impossible happen every day, no matter what. And that's what they do. That is why they come to work. That is why *I* come to work!

WORKING IN A CNO-COO POSITION

There are so many positives to working as a CNO-COO. This role allows me to step back and see a much bigger picture of healthcare and this facility. Years ago, nurses ran the first hospitals. Now we have come full circle and again, nurses are managing the day-to-day operations of many hospitals. Nurses understand the core business, and they understand what patients need when they come to the hospital. They are clear that patients come to the hospital for nursing care.

I believe that women bring a unique skill set to these leadership positions in which they encourage others to participate in decision making and focus on creating teams that address issues and solve problems. An RN in the COO position understands both the business side as well as the clinical needs for patients. And an RN is acutely aware of the critical nature of stabilizing the nursing workforce. Without a stable, skilled nursing workforce, the institution simply cannot survive.

The only potentially controversial side of the combined role is the perception that nursing will be positioned ahead of other employee groups. However, a nurse who is truly a transformational leader understands and has empathy for all employee groups and views them as equally vital contributors to the success of the institution. The nurse COO works diligently to create and sustain an inspirational spirit and pride among all the staff members who work in the institution.

Some may perceive the CNO-COO position as potentially two full-time jobs, but that is not my experience. If the CNO-COO surrounds herself with the best and the brightest team she can find, it is not difficult to integrate the multiple aspects of the position and focus on delivery of patient care at the point of service. It takes courage and wisdom to hire people more skilled than I am in particular specialties and then to put a team together in which strengths and weaknesses are balanced. The team recognizes the strengths of its individual members and the great potential of the team to achieve anything. The only time the joint responsibilities feel extremely challenging is when there is a vacant key position (such as one of the director positions) or if another director is experiencing major problems. At such times I can feel out of touch with the rest of my job and simply run out of time. However, that would happen in any position.

The senior administrative group is structured so that I have a VP for nursing. The CEO is a physician as is the chief of the medical staff. And of course there are other VPs such as finance, information systems, human resources, etc. Having a second nurse on the administrative team gives me added flexibility. There are times when I can actively speak for nursing and other times when, knowing that nursing is well represented, I can step back and consider the "big picture." The VP for nursing is a very strong leader and when there are issues critical to nursing, we can carefully and collaboratively plan how they will be presented.

If a graduate student were interested in pursuing a joint role such as mine, I would have several suggestions. It would be important to first eliminate any sense of awe and mystery about the job responsibilities. I would suggest that the student work in a non–prime-time administrative position such as the evening, night, or weekend supervisor. The supervisor is responsible for the entire house such as nutrition, materials management, and pharmacy, which do not have someone in-house during off-shifts. That is a microcosm of the COO's job. Handling these responsibilities would give the student a realistic understanding of how a system works as well as experience in managing crises. It is well known that, if there is a major problem, the "on call administrator" usually asks the supervisor for guidance. "So what do *you* think you should do?" There are no magic answers.

In addition, education is extremely important. It is imperative that a CNO-COO in a major tertiary facility have doctoral education along with some kind of business training from a leading program such as the Wharton School or Johnson & Johnson. And, the person must have the natural creativity to develop a vision.

I have a story to tell you about working in another facility: an inner-city hospital without many resources. I was attempting to quietly lead a process of transformation of the nursing culture. The organization had a very difficult year in which tens of millions of dollars were lost. There were wide-sweeping changes and reorganization. I knew that I would become responsible for some non-nursing areas and thought they would be patient care related. However, I was assigned to lead multiple support areas such as security, nutrition, and housekeeping. My immediate focus was on spending time in these departments getting to know their daily functions. What I discovered was that the work environments were terrible, and they had been completely ignored for years. I obtained funds for renovating the work areas and purchasing new uniforms. The morale increased in these areas but there was still a very limited sense of team between these employees and the more visible caregiver departments. It was clear to me that unless the staff from patient care areas walked in the shoes of these support people, there wouldn't be change. My position as CNO-COO enabled me to mandate change in both areas. We held off-campus retreats and redesigned the meaning of customer service. Then we organized a job exchange. I worked on the tray line in nutrition. Nurses shadowed with security out in the parking area. Security came into the patient care area and shadowed nurses. Nurses worked with the grounds crew and vice versa. The personal connections made though the job exchange changed the working relationships. The "walls" of the silos started to come down and the entire culture changed. Employees began to respect one another and especially the other person's job. Morale increased. Patient satisfaction increased dramatically. The physicians began to return to the hospital. My support departments became the stars of the institution. The entire culture of the facility changed and we became the lead hospital in the city. It was a huge success story! This CNO-COO position really works.

Chapter References

Aiken, L. H., Clarke, S. P., & Sloane, D. M. (2000). Hospital restructuring: Does it adversely affect care and outcomes? *Journal of Nursing Administration, 30*(10), 457-465.

American Nurses Association. (2004). *Scope and standards for nurse administrators* (2nd ed.). Washington, DC: American Nurses Association.

Berwick, D. M. (2004). *Escape fire: Designs for the future of health care.* San Francisco: John Wiley & Sons.

Centura Health. (2004). *Mission in motion, from the CEO Joe Swedish* (Special Edition) [Brochure]. Denver, CO: Author.

Doran, D. M. (Ed.). (2003). *Nursing-sensitive outcomes state of the science.* Sudbury, MA: Jones and Bartlett.

Gaskill, M. (2004, August 9). Trading places. *NurseWeek, 5,* 14.

Goode, C. J., & Piedalue, F. (1999). Evidence-based clinical practice. *Journal of Nursing Administration, 29*(6), 15-21.

Hertzberg, F. (1968). One more time: How do you motivate employees? *Harvard Business Review, 46,* 53-62.

Johnson, K. (2004). Keeping patients safe: An analysis of organizational culture and caregiver training. *Journal of Healthcare Management, 49*(3), 171-178.

Kenagy, J. W., Sundahl, D. L., & Udall, J. (2004). *Delivering on the promise: An adaptive approach to information technology in healthcare.* Retrieved June 1, 2004, from http://www.microsoft.com/Resources/Healthcare/adaptivedesign.aspx.

Kowalski, K. (2004). Growing future leaders: Developing perinatal managers from within. *Journal of Obstetric, Gynecological, and Neonatal Nursing, 33*(3), 362-380.

Krejci, J. W. (1999). Changing roles in nursing perceptions of nurse administrators. *Journal of Nursing Administration, 29*(3), 21-29.

The Leapfrog Group. (2004). *The Leapfrog Group: Survey results: Patient safety practices.* Retrieved August 18, 2004, from http://www.leapfroggroup.org/consumer_intro2.htm.

Matisoff, A. (2004). Chief nursing officers: A seat at the table. *HealthLeaders, VII*(4), 36-44.

McClure, M. L., & Hinshaw, A. S. (2002). *Magnet hospitals revisited.* Washington, DC: American Academy of Nursing.

Meleis, A. I., & Jennings, B. M. (1989). Theoretical nursing administration: Today's challenges, tomorrow's bridges. In B. Henry, C. Arndt, M. DiVincenti, &

A. Marriner-Tomey (Eds.), *Dimensions of nursing administration* (pp. 7-18). Boston: Blackwell Scientific Publications.

Otani, K., & Kurz, R. S. (2004). The impact of nursing care and other healthcare attributes on hospitalized patient satisfaction and behavioral intentions. *Journal of Healthcare Management, 49*(3), 181-196.

Page, A. (Ed.). (2004). *Keeping patients safe: Transforming the work environment of nurses.* Washington, DC: The National Academies Press.

Porter, M. E., & Teisberg, E. O. (2004, June). Redefining competition in health care. *Harvard Business Review,* 65-76.

Porter-O'Grady, T., & Malloch, K. (2002). *Quantum leadership.* Gaithersburg, MD: Aspen.

Reinertsen, J. L. (2004, January). *A theory of leadership for the transformation for health care organizations.* Retrieved April 19, 2004, from http://www.qualityhealthcare.org/ihi/Topics/Improvement/ImprovementMethods/Literature/ATheoryofLeadershipfortheTransformationforHealthCare Organizations.

Ritter-Teitel, J. (2002). The impact of restructuring on professional nursing practice. *Journal of Nursing Administration, 32*(1), 31-41.

Seago, J. A., Spetz, J., & Mitchell, S. (2004). Nursing staffing and hospital ownership in California. *Journal of Nursing Administration, 34*(5), 228-237.

Secretan, L. (2004). *Inspire!* Hoboken, NJ: John Wiley & Sons.

Sherman, V. C. (1993). *Creating the new American hospital: A time for greatness.* San Francisco: Jossey-Bass.

Sovie, M. D., & Jawad, A. F. (2001). Hospital restructuring and its impact on outcomes. *Journal of Nursing Administration, 31*(12), 588-600.

Studer, Q. (2003). *Hardwiring excellence.* Gulf Breeze, FL: Fire Starter.

Tucker, A. L., & Edmondson, A. C. (2003). Why hospitals don't learn from failures: Organizational and psychological dynamics that inhibit system change. *California Management Review, 45*(2), 55-72.

Weber, D. O. (1990). "Triad management" fosters productivity and financial gains at Moses H. Cone. *Healthcare Productivity Report, 3*(2), 1-6.

CHAPTER

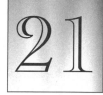 21 Creating Leadership Succession

Today's fast-changing world is demanding of its leaders—from the need for them to pursue seemingly impossible dreams to the importance of on-going training at all levels of an organization, to the opportunity that employees must be given to demonstrate their creativity and be a part of their organization's competitiveness. TOM PETERS

The nursing shortage is not limited to staff nurses; it extends to nursing specialty roles, nursing faculty, and nursing leadership. Because of the costs of recruiting senior nurse leaders and their limited availability, the issue must be considered from a different perspective: one of nurturing, training, educating, and coaching future leaders.

This chapter explores the strategies and benefits of leadership development at multiple levels of the organization, particularly related to nursing. The role of the chief nursing officer (CNO) in developing future nursing leaders is explored.

WHAT ARE NURSE LEADERS DOING TO TEACH, train, mentor, and nurture the future leaders of the profession? In view of the nursing shortage, some healthcare organizations have focused on leadership development and succession planning. A report from the American College of Healthcare Executives (ACHE) found that 21% of hospitals say they have implemented leadership succession planning in their organization. Nearly half of these organizations limited this planning to the CEO (ACHE, 2004). This means that 11% of hospitals nationally are active in succession planning for positions below the CEO level. Most of these facilities are seeking, or have recently obtained, Magnet status and have instituted leadership development and succession planning within the nursing division as a part of that process.

Succession planning is so important to nursing that the American Organization of Nurse Executives (AONE) (2005) included an entire section of the Nurse Executive Competencies on this topic. Their recommendations include promoting nursing management as a desirable specialty. They suggest that periodic organizational assessments be conducted to identify succession planning issues and to establish action plans for identified future leaders. The CNO must serve as a professional role model and mentor to future nursing leaders. The CNO should establish mechanisms that provide for early identification and mentoring of staff members with leadership potential. A succession plan for the CNO position is strongly encouraged.

SUCCESSION PLANNING: A DEFINITION

One of the first realizations for institutions seeking Magnet status is the critical nature of leadership. According to Noyes, McNally, Tourville, and Robinson (2002), clinical and financial outcomes are linked directly to the level of functioning found in the front-line leadership. The American Hospital Association (AHA) Commission on Workforce for Hospitals and Health Systems (2002) recommended the development of a succession plan for every supervisory position and that the most likely internal candidates for each position be identified before the position becomes vacant. Spitzer (2002) described her commitment to discovering methods that create a good succession management plan, which dictates, "Every leader **OWES** the employees and the organization" (p. 217). In other words, to preserve the integrity of the organization, minimally two or three possible replacement candidates must be identified for each leadership position, beginning at the nurse manager position and proceeding through the CNO. The institution is indebted to the nurse leaders for this kind of planning.

A succession plan is an ongoing process of identification, assessment, and development of talent within the organization that ensures leadership continuity for key positions. Garman and Glawe (2004) described a wide variety of activities that involve planning for key transitions within an organization. Early examples are power transitions within families such as royal families and family-owned business empires. Gradually this concept has taken root in the business world in the top positions and at various levels.

The key to the effective creation of a succession plan is the training and development of selected candidates before they are promoted into positions for which they are not prepared (Soares, 2002). Pulce (2002) wrote that internal development programs ensure that highly qualified people are available when positions in the organization become vacant. Such programs ensure continuity and development of the people within the organization in addition to enhancing retention, employee job satisfaction, commitment to work, and the organizational image.

LESSONS FROM THE BUSINESS WORLD

Fortune 500 companies and the business world are far ahead of healthcare in the establishment of programs to meet the needs of developing the future leaders for their organizations.

Even with internal leadership grooming, the business world has not always been successful. Conger and Fulmer (2003) discussed in considerable detail what has not worked in business and how business could improve. For example, Ivester was the chief financial officer (CFO) at Coca Cola for years and was the hand-picked successor. He was forced to resign in 2½ years because of a serious decline in share prices, bad public relations events, and poor handling of a European product contamination scare. Likewise, Mattel toys picked Barad as CEO because of her incredible success with the Barbie doll line. That success did not give her an understanding of finance or strategic planning for the entire company. Neither of these people had mastered the broad, general competencies needed as CEO. Broad, general competencies also are needed in healthcare and are not necessarily inherent in positions other than CEO.

At the same time Conger and Fulmer (2004) looked at successful CEO transitions, such as those at Eli Lilly and Bank of America. They developed some guidelines for success. First it is critical to focus on development. Development does not mean, "Send them off to a workshop." Even when participants return to work energized and enthusiastic, a few days in the "real world" brings them down to earth. Pairing classroom learning with real-life experience and exposing learners to multiple activities and committees is much more effective. "Action learning" pulls together a group of high-potential employees and assigns them to study and make recommendations on an important topic or critical issue for the organization. Leadership learning is stimulated through meaningful, relevant projects with the organization.

Earlier studies by Fulmer and Goldsmith (2001) focused on General Electric (GE), including the activities of the CEO, Jack Welch. Because of GE's success, many corporations have replicated GE's internal leadership development and leadership succession programs.

The business world has been interested in leader succession for some time. Peter Drucker (2002), one of the foremost business authors and researchers, stated that developing talent is business's most important task. This task is at the core of a knowledge-based economy. Likewise, in healthcare, the knowledgeable nurse at the bedside and those who facilitate the work done by staff nurses constitute the core of the healthcare business. The very survival of business and of healthcare institutions depends on the performance of the knowledge workforce (Drucker, 2002). This performance depends on the quality of nursing leadership and how the organizational structure supports and enables the nurse at the bedside to use professional judgment and problem solving to provide the best possible care.

The academic problem is that considerable articles and books address the "practice" of succession planning, but very few research studies exist on the subject, including practically no outcome data from implementation of succession planning programs. What little research that is available are primarily case studies (Garman & Glawe, 2004). Therefore, although succession planning is a great idea and logical for organizations, more research is needed.

One of the logical reasons for addressing succession planning comes from some existing data. Nelson (2002) surveyed 1500 employees to discover if any business incentives were more important to them than money. He reported in the *Washington Business Journal* that learning opportunities

topped the list. Learning translated into gaining additional skills and knowledge that added to the employees' worth and marketability. The generation X and Y workers were particularly interested in learning. They wanted to learn, grow, and develop. They also wanted to choose their work. Raines (1997) believes that people who are given choices often exceed performance expectations because of the power of choice. Therefore these young workers who chose specific work choices such as flexible hours and time off frequently exceeded performance expectations. In healthcare, this may be part of the motivation for the widespread use of 12-hour shifts.

The next group of responses indicated that employees wanted acknowledgment, including oral, public, and written praise. Workers also wanted increased autonomy and authority in their work. One of the more interesting findings indicated these young workers wanted time with their manager or leader. This request for time with a manager may be about the need for validation and inspiration in addition to the opportunity for a "teaching moment." That could include communicating, answering questions, or just listening to each other.

Most people are aware of the obvious success of GE. Since the early 1970s when Walt Mahler, Director of Executive Development, established the model for leadership development, the program has been tied to management responsibilities (Kehoe, 2001). In other words, the training has been action oriented and linked to important organizational projects and initiatives. The learning environment has been created through on-the-job experiences dedicated to solving real business problems. In studying GE and their internal leadership development program, Fulmer and Goldsmith (2001) discovered that Welch devoted as much as 30% of his time to leadership development. Such an approach exemplifies why Welch changed the 1960s GE motto, "Progress is our most important product," to "Leaders are our most important product." Before his retirement, Welch's replacement, as an inside candidate, had been groomed and developed to be CEO. The other two internal candidates were immediately hired by other Fortune 500 companies for CEO positions.

GE begins at the base of the pyramid, identifying leadership potential in its people. The guidelines for the development program are based on the GE values statement and are used by the development department to construct six courses. The beginning program focuses on entry-level employees and goes through the various levels to senior management. A key goal is behavioral change. Feedback/assessment tools completed by subordinates, peers, and supervisors are used before participants enter the courses, immediately after, and again at 6 months after the course to determine long-term effects. In addition to GE, other companies that have extensive internal development programs include Hewlett Packard, Shell Oil, Johnson & Johnson, and the World Bank.

From research conducted by Goldsmith and Morgan (2004), leadership development clearly is not focused on the importance of an "event" or an inspiration or transformation that occurs in a seminar or meeting. Rather, it involves a process that occurs over time and includes ongoing work and feedback. Goldsmith and Morgan have collected data on eight major companies, following these groups over time. The companies that excel at developing leaders also achieve higher long-term profitability. In addition, they found that leaders who asked for and received feedback from colleagues and peers were perceived to be changing their leadership in positive ways. Clearly, business is taking the leadership question very seriously and devoting time and significant monetary resources to the issue.

Many organizations begin development with identifying a pool of potential leaders, people who have some abilities and a desire for leadership. These companies also identify leadership competencies at each level. It is critical to know what the goal or objective is for leadership behaviors. Although learning may occur in groups, particularly at the entry levels, mentoring and coaching are primarily individual.

Structured leadership development programs are focused on improving the skills of front-line managers. Often this skill set is focused on such tasks as finances, budget preparation, interviewing and hiring, performance evaluations, and conducting quality reviews. These are very important skills and for the most part are focused on managing the status quo rather than leading into the future. In many business organizations, leadership skills are a more advanced level of preparation. In healthcare, fortunate new nurse managers find a mentor who will help, nurture, and support them in finding resources for leadership development. Even then, gaining skills and experience is often inconsistent or occurs through trial and error.

RATIONALE FOR INTERNAL DEVELOPMENT

The Cost of External Recruitment

If no concerted effort exists to institute programs for internal leadership development, replacements from outside of the institution must be recruited, and the recruiting firm costs for obtaining an experienced person are exceedingly high. Furthermore, if the newly recruited leader does not work out, the process begins again, while the costs are mounting and the responsibilities of that position suffer. Kosel and Olivo (2002) revealed in the Voluntary Hospitals of America (VHA) report that it costs approximately 100% of a staff nurse's salary to fill a vacant staff nurse position, and that translates into $45,000 to $65,000. Search firms charge from 30% to 50% of the first year's salary for placing a nurse executive of various levels. Using these figures as a guideline, it becomes clear how expensive it is to replace leadership people. If, instead, nurse leaders coach and train from the inside, the pros and cons of each leadership candidate are clear. It is often helpful to know strengths and weakness at the beginning of a venture rather than discovering major problems after the hiring and orienting have begun.

Nursing Shortages and Leadership Positions

An impending nursing shortage, fueled by an aging workforce and declining student enrollments, makes a strong business case for preparing for the future.
SMITH (2002, p. 237)

Leadership development, particularly within organizations, is especially critical in view of the nursing shortage. Most nurses are aware of the impact of the aging RN workforce during the next 5 to 15 years (Buerhaus, 2001). The RN workforce is aging more than twice as fast as other occupations in the U.S. workforce. From 1983 to 1998, the number of RNs under the age of 30 decreased by 41% compared with a 1% decrease in the workforce overall (Buerhaus, Staiger, & Auerbach, 2000). As all the nurses in their fifties begin to retire after 2010, the nursing shortage will reach crisis proportions. At the same time, the demand for nurses will continue to increase as the baby boomers retire and the need for services for this aging population increases. The demand for nurses will continue to increase because of general economic growth, policy changes that expand access to care, greater use of technology and the Internet, and expansion of the older population (particularly women) who are living longer than any previous generation (Buerhaus, 2001).

Although most of the nursing shortage data are more general and apply to nursing from a broad perspective, front-line and middle management positions experience proportional vacancies as exist for staff nurses. In addition many positions are filled temporarily or have been filled with "draftees," nurses who were begged to take the position. Some succumbed because they were willing to assume the position rather than for the position to continue vacant. In the Canadian Nurse Advisory Committee report (2002), staffing shortages and age of the workforce in Canada were found to be similar to those in the United States, whereas the age of Canadian front-line managers was similar to faculty ages in the United States.

Specific leadership data were not found for the United States but are, no doubt, very similar to Canada. This would suggest that RNs in leadership positions, because of their age, will retire nearly 5 years earlier than staff nurses, which makes the leadership crisis even more eminent. The business literature demonstrates that despite the economic difficulties, a 33% turnover is expected for management positions in the next 5 years in Fortune 500 companies, and in excess of one third of the positions are not expected to have suitable replacements (Clark, 2001). The projections certainly are no better for nursing.

Influence of Leadership on Staff Nurse Retention

The Joint Commission on Accreditation of Healthcare Organizations (JCAHO) report *Health Care at the Crossroads* (2002) and the report *Magnet Hospitals Revisited* (2002) make a strong case for the importance of front-line leadership in staff nurse retention. Abrams (2002) reports that *90%* of nurses who were dissatisfied with their leaders and managers were thinking seriously of leaving the unit or the facility. A recent survey of nurses conducted by the Bernard Hodes Group and *Nursing Spectrum* magazine, as reported by AHA News Now (2003), found these top three reasons for why nurses are working in their current facility: a better work schedule (46%), opportunities for growth (39%), and a shorter commute (31%). The respondents also were asked for the reasons they left their previous facilities, and they reported not feeling valued (39%), little or no growth potential (33%), not enough staff (33%), lack of confidence in management (31%), and lack of respect (30%). If units or areas of an institution have strong front-line leaders who interact with staff, support them, demonstrate good coaching and problem-solving skills, and are fair and help staff members in their own professional development, turnover is frequently low. If these front-line managers are growing and learning because that is the focus of the administrative leadership team, the entire milieu changes in the facility. Clearly, the cost of external recruiting, the difficulty in finding strong candidates for leadership positions, and the powerful influence they have over nurse retention mandate that internal leadership development be improved significantly. Even more important, the CNO must be the driving force in conceptualizing and implementing leadership development for his or her people.

FRONT-LINE COMPETENCIES

As competencies are being developed for leaders at all levels of organizations, one content area that is appearing in more and more position descriptions and lists of competencies is an area that addresses talent development. This is the area that will be most needed in the next decade. Many nurses chose administration because they have a commitment and passion for nurturing and supporting their nurses to grow, learn, and develop in the profession in addition to their clinical area of choice. To put this in perspective, the reader should consider the AHA publication *In Our Hands* (2002), which identifies 11 areas of leadership competency at the nurse executive level or senior service line manager level (Box 21-1). All of these areas of competency are important regardless of the level of leadership. Novice leaders are working toward competency in these areas.

In many organizations across the country, the traditional hierarchic nursing leadership structure is shifting its appearance. Some structures have a CNO and service line leaders in specialty areas such as women's services, oncology, and cardiac services. In many instances the service line leaders are responsible for development of their people. The necessary skills are the same as for other more traditional nurse executives and range from skilled communicator and change agent to personal integrity and talent development. Outlining these competency areas seems overwhelming. For a nurse executive to excel in all 11 areas seems more than overwhelming. However, one area that cannot be delegated and cannot be ignored or delayed is the area that focuses on developing the people

who report to the leader. This interest and concern in development improves morale and prepares the next generation of leaders for the organization. In addition, it provides strong help and support to those nurses who are learning leadership skills and who can then assist the leader in other areas.

The talent development competency includes such responsibilities for the CNO as providing a balanced and growth-oriented assessment of those reporting to the CNO. This involves matching employees' strengths with appropriate jobs, providing timely and constructive feedback, arranging appropriate special projects that promote learning new skills, providing support, and actively developing talent and career paths while addressing the long-term needs of the facility (Box 21-2). Although this list was originally created for the CNO level, many aspects apply to unit leaders working with charge nurses and staff members.

AONE (2005) established competencies that are critical for nursing leaders, and several competencies contribute to leadership succession. The areas of importance for which managers at all levels must demonstrate competency include communication and relationship building, knowledge and understanding of the healthcare environment, leadership, professional behaviors, and business skills.

The area of *communication and relationship building* focuses on effective communication particularly as it pertains to relationship development and maintenance with staff as well as with physicians, other professionals, and academic relationships. It also includes the ability to influence the behaviors of others and to honor issues of diversity. These skills can be demonstrated with community involvement.

Knowing and understanding the healthcare environment includes knowledge of clinical practice, patient care delivery models, healthcare economics, and healthcare policy. The leader understands issues of governance, evidence-based practice, and outcome data, particularly as it applies to patient safety concerns. The areas of utilization management, quality improvement, and risk management are also essential to improving the care environment.

Box 21-1   Leadership Competencies

Skilled Communicator: Creates an environment of mutual trust and respect; communicates both orally and in writing and demonstrates active listening; confronts communication breakdown skillfully; holds front-line managers and other professionals accountable for handling communication breakdowns in a nonjudgmental manner; models these same skills

Team Builder: Hires, retains, develops, and promotes talented people while building team spirit; unites the team with consensual and clearly defined mission, vision, and corresponding measurable goals

Agent for Change: Challenges traditional patient care practices and actively pursues positive changes; utilizes research-based and evidence-based practice; is current in clinical knowledge and aware of clinical and administrative advances; models desired behavior for staff and other leaders

Commitment to Service: Demonstrates a willingness to serve patients, staff, co-workers, physicians, the organization, and the community

Collaborative Relationships: Models collaboration with others; works in interdisciplinary teams for the benefit of the organization as a whole

Resource Management: Effectively manages human, financial, technologic, and other key resources of the organization

Results-Oriented: Has well developed business skills and acumen in managing for results in key areas such as clinical quality, service excellence, people management, and financial management

Analytic Thinking: Takes a step-by-step approach to problem solving; manages difficult situations by chunking them down into small pieces; performs systematic comparison

Personal Integrity: Demonstrates actions consistent with what she says or promises; communicates ideas and feelings openly and directly; demonstrates character, openness, and honesty, and requires the same from others

Talent Development: Demonstrates a genuine commitment to foster the growth and development of others in clinical, programmatic, and managerial ways

Leadership Effectiveness: Creates and acquires support for a shared vision and mission for the nursing division or the service area

Modified from American Hospital Association Commission on Workforce for Hospitals and Health Systems. (2002). *In our hands: How hospital leaders can build a thriving workforce.* Chicago, IL: Author. Reprinted with permission from American Hospital Association. Copyright © 2002.

Necessary *leadership skills* include the ability to think clearly and use systems approaches while effectively managing change. A key issue in this category is effective succession planning for the team. All of the competencies are dependent upon the leadership evident in initiating a personal journey of self-discovery and self-reflection.

The area of *professionalism* includes personal and professional accountability, career planning for self and other members of the team, demonstrable ethical decision making, evidence-based clinical and management practice, and advocacy for patients and nurses. The leader must be actively involved with professional associations.

Nurse leaders need *business skills*. They must understand healthcare financing, marketing, human resources management and development, and strategic planning and management. A clear understanding of the importance and function of information technology (IT) and its management becomes increasingly important with each passing year.

Box 21-2   KEY ELEMENTS IN THE TALENT DEVELOPMENT COMPETENCY FOR THOSE WORKING DIRECTLY WITH OR REPORTING TO THE CNO

Provides a balanced and realistic assessment of an individual's strengths and developmental needs and includes formal assessments such as a 360 review (one that seeks feedback about performance from those who report directly to the CNO, peers, and superiors)

Matches an employee's strengths with the needs of a position or task and makes assignments accordingly. This includes work that matches all the person's strengths and is easy for him/her, or it could be work that activates the full learning mode because the position is one in which the leader trainee has many areas requiring growth

Provides timely and specific suggestions as a part of feedback, with the intent of improving performance; acknowledges successes; and focuses on improvements;

this feedback may need to be more frequent if it is a task with a steep learning curve

Arranges appropriate and helpful stretch assignments, formal training, and other experiences such as specific projects for the purpose of fostering a person's growth and development

Provides needed support to buffer the individual from possible failure

Works with the immediate team to build long-term career plans

Participates in and fosters discussions aimed at developing talent to meet the long-term needs of the organization

Develops talent, including support for moving people to other areas of the organization to support their growth, even when doing so creates a stretch situation in the vacated position

Specific planning is critical if the list of behaviors associated with talent development or with AONE's general competencies is to be implemented effectively. The plan necessitates frequent, regular meetings with the immediate team. Many CNOs find it valuable to meet weekly or biweekly with these individuals. The meetings need to be conducted in a structured manner so that progress can be documented clearly. Numerous models and tools exist for facilitating these meetings. One example can be found in Box 21-3. In this format, the Personal Management Interview (PMI), each of the nine categories is reviewed and discussed. Comments ought to be made after each category, particularly if action items are associated with it. The initials of the person responsible for the action item go beside the designated action. The form can be replicated so that the leader and the nurse each have copies, or it could be computerized during the meeting and then sent to the other person. Either way, this series of written action items and

comments makes an annual evaluation a simple project. If ongoing discussion, interaction, teaching, and special projects are not documented in a timely manner, it is unclear how an annual evaluation can contribute to the personal and professional growth of the nurse.

EDUCATION AND TRAINING

Education plays a major role in the success of succession planning programs.
SMITH (2002, P. 238)

Soares (2002) reported on the development of succession planning at the North Bronx Healthcare Network. They first identified key leadership criteria, including skills and competencies and such objectives as customer satisfaction on the part of patients, physicians, and other staff members. Next they screened for future leaders through

Box **21-3**   Personal Management Interview (PMI)

A regularly scheduled meeting (weekly is preferred) occurs between the leader and each member of his/her team. These meetings are critical to the growth and development of each person. Detailed notes are kept on all action items. This is best done on a form that enables both people to have a copy of the items at the end of the meeting; action items can be entered via computer so that both have a copy.

The first few minutes of the meeting are devoted to follow up on the items from the previous meeting.

Areas of discussion include the following:

- Administrative and organizational problems (any resulting action plans are noted)
- Follow-up on the Developmental Action Form (progress reports on any activity devoted to or connected with the growth and development of the team member)
- Any interpersonal problems that may exist between the leader and the team member (open and honest discussion of any communication breakdowns, or other related problems)
- Information sharing (to bring both participants up to date)
- Any individual and organizational needs (for either person)
- Discussion of at least one success and/or achievement (by the team member)
- Any personal problems that affect either person
- Coaching session (leader coaching team member)
- Review staff coaching sessions (team member has had with his/her staff)

Detailed notes are kept on all action items and coaching. (See Chapter 11 for more detail.)

Modified from Boss, W. R. (1983). Team building and the problem of regression: The personal management interview as an intervention. *The Journal of Applied Behavioral Science, 19*(1), 67-83 and Kowalski, K. (2004). Growing future leaders: Developing perinatal managers from within. *Journal of Obstetric, Gynecologic and Neonatal Nursing, 33*(3), 362-370. Reprinted with permission.

understanding the staff member's talents, aptitudes, and interests. In many organizations, this is done with the assistance of human resources (Soares, 2002).

At the University of Pittsburgh Medical Center (Wolf, Bradle, & Nelson, 2005), they assess the readiness of nurses to enter the Beckwith Fellows Program through such testing as the Global Leadership Inventories battery and simulations of realistic leadership situations. These provide detailed performance analyses of the candidates. This results in a comprehensive, user-friendly development guide with specific activities, exercises, tips, and readings for how to improve performance. The entire process is based on identified competencies.

After candidates have been identified at the North Bronx Healthcare Network and the University of Pittsburgh Medical Center, education and practice experiences are aligned with the corporate culture and values. Generally speaking, it is important to measure results and to reinforce desired behavior through education and development wherever the succession planning efforts are proceeding.

In the business world, internal training and development are tied to projects so that learning is experiential. Soares (2002) describes some of the projects that evolved out of the leadership development efforts at the Bronx facility:

- Implementation of a follow-up process on patient complaints
- Implementation of policy, procedures, and guidelines for close observation
- Implementation of an improved patient discharge process

- Consolidation of corporate titles and job functions
- Implementation of an electronic medical record, including on-line
- Documentation of such tasks as nursing admission and order entry
- Revision of the critical care units' orientation process

The important aspect of this process is to use projects that are important to the facility in the development of leadership skills. These projects are not just busywork.

At the Beckwith Institute, Wolf et al. (2005) developed a core curriculum that is delivered over a 2-week period of intense classroom sessions and integrates didactic learning, dynamic role plays, case studies, and other interactive exercises designed to help learners apply new knowledge and skills to the work setting. The courses include content on transformational leadership, strategic planning, decision making, developing people, innovation and change, and healthcare economics.

In both of these programs a critical issue is follow-up and mentoring. Every effort has been made to follow these leadership learners, including a monthly 2-hour session that has presentations by the learners/fellows and impromptu or "on-the-spot" learning sessions by the instructors. The mentors are usually executive-level leaders and are selected on the basis of subject matter expertise. They guide from a behavioral and developmental perspective.

On a more general level, a tool that can be used to map the progress of the developing leader is found in Box 21-4. This development plan is divided into two parts: the plan and the results. Identifying the developmental goal for the learner that will be facilitated by this activity or project is helpful. By completing the form, the learner is encouraged to do more "in-depth" thinking and consideration of the plan and then the results as the person progressed through the plan toward the goal. If the form is completed on the computer, it is easy to change as additional thoughts and insights are developed. It is also easier to make notes on the results as progress or the process evolves.

Making certain the tool has been completed is one form of follow-up.

Follow-Up

Educational classes, workshops, a system-wide program such as the Beckwith Institute, or even a formal academic degree is appropriate and necessary. However, if nothing happens or no change results from the added knowledge, the process was likely a waste of time. As at the North Bronx Healthcare Network and the University of Pittsburgh Medical Center, the most powerful tool at the disposal of a teacher or leader is *follow-up*. According to Noyes et al. (2002), post-program connections can be maintained through advanced or follow-up classes. The ongoing relationship with a sponsor, mentor, or leader, as well as e-mail and telephone contact, are critical to success. During person-to-person follow-up sessions, the leader has the opportunity to assess how the knowledge or learning is being used to change behaviors, processes, or outcomes. In other words, how has the person put learning into practice? The leader can assess the use of learning through asking questions about implementation or having the learner tell a story or give an example about the application of new learning. More important, the expectation is established by the leader that new knowledge promotes personal growth and improves the work environment for other staff members and thus improves the quality of patient care.

Training Options

Smith, who is Director of Nursing Education at North Shore Long Island Jewish Health Systems, reports on the Center for Learning and Innovation and the effort to create a learning organization that focuses on leadership development as a major thrust in succession planning at all levels (2002). The development program is focused on the core values of excellence, teamwork, integrity, caring, innovation, and customer focus. This educational process plays a major role in the organization's succession planning just as it does in the North

Box 21-4 Sample Development Action Form*

Name: _____ Date: _____

Position/Title: _____

Department/Unit: _____

I. DEVELOPMENTAL PLAN

Goal. Identify one major developmental goal, such as a specific role challenge, organizational knowledge needed, competency, or a problem behavior. Add clarification and detail as needed. More than one goal can be listed if they can be addressed by the same action. Explain how development in this leadership skill or area will enhance success in your current position:

Descriptive Process. How will learning be obtained if required (e.g., coaching, observation, training program, advanced academic preparation, membership on a committee)?

Behavioral Description. Define the support needed to accomplish the learning.

Application. How will the development goal be applied in your current position? (Be specific [e.g., project, person(s), or group].)

Required Support. Define the support and follow-up needed to apply the developmental goal or learning.

Tracking. How will intermediate achievements or learning be tracked (if appropriate)? (When should the next meeting with the manager/mentor be held?)

Completion Plan. Specify the date for completing the application of the development goal or learning and describe how you will document accomplishment of learning.

II. DEVELOPMENTAL RESULTS

Acquisition. Evaluate the acquisition of the learning by both yourself and mentor/supervisor. If learning goals weren't met, list the reasons why.

Modified from Byham, W. C., Smith, A. B., & Paese, M. J. (2002). *Grow your own leaders: How to identify, develop, and retain leadership talent.* Upper Saddle River, NJ: Pearson Education.
*Because this format is open ended, it can be computerized and as much space as needed can be devoted to each question.

Continued

Box 21-4   Sample Development Action Form*—cont'd

Application. Evaluate the application of the behavior, skill, or knowledge. If application goals weren't met, list the reasons why.

Learning. What did you learn about developing your skills and knowledge or by changing your behavior?

Future Application. Probable future application of the newly learned behavior, skill, or knowledge:

Additional Learning. What additional knowledge or skills were obtained?

Process Evaluation. What could have been done to make the development process more efficient, effective, or rewarding?

Insights. What additional insights into leadership or management did you acquire?

Modified from Byham, W. C., Smith, A. B., & Paese, M. J. (2002). *Grow your own leaders: How to identify, develop, and retain leadership talent.* Upper Saddle River, NJ: Pearson Education.
*Because this format is open ended, it can be computerized and as much space as needed can be devoted to each question.

Bronx Healthcare Network and the Beckwith Institute in Pittsburgh.

Although the business world and the examples shared in this chapter have a structured and leveled approach to development, in which people are screened, trained, and then promoted, the nursing division of most facilities is not quite so organized or financially endowed in the approach to development. It might be helpful to extrapolate from business and these three healthcare models to design an example of a model for nursing services, using fewer resources.

A MODEL

This model* has four levels, beginning with an entry level for specified staff nurses and culminating in the nursing leaders who desire to be CNOs.

*The Span © (Succession Planning for Administration in Nursing). Copyright: 2005 by Kowalski, K., & Yoder-Wise, P.

Something like this may be appropriate for the CNO who is just beginning to work on succession planning for his or her division. The beginning-level classes may be taught by the CNO and the director group. This could increase the presentation skills of the leadership group and afford close interaction with some staff they may not otherwise see frequently.

Level I

Many facilities or systems have some type of entry-level management training program that includes the nuts and bolts of management. Such programs target charge nurses, new unit managers, or the team members of a more experienced leader, who is focused on facilitating the learning of the staff. For example, Krugman and Smith (2003) write about developing a permanent charge nurse role for which training was very specific, including many of the topics described here. Obviously, just sitting in the class for a couple of hours is not very useful. The most important part of the course and one that is frequently overlooked is coordination of classroom activities with experiential learning on the units. If these classes are structured in 2-hour sessions each week, there is an entire week in between classes for the participants to work with their leaders in practicing what was presented in class.

Examples of course content and experiential learning assignments are found in Table 21-1. The goal could be to have each class coordinated with the nurse manager/unit leader. Ongoing meetings could be scheduled between the class members, instructors, and unit leaders to assess how learning is progressing. Emphasis is on a skill set rather than a didactic lecture that produces questionable outcomes. In consideration of what is known about adult learning theory, assessing whether the participant remembers the content of the class is not useful. Rather, assessing how the content is put to constructive use is most helpful.

Level II

This might be a more advanced course and focus on a critical issue such as relationships. The workplace needs ever-improving relationship skills between staff and patients and families. Difficult patients and family members or very difficult situations, in which bad news must be delivered, are always a consideration. In addition, novice leaders need skills and tools to help with interstaff relationships, such as those between different shifts on the same unit, or between units who frequently transfer or receive patients from each other. Relationship issues can exist between nursing units and other departments such as pharmacy and radiology, or relationship issues can exist between staff and certain physicians. This kind of course could contain content such as the following:

- Advanced communication skills
- Active listening
- Models for communication and relationship building (e.g., differentiation model and triangulation model)

- Understanding of specific aspects of relationships that work and those that do not
- Conflict management
- Management of difficult people
- Communication of ideas in writing and verbally (the art of persuasion)
- Rules or agreements that support positive interactions: how they are created, how they are supported, and how others are held accountable

Again, the most important aspect of the course would not be the didactic content but the practice. It is critical to practice the skills and tools learned regarding all of the SPAN level topics. Unfortunately for the institution, communication and relationship breakdowns occur every day. Any of these problems or breakdowns can provide an opportunity to practice a different approach discussed in class. Such efforts would be reviewed in detail by the supervisor and the course participant with a focus on what worked and what did not, and what the next steps might be. Work on these issues can help a more advanced nurse (from the Level III program) by giving him or her an opportunity to coach the less-experienced nurse in these concepts and principles.

Level III

This could be a course that focuses on coaching. This can be a healthy, positive, and enabling process that develops the ability of staff members and front-line leaders to solve the problems in healthcare systems that frustrate and immobilize them. Coaching provides feedback regarding what has worked in communication and relationship development in addition to what did not work. It is possible to create a situation in which most professional staff members have a coach. Content could include the following*:

- The foundation for coaching: common knowledge and agreements

*Modified from Crane, T. G. (2002). *The heart of coaching: Using transformational coaching to create a high-performance culture.* (2nd ed.). San Diego: FTA Press.

Table 21-1 Succession Planning for Administration in Nursing: Level I Management Training Course

Class Content	Possible Assignments
Introduction to the course	
Identification of personality style in the workplace, using an acceptable tool (e.g., Personality Profile, Myers-Briggs)	People can complete the exercise and discuss results, and they can use a simple version of the tool for the rest of the staff
Interviewing skills	Organize and lead the next staff nurse interview process
	Prepare other staff members for the process

Basic budgeting and finance, including the following:
  Reading and understanding the monthly reports
  Gathering monthly data to submit
  Identifying potential problem areas
  Completing budget preparation
	Involve the trainee in reviewing next month's financial report, including data collected and sent and interpretation of results

What leaders do: An extensive discussion of what leaders do, including leader competencies	Assign one or two staff people to the trainee and have the trainees focus on the demonstration of leadership skills and competencies with these staff members
Discuss the practice of self-reflection	Have trainee practice self-reflection (perhaps through journaling) and discuss observations
Leaders vs. managers: Differentiate between the behaviors seen in the two skill sets	Have trainees write or discuss the differences between the two, giving observed examples of both; find the value in both skill sets
Evaluations and counseling skills	Have the trainee practice giving a hypothetical evaluation and then give an easy one to someone who would report to the trainee
	Discuss how to do a more difficult evaluation
Basic communication skills	Develop practice sessions to be done with each other (trainees)
	Practice with other staff members and report back or debrief with the instructor and classmates about how the exercise went (positive aspects and negative aspects)
Negotiation skills	Set up practice sessions for trainees, and after these sessions, have trainees attempt these skills with staff or other departments (leader should be with them for external departments or physician negotiations)
Required regulatory issues, such as JCAHO Medicare-Medicaid rules and regulations, DRGs, standards of care, practice guidelines	Have trainees chair subcommittees for these important areas
	Review standards and guidelines
	See how they apply to the unit
	Focus on any updates
Conducting creative staff meetings	Manage a staff meeting
	Create an agenda
	Emphasize creativity
	Learn something
	Have fun

- Criteria for selecting a coach
- The coach's job description
- Initial process: establishing the connection in the relationship; understanding any delegated responsibilities; observing performance; preparing for the coaching session
- Creation of mutual respect, learning, and insight, including requesting permission, offering feedback, actively listening, sharing personal experience, and using discussion to gain insight
- Construction of an action plan, including reinforcing positives, suggesting possible options, establishing specific follow-up behavior, obtaining an action commitment, and providing support
- Use of questions in the coaching session
- The value of compassion in coaching

Coaching supports a change in behaviors using identified skills and tools. Because most people come to work each day desiring to do their best, coaching provides a way in which the work environment can improve as staff members use these skills and appropriate feedback from the coach.

Level IV

This could be a course that focuses on self-development (what the leader does to develop himself or herself) and stress management. Possible content could include the following:

- The value of self-development
- Emotional intelligence
- Character development and leadership
- Commitment and connection
- Confidence and compassion
- Physical and emotional balance in your life
- Intellectual and spiritual balance in your life
- The power of journaling
- Creation of your own personal coach
- Identification of growth experiences

Considerable motivation is required to undertake this work. It requires the willingness to be vulnerable, to be open to feedback, and to devote time and energy in self-reflection and a commitment to heal old wounds in oneself and in others who have been hurt. It requires practice in demonstrating commitment and building relationships with people who would never be close friends. It requires increasing self-confidence and compassion for oneself and others. A focus on emotional intelligence and the humor, kindness, and availability to others that creates inclusiveness and caring is critical to success (Porter-O'Grady, 2003). This type of growth and development is a process and does not occur in an instant or in one course, but it happens over time with considerable support and encouragement. This is also the type of behavior and growth that creates a positive work environment.

TIME WITH THE LEADERS

Leaders who spend time with their direct team members and with staff members demonstrate the importance of each person as a human being. Experienced leaders at all levels also need to spend time with the leaders in training. Some meetings can be in groups, where more emphasis on team development can occur. One-on-one interaction needs to occur in an environment that supports truth, vulnerability, and caring and is structured to avoid interruptions. In addition, it is valuable for learners to have time with leaders higher up in the organization such as other unit leaders, directors, and the CNO. Suggestions for these interactions may include a journal club, or one of the leaders may teach a class or lead a discussion group. It gives leaders an opportunity to acknowledge staff members and to connect with them in a more personal way.

SUMMARY

Because of the nursing shortage and the expense and difficulty of recruiting and retaining staff nurses and nurse leaders, it is timely to focus on the time, money, and energy that could be devoted to internal leadership development. Some excellent models may be found in the literature to support other facilities to begin the process. However, a need clearly exists for additional research, including outcomes of the programs. Healthcare can take its cue from the business world, where efforts have been most productive. Significant advantages exist to internal programs, including more consistent follow-up and attention to supporting behavioral changes. The nursing profession is focused on caring and developing relationships with patients and their families. Consequently, continuing growth and development

in all aspects of life, leadership, and being human only increase the quality of the care provided. In addition, it creates an improved work environment, which supports better, safer patient care.

Key Points to Lead

1. Evaluate the current state of succession planning in the nursing division of your facility.
2. Analyze the needs of your division regarding succession planning.
3. Identify the other leaders in your organization who could help with leadership training, mentoring, coaching, or follow-up.

Literature Box

Most organizations struggle with leadership development. They promote the top performers, put them through a few workshops and seminars, and throw them to the wolves (and Griffin is from the financial industry). An amazing number of these people fail not because they wanted to but because most of the time the development program failed them. Griffin believes that at least in part this is because these training programs are not individualized. She divides new managers into four potential groups, including the reluctant leaders, who have skills but no confidence in their own success; arrogant leaders, who are the opposite, no skills, humility, or empathy and all the confidence; the unknown leaders, who have the right blend of skills but have failed to develop any network or relationships outside of their intimate group; and the workaholics, who have been rewarded for excessive hours at work but often lack the perspective and personality needed to lead.

THE PIPELINE PROBLEM

Because of poor selection and training, the organization described had few people promotable in the pipeline when senior leaders retired. So a cross-functional team was organized to discover

best "leadership" practices in the company and build a year-long program that included coaching, mentoring, observing others, and hands-on management experience. These classes were followed with regular feedback sessions and follow-up.

These programs were developed specifically to the four identified types:

1. *The reluctant leaders* were given help and support to change their assumptions and low self-esteem about being able to lead.
2. *The arrogant leaders* were supported to realize they were as insecure as the first group but covered it up by overcompensating for real self-concept. They were given very direct (sometimes harsh) feedback and hands-on practice in empathetic listening and teamwork and even threats of demotion or dismissal.
3. *The unknown leaders* were cautious and quiet but ambitious and highly competent. A 360-degree feedback was used with them and careful deconstruction of their beliefs about creating friends and networks being "glad handing" and a waste of time occurred. Working with this group required a lot of monitoring and support.

Literature Box—cont'd

4. *The workaholic leaders* had anxiety-driven, addictive personalities. Because employees respond better to more well-rounded managers, it was important to show this group that it was better to work smarter than harder. So workaholic behavior was punished rather than rewarded as it is in most companies.

This organization had some success with this approach and is expanding the model to the whole company.

Griffin, N. (2003). Personalize your management development. *Harvard Business Review, 81*(3), 113-120.

Contemplations

- What can be learned from examples outside of healthcare to foster and support the idea of succession planning?
- What is ongoing in your facility to grow an internal candidate to take your job, should you choose to leave?
- How many vacant nurse manager or director positions currently exist or are filled by someone who is serving on an interim or temporary basis?
- At what other levels in the nursing division does succession planning occur? How is it monitored? What are the results?

- What would it take to put an educational program together at any of the four levels of the SPAN model?
- How many of those nurse managers, reporting to you, would be able to help teach in a leadership development program?
- Would some of these nurses benefit from taking the program?
- What would be required to prepare this group adequately to help in a leadership development program?
- Is it possible to establish realistic objectives around creation of such a program?

LEADER STORY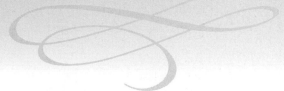

GAIL WOLF
CHIEF NURSING OFFICER
UNIVERSITY OF PITTSBURGH HEALTH SYSTEM
PITTSBURGH, PA

Leadership is both an art and a science. This has implications for teaching because students are frequently taught only the science, and without understanding how and when to apply that science, they fail. Others don't know the science but innately know the art, and they potentially succeed, although not as well as they could if they truly understood the science. So many things contribute to being a good leader, such as the ability to communicate through words and actions, the ability to develop trust, and the ability to demonstrate a real interest and concern for people.

I often talk about principles that are not usually taught in graduate programs. I refer to these concepts as "What's not in the books." For example, several years ago I heard an analogy of a butterfly, which still works today. A butterfly, after it hatches from the cocoon, needs at least a day for its wings to dry so that it can fly. It is a time of great vulnerability for the butterfly because it is defenseless and cannot yet fly. Ideas generated by our people in nursing are like the butterfly hatching; the ideas need some "wing drying" time. I try to eliminate the words, "That will never work!" If a leader says that, the nurse will probably never come to him or her again with an idea. There must be some "wing drying" time for all ideas while we consider the workability of the idea. I find that analogies like this one really help people remember a key concept.

Analogies or unusual events can really help people learn to look at something differently. When I was the VP for nursing at Shadyside, I talked all the time about innovation. Yet, it was difficult to get the staff to adopt innovative strategies. We had retreats, brought in speakers, did seminars, etc. And 3 days after the programs, the managers went back to their units and it was business as usual.

So, I decided to change strategies. One week, I sent all the managers a note that said to meet me in the hospital lobby at 3 PM on Friday. I told them to bring something with them that symbolized what they were willing to give up or leave behind in order to move forward with innovation. I marched them down the street to a funeral home. There was music, a casket, and the hospital chaplain was there. Each person had to put what he/she wanted to relinquish or leave behind in the casket. One manager brought a rock (that she said represented all the thinking and behavior that weighed her down and prevented innovation) while another manager brought a sign that read, "Fear of failure." We had a "funeral" for the things we brought, including a discussion on how hard it is to leave things that have been part of you for so long. People were still talking about the experience 15 years later.

The CNO position is sometimes very difficult because there are so many demands, and CNOs can't get out of the "muck." They have a wonderful idea over the weekend and then they go into the office, the phones are ringing and a crisis happens, and before they realize, they are consumed with all the tasks and meetings. Sometimes they confuse "busy" with accomplishment. I think this is one of the biggest mistakes CNOs make. In addition, our research has found that many nurse leaders do not know how to really operate strategically—to think futuristically about what strategic problems need to be addressed. They are seduced by the "busy" and repetitively deal with the same problems we've been dealing with for the past 40 years.

One of the major areas we need to focus on in nursing is leadership development. We would never send a nurse out to take care of patients without training, and yet we do that frequently with our managers and leaders. I put our first leadership course together 5 years ago. It was designed for the best and the brightest of our 35,000 employees. I was surprised at what they didn't know, although I shouldn't have been. I found that many folks understood the theory, but really didn't understand how to apply it effectively. We now spend a great deal of time in role play, case study, and experiential learning. For example, in our leadership academy, I meet once a month with the participants in a year-long clinical practicum after the classroom leadership content is completed. We talk about problems they are encountering with their projects and how to work through them. Making the learning focused on real life is the key for these learners.

Unfortunately, many faculty in our schools of nursing often don't have the skills and experience to teach leadership, especially given the challenges we are facing today. That is an issue we need to all own and jointly solve. To help address that problem, we have practicing VPs of Nursing from our system teaching in the leadership masters program at University of Pittsburgh. The response from the students, as well as the faculty, has been extremely positive.

If graduate students came to me for advice, I would tell them to get their graduate degree in nursing leadership, focus on understanding both the science and the art of leadership, and find a really strong mentor whom they can work with on a daily basis. What's not in the books is as important as what is in the books; applying it is the challenge facing us all.

Chapter References

Abrams, R. B. (2002, February 11). A nurse's viewpoint: A different course. Retrieved September 25, 2005, from http://www.HealthLeaders.com.

American College of Healthcare Executives. (2004, November 22). Succession planning routinely done by 21% of freestanding U.S. hospitals. Retrieved January 4, 2005, from http://www.ache.org/PUBS/Releases/112204_succession_release.cfm.

American Hospital Association Commission on Workforce for Hospitals and Health Systems. (2002). *In our hands: How hospital leaders can build a thriving workforce.* Chicago, IL: Author.

American Hospital Association News Now. (2003, May 23). Survey: Nurses want respect, better work schedules. Retrieved January 22, 2005, from www.ACHE.org/PUBS/Releases/112204_succession_release.cfm.

American Organization of Nurse Executives. (2005). AONE Nurse Executive Competencies. *Nurse Leader, 3*(2), 15-21.

Boss, W. R. (1983). Team building and the problem of regression: The personal management interview as an intervention. *The Journal of Applied Behavioral Science, 19*(1), 67-83.

Buerhaus, P. (2001). Expected near- and long-term changes in the registered nurse workforce. *Policy, Politics, & Nursing Practice, 2*(4), 254-270.

Buerhaus, P., Staiger, D., & Auerbach, D. (2000). Implications of a rapidly aging registered nurse workforce. *The Journal of the American Medical Association, 283*(22), 2948-2954.

Byham, W. C., Smith, A. B., & Paese, M. J. (2002). *Grow your own leaders: How to identify, develop, and retain leadership talent.* New York: Prentice-Hall.

Canadian Nurse Advisory Committee. (2002). Our health, our future: Creating quality workplaces for Canadian nurses. Retrieved January 4, 2005, from http://www.hc-sc.gc.ca.

Clark, R. L. (2001). Talent management nurtures future healthcare leaders. *Healthcare Financial Management, 55*(10), 16.

Conger, J., & Fulmer, R. (2003, December). Developing your leadership pipeline. *Harvard Business Review, 81,* 76–84.

Crane, T. G. (2002). *The heart of coaching: Using transformational coaching to create a high-performance culture.* San Diego: FTA Press.

Drucker, P. (2002). They're not employees, they're people. *Harvard Business Review, 80*(2), 70-77.

Fulmer, R. M., & Goldsmith, M. (2001). *The leadership investment: How the world's best organizations gain strategic advantage through leadership development.* New York: American Management Association.

Garman, A., & Glawe, J. (2004). Succession planning. *Consulting Psychology Journal: Practice and Research, 56*(2), 119-128.

Goldsmith, M., & Morgan, H. (2004, Fall). Leadership is a contact sport: The "follow-up factor" in management development. *Strategy + Business,* Retrieved January 4, 2005, from http://www.strategy-business.com.

Joint Commission on Accreditation of Healthcare Organizations. (2002). Health care at the crossroads: Strategies for addressing the evolving nursing crisis. Retrieved Date from http://www.jcaho.org.

Kehoe, J. K. (2001). The leadership pipeline: How to build the leadership-powered company. *Academy of Management Executive, 15*(2), 135-136.

Kosel, K., & Olivo, T. (2002, April). *The business case for workforce stability.* Irving, TX: Voluntary Hospitals of America.

Kowalski, K. (2004). Growing future leaders: Developing perinatal managers from within. *Journal of Obstetric, Gynecologic and Neonatal Nursing, 33*(3), 362-370.

Krugman, M., & Smith, V. (2003). Charge nurse leadership development and evaluation. *Journal of Nursing Administration, 33*(5), 284-292.

McClure, M. L., & Hinshaw, A. S. (2002). *Magnet hospitals revisited: Attraction and retention of professional nurses.* Washington, D. C.: American Nurses Publishing.

Nelson, B. (2002). What matters more than money to your employees. *Washington Business Journal.* Retrieved January 4, 2005, from http://www.bizjournals.com/washington/stories/2002/10/07/smallb5.html.

Noyes, B., McNally, K., Tourville, S., & Robinson, P. (2002). Preparing tomorrow's leaders through succession planning from the provider perspective. *Seminars for Nurse Leaders, 10*(4), 240-243.

Porter-O'Grady, T. (2003). A different age for leadership, part 1: New context, new content. *The Journal of Nursing Administration, 33*(2), 105-110.

Porter-O'Grady, T., & Malloch, K. (2002). *Quantum leadership: A textbook of new leadership.* Gaithersburg, MD: Aspen.

Pulce, R. (2002). Optimizing human capital through succession planning. *Seminars for Nurse Managers, 10*(4), 225–241.

Raines, C. (1997). Beyond generation X: A practical guide for managers. Menlo Park, CA: Crisp Publications.

Smith, E. L. (2002). Leadership development: The heart of succession planning. *Seminars for Nurse Managers, 10*(4), 234-239.

Soares, D. (2002). Developing a succession plan: The North Bronx Healthcare Network. *Seminars for Nurse Managers, 10*(4), 228-233.

Spitzer, R. (2002). Serendipity and Transition. *Seminars for Nurse Managers, 10*(4), 217.

Wolf, G., Bradle, J., & Nelson, G. (2005). Bridging the strategic leadership gap: A model program for transformational change. *Journal of Nursing Administration, 35*(2), 54-60.

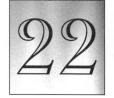

CHAPTER

22 Emerging and High-Stake Issues of the Workforce

Leadership is about making visions happen. LORRAINE MONROE

This chapter focuses on many issues that undergird most of the chapters in the book and that focus much of the attention of a chief nursing officer (CNO) in the operation of the nursing organization. These topics comprise special issues to which CNOs must attend if the issues are to be dealt with effectively. Each issue is, in its own right, a critical factor to the success of a nursing organization. However, the synergy of the issues creates a new way that CNOs must address how the organization deals with persistent issues that can prevent the organization from greatness. Specifically, this chapter focuses primarily on space and people issues: how to get them, how to keep them, and how to make them valuable and valued.

Work Environment of Nurses identified several issues. They chose ones that, if addressed effectively, could transform the work environment. The ones they cited could be viewed as a list of emerging/high-stake issues. These included using evidence-based practices, safe staffing levels, supporting clinical decision making, redesigning work processes and spaces, and enhancing interdisciplinary collaboration. Further, the *Nursing's Agenda for the Future* report (ANA, 2002) presented 10 domains critical for nursing to address for the future. These included delivery systems, professional/nursing culture, recruitment/retention, work environment, and diversity. Each set of issues represents topics of long duration. In the workplace, in some cases, the CNO does not control the issue or how it is addressed. An example of this is space consideration. In other cases, the CNO controls the issue and how it is addressed. An example of this may be recruitment of international nurses. In either case, however, the CNO must be engaged fully in the issues if any hope exists of resolution. Each of the issues cited has similar facets; all are important to be addressed by the CNO.

THE LIST OF ISSUES IN THE WORKFORCE IS not exhaustive. In fact, nurse administrators exist because of complex issues. If everything ran smoothly, few, if any, administrators would be needed. Just when progress with one issue is being made, several more pose challenges for the CNO. The Institute of Medicine (IOM, 2004) in its report *Keeping Patients Safe: Transforming the*

SPACE ALLOCATION AND DESIGN

At some time in a CNO's professional career, a building project will be looming on the horizon. Whether this is a new facility or a renovation, the CNO and related directors must be involved with the building design and testing. What looks

427

good on paper (blueprints) and meets code requirements may not address issues of patient care or nurse work. Because many existing hospitals were built in the 1950s and 1960s, many with the use of Hill Burton monies to accomplish the construction, many are now antiquated. In some cases it is not possible to renovate, either because of the extensive nature of the work to be done or because of exposure to environmental toxins that would result. If an organization has made building an ongoing priority, renovation may be possible. Regardless of which approach is taken, nursing needs to be involved.

When the CNO meets with staff members on the unit, they may express concerns about the physical space in which they do their work. Those comments usually relate to safety (texture or finishes that have worn), physical strain (location of materials and supplies needed to effect quality patient care), or general ambience (cleanliness, fabric integrity, or clearly outdated appearances). These are the concerns that need to be translated into design action. No matter who in nursing represents the department, people with the experience of direct care in the current setting, if such exists, need to be involved, especially during the design and mock-up phases.

The IOM (2004) identified three to four spaces in hospitals: the patient space (usually a room or a cubicle), the nursing station, the core space (where meeting rooms, equipment, and supplies are found), and the halls. Each of these spaces is important to nurses in their control of the environment, which Florence Nightingale would have defined as critically important to patient recovery.

Patient Spaces

Patient spaces vary widely across organizations and within organizations. Historically, hospitals had huge wards of patients. Over the years, however, these wards have transitioned to single or two- to four-bed units on medical-surgical units. Critical care areas also may be single rooms, but with clear glass in a large portion of the wall space

to ensure visualization of patients. When huge wards existed, the physical strain of moving from one end to the other was less than it is today because of the "in and out" movement through the various patient rooms and the need for more space to accommodate the same number of patients. When nurses need to cover miles in delivering patient care, the amount of "travel" time and the physical strain become an issue for the organization. If nurses are traveling up and down long halls, they are not available in patient rooms to provide care.

Nursing Stations

Nursing stations often are centralized and noisy. They are the communication hub of a nursing unit. It is the spot where staff members frequently congregate when not engaged in direct care activities. The number of people moving in and out of this space and the number of work transactions can contribute to a chaotic environment, which can be distracting to patients near the station and to anyone attempting to work in that space. Imagine trying to hear a telephone order while hearing multiple other conversations. The issue of patient confidentiality is an especially important concern in this space because of the professional dialogue that may be occurring without attention to the presence of others who are not engaged in patient care.

The Core Space

The core space could be the most hazardous to the nurse. It is where spills are likely to occur or where hazardous materials are not stored properly. Although many hospitals have made valiant efforts to ensure safety in this space, many physical restraints limit the possibilities for older facilities. Furthermore, a limited number of nurses could say they have seen and used a neat and orderly equipment room. These spaces usually have items jammed into any available space, and physical strain for the nurse obtaining the item in the back of the space becomes an issue.

The Hallway

Finally, the hallway is often a tempting "overflow" space for patients and equipment. It is where patients wait in transit from one place to another. This is where equipment is placed temporarily when it will not fit into a designated space. Many hospitals have long hallways, which require extreme organization of the nurse assigned to care for patients toward the end of those hallways. Otherwise, the number of trips back and forth between the core space and the patient rooms is a challenge. This area is also where nurses encounter a lot of other traffic: visitors and numerous other hospital personnel.

Changing the Space

According to the IOM (2004), "The majority of the nurses' time was spent walking between the patient rooms and the nursing unit core, or in the nursing station" (p. 251). This helps to explain how only 1.7 hours per 12-hour shift is the amount of time that all healthcare workers were in direct care situations (IOM, 2004). In addition, noise, lighting, and clutter interfere with nurses' ability to work effectively (Spath, 2000). Because of the importance of space to patients and nurses, space design becomes a high priority for nursing leaders.

The key is to use existing evidence about facility design to the organization's best advantage. According to Hamilton (2004), approximately 120 reliable studies indicate positive patient outcomes based on building designs. However, few healthcare professionals know about these studies or where to seek advice. In addition, design affects nurses. A building program provides an opportunity to improve hospital design to reduce staff stress and fatigue while improving patient-related issues (Ulrich, Quan, Zimring, Joseph, & Chaoudhary, 2004). Lindeke & Sieckert (2005) suggest three major points of consideration. The first has to do with space and equipment needs, including places for interdisciplinary interaction. The second is to state the space needs directly. The third is to change the existing space that includes places for interdisciplinary interaction in addition to work with patients and families.

> *Hospitals are held together, glued together, enabled to function…by the nurses and nobody else.*
> LEWIS THOMAS

Large organizations may have an architect who coordinates all of the ongoing activities related to the physical plant. In smaller organizations, it is usually necessary to contract with an architect for consulting and design services. If the contract architect does much healthcare design and construction, that person may be as savvy as the organizational architect. In either case, however, the CNO and directors need to understand in greater detail what the research suggests that betters patients' outcomes. As an example, the Center for Health Design* is a nonprofit organization that uses research-based findings. The report *Designing the 21st Century Hospital* is focused on integrating mind, body, and spirit needs in an evidence-based and cost-effective manner. Because so few hospitals today have used such an approach, the Center likely can provide invaluable service to nursing administration. Testing mock-up rooms to ensure sufficient space for equipment and movement is a practical way to evaluate research findings and prevent costly mistakes.

In addition, the *New York Times* reported on how hospital designs are created today to aid with healing (Alvarez, 2004). "The environment of a hospital contributes to the therapy of the patients," according to Tony Monk (¶ 5). He went on to say that the environment can help people feel good about what is happening and then focus on becoming well. The article further explained that key architects are quoting research that shows that seeing trees instead of cars helps people recover more quickly, and private rooms protect from infections and encourage visits from family and friends. Finally, as the baby boomers are retiring,

*http://www.healthdesign.org

they are pushing for reforms in healthcare, just as they did with other issues earlier in their lives. Among these reforms is the concern for a more patient-friendly environment.

Although nurses will not have the ultimate control, they clearly must have input into any patient care design process. Even building a "pilot" room can unearth problems before they emerge in actual patient care. For example, as obesity continues to remain a key concern in the United States, numerous implications for building design are present for ensuring safe and compassionate patient care. CNOs would be wise to test the space that accommodates heavier patients, any special equipment needed to render patient care, and how space and equipment work with each other before the building becomes a reality. These are the kinds of issues that nurse administrators must address from a patient and nurse safety perspective.

Space allocation and design are not decisions of the CNO. However, how a clinical unit is designed affects the workload, the morale, and the overall commitment of the workforce. In some cases, the design of space conveys value for the nursing staff and can support or detract from safety issues. Thus, without nursing's input, an organization unwittingly can omit some physical feature, which limits the ability of nurses to perform their best and function effectively. This issue is especially important because many hospitals have now reached an age at which they must be renovated or replaced. Although the physical space holds great importance, it pales in terms of the issues surrounding people. Getting enough of the right staff mix, keeping staff, and arranging for coverage of care needs are constant challenges for the CNO.

THE CHALLENGES OF THE WORKFORCE

Several factors form workforce challenges. The shortage of nurses is a challenge no responsible healthcare organization can ignore. The issues of recruiting and retaining quality staff are influenced by international recruitment efforts. Creating a workforce of cultural diversity is a challenge in any setting. Finally, basic coverage across units and shifts is a challenge in typical times and more so in times of healthcare shortages. Each of these factors requires the attention of the CNO so that movement toward better resolutions is always the focus. Each is explored in the following sections from the perspective of the CNO's primary concerns.

The Shortage

The shortage is really a series of shortages that have evolved over decades. Current CNOs probably recall the responses made to the shortage in the late 1980s. As schools of nursing released numerous new graduates into a stretched workforce, the full force of the HMO movement hit and many hospitals made drastic downsizing decisions. In addition to angering the nurses because of what seemed like a focus on money rather than care, these dramatic reductions had numerous negative effects on new graduates, students, and prospective students. Suddenly, the profession that had held a mantra of "You can always find work" faced unemployment. Although the reduction of positions seemed more dramatic than it was, not all nurses wanted to go where the new jobs were. Many nurses who were affected by organizational decisions made at this time did not want to work in non–acute care settings. However, home health care, pharmaceuticals, and day care services were expanding. The shortage that began in the late 1990s was more a factor of the increasing numbers of the aging population, the potential of the number of retirements within the profession, and the increasing acuity of patients needing care.

Again, schools are producing record numbers of graduates. Current graduates and those in practice, however, expect that they might work in settings other than acute care hospitals. They also expect that current nurse leaders have a better sense of where the industry is headed and thus have planned for major changes in a way that does not produce such dramatic swings in expectations as in the past. Regardless of the type of the next shortage, the CNO must be cognizant of the fact that in the future, more jobs will exist than people to fill them. That does not relate to nursing only; it relates to numerous disciplines because the number of new potential workers is smaller than the total demands of the workforce. To the savvy CNO, the prospect of a future shortage means that considerable attention needs to be made in restructuring the work of nurses, changing the workplace to accommodate a different workforce, addressing needs distinctive to an emerging workforce and a seasoned workforce, and recruiting and retaining a diverse workforce to meet the current and emerging needs of people who seek healthcare services. Wynne (2003, p. 104) states,

Macro-level incentives for economic reform have driven restructuring at the meso-organizational level in health care. Subsequent to this, clinical nurses at the micro-organizational level have had little involvement in the development of reform strategies despite implementing reform outcomes as a result of their role in patient care delivery.

In the context of the characteristics of the new graduate workforce, this would suggest that if staff nurses are not involved in the decisions about the future "reforms," they may be unwilling to stay within nursing. Wynne also advocates for the community to be involved in such discussions because they are the recipients of the resultant care.

If the CNO undertakes any restructuring of the work of nurses, it is clear that this must be done from a broad-based perspective. An example of a collaborative approach between service and education is the creation of the clinical nurse leader initiated by the American Association of Colleges of Nursing.* Whether this role fits within a specific organization is a matter for consideration about work restructuring within the organization. Other issues of restructuring include the way in which roles external to nursing are implemented. For example, if another department

*http://www.aacn.nche.edu/cnl/index.htm

creates a service requiring work from nurses, the CNO needs to think this change through to determine if it is appropriate for nursing to assume that additional work, or if it is necessary to create an assistive role to fulfill the expectation. Ideally, any discussion by any element of the organization would include representatives from other areas so that the best overall strategy is created. Further, having nurses who would be affected by a change would be those representatives for nursing. The work of nursing will change. How nursing work changes, while remaining true to our distinct core of caring, to use new approaches is the challenge that is most complex and holds the greatest potential to affect the availability of nursing care. Creating new ways to provide care without changing the workplace, however, will provide limited possibilities.

Changing the workplace to accommodate a different workforce goes beyond redesigning physical space. Issues of ergonomics and interpersonal relationships, especially with managers and physicians, are other examples. Another consideration for changing the workplace involves the increasing intensity of technologic devices and processes. Whether using bedside computers, personal digital assistants (PDAs), or wireless technology, nurses have the potential to streamline patient information and work flow in new ways. The ability to schedule events or page someone to secure equipment or supplies can lessen the number of trips needed or the number of unproductive events. This is especially beneficial to nurses with physical limitations.

Creating the right climate is obviously important to enable nurses and others to remain committed to the organization. Although the manager is the key influence on the climate, the CNO sets the tone of how important the organizational climate is. How tolerant nurses will be of verbal, and sometimes physical, abuse is an example. A universal zero tolerance policy is an example of how the workplace can be changed in a positive manner. It is equally unacceptable to tolerate verbal abuse from peers as it is from physicians or others.

In addressing these various considerations, the CNO has to engage the workforce in the discussion about what needs to change. Some conversations have to focus on how to implement decisions because the decisions are firm. In other cases, the discussions can focus on what decision to make and what is best for the members of the workforce and the patient receiving care. Being well informed about changes under consideration, knowing what forecasts are probable, and knowing who the political players are and their motivation for their positions are examples of information valuable to those discussing changes in the workplace. Some changes relate directly to the nature of the generational differences in the workforce today. Although other areas of a healthcare organization have the same kinds of age diversity, nursing by virtue of numbers has an intense need to address and resolve the needs of an established and emerging workforce.

In addition to understanding the common information about the differences in how older and younger people approach work and using that to make changes in the way current staff members work with new staff members, the CNO will need to be the champion of creating benefits options and scheduling options. Traditional views of what benefits comprise and how all employees receive comparable benefits have evolved over recent years so that most places have at least some of their benefits available in a "cafeteria" type plan. The employee option to choose allows each individual to select the use of benefits to best meet his or her needs. Having the option of additional time off versus additional money for working any overtime may attract people who value time over money. Ways to acknowledge successes may differ, too. One person may want a plaque; another may want a donation to a favorite charity. If the person in charge of the largest number of employees presses for such considerations, such discussion becomes a greater organizational priority.

To address the near future needs, the CNO needs to have a plan that encourages and supports hospital employees to secure additional education.

The idea of a ladder program of some ilk could address how an individual may move from nursing assistant to licensed practical nurse to registered nurse to nurse practitioner/educator/administrator/researcher.

The CNO needs to forecast what will be needed in the future and to work with schools of nursing to create the graduate that will be needed. The CNO has to pay even more attention to the work of the institution's staff development program to ensure that current needs are being addressed. Building the workforce skills needed in the future is critical to the use of experienced talent that the organization has developed already to help solve the issues of changing needs and services. In doing all of this, the CNO needs to be skilled in ensuring the voice of the entire staff so that each aspect of care is moving forward with the organization's evolution. Recruiting the talent needed for changing the workplace and retaining those who can sustain and grow the efforts of the nursing enterprise are key challenges to addressing these issues.

Recruitment and Retention

Without nurses to provide care, few other issues can be addressed, and certainly the mission of the healthcare organization will fail. The IOM (2004) report on transforming nurses' work environment identified five key ways in which nurses directly contribute to patient care. Box 22-1 explicates

---

Box 22-1   How Nurses Contribute to Patient Care

Monitoring patient status
Providing physiologic therapy
Helping patients compensate for
  loss of functioning
Providing emotional support
Educating patients and families

From Institute of Medicine. (2004). *Keeping patients safe: Transforming the work environment of nurses.* Washington, DC: The National Academies Press.

these ways. The additional related activities are defined as integration of care, documentation, and supervision. These are all critical functions of a nursing service. Thus determining how to recruit and retain nurses is a critical factor. Securing and holding the right number and quality of nurses allows the organization to meet the demands of care. The public agrees: Hudson Healthcare reported that 39% of patients surveyed and 41% of family members surveyed stated that the most positive impact on quality of care would be adding more nursing staff (2004). Affecting the quality of care through having more nurses available to provide care implies that recruitment and retention are critical to the success of an organization. Further, creating the culture of a desirable place to work affects financial aspects in major ways. For example, one hospital reported a budget savings (cost avoidance) of $8 million through successful recruitment and avoidance of using temporary nursing services (Georgetown University, 2004).

Various studies, starting with the original work of Kramer and Schmalenberg (1977) have described factors related to recruitment and retention. Schumacher and Nathanson (2004) reported on the six factors that emerged from the study conducted by McManis and Monsalve Associates in partnership with the American Organization of Nurse Executives (AONE). These factors seemed to be especially important to the success of an organization: leadership development and effectiveness, empowered and collaborative decision making, work design and service delivery innovation, values-driven organizational culture, recognition and reward systems, and professional growth and accountability. So, nurses clearly are important.

Current increases in the number of professionals create an interesting picture. Buerhaus, Staiger, & Auerbach (2004) found that older women and foreign-educated nurses contributed to the greatest amount of employment increases in nursing. Most younger nurses are entering employment with an associate degree. Many foreign-educated nurses enter practice in the United States with a bachelor's degree. Although no source seems to

have identified the number of ethnic minority nurses in leadership roles, more than half of the nursing population holds less than a baccalaureate degree (National Advisory Council on Nurse Education and Practice, 2000). These data suggest that the CNO must remain concerned about the workplace and how to accommodate the needs of the older nurse, how to balance the needs and interests of a seasoned and emerging workforce simultaneously, and how to advance formal educational preparation of the staff.

One of the common ways to recruit is to create incentives to join an organization. Although this creates more prospective employees, it also is disconcerting to those currently employed. In addition, other similar healthcare organizations match the incentives and "musical chairs" results. Moving nurses from one organization to another obviously does not increase the overall quantity of care available. Unfortunately, this approach is disruptive to ongoing initiatives. Long-time employees become discontented because their new counterparts are compensated in fairly comparable ways. The CNO has the challenge of competing with other community facilities in matching or exceeding the total benefits packages while not ignoring the needs of long-term and loyal employees. Further, the CNO has to contend with internal migration issues. The International Council of Nurses (2005) defined a need to address the concerns of internal migration, which they describe as shifts from rural to urban, from public to private, and from nursing to non-nursing or no employment.

At the same time the organization is looking to recruit for tomorrow, it also must be concerned with the subsequent years. Thus holding discussions about how the values of the current organization articulate with those of subsequent generations (the source of nurses for the future) can create a sustainable supply of nurses by relating to the world at large. This activity may require creating new and different relationships with the schools of nursing and the public system. If children are expected to choose their educational track in junior high, they need to know before then what it takes to be a nurse and why they would want to be prepared for such a career option. Creating opportunities for nurses to tell the story of their profession can generate excitement about becoming a nurse; this is a challenge for the CNO.

> *Value people. Praise effort. Reward performance.*
> JOHN C. MAXWELL

International Recruitment of Nurses

Another challenge CNOs face is how to recruit, acculturate, and retain foreign nurse graduates (FNGs). In fact, many solutions for the nursing shortage involve the recruitment of FNGs. The Literature box describes various aspects of international nurse migration. FNGs derive from several countries, although the Phillipines is the primary country that produces nurses for exportation to other countries. The United Kingdom and Canada exceed the United States in importing nurses from other countries, but as countries with limited numbers of nurses to provide care for their own citizens became "targets" for recruiting, concern about the number of nurses from other countries became a major issue. In other words, recruiting from countries with their own shortages creates incredible ethical concerns. Is it helpful to encourage people who already wish to leave their country to do so? Is it better to ignore their personal desires or to evaluate them before determining whether to recruit?

The real influx initially began in the mid 1960s when the United States Immigration Act (1965) was created (Brush & Berger, 2002). Many hospitals and nursing homes, the primary employers of FNGs, have said repeatedly over the years that they could not survive without these dedicated nurses. This is especially true for nursing homes, where, according to Crawford (2004), the number of foreign-educated nurses is almost five times the number of U.S.–educated nurses (21.6% compared with 4.4%, respectively). In addition, the percentages are almost equal in medical/surgical units (41.4% foreign-educated nurses compared with 42.7% U.S. educated).

According to the World Health Organization, the International Council of Nurses, and the Royal College of Nursing* (United Kingdom), working conditions are the major factor driving nurse migration. When FNGs seek employment external to their country, it is often because of higher pay, better working conditions, and greater career opportunities. Alexis and Chambers (2003) suggest that the United Kingdom, the greatest importer of nurses worldwide, needs to address issues relating to valuing FNGs if they wish to keep them in their system. The FNGs need to feel valued in their contributions to healthcare. Many U.S. states require that FNGs pass the Commission on Graduates of Foreign Nursing Schools (CGFNS) examination and most nurses are recruited from countries where English is a prominent language. The process of validating credentials is complex and frequently takes considerable time to complete.

The 2000 regulations pertaining to FNGs require a variety of actions or documentations. One of the keys is that organizations must document that they have made deliberate efforts to recruit nurses within the United States before seeking nurses externally. Payment (salaries or hourly rates) cannot be less than that offered to nurses in the United States. In addition, organizations must attest to the fact that employing nurses outside the United States will not lessen wages or working conditions already enjoyed by the current workforce. Internally, the organization must let the current staff know that it is recruiting from other countries and where it intends to place any recruited FNGs. The North American Free Trade Agreement created special considerations for Canada and Mexico, but the latter seldom seek practice in the United States, primarily because of a disparate educational system. The freedom to travel back and forth across international borders has, however, changed based on the Homeland

*http://www.icn.ch/PR22_03.htm

Security Act. All of this becomes even more complex when a nurse from another country is immigrating to the United States and was educated in a third country and became licensed through an immigration procedure in the current country of employment. Needless to say, employing nurses from other countries is a complex situation, one that usually involves the organization's attorneys to validate that all requirements are being met.

Meanwhile, the CNO must attend to how any FNGs are introduced into the environment, even when a cadre already exists in the organization. The CNO also needs to be concerned with ensuring that the conditions are not altered to accommodate an FNG in the practice setting. As Thompson (2004) says

As leaders sort through the current environment of ambiguity, the temptation is to find answers quickly so as to end the sense of uncertainty. The better choice, though, is to explore the ambiguous situations from multiple perspectives, to consider the many options to the fullest extent possible. (p. 195)

This statement seems applicable to various issues of cultural diversity; creating or considering multiple options creates the best opportunity for success.

Cultural Competence and Considerations

Whether the discipline is medicine (Betancourt, 2004; Genao, Bussey-Jones, Brady, Branch, & Corbie-Smith, 2003), nutrition (Ruel, 2003), or nursing (Swanson, 2004; Washington, Erickson, & Ditomassi, 2004), healthcare professionals are concerned about cultural diversity. All disciplines see the changing population of patients seeking service, and they see the lack of diversity as they look among their peers.

The issue of cultural diversity is three pronged. The first part is how to develop the current workforce, which, in nursing, is predominantly white, female, Christian, and middle class, to work with patients who do not necessarily reflect any of these characteristics. The second relates to how to help the current workforce embrace new nurses who also do not reflect these characteristics. The third is recruiting a more broadly diverse population into nursing and subsequently into an organization. Preparing a predominantly white professional workforce (Bureau of Health Professions, 2002) to work effectively with others of diverse cultural backgrounds is one challenge. To that add the challenge of working with a culturally diverse patient population. Furthermore, to those add the idea of developing ethnic minority nurses for leadership roles.

Numerous articles and speeches have focused on the need for nurses to be competent in working with others and providing care to patients of differing cultural backgrounds. Frusti, Niesen, and Campion (2003), for example, created a diversity competency model and strategic plan that included developing current staff, recruiting and retaining diverse staff, and working with a diverse patient population to address the multiple aspects of creating a culturally competent organization. This issue has tremendous implications for nurse leaders.

The issue of care to patients of a minority population is not limited to the predominant ones that come to mind: African Americans, Hispanics, and Native Americans. For example, Cortis (2004) reported about nurses' interactions with members of a Pakistani community. In essence, the concept of holism was implemented inadequately. In another article by Cortis (2003), differences between English and Scottish people are used as an example of cultural diversity. Both of these illustrate the complexity of cultural diversity.

Bessent and Fleming (2003) suggested that five basic elements are "key to the enhancement and development of leadership and essential for nurses in educational settings who are committed to working in diverse environments nationally and internationally" (p. 258). The five elements are knowledge of self, integrity, vision, communication, and collaboration. The model they developed is designed to take one's insight into self as the foundation on which to use integrity (being responsible and credible) and to move to creativity. Communication allows for feedback in development, and collaboration allows for ways to strengthen each individual's potential. This comprehensive approach to developing leadership in diverse environments takes a commitment of the nursing leadership and considerable effort on the part of numerous members of the entire organization to invest the needed energy and resources.

> *Diversity doesn't necessarily concern gender, ethnicity or culture. Rather, diversity means cultivating difference and puncturing conformity.*
> CHARLES FISHMAN

During the work of *Nursing's Agenda for the Future* (ANA, 2002), an effort by more than 60 nursing organizations, an attempt was made to reduce the focus from 10 domains (areas to be addressed) to the key drivers in the system. Although the key drivers were economic value and delivery systems, inherent in this result and all other domains was the domain of diversity. In other words, diversity is critical to each of the other domains; it is a theme that is interwoven in all of the other domains. The Desired Future Statement (Vision) states,

Nursing increasingly reflects the population it serves. Our profession derives strength from its ethnic, cultural, social, economic and gender diversity, thereby enhancing its capacity to respond to the healthcare needs of a diverse nation. Nursing is a model for other professions in demonstrating the value of diversity. The primary strategy to achieve this vision is to increase health system leadership that reflects and values diversity.

The total work of this collaboration is projected to be complete by 2010. How this work moves to conclusion is important to watch because it is nurses working together to create cases and solutions.

Without diversity, limitations will be imposed on nursing in relation to how well it connects with the population it serves. The good news is that the Sullivan Commission report regarding

diversification of the U.S. healthcare workforce indicates that college campuses clearly will be more ethnically diverse in the future.* The work of the commission focused on means of ensuring a more diverse group of professionals. The work included examining admission criteria and taxpayer funding for students entering health professions. It also included training and mentoring programs and embraced the concept of community service expectations. One of the glaring statistics the Commission provided was that 25% of the U.S. population is African American, Hispanic American, and American Indian, but only 9% of the nurses derives from these minority populations (Sullivan Commission, 2004, p. 2). A specific recommendation with major implications for the CNO is found in the set dealing with accountability. "Health professions schools and health systems should have strategic plans that outline specific goals, standards, policies and accountability mechanisms to ensure institutional diversity and cultural competence" (p. 10).

The effects of the Sullivan Commission may be long range. Even if schools act on the recommendations immediately, a period of time will elapse before the effects of these efforts are felt in healthcare organizations. Meanwhile, organizations can do considerable work to change the knowledge level of today's nurses. Through specific efforts, even attitudes can change.

Although efforts are underway to increase the total number of ethnically diverse nurses, the key is that currently the field of nursing is not ethnically diverse. What is worse is that in some situations nurses of an ethnic minority background (and nurses of other cultural minority factors) suggest that they do not feel welcome. That *must* change.

The good news is that immediate steps can be taken to change the work environment for cultural sensitivity, if this has not been done already. It is unnecessary to wait for a basic nursing education program to produce new graduates. For example, the Center for the Health Professions (2002)

---

*http://admissions.duhs.duke.edu/sullivancommission

created a curriculum to be used by various groups to gain the knowledge and skills to provide care in an increasingly diverse workplace. Current steps will influence the perception of future work settings. Whether the CNO's goal is to increase the diversity of the nursing workforce or whether community pressure exists to do so, the key is that it must happen in almost all settings if health disparities are to diminish. This issue for ethnic diversity becomes even more pressing in consideration of the changing demographics in the United States. Majumdar, Browne, Roberts, and Carpio (2004) suggest that appropriate education created more open-mindedness and cultural awareness, better understanding of multiculturalism, and a better ability to communicate with people from minority groups. As a result of this effort, patients had better outcomes.

Cultural diversity is not a simple issue that can be addressed easily, but it is clear that it won't improve unless there is clear commitment by the current majority workforce. Stereotypes of any ethnic group are unacceptable. Rather, groups of one ethnic background must engage with individuals of other backgrounds to enhance greater understanding of individual perspectives. Not every Native American eats Indian bread; and no one should leap to that conclusion. If an organization really wants to attend to the issue, placing a goal of cultural diversity in the strategic plan is beneficial. Biggerstaff and Hamby (2004, p. 31) describe how their organization addressed the issue: Meeting these goals involved holding additional staff training, customizing diets, and developing practices sensitive to cultural differences related to birth, sickness, and death. Another example they cited is the financial commitment to be more responsive, for example, with providing signage in Spanish and Hmong, the two leading non-English languages in their patient population.

"Culture does not determine behavior, but affords group members a repertoire of ideas and possible actions, providing the framework through which they understand themselves, their environment, and their experiences" (Hunt, 2004, ¶ 5).

Thus a nursing culture exists, as does a gender culture, as does an ethnic culture, as does a generational culture. So, the 35-year-old male Hispanic nurse is influenced by each of these cultures as he provides care to the 65-year-old Jewish female. The key again is to focus on the individual and not make assumptions based on stereotypes. These cultural "norms," however, provide a starting point for thinking about the range of considerations in interacting with someone else. "Culture is neither a blueprint nor an identity; individuals choose between various cultural options..." (Hunt, 2004, ¶ 6).

The What I Do on New Year's Eve strategy is a great way to help see the differences in *people* not in *cultures* (Allison et al., 2004). Basically each person in a small group tells what he or she does to celebrate New Year's Eve. Even those of apparently same cultural groups typically have different traditions. For example, at one meeting in which the group discussed the foods to eat in celebration, sushi, sausage, pork, cabbage, sauerkraut, and black-eyed peas were mentioned as the thing to bring good luck for the new year.

Whether the CNO is involved directly in a particular issue related to the cultural competence and diversity of the workforce, the CNO sets the tone and encourages the focus on this important issue. Cultural considerations affect who will be nurses, how diverse nurses are incorporated into the organizational culture, and how they, in turn, convey values of diversity to the patients they serve.

Staffing Dilemmas

Staffing discussions have evolved from the general topic of mix (the number of unlicensed assistive nursing personnel, licensed practical/vocational nurses [LP/VN], and registered nurses [RN]) to the educational preparation of the registered nurse workforce and the consideration of whether a specified ratio of registered nurses to patients should be used. Mix in some organizations is used to mean unlicensed to licensed personnel ratios. For example, according to a 2003 survey by the

National Council of State Boards of Nursing (Smith, 2003), some nurses and employers do not distinguish between LP/VNs and RNs, which of course is a concern from the standpoint of the legally defined scope of practice statements legislated in various states. Other organizations distinguish, and correctly so, between LP/VNs and RNs and between the educational and experiential qualifications within the registered nurse population. Where staffing ratios are mandated, the CNO must use those legal requirements of the numbers.

Where staffing is required to be planned on a unit-by-unit basis, such as the approach proposed by the American Nurses Association (1999), the CNO has to design a system that integrates numerous factors. The factors, which appear in Table 22-1, intertwine to create a logical staffing plan. The issues encompass various factors from the number of patients and their characteristics to the geographic environment and abilities of the staff. Some of the factors vary daily: for example, the number and characteristics of patients. Others may never vary: for example, the geography of the unit.

Aiken, Clarke, Sloan, Sochalski, and Silber (2002) found that the numbers of registered nurses made an impressive difference in failure-to-rescue. In looking at 168 Pennsylvania hospitals, they found that adding patients to the registered nurses' workload resulted in a 7% increase in risk of death for each patient with complications. Also a 23% and 15% increase occurred in risks of burnout and job satisfaction, respectively, for nurses in hospitals for every additional patient per nurse. These data cannot be ignored. The CNO needs to ensure the nursing organization has sufficient resources to obtain these types of data and to create the systems that provide for the best possible staffing that reflects safe care. Furthermore, creating a culture of caring attracts and retains staff.

Aiken, Clarke, Cheung, Sloane, and Silber (2003) found that hospitals (surgical units) with higher proportions of nurses holding bachelor's degrees in nursing had lower surgical mortality and failure-to-rescue rates. Thus, for organizations that are driven by data, the emerging research can influence how staffing is approached. This study suggests that the CNO needs to ensure that some system that fosters additional academic education is in place in the professional development program. Rogers, Hwang, Scott, Aiken, and Dinges (2004) reported findings similar to other areas of work external to healthcare in terms of the number of hours per day that an individual seems to be able to work effectively. One of the most important findings was this: "The likelihood of making

Table **22-1** KEY FACTORS INFLUENCING NURSE STAFFING DECISIONS

Area of Consideration	Example(s)
Patient care unit	Number of patients
	Architecture and geography of environment
Staff	Experience with patient population
	Language skills
	Number and skills of those who support the RN's work
Institution/organization	Presence and effectiveness of non-nursing services
	Readily available information
	Method for determining staffing needs
Evaluation	Analysis of trends (turnover, overtime, levels of staff satisfaction)

From American Nurses Association. (1999). *Principles for nurse staffing*. Washington, DC: The Association.

an error increased with longer work hours and was three times higher when nurses worked shifts lasting 12.5 hours or more" (p. 206). In addition, "Working overtime increased the odds of making at least one error, regardless of how long the shift was originally scheduled" (p. 206). These findings suggest that the CNO would be wise to spend time on the issue of overtime and the issue of length of shifts. The sentiment among staff nurses seems to be that the first issue has their support; they do not want mandatory overtime. Changing the length of the shift and thus the number of days worked per week has less support. Who would want to commit to another day per week, especially if assurance of being limited to 8 hours of work per day did not exist?

All of these issues surrounding staffing may cause anxiety about how to pay for additional staff. However, McCue, Mark, and Harless (2003) suggest that just as much profit (or income in excess of expenses) can be made with higher staffing levels. Four hundred fifty five (455) hospitals' financial records from 1990 to 1995 were analyzed and showed a statistically significant increase in operating costs when registered nurse levels increased. However, no statistically significant decrease in profit occurred. In essence, the greater numbers of registered nurses were able to handle more complex patients more quickly.

A political approach to increasing the number of registered nurses can be found at the Michigan Nurses Association web site.* The Michigan Nurses Association created a specific model to address that state's need for hiring more registered nurses in a cost-effective manner. The CNO's commitment to safe staffing can be demonstrated through an economic model. Thus the way in which the CNO gathers data, interprets it, and presents it in terms of staffing needs is critical to securing funding for positions. The CNO can set the tone for managing staffing issues, but more importantly the CNO can make a substantive business case for increasing the size of the staff.

*http://www.minurses.org/spc/MandatoryOvertimeforNurses FinalReport.pdf

EXITING THE POSITION

One final special issue for a CNO that certainly has high stakes is that of exiting the position. Failure in addressing emergent or high-stake issues often leads to the need to exit. Even success with these complex issues can precipitate discomfort—too much change or change too rapidly.

Although exiting a position is not necessarily an aspect one normally considers from the point of an initial interview, thinking about how one might leave is probably good strategy. Putting the right people in place so that some line of succession occurs takes time; thus from the moment of employment, the CNO should think about how to exit the position.

CNOs are among those groups with limited tenure in major medical centers. Sometimes the exit is voluntary and other times it is not. In situations in which the CNO believes that termination is imminent, it is wise to secure personal legal counsel (not the hospital attorney or a board member) to ensure that personal benefits are protected and that the CNO has an official spokesperson. Because this situation usually provides little warning, the CNO probably should think of this option going into the position. At the 2004 AONE meeting, some former CNOs told their stories about being terminated. One of the themes was the unbelievability of the situation in which they found themselves. In other words, even very experienced CNOs were still unable to believe the complexity of the situation in which they found themselves. Unfortunately, some current CNOs are being told that they are to "get Magnet" or they will be terminated. The best of what Magnet is intended to be has been diminished by this attitude of its being another indicator of care to display on a wall to increase the organization's business. With messages such as these, it is clear that thinking about leaving without a specific desire to do so may in fact be possible.

In other situations, the CNO decides to leave. Leaving may be due to lack of interest in administration, it may be related to a new CEO whose values do not fit with those of the CNO, or it may be a new opportunity (either internally or externally). Regardless of what the next step is, the way in which the CNO deals with leaving the position and the team of supporters is critical to the CNO's future and to the team left behind. Although it is useful to use some method that lets most people know simultaneously, the people closest to the CNO expect to hear the message directly. After all, that group has committed to the CNO's vision and leadership. That group should be given the same written message so that they know what others are getting. Staff members who have been especially devoted, regardless of position, also will want to hear something directly. So, before actually announcing a decision, the CNO needs to know who will expect a personal message.

The CNO should spend some time before resigning clearing files of any irrelevant materials, making certain that the critical documents are readily available for the successor, and providing a list of the key community leaders who have been supportive of nursing. Timelines of events (such as what happens in a particular month) also can be exceedingly useful.

In some situations the transition between the current CNO and a successor will be smooth, as in when effective succession planning has occurred. In other cases, the CNO may be expected in a new position external to the organization before a replacement can be found. In that case, the CNO should be sure that the immediate team of directors or supervisors knows whether they may call the departing CNO for advice. They also need to know any concerns that may require follow through before a successor arrives. If the CNO is moving into a new position within the organization, such as

the chief operating officer (COO) or the CEO position, it is important to determine how quickly the CNO role can be filled or if temporary adjustments need to be made until a successor is found. If the CNO is accountable for two roles, combining tasks and shifting some responsibilities may be the best and most immediate strategy.

SUMMARY

The CNO's strategies to keep abreast of these critical issues and the plans to address them effectively are critical to the success of the CNO and the nursing organization. The challenges may evolve, but space and people always will be two key issues that require considerable thought. Although others may be involved in making decisions or implementing plans associated with these issues, the CNO has to remain committed to these issues as ones that require ongoing attention and reporting. Without that commitment, nursing services suffer.

KEY POINTS TO LEAD

1. Evaluate a local hospital to determine if evidence of using the research about hospital design exists.
2. Assess the involvement of the CNO with community nursing education programs.
3. Evaluate the local recruitment and retention programs to determine the strategy that is employed to address issues about this aspect of the workforce.
4. Determine if a foreign nurse recruitment program exists and how new FNGs are acculturated into the workforce.
5. Discuss key considerations for a CNO in exiting a position.

Literature Box

This study looked at six countries, all English-speaking, that were recruiting nurses from developing countries. The countries were the United States, Canada, United Kingdom, Iceland, Australia, and New Zealand. Currently 4% (n = approximately 90,000) of the registered nurses in the United States are foreign-trained. However, that percentage may double if the United States follows what the United Kingdom and Ireland have done in the years preceding this study.

Recruiting countries had almost twice as many nurses per population as did the source countries.

In spite of the needs within some countries for nurses, they are unable to create enough positions to retain the nurses in their home countries. The "push" factors (those that force nurses out of their country) included poor wages, risk of AIDS, and safety concerns. The "pull" factors (those that attract nurses to more developed countries) included better wages, opportunities to advance their education, and better working conditions.

U.S. requirements for licensure and immigration have limited the number of nurses entering the United States from other countries. Even with NAFTA, few nurses immigrate from Mexico because their system is so different from that of the United States and few nurses speak English, a requirement for migration to the United States.

The United Kingdom, the largest importer of nurses, in 2002 actually exceeded the number of nurses educated in Britain through its immigration of nurses from other countries. Immigration became such a concern that the U.K. Department of Health created an ethics code in 1999 to prevent further drain on nurses from Africa, a common source of U.K.'s immigrant nurses. Currently little movement of nurses occurs among the countries in the European Union, but that is expected to change as countries with fewer resources join the EU.

Ireland, like the UK, is importing more nurses than it is producing. Furthermore, many nurses from the United Kingdom are now immigrating to Ireland.

The Phillipines, the largest source of registered nurse exportation, reported that in 1993 more than $800 million was sent home to support the local economy. The authors found that about 85% of Filipino nurses are working internationally.

Part of this global situation is due to the fact that developed countries have not addressed their own workforce production adequately. Further, many deficits in developing countries are easily correctable. Stabilizing migration can benefit developing and established countries.

Aiken, L. H., Buchan, J., Sochalski, J., Nichols, B., & Powell, M. (2004). Trends in international nurse migration. *Health Affairs, 23*(3), 69-77.

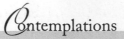

Contemplations

- What physical attributes of your healthcare organization facilitate or impede the effective functioning of the nursing staff?
- What evidence in your healthcare organization suggests it is consistent with some building design research?
- How does your healthcare organization enhance cultural diversity?
- What specific professional development activities are geared to enhancing cultural diversity?
- What social interactions exist that reflect a willingness to understand and/or value a culture different from the majority of the employees?
- How is the recruitment plan affected by the number and type of new graduates produced in the geographic area?

- How were international nurses, if they are present, recruited? How were they incorporated into the culture? How did their culture affect the majority culture?
- What is the biggest staffing issue in your healthcare organization? How is it being addressed? Are those most affected (staff nurses/a specific unit/a specific shift) involved in creating the solution?
- What would your letter of resignation say that suggests you understand the need for careful transitions?

LEADER STORY ❧

PHYLLIS BECK KRITEK

COURAGE

CONFLICT TRANSFORMATION CONSULTATION,

TRAINING, COACHING, AND MEDIATION SERVICES

CREATING COMMON CAUSE

RICHMOND, VA

I learned the most about cultural competence when I was involved in starting a community clinic. There are a lot of interesting lessons in this work. Talking about cultural competence makes most people anxious. We know we aren't supposed to be racist or dumb about these things, but that doesn't make us knowledgeable. There is some inherent discomfort. Additionally, organizations give lip service to the importance of cultural competence but aren't real sure what they're supposed to do with it. In healthcare environments, that involves people who were raised in the dominant cultures. The same problems exist when you are trying to integrate immigrant nurses into your healthcare system. You want to do it right, but there is enormous discomfort because we don't know what doing it right looks like.

The first obstacle I had with the clinic was trying to figure out what this community needed. We have a natural tendency to go to the nursing process, so we tend to go to an assessment. We started with kids in the area. From the dominant culture viewpoint, we assumed priorities would be something like immunizations and nutrition. What the kids told us was their biggest need, however, was getting home safely after school without getting shot. It was one of those startling moments when you realize that your presumptions from a dominant culture perspective were incorrect. The same kind of thing happened with trying to figure out the needs of immigrating nurses. We thought they might have needs related to medical terminology. The bigger issue, however, is about the slang and colloquialisms we use. One of the most interesting and amusing is our colloquialisms about elimination. We must be

uncomfortable talking about elimination because we have all these words we make up for it. Someone coming into our culture doesn't have any idea what these words mean. The very fact that we use all of these terms says that we are uncomfortable so it is a challenge to deliver a message to the dominant culture that helps them help people coming into the culture.

The violence issue for the kids was a real challenge. We had to go to the drawing board to look at what our assumptions were. It would be difficult to tell people about getting immunizations and helping them with nutrition when the primary issue was safety in the community. For me the lesson was that I had to be a student if I wanted to be culturally competent. I learned I couldn't go into another culture without being fairly self-critical and self-reflective. I couldn't presume I understood a culture I didn't understand.

I was faced with a critical question of how you secure resources for an unpopular initiative. This was a community where all of the essential health services had been stripped away. The whole question was about how to get enough money for an effort the culture has already decided to underinvest in. I got $60,000 from the local health department that had gotten money from the state health department that had gotten it from the federal government. There was a continuous subtext that devalued what I would put together for the service. The presupposition was, How could you, coming from the dominant culture, being imbedded in a dominant culture institution that had not done this kind of work, possibly do this kind of work? Building coalitions within the community became a big issue. I worked with an African-American colleague who was very credible in the community, and she became my colleague in these negotiations. We learned to go negotiate together. So, first we had to craft our own relationship and how that would work before we could figure out how to go forward in the community. She was very frustrated with the amount of money available. At times she would decide that she just didn't want to do any more for such a small amount of money. That would make me rethink the situation, and I always decided that some money was better than no money, and so I would say that I was going ahead even if it had to be without her. I also made clear that I much preferred having her with me.

The next piece that was really interesting to me was the support from my home institution. This relates to what happens when you really want to do something that is important within your terrain and the larger community of which you are a member (or a member of the leadership team) is not supportive. I saw this clinic as totally congruent with the mission and I would always argue that if you read our mission statement, the unit that was most clearly aligned was nursing. The direct link between the mission statement in hospitals and what people are doing for a living is most intensely demonstrable in nursing. I always argue for mission. Nursing is particularly advantaged. We tend to be almost archetypical in matching the mission. I knew what we were doing was the right thing to do. Everyone knew this work was risky, so rather than asking them to do it with me, I essentially said I was going to do this because it is part of the mission and let them decide if they were going to stop our work. It would be pretty hard to say, "No, don't do it." What I had to let go of was the hope that they would back me, either publicly or privately, to achieve this clinic. Part of making change is being willing to be up front. Sometimes change that is worth making requires that you just have to go it alone. Everyone wanted me to succeed, but no one said, "And, I too have signed on." Fears keep us trapped. Other people's fear is theirs to deal with, but I can't use that to limit what I might do. This

was an important lesson for me. I had to face my fears and own them and acknowledge there was no cheering section.

The proposal from the community (and from my colleague who was very much a part of the community) was if you really want to help us, you'd want us to control our healthcare. Therefore, you would want to create an ideal model using the institution's infrastructure and startup abilities and then allow the community to eventually take over the clinic. That was pretty scary...the institution would provide the initial support and then the community would control it. I was faced with a huge insight: Does the dominant culture really want communities to control their own fate or does it prefer to have dependent communities? There is great risk when you don't operate from a place of entitlement. The issues are often around control. Very often control issues stem from our desire to protect ourselves from failure. We put together a community-based advisory board that actually started before the clinic did. This provided me a great chance to explore what I would call "white guilt"...I wanted them to trust me and their prior experiences suggested they should be very leery of someone who wanted to "come in" and help. I made the commitment to work with the community. We wanted to get communities of healthcare providers to engage with the work of the clinic. We wanted to create it as a teaching site and I was surprised that it was dentistry that stepped up. One of the things that taught me was that you never know which door will open up. We had access to an old school that had been turned over to the community and they said that was where they wanted the clinic. There was a strange mix of services there, but the community wanted a one-stop shop. Another top priority was AIDS testing for men, and the only service available to them was in a setting where everyone knew what you were being tested for based on the physical setup. AIDS is a very charged disease in the African-American community...it has overtones of homosexuality and Africa and monkeys with the disease. They basically said that the only way that it was safe to get AIDS testing was if they controlled it. It was a great example for me of being culturally incompetent...I had to be taught all of that. Reading an article is different from having a community group tell you the story. What I learned from this was that you find out what the community tells you are its first needs. You don't go in with what you wish they had. Part of why healthcare isn't fitting other cultures is because we tell other cultures what they should have. Don't give the appearance of having voice if they don't.

One of the next things they said is that there is nothing about African-American male health. Because women were used to getting care for the family, they had figured out ways to work the system. Sometimes that might involve three bus transfers; that just wasn't going to work for males. Where do you get money for that? What we learned to do was approach foundations with single-focused health problem issues. We built our base this way. Being candid is more uncomfortable for some groups than others. We decided to be innovative and do what is possible and build on that to the next possible level.

We had a grand opening and all of the institutional leaders showed up. Suddenly it was the institution's work. All of the right things were voiced: our commitment, we value diversity, etc. If you are doing something really important, don't wait for the confetti...just keep on moving. What was interesting was the fact that the community didn't have to "make nice," they could genuinely accept or reject those who wanted to interact with them. Do I want to work with issues that don't sustain the disadvantage? That is a critical question to ask yourself.

This is so similar to my work with international nurses. They are seen as just as competent, but they are less likely to have promotional and developmental opportunities. They are very focused on managing the culture. We provide rapid acculturation programs, but we need to come at that as learners...what do they bring to help us understand the world? There is a schism

between comfort and science and most commonly the ones who are providing comfort are people of color. We have lost our focus on comfort; we are too scientific.

One of the big pieces we miss is the sacrifice of the women who come from other countries and leave their families and husbands at home. We are attracting middle and upper class to move to the United States. In general, many of the women are generating resources to be sent home to families. We essentially support them ghettoizing...here are the other X type nurses. We have often excluded the immigrant nurse in a lot of what we do. As you look at demographics of the country, workers will be augmented by nurses from elsewhere. The dominant culture is changing and is already becoming a minority. The dominant culture has no minority skills, and they do have the concept of entitlement. The United States will be increasingly minority. The dominant culture tends to decide there is a right answer and then they make up a story about the right answer. You have to put yourself in an uncomfortable position and be willing to listen if you want to make a difference. You also need to know that you will make a mistake.

One of the issues of Hispanic nurses is the mastery of English language. That is a dialogue that needs to happen. Do we want to be helpful? Does some group or organization want to assume some part of the solution?

One of the examples of language as an important factor is the limitation of access to the country by certain other countries. As a result there is sudden interest in recruiting from the Caribbean. One of their advantages is that they are bilingual; and we need bilingual nurses!

I have a theory: the Kritek Theory of Creating Competence. My theory is that white women are pivotal. They have the advantage of being dominant in ethnicity. They have the disadvantage of gender...they are in the minority. White women understand both sides. The other protocol group is black men. We both are bicultural, we are the translators, the bridge builders. Men in nursing understand this too. Nursing is the most promising community to effect a broad change. We also need to know that the disadvantaged don't necessarily thank us. We are more equipped than the average person in our society....

There are all sorts of possible responses to the issues in healthcare if we are going to address those issues. We are the most promising community!

Chapter References

Aiken, L. H., Buchan, J., Sochalski, J., Nichols, B., & Powell, M. (2004). Trends in international nurse migration. *Health Affairs, 23*(3), 69-77.

Aiken, L. H., Clarke, S. P., Cheung, R. B., Sloane, D. M., & Silber, J. H. (2003). Educational levels of hospital nurses and surgical patient mortality. *The Journal of the American Medical Association, 29*, 1617-1623.

Aiken, L. H., Clarke, S. P., Sloane, D. M., Sochalski, J., & Silber, J. H. (2002). Hospital nurse staffing and patient mortality, nurse burnout and job satisfaction. *The Journal of the American Medical Association, 288*, 1987-1993.

Alexis, O., & Chambers, C. (2003). Exploring Alexis' model: Part one: Valuing resources. *Nursing Management, 10*(4), 29-33.

Allison, V., Bradley, S.G., Chavez, J., Gallegos, B., Rowin, A., Welch, G., & Yoder-Wise, P. S. (2004). Unleashing creativity: Seven strategies for successful learning. *Nurse Educator, 29*(3), 95-96.

Alvarez, L.. Where the healing touch starts with the hospital design. Retrieved September 7, 2004, from *New York Times*, http://www.nytimes.com.

American Nurses Association. (2002). *Nursing's agenda for the future*. Washington, DC: The Association.

American Nurses Association. (1999). *Principles for nurse staffing*. Washington, DC: The Association.

Bessent, H., & Fleming, J. (2003). The leadership enhancement and development (LEAD) project for minority nurses in the new millennium model. *Nursing Outlook, 51*, 255-260.

Betancourt, J. R. (2004). Becoming a physician: Cultural competence—Marginal or mainstream movement. *The New England Journal of Medicine, 351*(10), 953-955.

Biggerstaff, G., & Hamby, L. (2004, August). Diversity—An evolving leadership initiative. *Nurse Leader*, 30-32.

Brush, B. L., & Berger, A. M. (2002). Sending for nurses: Foreign nurse migration, 1965-2002. *Nursing and Health Policy Review, 1*, 103-115.

Bureau of Health Professions. (2002). *The registered nurse population: Findings from the 2000 national sample survey*. Washington, DC: Health Resources and Services Administration.

Buerhaus, P. I., Staiger, D. O., & Auerbach, D. I. (2004). New signs of a strengthening U.S. nurse labor market? *Health Affairs*, 526-533.

Center for the Health Professions. (2002). *Toward culturally competent care: A toolbox for teaching communication strategies*. San Francisco: Center University of California.

Cortis, J. D. (2004). Meeting the needs of minority ethnic patients. *Journal of Advanced Nursing, 48*(1), 51-58.

Cortis, J. D. (2003). Managing society's difference and diversity. *Nursing Standard, 18*(24), 33-39.

Crawford, L. (2004). Nurses educated in other countries: Coming to America. *Journal of Nursing Administration, 6*(3), 66-68.

Frusti, D. K., Niesen, K. M., & Campion, J. K. (2003). Creating a culturally competent organization: Use of the diversity competency model. *Journal of Nursing Administration, 33*(1), 31-38.

Genao, I., Bussey-Jones, J., Brady, D., Branch, Jr., W. T., & Corbie-Smith, G. (2003). Building the case for cultural competence. *The American Journal of Medical Sciences, 326*(3), 136-140.

Georgetown University. (2004, January-February). GUH nurses, staff honored with prestigious "Magnet status" award. *The Star*, p. 1.

Hamilton, D. K. (2004). *A better building*. Retrieved on March 26, 2004, from http://www.hospitalconnect.com/

hhnmag/jsp/articledisplay.jsp?dcrpath=AHA/PubsNews Article/data/040323HHN_Online_Hamilton&domain= HHNMAG.

Hudson Healthcare. (2004). *Symptoms of the nursing shortage affect patients and their families.* Retrieved September 16, 2004, from http://www.Hudson.com.

Hunt, L. M. (2004). *Beyond cultural competence: Applying humility to clinical settings.* Retrieved May 1, 2004, from http://www.parkridgecenter.org/Page1882.html.

Institute of Medicine. (2004). *Keeping patients safe: Transforming the work environment of nurses.* Washington, DC: The National Academies Press.

International Council of Nurses. (2005). *The global shortage of registered nurses.* Geneva, Switzerland: The Council.

Kramer, M., & Schmalenberg, C. (1977). *Path to biculturalism.* Wakefield, MA: Contemporary Publishing.

Lindeke, L. L., & Sieckert, A. M. (2005). *Nurse-physician workplace collaboration.* Retrieved February 3, 2005, from http://www.nursingworld.org/ojin/topic26/tpc26_4.htm.

Majumdar, B., Browne, G., Roberts, J., & Carpio, B. (2004). Effects of cultural sensitivity training on health care provider attitudes and patient outcomes. *Journal of Nursing Scholarship, 36*(2), 161-166.

McCue, M., Mark, B. A., & Harless, D. W. (2003). Nurse staffing, quality and financial performance. *Journal of Health Care Financing, 29*(4), 54-76.

National Advisory Council on Nurse Education and Practice. (2000). Report to the Secretary of Health and Human Services and Congress: A National Agenda for Nursing Workforce Racial/Ethnic Diversity. U. S. Department of Health and Human Services, Health Resources and Services Administration, Bureau of Health Professions, Division of Nursing.

Rogers, A. E., Hwang, W., Scott, L. D., Aiken, L. H., & Dinges, D. F. (2004). The working hours of hospital staff nurses and patient safety. *Health Affairs, 23,* 202-212.

Ruel, M. T. (2003). Operationalizing dietary diversity: A review of measurement issues and research priorities. *Journal of Nutrition, 133*(11): 3911S-3926S.

Schumacher, E. J., & Nathanson, P. (2004). *What nurses want.* Retrieved February 3, 2004, from http://www.hospitalconnect. com/hhnmag/jsp/articledisplay.jsp?dcrpath=AHA/PubsNe wsArticle/data/040203HHN_Online_Schumacher& domain-HHNMAG.

Smith, J. (2003). *The practice of LP/VNs: NCSBN research findings.* Paper presented at NCSBN Annual Meeting, August 3-6, 2004, Kansas City, MO.

Spath, P. (2000). Reducing errors through work system improvements. In P. Spath (Ed.), *Error reduction in health care.* San Francisco: Jossey-Bass.

Sullivan Commission. (2004). *Missing persons: Minorities in the health professions: A report of the Sullivan Commission on diversity in the healthcare workforce.* Retrieved June 15, 2005, from http://admissions.duhs.duke.edu/sullivancommission/ documents/Sullivan_Final_Report_ØØØ.pdf.

Swanson, J. (2004). Diversity: Creating an environment of inclusiveness. *Nursing Administration Quarterly, 28*(3), 207-211.

Thompson, P. A. (2004). Leadership from an international perspective. *Nursing Administration Quarterly, 28*(3), 191-198.

Ulrich, R., Quan, X., Zimring, C., Joseph, A., & Choudhary, R. (2004). *The role of the physical environment in the hospital of the 21st century: A once-in-a-lifetime opportunity.* Retrieved March 8, 2005, from The Center for Health Design, http://www.healthdesign.org/research/reports/physical_ environ.php.

Washington, D., Erickson, J. I., & Ditomassi, M. (2004). Mentoring the minority nurse leader of tomorrow. *Nursing Administration Quarterly, 28*(3), 165-169.

Wynne, R. (2003). Clinical nurses' response to an environment of health care reform and organizational restructuring. *Journal of Nursing Management, 11,* 98-106.

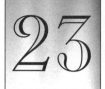

The Chief Nursing Officer and the External World

All that is necessary for the triumph of evil is that good men do nothing. EDMUND BURKE

This chapter focuses on the role of the chief nursing officer (CNO) beyond the place of employment and its related obligations. Creating networks of support and influence and developing levels of influence are important to expanding nursing's influence beyond the organization. A model identifies levels and types of connections important for connecting to the world external to the employing organization.

MOST OF THE TIME AND EFFORT A CHIEF nursing officer puts into work focuses primarily on the internal demands of the role. What the CNO accomplishes within the organization and as an official representative of the organization determines the success of the CNO and of nursing. That work is critical and time consuming. Depending on the role span and the number and abilities of assistive staff, the CNO can feel as if little, if any, time remains for other activities. Even though the internal role can be all-consuming, CNOs have an even broader potential and accountability as leaders in the profession. The connection to the larger world allows the CNO and the nursing service organization to influence that larger world, hopefully for the better.

CNOs typically are seasoned nurses. They have had careers that include increasing accountability,

and they have had external collegial experiences. Sometimes the increase in accountability happens quickly. For example, in nursing homes, staff nurses may become CNOs overnight. Most often, however, the career progression to CNO is one of hierarchic and lateral moves that increase the span of control. As a nurse moves into positions of higher levels of administration, fewer internal peers are available until the solitary CNO level is reached. This diminishing of a peer group within the organization means that CNOs must look to the external world for peers. Thus instead of coaching and supporting peers, top nurse administrators are looking for external colleagues to coach and counsel them. As CNOs become more seasoned, they seek opportunities to provide support to external peers. How CNOs combine these elements to be personally rewarding, to model for those who observe what they do, and to benefit the profession is critical to their future and that of nursing. Looking beyond employment settings and roles allows CNOs and others the opportunity to influence nurses and others and the local community, the state, the nation, and other nations.

After decades of educational programs drilling professional involvement into new graduates, over the past several decades schools have focused heavily on clinical abilities, sometimes to the extent that professional involvement was mentioned briefly and without connection to why it could be valuable. To develop subsequent generations of nurses who will deal with broad policy issues of the profession, the CNO also has to convey the importance of involvement beyond the employment setting. One clear way is to model that important behavior.

The American Organization of Nurse Executives (AONE) Nurse Executive Competencies (2005) address the external nature of the role of the CNO. These competencies include an expectation of organizational involvement, from membership in professional organizations to legislative involvement. They also, for example, address the need for obtaining mentorship from a respected colleague. These competencies form the basis for interpreting what CNOs can do with their careers to support the further development of the profession through work beyond the organization at which they are employed.

INVOLVEMENT IN THE PROFESSION

Organizational views and commitments often change as a new graduate moves toward seasoned professional. One way to think of this involvement is one of evolution. Figure 23-1 suggests a four-phase process. In early stages of new careers, nurses

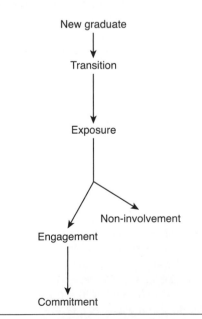

Figure 23-1 Involvement in the profession.

have minimal, if any, involvement in professional organizations, or any other organizations for that matter. Their focus is on transitioning to the world of work and moving from being a novice nurse to a more confident nurse. If they had student loans, they are trying to pay those debts. They are focused on relationship formations, either as young adults or as new nurses, or both. Nurses at this stage of their careers often connect with professional organizations via their web sites and occasionally through a meeting. This phase of professional involvement could be described as *Transitional*.

The next phase of professional involvement could be described as *Exposure*. In other words, these nurses may have connections with an active member of a professional or voluntary organization. They may attend meetings but usually do not do so on a regular basis. They also may become involved in community projects, especially those associated with what their work unit assumes is a worthwhile project. For example, hospitals that are members of Children's Miracle Network often engage their pediatric and neonatal nurses in work associated with that fund-raising endeavor. Professional organizations often are viewed at this point in context of the specific experience the nurses had in any prior involvement. In other words, nurses in this professional phase may move to the next level or they may move to continued (no change) or diminished involvement. Thus this phase influences nurses in their decisions to become more involved or not.

Engagement is the next phase. In this phase, nurses join an organization(s) and at least pay dues. They also begin to experience additional benefits of membership, especially those beyond the educational benefits. They may volunteer for some activity, or they may consider seeking elective office. They also may determine that the effort they can afford is only financial.

Finally, the *Commitment* phase occurs when nurses assume leadership roles by increasing service on committees, seeking elected office, and influencing policy. The commitment level is portrayed by individuals who dedicate a portion of their time for improving the profession at large, not just nursing within the employment settings. These nurses are concerned with and engaged in work that improves the profession or healthcare or both.

It is the responsibility of the CNO to take advantage of external opportunities and to help create situations in which others can gain important external exposures so that their work within the organization benefits.

CREATING NETWORKS

One of the key external involvements that CNOs should have is networks. Several types of networks exist, but all serve important purposes. Gary (2004) defined a developmental network as the group of career advisors on whom one can rely. Gary also identified that it is frequently difficult, if not impossible, to find the full combination of skills in one person. Table 23-1 defines four subnetworks and the functions and values of each.

Receptive networking, just by its name, suggests that little energy has to be expended. It is passive and the networking is almost imposed on the person. In this network, limited personal connection occurs; it is the weakest of the networks.

Traditional networking is often organizationally based. Members of this type of network often are committed to each other and to the organization.

This type of networking comprises loyalty and camaraderie. The challenge may be to help these individuals see beyond the organization for opportunities to connect to broader issues.

Opportunistic networking can be unsatisfactory, because this network can create a sense of "being used." In this case, the member with a need is the one who reaches out to others and usually is asking for direct assistance. Members on the other end of this interchange may feel as if they always are being asked to provide rather than having someone share benefits with them. Little professional development is sought. In other words, "user" members usually are asking for an answer or a favor, not advice and insight.

At the other end of the spectrum is *entrepreneurial* networking. The individual can determine how this network is constructed based on specific, desired learning goals. In addition to the broader connections to people inherent in this type of network, the potential also exists for connection with broader issues. This network focuses on developing loose, lasting relationships. It is designed to provide advice, insight, and connections. This network comprises peers (and others) who could be described as "loyal to me." Regardless of the network type, networks become important.

Another way to think about networking is forming a circle of advisors. These typically are

Table 23-1 Subnetworks That Support Careers

Types	Function/Value
Receptive	Narrow-range networking, low relationships *Little energy expended*
Traditional	Narrow-range networking, high relationships *High level of organizational commitment*
Opportunistic	Wide-range networking, low relationships *Accessing experts for short-term needs*
Entrepreneurial	Wide-range networking, close relationships *High learning potential*

From Gary, L. (2004). The science of networking. *Harvard Management Update*. Article reprint U0401F.

people who can provide the best advice to emerging and established leaders and who trust and are trusted by these individuals. Advisors can assist in creating support for professional learning, career advancement, and work advisement. For example, multiple professional development programs exist. Which is the best "fit" may be determined through discussions with members of a circle of advisors. They may not be the career advancement advisors, but they are always people who are linked to the individual. These people can provide information, which individuals and groups use as connections. No one element is more important than another, and no specific pattern in terms of the advice would be helpful. So, the strategy is to have a network for each of the three areas. If an advisor overlaps in two or more networks, it is even more advantageous.

Professional learning networks are those advisors who can guide the nature of the learning most valuable to a career path and serve as a sounding board about the learning that occurs throughout one's career. For example, knowing which groups are "must connections" is valuable information for nurse leaders who wish to advance their careers. Professional learning consists of more than formal continuing education. Professional learning is an attitude that involves formal educational opportunities in addition to others such as reading publications from other fields and testing ideas in nursing. It may involve attending formal developmental activities, such as the Robert Wood Johnson Nurse Executive Fellows Program. It also may include connecting with a CNO from a comparable organization in a different system, city, or state. Hopefully, it also involves finding a confidant with whom to share ideas about personal learning to gain additional insight and to invest professional development time and money wisely.

Career advancement is another area in which a circle of advisors can help. This circle may be compared with Gary's developmental network described earlier. Career advancement is designed with the intent of having people who are well informed and well connected to serve as advisors.

Although many employment positions are advertised openly, some candidates have advantages because they are connected with prospective positions and key people. People in this career advancement circle provide referrals to others in their group and to organizations for members of the circle. These people are well enough connected with other networks that they know how to analyze potential positions and organizations to determine best fits. They also may know others who know what the issues are in a particular position. In the business world, this network often is referred to as the "old boys" network. Often it is based on place of education and social groups. Nurses, in part because of their massive career potential, often do not capitalize on their first networks: classmates. However, classmates can be valuable, especially if they have followed similar career goals. In addition, some professional organizations even provide specific career counseling.

Work advisement can be therapeutic (most common) or preventive. This circle of advisors is especially useful in providing advice about how to extricate oneself from difficult or impossible situations or from major mistakes. Therapeutic advisement consists of how to handle extremely difficult employees, how to avoid run-ins with physicians, how to handle issues of gender discrimination or inappropriate behavior in the workplace, or how to refute personal rumors. Each of these examples represents situations that most do not think about in advance. In other words, nurses often have not thought about prevention. Often nurse leaders have not considered how to handle finding two employees fighting in an empty patient room or how to handle finding an employee asleep in a back room. Rather, they find the situation and then wonder how to handle it; or they handle it and then wonder if what they did was best. That is what this circle does in a therapeutic manner. After a few exposures to such situations, the smart, emerging nurse leader often seeks preventive advice and forms several "what if" scenarios to ask others in this network so as to be prepared for these difficult challenges. No matter how bizarre something is, probably someone has experienced the same or a comparable situation. Although that person may not be in the nurse's circle of advisors, one of the members may know the right person. That is what a circle of advisors does. It is not static; it evolves as needs and issues arise and as new members are incorporated into the circle.

Several questions can shape the nature of the networking in which a nurse engages. Some of the key questions are the following:
- Who should be in my network?
- How can I expand an established network?
- What is the value of networking outside of my "profile"? (*Profile* refers to how you describe yourself, e.g., nurse, woman, mature, and so forth.)
- How can I improve my current networks? (Yoder-Wise, 2003)

The answers to the questions help shape the nature of a group with which one engages and makes clear why a particular group is valuable. Maintaining relationships takes work, however. Ferrazzi (2005) offers a number of suggestions. For example, "pinging" members of a network is important. This term refers to staying in touch with network members on a regular basis so that members are not strangers to each other when help is needed. Another tip is to not keep score; networks are not as useful as they could be if someone is keeping score regarding who owes what to whom. Doing something as simple as forwarding an important news item can keep a relationship valuable for another member of the group.

Relationships are all there is.
MARGARET WHEATLEY

These networks operate *for* nurse leaders and *by* nurse leaders. In other words, the same general approaches apply whether the person is the recipient or giver of this support. One of the obligations of a CNO is to help others find or create their own circles of advisors.

SPHERES OF EXTERNAL INFLUENCE

Covey (1989) advocates strongly for an attitude of service as one fulfills any leader role. Service, in this sense, refers to providing support to others in their movement toward goals. Service to others is the way to be highly successful, and using that attitude beyond the organization increases the CNO's sphere of influence. Further, Covey's eighth habit, finding your voice and helping others find theirs, is exemplified in the work CNOs do beyond their organizations (2004).

CNOs already have reasons to connect with external groups. Figure 23-2 indicates the complexity of external influences. External influences can range from the local level all the way through international connections. Each circle in Figure 23-2 represents a growing type of influence. Further, the types of interactions can relate to community, nursing, healthcare, or society. Each quadrant represents a wedge of influence. The interaction of levels and types produces multiple ways that a CNO influences others. In each of the various venues, the CNO has the potential to work from local through international levels. It is the "wedge" that allows for depth and intensity, and it is the

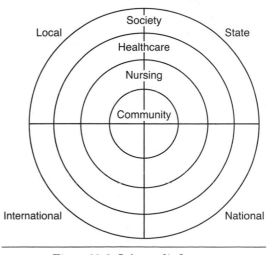

Figure 23-2 Sphere of influence.

circle that allows for the breadth of influence. Although the following information refers to the CNO, it can apply equally well to the connections and support that the CNO uses to assist nurses to attain comparable involvement.

Levels of Connections

Levels of connections also suggest an ever-increasing sphere of influence. These relate to an ever-broadening potential for influence. Generally speaking, during a nurse's career, influence is likely to start with local involvement and move "up" the levels of connections. Whenever the CNO relocates to a new community, a need exists to reestablish local connections even though the higher levels remain. In other words, a CNO may continue to hold a state-elected office even though he or she moves from one city to another. The state connections remain strong even though new local relationships are being established. Taking time to create new local relationships provides intense opportunities to understand how the work of the organization translates to the new community. Using those strengths, the CNO can connect to state, national, and even international levels.

Local Level

As a member of a geographic community, a CNO has the right and simultaneous obligation to be involved in the community. This involvement may be related to the organization, such as serving on a committee of the local board of health. This involvement, which also illustrates commitment to community, could even be serving on the symphony board. One board membership may be better than another, but not necessarily. Any group involvement requires skills such as exquisite listening skills, negotiation, and setting priorities. These are strengths a CNO brings to the job and to the larger world. Although clinical expertise also is captured through the prior board of health example, other benefits can be derived by working with groups external to the field. For example, groups such as the Junior League seek service

opportunities, and the CNO may have a need for such service. Approaching an organization's president when the CNO and president are members of a mutual service organization creates a different entry than if they knew little or nothing about each other. Regardless of the nature of the external involvement as a professional, the point is that external involvement does exist.

State Level

These opportunities can vary widely from serving on a task force of the state nurses association to holding elective office in a nursing or governmental organization. Some CNOs choose to be engaged in some manner at the state level to influence policies that eventually will influence their workplace. For example, service on a state board of nursing could provide opportunities to create blame-free environments as a strategy to improve patient safety.

Sometimes governmental task forces and committees are appointed based on expertise, sometimes on type of organization represented, and sometimes on geographic area. Vetting through the governor's office may be a requirement of appointment, and thus an expectation exists that people beyond the employing organization are familiar with the prospective appointee. Often political involvement assists in this endeavor. Being a registered voter, and voting, is the minimal expectation. Providing contributions or working in campaigns further enhances the prospect for major appointments. This is another reason for being involved in the world external to the employing organization.

National Level

Few nurses have the opportunity to hold national offices in various organizations; however, every CNO can belong to and attend meetings of national groups. Although this involvement creates new networks, it also holds the expectation that the learning potentials are expanded greatly. Now the circle of advisors should include people from various states. Often this level provides exposure to major nursing, healthcare, and political leaders.

Each poses an opportunity to shape others' opinions about relevant issues and to hear even more diverse issues. These connections allow the CNO to exert even more influence in health and public policy.

International Level

Not every CNO will be affiliated with an organization that has an interest in and commitment to international work. For those who do, the relationship may involve sharing older equipment with a developing country. It can involve groups such as Doctors Without Borders, an interdisciplinary group devoted to charitable care of victims worldwide. It also can involve serving as a "sister" hospital to a hospital with greater healthcare needs than those found in the United States. For example, the hospitals in Russia and Armenia that were interested in the Magnet concept were linked with U.S. Magnet facilities to support their work in undertaking a journey to excellence. In recognition of their efforts, these international hospitals received recognition from the American Nurses Credentialing Center (ANCC) for their work. This involvement takes additional effort to be culturally sensitive to the differences between countries in addition to the differences between nursing and healthcare.

Types of Connections

The four different types of connections or interactions suggest an ever-increasing sphere of influence.

Community

The community may be defined roughly as the service area. Therefore in a rural Utah area, the community may encompass several towns. In New York City, the community may represent only a small portion of a borough. Although few reasons exist to have a specific definition of community, the key is it is the core relational basis for the CNO.

Community also can refer to a larger "service area": for example, the usual referral network or a global population group. That may encompass hundreds of miles and millions of consumers. In such cases, the CNO again represents the organization to people who may or may not be familiar with the healthcare organization.

Community also can be seen as the citizen of the health plan, the state, or the region, depending on how the organization defines itself in its mission. In fact, some organizations clearly define themselves as world-class organizations with the expectation that people seeking the best healthcare from any place in the world might connect with them.

Because CNOs are members of communities, CNOs automatically have connections with the community. What the CNO does with those connections is what matters in networking. For example, part of a marketing strategy relates to the way in which the organization and its representatives connect with the community. As the chief of the core service, nursing, the CNO has a remarkable opportunity to engage with others outside the organization. The CNO can "tell the story" in a different way than other executives because, if he or she has done the job right, involvement in care issues is a part of everyday work. These rich exposures provide an abundance of stories. In addition to discussing real healthcare problems, the CNO can share the humanity of caring, and that is a key element in creating personal connections with the healthcare organization. So, whether the group is the Junior League, the Kiwanis, the Fraternal Order of Eagles, a school board, a group of retired citizens, or a church group, the CNO can connect the group to the healthcare organization's mission. Joining such groups or serving on a committee can be even more influential than giving a speech. No matter where the CNO is or what the CNO is doing, the CNO represents himself or herself, the profession, and the organization. Linking with the community provides new connections for influence.

Nursing

Nursing can be the most pervasive external relationship because that is what the CNO is—a nurse.

Nursing connections occur most commonly through professional organizations. Providing expert leadership through the broad professional organization, the American Nurses Association (ANA) or one of its member organizations; or through a clinical specialty organization, such as the American Association of Critical Care Nurses (AACCN); or through a role-specific organization, such as AONE, allows the CNO to influence the broader nursing community. Box 23-1 highlights AONE.

More than 90 nursing organizations exist in the United States, which makes the low percentage of nurse membership in any professional organization difficult to understand. The CNO can help change this by modeling professional involvement, creating opportunities for others to participate in external events, and supporting policies that enhance the potential for others to engage in such opportunities.

Sometimes the CNO is in a nursing meeting as the spokesperson or representative for the nursing service organization; other times, the CNO is involved as an individual expert. Either way, the CNO is linking the organization with the larger world of nursing.

Healthcare

Everything that can be said about nursing can be said about healthcare involvement; the groups merely change. Therefore groups such as the American Hospital Association (AHA) and its state groups, the Joint Commission on Accreditation of Healthcare Organizations (JCAHO), or the numerous governmental panels (city, county, state, and national) that incorporate disciplines other than nursing are representative. In these situations, CNOs may be representing the organization of employment or the profession of nursing. However, despite how the CNO arrived at one of these tables, he or she remains a nurse. Pam Thompson's story (see the Leader Story) illustrates this point.

Society

Once again, the type of involvement may be the same, as previously described, but the groups change. When CNOs are involved at societal levels, they may be representing an organization through a professional or employment capacity or they may be representing themselves. In other words, sometimes a CNO is selected because he is a nurse or because he represents the city or county hospital. Other times, the CNO is selected because she is who she is; Florence Nightingale would be a perfect historical example of this selection.

Societal involvement may be related to activities such as forming policy recommendations or testifying before groups to improve healthcare. Influencing governmental agencies and Congress are probably the ultimate activities in creating far-reaching effects for society. Serving in think tanks related to healthcare is another example. Furthermore, each of these illustrates ways in which CNOs can influence society.

Box 23-1   American Organization of Nurse Executives (AONE)

AONE is a subsidiary of the AHA and represents nurses who are leaders in the design and delivery of nursing care.

According to the AONE web site, the organization provides leadership, professional development, advocacy, and research to advance nursing practice and patient care, promote nursing leadership excellence, and shape healthcare public policy. The organization is divided into regions. More than 45 chapters exist, and they provide services and networking opportunities in the states or regions they comprise. The organization holds an annual meeting in the spring and numerous other meetings throughout the year. *Nurse Leader*, the official publication of AONE, began in January 2003.

SUMMARY

Extending talents beyond the organization is a way that CNOs can influence the broader world. Carefully honing talents typically allows exercise of more influence than often benefits the organization. Involvement in ever-expanding levels of influence creates broader levels of influence. Being involved in more than nursing also expands the types of influence a CNO can have. Networking with other CNOs often creates or supports these expanding opportunities. Concomitantly, the CNO

can encourage development of networks for others within the organization so that they too have greater influence.

KEY POINTS TO LEAD

1. Evaluate your network, using Table 23-1.
2. Create a plan to expand the level and/or type of influence you have in the external world.
3. Attend a local, state, or national meeting with the goal of creating a broader circle of advisors.

Literature Box

In addition to more demands on the current workforce, the level of volunteerism has declined over the past few years. This article describes a leadership fellows program to develop new leaders and to provide personal development opportunities. The New York State Nurses Association (NYSNA) created such a program with an anticipated cost of under $20,000 per class. The focus on selecting fellows was the potential for leadership, not recognition of veteran leaders. The program is designed to be a "risk-free observational and experiential" one (p. 82). In addition to other activities, the Myers-Briggs Type Indicator is used as the basis for a team-building workshop that is part of this program.

The outcomes of the work reported in this article are profound. Of the 36 fellows (who had completed the program at the time of this article's publication), 32 held leadership positions at the

national, state, or local levels. Many had received awards for work they had accomplished. In addition to geographic diversity, the fellows represented direct practice, management, and education. Concomitantly, NYSNA created a Leadership Institute to recognize veteran leaders as a way to simultaneously acknowledge "faithful" leaders. Finally, the program includes a formal mentoring role.

To address broad issues within the profession, developing future leaders is critical. This program is one example of how such formal support is available.

Barrett, B., & Orr, M. L. (1999, January). Developing future leaders: How one association uses a fellowship program to attract and develop new volunteer leaders. *Association Management*, 80-83.

Contemplations

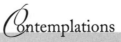

- What core elements exist among all of the various expectations for the role of the CNO?
- How is it possible to juggle the daily focus of being a manager with the long-range view of being a leader?

- Who are the best role models in the organization? How do they balance their subroles within the administrative role? How do they balance their work role with their personal life?
- How can the CNO best balance all of the demands and expectations of the role?

LEADER STORY ❧

Pamela Austin Thompson
CEO, American Organization of Nurse
Executives
Washington, DC

After I completed my master's degree, I held several positions before I interviewed at Dartmouth-Hitchcock Medical Center in Lebanon, New Hampshire. Up until that point, I hadn't been active in professional organizations. During this time, I had been trying out different roles to see if I could find out which role suited me best. I had both a strong education and administrative preparation in my master's program. So, I worked in education and then management. I even negotiated the creation of a different position to combine my manager role and a clinical nurse specialist (CNS) role. I was really exploring what arena I wanted to practice in. I was busy testing these various roles and too focused on deciding what direction to take. I had no focus on association involvement. During my interview at Dartmouth, one of the interviewers asked about my lack of professional association involvement and then told me that she expected that I would become involved if I accepted the position. She shared with me that she liked my professional resume but that she didn't think my professional life would be complete without external involvement. So, when I became the Director of Maternal Child Health and Psychiatric Services, becoming active in a professional association was one of my goals. In New Hampshire that was the New Hampshire Organization of Nurse Executives (NHONE). So I joined and served on several task forces. Then, I ran for office and was elected Secretary and then President.

As part of my role as President of NHONE, I also became involved with the New Hampshire Hospital Association (NHHA) and eventually was elected Chair of their Board of Trustees. I was the first nurse executive ever to be elected

Chairman of the Board and the NHHA staff believed that I was also the first nurse executive nationwide to do so. We were very excited about that. It was a wonderful story of building relationships within associations and having the value of the nurse leader's perspective at the table and included. I was able to bring both the nursing and the patient care perspective to the work we did at the hospital association.

While serving on the NHHA Board, I ran for office of AONE and was elected as the Board representative from the New England region. In this role, I attended regional hospital association meetings representing AONE. However, the region knew me as Chair of the NHHA Board and yet I was at these regional meetings because I was representing AONE. This time allowed me to walk among different circles and interweave the work. I found that I really loved what I was doing, working within associations for the profession.

That experience really evolved into the position I have now. The former Executive Director of AONE retired and someone asked if I were going to apply. I laughed! I thought, "Why on earth would I do that?" My career track at the time was to be either a CNO of a larger healthcare organization or the CEO of a small rural hospital. That's what I thought I really wanted. That's what I thought my career would be. The idea of association management had never even been considered. But, because I wanted to explore the possibilities, and I respected my colleague's suggestion that I should consider it, I bought a book on "Successful Association Management." As I was reading, I realized that everything I loved in my professional volunteer life would be my paid job. It was as though I had been preparing myself for that job for years, without even knowing it. And then I knew why on earth I really wanted to try for this job—it was a perfect match to what I loved to do. So, I applied and the association leadership was willing to take a chance with me. It was one of the best decisions I ever made. It tapped my passion and joy in a way that I could never have constructed a deliberate path to achieve it.

Relationship management was one of the most important skills I developed through all of this. During another volunteer experience, I served on a board where I was the only nurse, the only female, and one of only two hospital employees. Everyone else was from community mental health centers. I had to learn how to "cross talk." Working with colleagues from different backgrounds provided me with the opportunity to translate my perspective to others and educate them at the same time. Often, because of my hospital clinical perspective, I was the one with a diverse opinion, and I didn't approach the issues the same as the rest who were serving on this board. If I wanted to be heard, I had to understand how to bring forth a different perspective that they would hear. That allowed me to gain credibility and respect. The same thing was true for the hospital association. There were limited opportunities for a nurse to be engaged with the board except as a guest. To be present with a decision-making capacity, I had a responsibility to articulate positions so that they were understood by others on the board. I had to be able to understand the perspective of the other person so that I would know what is important to them. Sometimes, it is almost as if you speak different languages. But the common goal was always patient care.

You have to listen to the other person's language and translate your message. You have to listen to what is important to others. If you were to ask most CEOs if they value patient care, the answer would be yes. They just approach it from a different perspective. Part of the listening is to understand the language, but the other part is to determine what the common goals are. Once you know what the common goals are, you can align

your message and then different opinions don't seem so diverse. Listen to align…it's very subtle. If there isn't agreement, at least you are bringing the disagreement to the table so that you are all talking with a common understanding.

Watch what you do and learn from it. It gave me insight into when I was successful and when I wasn't. I really tried to understand what was happening in any situation, and part of how I gained that insight stemmed from people asking me to reflect on an event or exchange. For example, people asked me how I came to be elected president of the hospital association. Well, part of it was hard work…you have to volunteer. You can't wait for people to come to you. You can't sit on the sidelines. When you produce the work and engage in the conversation, that helps create your credibility.

I also took advantage of opportunities to teach. For example, I had gone to a conference on chaos theory when this was a new topic in healthcare. Several months later, I was at a hospital association retreat and I mentioned that I had learned how to teach chaos theory with a tennis ball and a balloon. They were intrigued. They wanted to know what I meant. So, they got the tennis ball and balloon and I taught them that the tennis ball was like linear thought. You bounce the ball and depending on where you aim it, you can predict where it will bounce. It is not affected by the more subtle variables in the environment. However, take a blown-up balloon. If you point it in a direction and release it, who knows where it will go even when aimed in somewhat the same direction as the tennis ball? It behaves in a nonlinear way. They both take a path, one predictable, one not, one linear, one more like chaos theory. That changed our conversation; I became the teacher. I took advantage of as many of those conversations as I could. That ability to be a participant and a part of bringing new knowledge to the table made a difference. We shouldn't discredit what we know, and we should share what we know.

Another major thing I learned is a harder conversation for us. In these non-nursing board rooms, nursing was often seen as being in a "needy state."

Hearing our messages described that way taught me an important lesson. We have to be careful about how we put our message forward. What some people shared with me was that they had a very negative reaction to the position of "always needing." I got that advice early on, and I was very attentive to not presenting ideas from that perspective. I could present the same information and the same needed solution, but I could be sensitive to what in the message might be perceived in a way that blocked my message from being heard. It was a learning that I incorporated and tried to work with. You still deliver the message of what is needed; you just have to frame it differently. It is all about the language and how we use it. That's why I see that so much of this is about relationships and communication.

Some may think that I sought these experiences so I could say that I was president of various groups. I don't think that is the case. I didn't have a master plan of what I would do; the opportunities just presented themselves and I acted on them. I do believe I saw how much my learning about leadership was enhanced with these experiences. That became the motivation to seek additional opportunities. They kept me fueled and made me better. Much of personal leadership development comes from experience and the learning gained by reflection.

I think we have some specific obligations to the next generation of leaders in nursing. I think they come with much stronger business skills and they will put those skills to use by creating a business case for patient care. I think they don't have good life balance skills…and neither do we. It is very hard right now to create a balance. Sometimes you feel as if you don't have time to do what's really important. Too many priorities pose a dilemma. You have to do both. Nurse leaders are pressured by staff and by CEOs and there seem to be limited options. The multitude of competing demands in healthcare seem to be one of the most stressful situations people face. And, on top of that, we live in a society that is also too fast-paced. However, I think many exciting things are happening and the real key is to find your passion. For me, I loved my volunteer work. It took me out of the four walls of the hospital and revealed a bigger picture of nursing leadership. Now, I am deliberately crafting my work around that passion.

So, make sure you identify and pursue what you love to do. But most important of all, be open for the surprise. You never know where it might take you.

Chapter References

American Organization of Nurse Executives. (2005). AONE Nurse Executive Competencies. *Nurse Leader, 3*(1), 15-21.

Barrett, B., & Orr, M. L. (1999, January). Developing future leaders: How one association uses a fellowship program to attract and develop new volunteer leaders. *Association Management,* 80-83.

Covey, S. R. (1989). *The seven habits of highly effective people: Powerful lessons in personal change.* New York: Simon and Schuster.

Covey, S. R. (2004). *The 8th habit: From effectiveness to greatness.* New York: Simon and Schuster.

Ferrazzi, K. (2005). *Never eat alone: And other secrets to success, one relationship at a time.* New York: Doubleday.

Gary, L. (2004). The science of networking. *Harvard Management Update.* Article reprint U0401F.

Yoder-Wise, P. S. (2003). Networking. In L. J. Shinn (Ed.), *Conversations in leadership in professional nursing associations.* Pensacola, FL: Pohl Publishing.

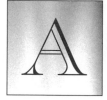

Leadership and Management Concepts: A Brief Overview

Nurses who approach higher levels of nursing positions in healthcare organizations have read about, discussed, and used leadership, management, and related theories and concepts. Sometimes, however, the focus has been on the practicality of a theory or concept rather than the core elements of what it comprises. Therefore this appendix provides a brief overview of key theories and leadership and management thought as a quick reference.

ABILENE PARADOX

This famous 1974 article by Jerry Harvey conveys a story about a family taking a trip to Abilene for dinner. The gist is that no one wanted to get in the car on a hot Texas afternoon, but they all did because they thought someone else wanted to go. "Organizations frequently take actions in contradiction to what they really want to do and therefore defeat the very purposes they are trying to achieve" (p. 129). The key point is that being able to secure disagreement and manage agreement is important to an organization's survival.

Harvey, J. B. (1974, Summer). The Abilene paradox: The management of agreement. *Organizational Dynamics*, 128-146.

ACCOUNTING PRINCIPLES

The rules by which the budget is analyzed for the purpose of audits are controlled by federal standards, which have tightened since the late 1990s. The principles are numerous, but the most dramatic

recent ones are referred to as Sarbanes-Oxley. Among those provisions is the equivalent of a CEO affidavit that the financial status is as depicted in the audit. Although Sarbanes-Oxley applies only to for-profit organizations, many not-for-profit organizations use the principles to guide their performance.

ALBRECHT'S ORGANIZATIONAL POLITICS ANALYSIS

Each of the following five categories represents possible political influences within an organization:
- Inner-circle relationships: existence of special groups with the potential for more influence than another group
- Axis of influence: connection to the executive level offices that enhance an individual's influence over others
- Informal power centers: influential groups or departments, which may be related to expertise, control of resources, or special relationships with influential others
- Polarizing elements: competitive or negative relationships
- Informal coalitions: groups that tend to side together in disputes or for a specific purpose, but not necessarily in ongoing relationships

Albrecht, K. (1983). *Organization development: A total systems approach to positive change in any business organization*. Englewood Cliffs, NJ: Prentice Hall.

AUTOCRATIC LEADERSHIP STYLE

See Leadership Styles.

BENCHMARKING

This term refers to a process of comparing practices at one place with the best practices of another comparable organization. It uses Deming's *plan, do, check, act* process. The first step involves such decisions as determining if your organization is able to conduct a benchmark by itself or if it needs to secure external assistance. This step also involves determining with whom to benchmark. The second step is to determine as much as possible about the organization with which you want to benchmark. The third step involves analyzing the findings of the gaps between your organization and the benchmarked organization. The final step is the actual action to take on the findings. What should be changed and how? Bias for action is built in, which creates an improvement-driven approach.

BENNIS

Warren Bennis has been influential in management and leadership work for years. He is a distinguished professor of business administration at the University of Southern California. He is best noted for his work with leadership.

BLAKE AND MOUTON

Blake and Mouton created the Managerial Grid, which plots production and people concerns on axes. Because the two axes are independent, it is possible for an individual to be high or low or mixed on both factors. After completing an assessment, individuals are able to plot their results on the grid. The result is one of five key management styles. Thus a person can range from minimal concern for people or production all the way to a highly productive, people-oriented style.

THE MANAGERIAL GRID (BLAKE AND MOUTON)

Name of Style	Description	Concern for People	Concern for Production
Country Club Management	Friendly work environment based on attention to relationships	High	Low
Team Management	Common mission and relationships of trust and respect	High	High
Task Management	Balance between productivity and maintenance of morale	Mid level	Mid level
Impoverished Management	Minimal interaction and performance	Low	Low
Middle of the Road Management	Focus on production with minimal concern for human element	Low	High

Modified from The Leadership Grid® figure by Robert R. Blake and Anne Adams McCanse (Formerly the Managerial Grid by Robert R. Blake and Jane S. Mouton). Houston: Gulf Publishing Company. © 1991 by Scientific Methods. Inc. Reproduced by permission of the owners.

BLEICH'S TASK OF MANAGEMENT AND FOLLOWERSHIP

Aspect	Management	Followership
Systems and processes	Identifies those for which management is responsible and accountable	Works within defined systems and processes; is individually accountable
Standards	Verifies expectations for staff achievement	Abides by the standards
Knowledge, skills, and abilities	Validates and capitalizes on these in staff and strengthens development	Offers these to accomplish work
Plan of work	Communicates comprehensive plan of work	Collaborates to achieve work
Work effectiveness	Eliminates barriers and obstacles	Contributes to effectiveness through data collection for outcome measures
Individual effectiveness	Evaluates equity in work	Demonstrates accountability for self
Change	Provides rewards for individuals and teams	Assumes reasonable risks
Improvement	Recommends system and process improvements	Provides feedback
Culture	Includes others in decisions as appropriate	Enhances culture through feedback

From Bleich, M. R. (2003). Managing, leading, and following. In P. S. Yoder-Wise (Ed.), *Leading and managing in nursing.* St. Louis: Mosby.

BRAINSTORMING

This strategy is designed to produce as many ideas as possible for a problem or issue. A session can last a few minutes or several hours.

The Process

- Develop a clear problem statement.
- Introduce statement to group (usually a small group of 6 to 12).
- Share the rules.
- Record all ideas on chalkboard or flip chart.
- Review the list to select a key idea for implementation.

The Rules

- No criticism of ideas is allowed. (Note: This is what happens in the review stage.)
- Wild ideas are welcome!
- Quantity, not quality, is the goal.
- No proprietary ideas are allowed. (Build on or combine others.)

Osborn, A. F. (1963). *Applied imagination* (3rd ed.). New York: Scribner's.

BUNDLING

Bundling involves grouping several products or services together. In nursing, the "fee" for services is included in a daily charge for the basic room and services. The criticism of this practice is that clients do not see the costs of the care they receive from the nursing staff. In addition, because the charge typically varies by clinical site not intensity of care, the room charge often does not reflect the actual level of care provided.

BUSINESS WARNING SIGNALS

Although most CNOs do not have direct accountability for the financial viability of an organization, they do need to know signals of difficulty.

- Financial reports are late or unavailable or require major adjustments.
- Deposits are limited and overdrafts or returned checks are more common.
- Accruals are increasing.
- Loan payments are late.
- Services are late or substandard.
- Inventory is not replaced.
- Key business operations are not timely.
- Scheduling meetings is difficult.
- Legal actions are instituted.
- Negative talk from customers and competitors increases.

CAPACITY

This term refers to the potential outcome of any work endeavor. It involves availability of staff and services that could be expanded to meet a need. For example, *staff capacity* refers to how much actual provision of care is possible.

CASH COW

This term refers to a service or product that produces more than sufficient income to offset the costs of producing that service or product. Although reasons may exist not to pursue cash cows, if they are consistent with the mission, they can provide financial support for endeavors that are important but not financially productive.

CHANGE PHASES

One of the literature's frequently referenced sets of words pertains to the way change occurs. Multiple people have been given credit for actually coining the terms. The four phases are the following:

1. *Forming:* Forming refers to the results of a forecasting process: what needs to change and how. Clear goals are set.
2. *Storming:* Storming refers to the intense process of the change itself.
3. *Norming:* Norming refers to the strategy of "fixing" the change. Although cultural shift occurred in both of the prior phases, this step makes clear that "this is the new expectation," and thus the new performance is now the new culture.
4. *Performing:* Performing refers to the actual integration of the new performance into everyday practice to the extent that minimal or little "backsliding" occurs to the prior standard or performance.

Herman, S. M., Te Ching, L. T. T., & De Jing, L. D. (1994). *Tao at work: On leading and following.* San Francisco: Jossey Bass.

CHERRY PICKING

This term refers to selecting only certain elements of services and products frequently seen as the best. Similar to eating cherries, you discard the less than desirable and choose only the most desirable.

COGNITIVE DISSONANCE

This theory is based on an attempt to maintain consistency or balance among knowledge, viewpoints, and values. When they are inconsistent, dissonance occurs.

CONTINGENCY THEORY

This theory focuses on matching the leader's style to the context of the situation. It is about the "fit" of the leader's actions with the situation, which includes many factors, such as the sophistication of the follower in relation to a specific task.

CORPORATE CULTURE

Simplistically, this term refers to the general feel or overall style of an organization. It refers to such aspects as formal or informal, patient-centered or not.

COST-BENEFIT ANALYSIS

This analysis refers to comparison of the total costs of performing a service (or producing a product) with the benefits, which may include income, good will, creation of a market niche, and so forth.

COST CENTER

A unit or division to which costs (and income) can be attributed makes up a cost center. Most nursing units and specialized services are cost centers.

COVEY

Although Covey did not invent the concept of servant leader, he certainly is the individual who popularized the phrase and the concept. He is best known for his book *The 7 Habits of Highly Effective People.*

Covey's seven habits of highly effective people are as follows:

1. Be proactive.
2. Begin with the end in mind.
3. Put first things first.
4. Think win/win.
5. Seek first to understand, then to be understood.
6. Synergize.
7. Sharpen the saw.

Covey, S. R. (1989). *The 7 habits of highly effective people.* New York: Simon & Schuster.

His eighth habit, published in 2004, is to find your voice and encourage others to find theirs.

Covey, S. R. (2004). *The 8th habit: From effectiveness to greatness.* New York: Simon & Schuster.

DECISION TREE ANALYSIS

A decision tree analysis is designed to show options and outcomes of a decision and subsequent decisions. Adding financial information and the probabilities of success helps leaders to focus on selecting the best decision.

1. Select the options available for addressing an issue.
2. Draw a decision tree.
3. Enter the projected costs of each decision.
4. Enter the probabilities of success.

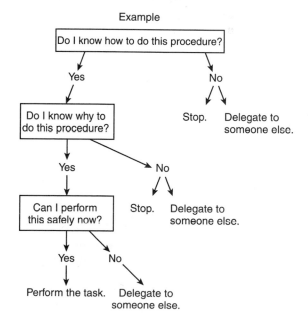

Decision Tree Analysis

Example

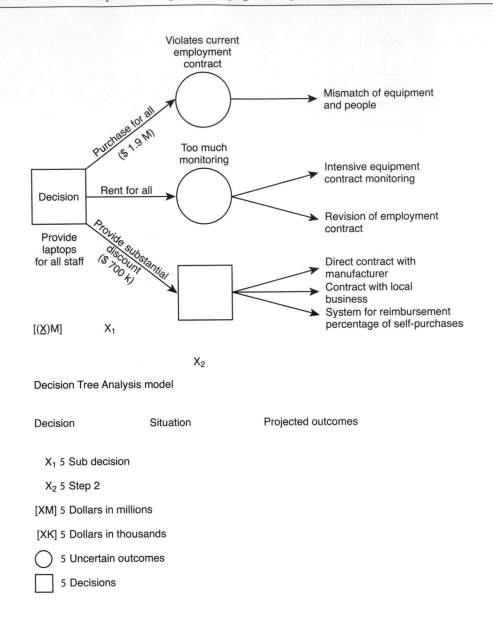

Decision Tree Analysis model

Decision	Situation	Projected outcomes

X_1 5 Sub decision

X_2 5 Step 2

[XM] 5 Dollars in millions

[XK] 5 Dollars in thousands

◯ 5 Uncertain outcomes

▢ 5 Decisions

DELPHI TECHNIQUE

Developed by the Rand Corporation, this strategy is designed to capitalize on individuals' thinking even when they are in remote places. It originally was designed as a forecasting technique but is now used in numerous ways when a group is attempting to reach a reasonable consensus. Generally a group of experts is used as the responders. The following are the general steps to follow:

1. Leader creates a factual briefing.
2. Leader sends the briefing to all.
3. Each member generates a list of ideas related to the topic.

4. Leader reviews the ideas and creates a listing of all.
5. Leader sends out a second round (ideas, responses, questions).
6. Leader repeats the review and listing and resolicitation until no new ideas emerge.
7. Leader creates a resolution. This may be from a clear consensus or on the merit of the ideas or an actual "final" round where voting is conducted.

Sackman, H. (1974). *Delphi assessment: Expert opinion, forecasting and group process.* Santa Monica, CA: The Rand Corporation.

DEMING'S 14 POINTS OF QUALITY MANAGEMENT

1. Create constancy of purpose for improvement of product and service.
2. Adopt the new philosophy.
3. Cease dependence on inspection to achieve quality.
4. End the practice of awarding business on the basis of price tag.
5. Improve constantly and forever the systems of production and service.
6. Institute training on the job.
7. Institute leadership.
8. Drive out fear.
9. Break down barriers between departments.
10. Eliminate slogans, exhortations, and targets for the workforce.
11. Eliminate numerical quotas for the workforce and numerical goals for management.
12. Remove barriers that rob people of pride and workmanship.
13. Institute a vigorous program of education and self-improvement for everyone.
14. Put everyone in the company to work to accomplish the transformation.

Deming, W. E. (1986). *Out of the crisis.* Cambridge, MA: Massachusetts Institute of Technology. Reprinted with permission.

DEMOCRATIC LEADERSHIP STYLE

See Leadership Styles.

DRUCKER

Peter Drucker is a name commonly associated with organizational leadership. He often is considered the father of modern management. His 35 books span numerous management issues. *See Management by Objectives.*

DUN AND BRADSTREET

This organization produces reports that frequently result in an organization's credit rating. This in turn affects the organization's ability to secure loans, seek advancements on cash, and so forth.

ECONOMIES OF SCALE

Basically this concept refers to lowering costs by producing or including more. It is associated with such aspects of healthcare as specific specialties for which the costs of personnel and equipment are readily offset by the number of clients needing the service and the rate of reimbursement or payment for the service. The greater the quantity is, the lower the per-unit cost is.

EMOTIONAL INTELLIGENCE

Emotional intelligence is focused on the social skills or interpersonal competencies that lead to positive working relationships. The idea of psychologic maturity allows people to interact in positive ways and focus on the goal of the work rather than on negative feelings about another. Having self-insight is one of the key factors in this concept. That theoretically is the basis for controlling our emotions, being positive in interactions with others, and being empathetic.

Goleman, D. P. (1995). *Working with emotional intelligence.* New York: Bantam Books.

EXPECTANCY THEORY

Expectancy theory is based on force field analysis. Thus it is based on the number of people who need or want something to be or to exist. The actual drive to achieve this something is based also on the likelihood of being able to achieve it. Therefore expectancy is both how many want something and how realistic/attainable something is. The thought then is that something that is more easily attained does not take the same force of people wanting it as would something less attainable. Like force field analysis, the use of negatives (−1) and positives (+1) suggests in which direction the expected force exists.

−1 _____ +1

Negative   Positive
expectation   expectation

    Place an x on the line. For example, how many people support an idea (decision, goal, etc.)? How realistic is attainment of the idea?

Vroom, V. (1964). *Work and motivation*. New York: Wiley.

FAYOL

Henri Fayol is known as the father of the management process: planning, organizing, coordinating, and controlling. Like others, he was a devotee of specialization. He also advocated for worker stability and equal treatment. He was widely influential at the turn of the 20th century.

FIXED ASSET

Fixed assets usually appear as a part of the balance sheet of an organization. They represent such aspects of businesses as buildings, land, and major equipment.

FOCUS GROUP

This type of research consists of forming a small group (usually 8 to 12 people) that is then interviewed as a group for the purpose of exchange of ideas and elaboration on points. This kind of approach could be done, for example, with a specific type of patient group to determine what they valued (or not) about current services. It is used in numerous businesses that provide services and products to the public.

FORCE FIELD THEORY

Kurt Lewin (pronounced loo-vin) studied group forces and concluded that group pressure was more effective than individual influence. His theory typically is represented by a series of factors above or below a line (where the line represents no change) and plus or minus indicators with numbers to show the strength of an influence on a proposed change. The following example reflects positive movement toward supporting a change in the way in which medications are administered.

Supervisor's support	Physician's support	Staff support	
+1	+2	+4	Positive factors ↑
−3	−2		Negative factors ↓
Cost	Pharmacy support		

    Numbers noted in the above example represent relative values, with higher numbers representing more of the factor.

Lewin, K. (1951). *Field theory in social sciences*. New York: Harper & Row.

FOUR Ps

This classic terminology represents product, price, place, and promotion. Those are the four key areas of marketing concerns.

GANTT CHARTS

Gantt charts comprise two axes. On one, the work plan appears; on the other, the amount of time. Each step of the work plan appears and is noted in terms of when it is to occur.

GANTT CHART EXAMPLE

Work Plans

Steps	Weeks				
	1	2	3	4	5
Develop	X				
Implement Phase 1		X			
Implement Phase 2			X		
Monitor Phase 1			X	X	
Monitor Phase 2				X	
Evaluate data					X

X, Number of weeks to achieve work plan.

GARDNER'S TASKS OF LEADERSHIP

- Envisioning goals
- Affirming values
- Motivating
- Managing
- Achieving workable unity
- Developing trust
- Explaining
- Serving as symbol
- Representing the group
- Renewing

Gardner, J. W. (Copyright © 1990). *On leadership.* New York: Free Press, a Division of Simon & Schuster Adult Publishing Group. All rights reserved.

GILBRETH'S TIME AND MOTION

Frank and Lillian Gilbreth focused on time and motion and increasing efficiency. They also originated flow charts to diagram work and were the first to look at fatigue in repetitive work. The book and movie *Cheaper by the Dozen* was based on their lives and illustrates their commitment to efficiency in all aspects of life, including how they managed their family.

Gilbreth, R. B., & Gilbreth, L. M. (1917). *Applied motion study.* New York: Sturgis & Walton.

GREAT MAN THEORY OF LEADERSHIP

This theory of leadership operates on the belief that leaders are born. Most literature sources may cite this theory yet focus more on the concept that leaders are developed.

GREENLEAF'S SERVANT LEADERSHIP

The idea of servant leadership was first described by Greenleaf. This is the basis for Covey's later work. The idea of serving the group is core to the group's focus and cohesiveness in purpose. The Greenleaf Center for Servant-Leadership is accessible at http://www.greenleaf.org.

Greenleaf, R. K. (1977). *Servant leadership.* New York: Warner Books.

GROUP NORMS

Group norms are the standards of acceptable behavior within a defined group. One individual may experience various group norms based on the number of groups in which he or she interacts. The norms may include clothing expectations, formalities, location of meetings, specific behaviors, the style of communication, and the use of "in" terms.

GROWTH SHARE MATRIX

The Boston Consulting Group is a recognized source for the matrix of comparing market growth potential with competitors (share).

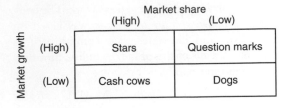

Relative Market Share

Stars: High growth and share. Rapid growth potential.

Question marks: Low share. Weak cash flow. Considerable cash needed to maintain share.

Cash cows: Dominant products in mature market.

Dogs: Low share and slow growth. If cash infusion is needed, consider divesting and reallocate funds and efforts to question marks or stars.

The Boston Consulting Group, 1973.

HAWTHORNE EFFECT

The Hawthorne Effect became the standard term for the different behavior of workers when they were observed. When Hawthorne conducted studies about the effects of light in the workplace, using a control and experimental group, both groups increased their productivity. In essence, the increased production was due to the fact that the workers were engaged in a process that was being observed.

http://www.accel-team.com/motivation/hawthorne_02.html

HERSEY AND BLANCHARD

These researchers' work includes a balance of tasks and relationships and adds the factor of the maturity of the worker (in terms of the work to be performed). The idea is that the more sophisticated the worker is in relation to the work, the less task orientation the leader will have.

HERZBERG'S MOTIVATION-HYGIENE THEORY

Frederick Herzberg looked at what motivated people. He was exceedingly influential in his view of management and his theory of motivation. Factors causing dissatisfaction are different from those causing satisfaction. So a certain level of salary has to be present or dissatisfaction occurs, but a higher level salary does not necessarily create satisfaction (see *Motivation-Hygiene Theory*).

INDIRECT COST

Any cost that cannot be attributed to a specific unit or service is called *indirect*. This cost frequently includes management salaries, utilities, taxes, and rent. These costs also may be termed *overhead* or *administrative fees*.

JOHARI WINDOW

The Johari Window, created by Joseph (Jo) Luft and Harry (har) Ingham (i), was designed to depict human interaction. It consists of self and others as the two key factors and whether something is known. This "window" (seeing into a relationship) consists of four panels ranging from openness (both parties are aware of elements in this box) to hidden (the individual does not share this) to blind (others know but the individual does not) to unknown (neither party has insight into these elements).

	Known to self	Not known to self
Known to others	Open	Blind
Not known to others	Hidden	Unknown

Luft, J. (1969). *Of human interaction*. Palo Alto, CA: National Press.

JOINT VENTURE

Joint ventures may occur between similar organizations to enhance an existing service or between dissimilar organizations with common goals to create or enhance a service.

JUST-IN-TIME

Just as this terms sounds, this is an approach to ensuring that money is not tied up in excessive inventories. The idea is that the supplier assumes the burden of producing the needed quantities just in time for their use. It also refers to services—they emerge as needed.

KAIZEN

This is the Japanese term for continual improvement.

KOUZES AND POSNER

James Kouzes and Barry Posner are best known for their work that culminates in *The Leadership Challenge.* This is a practical guide for leaders at all levels of an organization, and their beliefs of the Five Practices reflect how important it is to lead people, not tasks.

The Five Practices

1. Model the way.
2. Inspire a shared vision.
3. Challenge the process.
4. Enable others to act.
5. Encourage the heart.

Kouzes, J. M., & Posner, B. Z. (2002). *The leadership challenge.* San Francisco: Jossey Bass.

LAISSEZ-FAIRE LEADERSHIP STYLE

See Leadership Styles.

LEADER-MEMBER EXCHANGE THEORY

The main focus of this theory is that the interaction between the manager and the worker creates the way in which further interaction occurs. Unlike approaches that are geared to groups, this theory is about the individuals as individuals or dyads. The idea of in-groups suggested those dyads with positive relationships were based on being in relationship with another person. The idea of out-groups suggested those dyads with formal relationships were based on the need for communication rather than on relationships.

Dansereau, F., Graen, G. G., & Haga, W. (1975). A vertical dyad linkage approach to leadership in formal organizations. *Organizational Behavior and Human Performance, 13,* 46-78.

LEADERSHIP STYLES

The three traditional leadership styles are seen as autocratic, democratic, and laissez-faire. Each has advantages and disadvantages, and each has application in some situations. Autocratic refers to the take-charge style. Little, if any, input is sought. The autocratic leader makes pronouncements about what will be. Democratic styles seek considerable input and may even look weak. This style supports independence of workers and consensus building. Laissez-faire can best be described as uninvolved and indecisive. This is a hands-off style. Although this style may seem unacceptable, it is useful in some situations in which the outcome is inconsequential. *See also Situational, Leadership, Transactional Leadership, and Transformational Leadership.*

LEADERSHIP VERSUS MANAGEMENT

Although these terms have been used interchangeably, they are different. The key difference has to do with focus, position, and outcomes. Frequently, the difference is described with the statement of doing the right thing (leadership) versus doing things right (management). The key is that neither can exist in isolation of the other.

Aspect	Leadership	Management
Focus—time	Future	Present
Focus—work	Change	Compliance
Focus—questions	What does this mean?	Who can do this better? How can we do it better?
Position	Leadership (official or nonofficial position)	Headship (official position)
Outcomes	Improvement	Compliance

LEARNING ORGANIZATIONS

This concept refers to the fact that organizations must learn constantly if they plan to survive. Organizations that do not learn are not merely maintaining status quo, they are falling behind. This term refers to individual development and accumulated organizational knowledge.

Senge, P. (1990). *The fifth discipline: The art and practice of the learning organization.* New York: Doubleday.

LEVERAGED BUYOUT

This is one form in which two organizations unite. It is the purchase of the controlling interest of an organization using debt collateralization to fund most of the purchase price.

LEWIN'S FIELD THEORY

See Force Field Theory.

LIKERT

Although Likert had numerous ideas about management and defined four distinct systems, he is best known for the scale he originated. A Likert scale consists of a range of values showing dichotomies. The scale frequently is a five-point scale, ranging from strongly agree to strongly disagree.

www.socialresearchmethods.net/kb/scallik.htm

LIQUIDITY

This accounting term refers to the ability of the current assets to meet the current liabilities.

LOSS LEADER

This marketing term refers to assigning a low price on selected goods or services to attract clients. This may be used in healthcare to undercost (charge less than cost) a service to a targeted group of patients so that they develop organizational loyalty and choose that organization for a service that produces a high payoff.

MANAGEMENT BY OBJECTIVES

Although Drucker is known for many managerial concepts, one of the key ones is management by objectives. The idea is that the objectives are mutually agreed to by the individual and the manager, and the work is evaluated based on progress toward or attainment of objectives.

MARKET EXPANSION

Market expansion occurs in one of four ways. It is a result of the intersection of products and markets and whether they are new or current. The result is, for example, if the current products and current markets intersect, penetration is the approach to use. If, on the other hand, an organization is creating new products and new markets, diversification is needed.

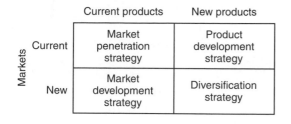

MARKET SEGMENTATION

Segmenting a market is designed to take a larger group and narrow it into a more homogenous group. The idea is that then targeted marketing for this smaller group will produce better results than more generalized marketing.

MARKET SHARE

Share is usually expressed in dollars or percent of a client population, and it refers to the portion of a given market (e.g., all patients, all coronary artery bypass patients) targeted by an organization.

MASLOW'S HIERARCHY OF NEEDS

For decades, nursing students and others have learned the pyramid of ascending human needs. The basis of the theory is that the lower-level needs must be met before higher-level needs are met. The basic five levels, in *ascending order*, are basic physiologic needs, safety and security needs, social and belonging needs, esteem needs, and self-actualization needs. (See table at top right.)

MATRIX STRUCTURE

This is a formal organizational structure that involves dual authority, typically service and discipline. For example, a nursing manager of the emergency department may report to the CNO and the emergency room medical director.

MASLOW'S HIERARCHY OF NEEDS

Need	Examples
Self-actualization	Absolute security in oneself, feelings of mastery, major accomplishments, self-growth
Esteem	Competence, achievement, prestige, respect, praise, and recognition
Social and belonging (love)	Affiliation with others, acceptance in a group, recognition, friendship and value of/by co-workers
Safety and security	Stable environment, freedom from worry about personal and professional safety
Physiologic	Water, air, food, shelter, exercise, elimination

Maslow, A. H. (1954). *Motivation and personality.* New York: Harper & Row.

McGREGOR

Douglas McGregor proposed Theory X and Theory Y in the early 1960s. He was a social psychologist interested in people's motivation.
See Theory X/Theory Y.

MINIMAX/MAXIMAX

This strategy is designed to construct a payoff table to identify options from various strategies. Minimax represents the conservative approach (maximizing the minimum payoffs); Maximax represents the optimistic approach (maximizing the maximum payoffs). To reach a decision using this strategy, the following information is needed: the options, costs, and capacity for each and then a stated, desired payoff with the probability that the payoff will be reached. Each maximum payoff, from a conservative and optimist perspective, is then the two best choices depending on the perspective selected.

MOTIVATION-HYGIENE THEORY

The idea of this theory is that these factors are not a continuum; the addition of more motivation factors does not eliminate the need for basic maintenance factors. Motivators, or satisfiers, consist of factors such as positive feedback, the opportunity to develop new skills, and the potential to work at higher levels of performance. Maintainers, or dissatisfiers or hygiene, consist of such factors as pay, benefits, job security, and supervision. Workers need to feel they are being paid well, but adding more money in the absence of motivators will not make someone feel satisfied at work.

Hertzberg, F. (1968). One more time: How do you motivate employees? *Harvard Business Review, 46,* 53-62.

MYERS-BRIGGS TYPE INDICATOR

This personality test is used widely in numerous disciplines, including those found in healthcare. It is designed to indicate how people behave in various situations. Such tools as the Myers- Briggs are used to determine the best fit of employees' skills to available jobs. This test can be used to capitalize their strengths in group work.

http://www.myersbriggs.org

NEGOTIATION

Principles

- Separate the people from the problem.
- Focus on interests, not positions.
- Invent options for mutual gains.
- Insist on objective criteria.

Fisher, R., & Wry, W. (1981) *Getting to yes.* New York: Houghton Mifflin.

Tactics

The following list represents some of the most commonly used strategies in any negotiation situation.

Best and Final: This offer is usually not offered early in the process. This is the "bottom, bottom line" and thus terminates further negotiation.

Devil's Advocate: Saying, "To play the devil's advocate…" allows for challenging the opponent's viewpoint indirectly. It also allows for pointing out the potential down sides of the proposed solution.

Divide and Conquer: This approach involves separating one person or small group from the larger group and using him/her/them to gain your objective.

Emotional Intensity: Ratcheting up the message with emotional overtones and behaviors intensifies the message.

Left-Fielders: Sudden and unexpected shifts in tactics are designed to keep opponents from predicting your strategy.

Limited Authority: References are made about needing to check with someone else, thus allowing time for rethinking and for good faith bargaining.

Outwait: Remaining silent rather than commenting usually creates a need to talk for the other person. Not being eager to settle a disagreement creates a desire of the other person to reach a settlement.

Poker Face: The negotiator provides no feedback to proposals or statements and therefore does not reveal information or his/her position.

Referent Power: The negotiator aligns with a powerful person, dropping that person's name at appropriate times. This "powerful person" may be seen as the person to be brought in if agreement is not reached now or as someone who will be disappointed in the outcome if expectations are not met.

Split the Difference: This statement is usually said by the party with the least to lose. It is designed to get to a quick decision.

Timing: Timing refers to stalling for time to wait for messages to be clear or for some new development. An example is meeting until late hours with the intent that people will finally agree to something just to be able to leave the situation.

Trial Balloon: A statement designed to assess the reaction to an idea without its being a formal proposal is a trial balloon.

Whipsaw/Auction: Negotiating with several competitors increases the tension of how each competitor can best meet the proposer's needs.

NICHE MARKETING

This term refers to focusing on a special segment of a market to develop a specialty service for that segment.

NOMINAL GROUP TECHNIQUE

This process is designed to neutralize political statements and dominating speakers to obtain multiple ideas. The process is highly structured.

1. Leader prepares a formal statement of a problem/issue after defining the process to be used. (Note: The more narrowly defined the statement, the more likely is having a higher-quality result.)
2. Members write ideas on paper without any interaction (about 5 to 10 minutes).
3. Members read ideas one at a time, in turn and without discussion, until no additional ideas are offered.
4. Leader writes each idea on chalkboard or flip chart, keeping idea and number visible throughout this phase.
5. Leader opens discussion of each idea to clarify all and define assumptions related to the ideas. (Note that this should be open discussion to seek clarification not to create pro and con camps for the idea.)
6. Members vote for their top five (or so) favorites by recording the number from the list of ideas on an individual file card (1 is high, 5 is low).
7. Leader tallies the votes and summarizes results.
8. Leader clarifies any ties to determine if on another vote a clear priority can be described.

Debecq, A. L. , & Van de Ven, A. H. (1971). A group process model for problem identification and program planning. *Journal of Applied Behavioral Science, 7,* 466-492.

OPINION LEADERS

These leaders are frequently influential community citizens with a major believability with the group they influence. They are seen as shaping others' opinions.

OPPORTUNITY COST

This cost refers to what was sacrificed or lost because one selection was made over another. In other words, we typically sacrifice one opportunity to pursue another.

ORGANIZATIONAL POLITICS

This term refers to the influence within an organization that is evident in how things get done. This may encompass spreading rumors, exchanging favors, or favoring one person over another.

OVERHEAD

See Indirect Cost.

PARETO PRINCIPLE

The Pareto (Pah-RET-toe) Principle has been used to illustrate numerous outcomes in various aspects of working with people. In general, the principle means that 80% of the outcomes derive from 20% of the efforts. For example, this could mean that 20% of the customers account for 80% of sales; 20% of workers account for 80% of the results; or 20% of the people in a group create 80% of the group's problems.

Koch, R. (1998). *The 80/20 principle: The secret to success by achieving more with less.* New York: Doubleday.

PATH-GOAL THEORY

The key role of the manager in the path-goal theoretic perspective is to facilitate the employees' attainment of their goals. The manager therefore manages the environment and the process in the workplace that interferes with goal attainment. "Clearing the path" is the key activity.

Evans, M. G. (1996). R.J. House's "A path-goal theory of leader effectiveness." *Leadership Quarterly, 7,* 305-309.

PEARSON'S FIVE STRATEGIES FOR INNOVATION

1. Commit to the right mind-set. (commitment to change)
2. Unsettle the organization. (task forces, spinoffs, out-of-the-box thinking, and action)
3. Focus and strategize. (being focused)
4. Analyze the current. (knowing the business)
5. Persist! (choosing a few strategies and focusing on them)

Pearson, A. E. (1988, May-June). Tough-minded ways to get innovative. *Harvard Business Review, 66,* 99-106.

PERT

Program evaluation and review technique (PERT) refers to a scheduling and control plan, usually represented as a chart, to ensure that elements of a project are achieved in a timely manner.

PETERS

Tom Peters is one of the most prolific, contemporary authors in management. He is most known for his work on excellence and chaos in organizations. Two key themes associated with Peters are being close to customers and having a passion for what you do.

Peters, T., & Waterman, R. H. (1982). *In search of excellence.* New York: Harper & Row.
Peters, T. (1987). *Thriving on chaos.* New York: Harper & Row.

PSYCHODYNAMIC APPROACH

This approach to leadership suggests that the key is to have self-insight and also interpret others' responses based on knowledge of self. In other words, this approach would seem to reflect the concept of emotional intelligence. Thus it does not matter what traits the leader has so long as the leader understands that basis for leadership approaches. In general, to be effective, it is equally important for followers to have insight into their own approaches. An assumption of this approach is that characteristics are fairly well formed by the time someone becomes employed and then assumes a leadership position.

Zaleznik, A. (1977, May-June). Managers and leaders: Are they different? *Harvard Business Review, 55,* 67-68.

PUSH-PULL STRATEGY

These two strategies are marketing approaches. The push strategy is focused directly on the customers (think of the television ads for various medications) versus the pull strategy, which is focused on the "distribution channels" (frequently the physicians) to have them promote the product.

QUALIFIED OPINION

This accounting terms means that the auditor has found that not all elements are in compliance with accepted accounting principles. Varying degrees of issues of noncompliance exist. This standard derives from generally accepted accounting principles.

ROLLOUT MARKET

This is a strategy for introducing a new product or service. It refers to the launch period and allows for spreading the cost over a period of time.

SENGE

Peter Senge (pronounced "sen-gay") was the first person attributed with designating the concept of the whole organization learning.
See Learning Organizations.

SERVANT LEADERSHIP

See Covey; Greenleaf's Servant Leadership.

SITUATIONAL LEADERSHIP

See Hersey and Blanchard.
　　The axes of situational leadership are focused on relationship and task. The range of options can extend from low on both axes to high on both. The maturity of the worker is represented under the horizontal axis with movement from high to low on that element.

Hersey, P., & Blanchard, K. (1969). *Management of organizational behavior: Utilizing human resources.* Parmus, NJ: Prentice Hall.

SLIP TECHNIQUE

The slip technique is a strategy for obtaining ideas from a large group without influence of other participants. Slips of paper (thus the name for this strategy) or index cards are distributed to each participant. Allowing 20 to 30 cards per participant and about 5 to 10 minutes is usually sufficient. Propose the topic/issue/problem and ask all to write down one idea on each of the slips of paper. One person (the group leader or a designated assistant) or a small group then collects all slips and categorizes them. The categorized ideas can then be used to form topics of discussion to address the original topic/issue/problem. This discussion can be held immediately or at a subsequent point of discussion.

Hospital Research and Educational Trust. (1970). *Training and continuing education.* Chicago: The Trust.

SPINOFFS

A spinoff is a formal process of divesting one organization of a service or product so that it becomes a free-standing but related entity. The parent company retains overall control, and the organization that was spun off has various tax and liability advantages while still being affiliated with the parent organization.

SWOT

SWOT is the acronym for strengths, weaknesses, opportunities, and threats: the key elements in the strategic planning process. This set of words is designed to provide a comprehensive approach to strategic planning. The use of threats, opportunities, weaknesses, and strengths (TOWS) is designed to convert the less desirable elements (threats and weaknesses) into the more positive ones (opportunities and strengths). The point of this second component is to determine what strategic decisions could be made to enhance positive outcomes.

TAYLOR'S TIME AND MOTION

The father of scientific management, Taylor focused on time and motion studies to create greater efficiency. His focus was on management's accountability for planning. Everything was standardized, and workers were specifically selected for specific work.

Taylor, F. W. (1911). *The principles of scientific management*. New York: Harper & Brothers.

THEORY X/THEORY Y

This theory focuses on the motivation of people. X suggests that people have to be forced to work, that it is the manager's job to make the worker work. Theory Y, on the other hand, suggests that work is intrinsic and people want support from the manager to accomplish the work. That people shun responsibility, are motivated by money, and lack the desire to improve are typical thoughts associated with Theory X. Theory Y suggests that people enjoy responsibility; that they are motivated by acceptance; and that although they need money, they want more than that from a position, including the improvement of quality within the organization (see table on p. 481).

THEORY Z

Several names have been associated with this theory about Japanese participative management. Small units are composed of life-long workers who work within the unit. The benefit to the group is stressed; collective decisions are made and cooperation is a highlight of these units. They focus on quality circles to improve what they do and are focused on the future. This theory suggests that workers are highly committed to their work and the improvement of it.

Ouchi, W. G. (1981). *How American business can meet the Japanese challenge*. Reading, MA: Addison-Wesley.

TICHY

Noel Tichy, a professor of organizational behavior and human resource management at the University of Michigan, has focused considerable research on the context of winners and losers. His emphasis has been on a teachable point of view, a story, and specific coaching strategies. His work underpins the ideas of succession planning.

TIPPING POINT

The three characteristics of dramatic changes are contagiousness (others buy in), little causes can have big effects (it is easy to make the first step toward change), and change happens at one dramatic moment (when the timing is right). Although the tipping point can be negative or positive, from a leadership perspective, the focus is on creating the positive elements to interact to energize the group to move to even higher levels of accomplishments.

Gladwell, M. (2000). *The tipping point: How little things can make a big difference*. Boston: Little, Brown & Company.

TOWS

See SWOT.

TRANSACTIONAL LEADERSHIP

Transactional leadership suggests that the manager focuses on the transaction of work. The manager sets goals and provides rewards for attainment of those goals. The focus is on daily work and is fairly focused on tasks and hierarchy. The ongoing monitoring of what is happening is designed to allow for interventions on a management-by-exception approach.

Burns, J. M. (1978). *Leadership*. New York: Harper & Row.

COMPARISON OF THEORY X AND THEORY Y

X	Y
Workers hate work.	Work is natural.
The manager's job is to make the worker work.	The manager's job is to create the climate in which work is accomplished.
Workers need considerable guidance.	Workers are self-directed.
Workers avoid responsibility.	Workers enjoy responsibility.
Money is the motivator.	Money is one of many factors.
Workers lack interest in improving quality.	Workers want to improve quality.

McGregor, D. M. (1960). *The human side of enterprise.* New York: Harper & Row.

TRANSFORMATIONAL LEADERSHIP

Transformational leadership is focused on charisma, inspiration, relationships, and knowledge. The focus of the manager is longer term in the sense that development of employees is key. It is process oriented and is driven by the needs of the workers. The manager focuses on creating the vision and supporting movement toward that vision. Encouragement strategies and creating influence are important elements.

Bass, B. (1998). *Transformational leadership: Industry, military, and educational impact.* Mahwah, NJ: Lawrence Erlbaum Associates.

TWO FACTOR THEORY

See Herzberg's Motivation-Hygiene Theory.

VROOM'S EXPECTANCY THEORY

See Expectancy Theory.

VROOM-YETTON DECISION STRATEGY TREE

This research-based strategy is used to define the level of staff involvement, for example, to determine if a decision should be delegated or to call a meeting. The goal is to create a fast and easy decision-making approach. Seven key areas for consideration form the yes-no flow to reach a conclusion (one of five strategies).

Nature of Decision (answered with yes/no options)
1. Quality importance.
2. Manager expertise and information.
3. Type of problem: structured or ambiguous.
4. Importance of acceptance.
5. Acceptance of autocratic decision by employees.
6. Shared goals of organization (manager and employees).
7. Likeliness of conflict.

Decision Strategy Options
1. Manager makes decision alone.
2. Manager requests information and then makes decision alone.
3. Manager requests information and opinions in one-on-one meetings but makes decision alone.
4. Manager holds group meeting to discuss problem and then makes decision alone.
5. Manager holds group meeting to discuss problem, and group makes decision.

Vroom, V. H., & Yetton, P. W. (1973). *Leadership and decision-making.* Pittsburg: University of Pittsburg Press.

WORK IN PROCESS

This term refers to any partially completed effort. It also can convey the complexity of a process, or it can be a delaying tactic because some processes continue to evolve.

WRITE-OFF

This accounting term refers to acknowledging an asset is not going to be recouped. It may be designated as an expense or as a loss.

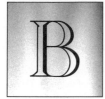

Additional References

BALDRIGE

The Malcolm Baldrige National Quality Award. Retrieved February 23, 2005, from http://www.cmwf.org/publications/publications_show.htm?doc_id=261096.

Case study: Using Baldrige criteria to achieve performance excellence at the Robert Wood Johnson University Hospital Hamilton. Retrieved February 23, 2005, from http://www.cmwf.org/publications/publications_show.htm?doc_id=261096.

BEST PRACTICES AND EVIDENCE-BASED PRACTICE

Dykes, P. C. (2003). Practice guidelines and measurement: State-of-the-science. *Nursing Outlook, 51*, 65-69.

Koloroutis, M., & Moe, J. K. (2000). Assessment: The first step in creating a more integrated system-wide approach to nursing practice. *The Journal of Nursing Administration, 30*(2), 97-103.

CARING

Authier, P. (2004). Being present—The choice that reinstills caring. *Nursing Administration Quarterly, 28*(4), 276-279.

Knapp, B. (2004). Competency: An essential component of caring in nursing. *Nursing Administration Quarterly, 28*(4), 285-287.

COACHING

Berglas, S. (2002, June). The very real dangers of executive coaching. *Harvard Business Review, 80*(6), 86-92, 153.

Goldsmith, M., Lyons, L., & Freas, A. (2000). *Coaching for leadership: How the world's greatest coaches help leaders learn.* San Francisco: Jossey-Bass/Pfeiffer.

Ludeman, K., & Erlandson, E. (2004). Coaching the alpha male. *Harvard Business Review, 82*(5), 58-68.

Porche, G., & Niederer, J. (2001). *Coach anyone about anything: How to help people succeed in business and life.* Del Mar, CA: Wharton.

Stern, L. (2004). Executive coaching: A working definition. *Consulting Psychology Journal: Practice and Research, 56*(3), 154-162.

von Hoffman, C. (1999). *Coaching: The ten killer myths.* Harvard Management Update. Boston: Harvard Business School.

Wales, S. (2003). Why coaching? *Journal of Change Management, 3*(3), 275-282.

COMMUNICATION

Clark, E. (2004). *Around the corporate campfire: How great leaders use stories to inspire success.* Sevierville, TN: Insight.

Patterson, K., Grenny, J., McMillan, R., & Switzler, A. (2002). *Crucial conversations: Tools for talking when stakes are high.* New York: McGraw-Hill.

CONFLICT AND NEGOTIATIONS

Camp, J. (2002). *Start with no.* New York: Crown Business.

Cleary, T. (1988). *The art of war.* (Translation by Sun Tzu). Boston: Shambhala.

Fisher, R., & Ury, W. (1991). *Getting to yes: Negotiating agreement without giving in* (2nd ed.). New York: Penguin Books.

Heim, P., & Murphy, S. (2001). *In the company of women: Turning workplace conflict into powerful alliances.* New York: Tarcher/Putnam.

Kritek, P. B. (2002). *Negotiating at an uneven table: Developing moral courage in resolving our conflicts* (2nd ed.). San Francisco: Jossey-Bass.

Patterson, K., Grenny, J., McMillan, R., & Switzler, A. (2002). *Crucial conversations: Tools for talking when stakes are high.* New York: McGraw-Hill.

CULTURE AND DIVERSITY

Crowell, D. M. (2005, Winter). Transforming the work environment of nurses. *ANA-Maine Journal,* 6-7.

Earley, P., & Mosakowski, E. (2004). Cultural intelligence. *Harvard Business Review, 82*(10), 139-147.

Georges, C. A. (2004). African American nurse leadership: Pathways and opportunities. *Nursing Administration Quarterly, 28*(3), 170-172.

Lee, F. (2004). *If Disney ran your hospital: 9 ½ things you would do differently.* Bozeman, MT: Second River Healthcare.

Swanson, J. W. (2004). Diversity: Creating an environment of inclusiveness. *Nursing Administration Quarterly, 28*(3), 207-211.

Villarruel, A. M., & Peragallo, N. (2004). Leadership development of Hispanic nurses. *Nursing Administration Quarterly, 28*(3), 173-180.

Washington, D., Erickson, J. I., & Ditomassi, M. (2004). Mentoring the minority nurse leader of tomorrow. *Nursing Administration Quarterly, 28*(3), 165-169.

FINANCES

Chang, C. F., Price, S. A., & Pfoutz, S. K. (2001). *Economics and nursing: Critical professional issues.* Philadelphia: F. A. Davis.

Dunham-Taylor, J., & Pinczuk, J. Z. (2006). *Health care financial management for nurse managers: Merging the heart with the dollar.* Sudbury, MA: Jones and Bartlett.

Finkler, S. A., & Kovner, C. T. (2000). *Financial management for nurse managers and executives* (2nd ed.). Philadelphia: W.B. Saunders.

Kritek, P. B. (2002). *Negotiating at an uneven table* (2nd ed.). San Francisco: Jossey-Bass.

Marriner Tomey, A. (2004). *Guide to nursing management and leadership* (7th ed.). St. Louis: Mosby.

Murray, M. E., Brennan, S. F., & Moore, S. M. (2003). A model of economic analysis. *Nursing Economics, 21*, 280-287.

Pfoutz, S. K., Price, S. A., & Chang, C. F. (2002). Health economics. In D. J. Mason, J. K. Leavitt, & M. W. Chaffee (Eds.), *Policy & politics in nursing and health care* (4th ed., pp. 229-239). St. Louis: W.B. Saunders.

Serb, C. (2003, January). Medicare+Choice: Health plans flee, enrollment drops. What went wrong? Can we fix it? *Hospitals and Healthcare Networks*, pp. 42-44.

Thrall, T. H., & Scalise, D. (2002, November). America's uninsured. *Hospitals and Healthcare Networks*, pp. 30-32, 34, 36, 38, 40.

Van Slyck, A. (2000). Patient classification systems: Not a proxy for nurse "busyness." *Nursing Administration Quarterly, 24*(4), 60-65.

Whetsell, G. W. (1999). The history and evolution of hospital payment systems: How did we get here? *Nursing Administration Quarterly, 23*(4), 1-15.

FORECASTING

Center for the Health Professions. Centering on... It's the practice model, stupid. Retrieved March 2, 2004, from http//futurehealth.ucsf.edu/from_the_director_0304.html.

Christman, L. P. (2000). Management adjustment: A glimpse into the future structure of care. *Nursing Administration Quarterly, 25*(1), 14-17.

Drenkard, K. N. (2001). Creating a future worth experiencing, *Journal of Nursing Administration, 31*(7/8), 364-376.

Ellis, D. (2004, August). What if... (The consequences of innovation). *Hospitals & Health Networks*, 38-42.

Forecasts for Management Decision Making (2003, November 26). *Kiplinger Letter,* Washington, DC: The Kiplinger Washington Editors.

Grossman, S., & Valiga, T. M. (2000). *The new leadership challenge: Creating the future of nursing.* Philadelphia: F.A. Davis.

Hill, S. (2002). *60 Trends in 60 minutes.* Hoboken, NJ: John Wiley & Sons, Inc.

Holmes, W. (2004, September-October). Our microtech future. *The Futurist*, 51-56.

Institute of Medicine. (2000). *Informing the future: Critical issues in health.* Washington, DC: The Institute.

Irvin, II, N. (2004, March/April). The arrival of the thrivals. *The Futurist*, 16-23.

Kiplinger Letter. (2003). *What's ahead for 2004 and what you can do about it.* Washington, DC: Kiplinger Publications.

Laermer, R. (2002). *Trend spotting.* New York: The Berkley Publishing Group.

Lancaster, L. C., & Stillman, D. (2002). *When generations collide: Who they are, why they clash: How to solve the generational puzzle at work.* New York: Harper Books.

Mastorvich, M. J., & Drenkard, K. N. (2000). Nursing future search: Building a community of nurses in an integrated healthcare system. *Journal of Nursing Administration, 30*(4), 173-179.

McClure, M. L. (2000). A look back and a look ahead. *Nursing Administration Quarterly, 25*(1), 107-114.

Rosenhead, J. *Complexity theory and management practice.* Retrieved July 6, 2004, from http://human-nature.com/science-as-culture/rosenhead.html.

Roy, C. (2000). A theorist envisions the future and speaks to nursing administrators. *Nursing Administration Quarterly, 24*(2), 1-12.

Roy, C. (2000). The visible and invisible fields that shape the future of the nursing care system. *Nursing Administration Quarterly, 25*(1), 119-131.

Shorr, A. S. (2000). Has nursing lost its professional focus? *Nursing Administration Quarterly, 25*(1), 89-94.

Stedron, B. (2004, March/April). Forecasts for artificial intelligence. *The Futurist*, 24-25.

Strauss, W., & Howe, N. (2000). *Millennials rising: The next great generation.* New York: Vintage Books.

Wacker, W., & Taylor, J. (2000). *The visionary's handbook: Nine paradoxes that will shape the future of your business.* New York: HarperBusiness.

FOREIGN-EDUCATED NURSES

Gerrish, K., Griffith, V. (2004). Integration of overseas registered nurses: Evaluation of an adaptation programme. *Journal of Advanced Nursing, 45*(6), 579-587.

Simpson, R. (2004). Recruit, retain, assess: Technology's role in diversity. *Nursing Administration Quarterly, 28*(3), 217-220.

GOVERNANCE

Conduff, M. A. (2000). Sustaining policy governance. *Board Leadership, 51,* 1-2, 7.

Genovich-Richards, J., Gorenberg, B., & Deremo, D. E. (2000). The role of governance in improving clinical outcomes: Opportunities for nurses. *Nursing Administration Quarterly, 24*(2), 62-71.

Ingram, R. T. (n.d.) *Ten basic responsiblities of nonprofit boards.* Washington, DC: National Center for Nonprofit Boards.

Matisoff-Li, A. (2004, April). Chief nursing officers: A seat at the table. *HealthLeaders,* 36-44.

Nadler, D. A. (2004, May). Building better boards. *Harvard Business Review,* 102-111.

KNOWING YOURSELF

Bunker, K., Kram, K., & Ting, S. (2002). The young and the clueless. *Harvard Business Review, 80*(12), 80-88.

Cialdini, R. (2001). *Influence: science and practice* (4th ed.). Boston: Allyn and Bacon.

Cummings, G., Hayduk, L., & Estabrooks, C. (2005). Mitigating the impact of hospital restructuring on nurses: The responsibility of emotionally intelligent leadership. *Nursing Research, 54*(1), 2-12.

Denning, S. (2004). Telling tales. *Harvard Business Review 82*(5), 122-128.

Evans, R., & Reiser, D. (2004). Role transitions for clinical leaders in perinatal practice. *Journal of Obstetric, Gynecologic, and Neonatal Nursing, 33*(3), 355-361.

Galford, R., & Drapeau, A. (2003). The enemies of trust. *Harvard Business Review, 81*(2), 88-96.

Garvin, D., & Roberto, M. (2005). Change through persuasion. *Harvard Management Update.* Boston: Harvard Business School.

Ghiselin, B. (1987, Fall). Images. *Issues and Observations, 7*(4), 8-9.

Goldsmith, B. (2002). Inside-out leadership: Learning to manage from the core. *Office Solutions, 19*(4).

Hesselbein, F., Goldsmith, M., & Bechard, R. (1997). *The organization of the future.* New York: The Peter F. Drucker Foundation for Non-Profit Management.

Mackoff, B., & Wenet, G. (2005). *Leadership as a habit of mind.* New York: Authors Choice Press.

Maxwell, J. (2001). *The right to lead: A study in character and courage.* Nashville, TN: Thomas Nelson.

Maxwell, J. (1993). *The winning attitude.* Nashville, TN: Thomas Nelson.

Moss, M. (2005). The emotionally intelligent nurse leader. San Francisco: Jossey-Bass/Wiley.

Pitman, B. (2003). Leading for value. *Harvard Business Review, 81*(4), 41-47.

Stewart, T. (2004). Winning attitudes. *Harvard Business Review, 82*(4), 10.

Sull, D. (2003). Managing by commitments. *Harvard Business Review, 81*(6), 82-92.

LEADERSHIP AND MANAGEMENT

Atson, R. A., & Brown, B. (2001). *The most effective organization in the U.S.: Leadership secrets of the Salvation Army.* New York: Crown Business.

Bennis, W. (2004). The seven ages of the leader. *Harvard Business Review, 82*(1), 46-53.

Buchanan, L. (2004). The things they do for love. *Harvard Business Review, 82*(12), 19-21.

Buckingham, M., & Clifton, D. O. (2001). *Now, discover your strengths.* New York: The Free Press.

Buckingham, M. (2005). *The one thing you need to know...about great managing, great leading, and sustained individual success.* New York: Free Press.

Buckingham, M. (2005). What great managers do. *Harvard Business Review, 83*(3), 70-79.

Cairo, P., Dotlich, D., & Rhinesmith, S. (2005, March). The unnatural leader. *Training and Development,* 24-41.

Connellan, T. K. (2003). *Bringing out the best in others.* Austin, TX: Bard Press.

Coutu, D. (2004). Putting leaders on the couch. *Harvard Business Review, 82*(1), 65-71.

DePree, M. (1992). *Leadership jazz.* New York: Dell Publishing.

Drucker, P. (2004). What makes an effective executive. *Harvard Business Review, 82*(60), 58-63.

Gerber, R. (2002). *Leadership the Eleanor Roosevelt way: Timeless strategies from the First Lady of courage.* New York: Prentice Hall.

Goleman, D., Boyatzis, R., & McKee, A. (2002). *Primal leadership: Realizing the power of emotional intelligence.* Boston: Harvard Business School Press.

Goleman, D. (2004). What makes a leader? *Harvard Business Review,* Best of HBR (1998), *82*(1), 82-91.

Hamel, G. (2003). The quest for resilience. *Harvard Business Review, 81*(9), 52-64.

Hintze, J. (2003). What should a leader be? *Harvard Management Update, Harvard Business School Publishing,* EBSCO publishing.

Kanter, R. (2003). Leadership and the psychology of turnarounds. *Harvard Business Review, 81*(6), 58-68.

Kanter, R. (2004). The middle manager as innovator. *Harvard Business Review, 82*(7/8), 150-161.

Kellerman, B. (2004). Leadership, warts and all. *Harvard Business Review, 82*(1), 40-45.

Kim, W. C., & Mauborgne, R. (2003, April). Tipping point leadership. *Harvard Business Review,* 60-69.

Kouzes, J. M., & Posner, B. Z. (2002). *The leadership challenge.* San Francisco: Jossey-Bass.

Lencioni, P. (2000). *The four obsessions of an extraordinary executive: A leadership fable.* San Francisco: Jossey-Bass.

Lencioni, P. (2004). *Death by meeting: A leadership fable.* San Francisco: Jossey-Bass.

Loehr, J., & Schwartz, T. (2003). *The power of full engagement: Managing energy, not time, is the key to high performance and personal renewal.* New York: Free Press.

Magee, M. (2000). *Positive leadership.* New York: Spencer Books.

Maxwell, J. C. (1999). *The 21 indisputable qualities of a leader: Becoming the person others will want to follow.* Nashville, TN: Thomas Nelson Publishers.

Maxwell, J. C. (2000). *Failing forward: Turning mistakes into stepping stones for success.* Nashville, TN: Thomas Nelson.

Maxwell, J. C. (2001). *The 17 indisputable laws of teamwork: Embrace them and empower your team.* Nashville, TN: Thomas Nelson.

Maxwell, J. C. (2003). *Thinking for a change: 11 ways highly successful people approach life and work.* New York: Warner Business Books.

Northouse, P. G. (2001). *Leadership: Theory and practice* (2nd ed.). Thousand Oaks, CA: Sage Publications.

Norwood, S. L. (2003). *Nursing consultation: A framework for working with communities* (2nd ed.). Upper Saddle River, NJ: Prentice Hall.

Offerman, L. (2004). When followers become toxic. *Harvard Business Review, 82*(1), 54-61.

Peters, T. (1987). *Thriving on chaos: Handbook for a management revolution.* New York: Harper and Row.

Porter, M., Lorsch, J., & Nohria, N. (2004). Seven surprises for new CEOs. *Harvard Business Review, 82*(10), 62-72.

Porter-O'Grady, T. (2003). A different age for leadership, part 1: New context, new content. *Journal of Nursing Administration, 33*(2), 105-110.

Porter-O'Grady, T. (2003). A different age for leadership, part 2: New rules, new roles. *Journal of Nursing Administration, 33*(3), 173-178.

Porter-O'Grady, T., & Malloch, K. (2002). *Quantum leadership: A textbook of new leadership.* Gaithersburg, MD: Aspen.

Prentice, W. (2004). Understanding leadership. *Harvard Business Review,* Best of HBR (1961) 82(1), 102-109.

Reno, K. (2005). Management skill training: The top 10 lessons learned. *Nurse Leader, 3*(2), 28-30.

Schaffer, M. (2003). Leading the way: Seeing the possibilities. *Gastroenterology Nursing, 26*(6), 269-270.

Stewart, T. (2004). The highway of the mind. *Harvard Business Review, 82*(1), 116.

Studer, Q. (2003). *Hardwiring excellence: Purpose, worthwhile work, making a difference.* Gulf Breeze, FL: Fire Starter Publishing.

Tecker, G., Eide, K. M., & Frankel, J. S. (1997). *Building knowledge-based culture: Using twenty-first century work and decision-making systems in associations.* Washington, DC: American Society of Association Executives.

Thyer, G. (2003). Dare to be different: Transformational leadership may hold the key to reducing the nursing shortage. *Nursing Management, 11*(2), 73-79.

Walker, C. (2002). Saving your rookie managers from themselves. *Harvard Business Review, 80*(4), 97-103.

Wheatley, M. J. (1999). *Leadership and the new science: Discovering order in a chaotic world.* San Francisco: Berrett-Koehler.

Zander, R. S., & Zander, B. (2000). *The art of possibility: Transforming professional and personal life.* New York: Penguin Books.

LEARNING

Barker, A. (2004). Using online learning technology to develop nurse leaders. *Nurse Leader, 2*(5), 32-35.

Berke, W. J., & Wiseman, R. L. (2004). The e-learning answer. *Critical Care Nurse, 24*(2), 80-84.

Drenkard, K. N., & Gesh, B. (2004). Innovation in nurse executive development: Computer simulation. *Nurse Leader, 2*(5), 36-38.

MAGNET

American Association of Colleges of Nursing. (2002, September-October). The hallmarks of the professional nursing practice environment. *Journal of Professional Nursing, 18*(5), 295-304.

American Nurses Credentialing Center. (2004). *Magnet: Best practices in today's healthcare environment.* Silver Spring, MD: ANCC.

Armiger, M. (2002, March). Drawn to the Magnet series. *Nursing Management, 33*(3), 6.

Buchan, J. (2002, April 24-30). Work force. *Nursing Standard, 16*(32), 26.

Bumgarner, S. D., & Beard, Jr., E. L. (2003). The Magnet application: Pitfalls to avoid. *Journal of Nursing Administration, 33,* 603-606.

Carol, R. (2002, Spring). Career magnetism: Magnet hospitals are more than just great places for nurses to work—they're also employers with an exceptional commitment to helping minority nurses advance their careers. *Minority Nurse,* 32-28.

Dean-Barr, S. (2003, March-April). Magnet Recognition program illuminates nursing roles. *Rehabilitation Nurse, 28*(2), 38.

Dinsdale, P. (2003, January). More trusts interested in Magnet hospital scheme, *Nursing Standards, 17*(17), 9.

Frazier, S. C. (2003, September). Magnet home care agencies: A professional way to impact quality and retention. *Home Health Nurse, 21*(9), 603-610.

Gasda, K. A. (2002, October). The magnetic pull: Nursing's highest honor draws additional recipients…fourth of an ongoing series. *Nursing Management, 33*(10), 60, 62-63.

Goldsmith, J. (2003, April). Eastern European hospitals pursue Magnet status: Russian and Armenian hospitals to get help from U.S. partners. *American Journal of Nursing, 103*(4), 21.

Goldsmith, J. (2003, May). Winning and losing Magnet designation: The ANCC gets tough. *American Journal of Nursing, 103*(5), 25.

Graf, E., & Halfer, D. (2002, November-December). Creating great places for nurses to work: Magnet award for excellence in nursing services sets standards. *Chart 99*(6), 4, 6.

Havens, D. S., Labov, T. G., Faura, T., & Aiken, L. H. (2002, January-February). The clinical environment of hospital nursing (Spanish). *Enfermedades Infecciosas y Microbiologia Clinic, 12*(1), 13-21.

Kramer, M., & Schmalenberg, C. (2003). Securing "good" nurse physician relationships. *Nurse Management, 34*(7), 34-38.

Kramer, M., & Schmalenberg, C. (2003, January-February). Magnet hospital staff nurses describe clinical autonomy. *Nursing Outlook, 51*(1), 13-19.

Kramer, M., & Schmalenberg, C. (2003, June). Magnet hospital nurses describe control over nursing practice. *Western Journal of Nursing Research (West) 25*(4), 434-452.

Laschinger, H K., Almost, J., Tuer-Hodes, D. (2003, July/August). Workplace empowerment and Magnet hospital characteristics. *Journal of Nursing Administration, 33*(7/8), 410-422.

Monarch, K. (2003, January). Making informed employment decisions: Questions to ask and issues to consider. *American Journal of Nursing* (Part 2): (Career Guide 2003), 29-32, 38-39.

Mueller, C. (2002). Demonstrating excellence, attaining Magnet status. *Creative Nurse, 8*(2), 7-8.

Pinkerton, S. (2002, September-October). Retention and recruitment. Payoffs from investments: Improving, transforming and building skills. *Nursing Economics, 20*(5), 244, 248.

Porter-O'Grady, T. (2002, January). Let nurses play governance role...your piece on the nursing shortage. *Modern Healthcare, 32*(2), 21.

Smith, A. P. (2003, May-June). Magnet and Baldrige: SSM Health Care's journey for excellence (part II of II). *Nursing Economics, 21*(3), 127-129.

Stechmiller, J. K. (2002, November). The nursing shortage in acute and critical care settings. *AACN Clinical Issues Advance Practice Acute Critical Care, 13*(4), 577-558.

Stolzenberger, M. (2003, October). Beyond the Magnet award. *Journal of Nursing Administration, 33*(10), 522-531.

Taylor, N. T. (2003, October). The magnetic pull. *Nurse Management, 34*(10), 63-64, 66, 68, 70, 72-73.

Taylor, N. T. (2004, April). The Magnetic pull. *Nursing Management, 34*(4), 59-64.

Thompson, E. (2002-2003, December-January). Becoming a Magnet Hospital. *Kai Tiaki Nurse New Zealand, 8*(11), 13.

Upenieks, V. (2003, January-February). Recruitment and retention strategies: A Magnet hospital prevention model. *Nursing Economics, 21*(1), 7-13, 23.

Upenieks, V. (2003, February). What's the attraction to Magnet hospitals? *Nurse Management, 34*(2 part 1), 43-44.

Upenieks, V. (2003, April-June). The Interrelationship of organizational characteristics of Magnet hospitals, nursing leadership, and nursing job satisfaction. *Health Care Manager, 22*(2), 83-98.

Upenieks, V. (2003, April-June). Nurse leaders' perceptions of what compromises successful leadership in today's acute inpatient environment. *Nurse Administrator Quarterly, 27*(2), 140-152.

Upenieks, V. V. (2003). What constitutes effective leadership? Perceptions of Magnet and non Magnet nurse leaders. *Journal of Nursing Administration, 33*(9), 456-467.

MARKETING

Cialdini, R. B. (2001). *Influence: Science and practice* (4th ed.). Boston: Allyn and Bacon.

Herzlinger, R. E. (2002, July). Let's put consumers in charge of health care. *Harvard Business Review*, 44-55.

Nash, M., & Gremillion, C. (2004). Globalization impacts the healthcare organization of the 21st century: Demanding new ways to market product lines successfully. *Nursing Administration Quarterly, 28*(2), 86-91.

Reinartz, W., & Kumar, V. (2002, July). The mismanagement of customer loyalty. *Harvard Business Review*, 86-94.

Rust, R. T., Zeithaml, V. A., & Lemon, K. N. (2004, September). Customer-centered brand management. *Harvard Business Review*, 110-118.

Smith, A. P. (2003). Market power: An interview with Miles Snowden of Delta Air Lines and the Leapfrog Group. *Nursing Economics, 21*(1), 20-23.

Stokamer, C. L. (2003). Pharmaceutical gift giving: Analysis of an ethical dilemma. *Journal of Nursing Administration, 33*(1), 48-51.

Vollman, K. M. (2004). Nurse entrepreneurship: Taking an invention from birth to the marketplace. *Clinical Nurse Specialist, 18*(2), 68-71.

Woods, D. K. (2002). Realizing your marketing influence, Part 1: Meeting patient needs through collaboration. *Journal of Nursing Administration, 32*, 189-195.

Woods, D. K. (2002). Realizing your marketing influence, Part 3: Professional certification as a marketing tool. *Journal of Nursing Administration, 32*, 379-386.

Woods, D. K., & Cardin, S. (2002). Realizing your marketing influence, Part 2: Marketing from the inside out. *Journal of Nursing Administration, 32*, 323-330.

NANDA, NIC, AND NOC

Dochterman, J. M., & Jones, D. A. (Eds.). (2003). *Unifying nursing languages: The harmonization of NANDA, NIC, and NOC.* Washington, DC: The American Nurses Association.

NETWORKING

LaCoursiere, S. P. (2001). A theory of online support. *Advances in Nursing Science, 24*(1), 60-77.

Restifo, V. (2002). *Networking for career advancement*. King of Prussia, PA: Nursing Spectrum.

ORGANIZATIONS

Ponte, P. R. (2004). The American health care system at a crossroads: an overview of the American Organization of Nurse Executives. *Online Journal of Issues in Nursing*. Retrieved on June 13, 2004, from http://www.nursing-world.org/ojin.

Thorman, K. (2003). Nursing leadership in the boardroom. *Journal of Obstetric, Gynecologic, and Neonatal Nursing, 33*(3), 381-387.

QUALITY

Gillem, T. R. (1988). Deming's 14 points and hospital quality: Responding to the consumer's demand for the best value health care. *Journal of Nursing Quality Assurance, 2*(3), 70-78.

Pui-Mun, L. (2002). Sustaining business excellence through a framework of best practices in TQM. *The TQM Magazine, 14*, 3.

Rantz, M., Bostick, J., & Riggs, C. J. (2002). *Nursing quality measurement: A review of nursing studies. 1995-2000.* Washington, DC: The American Nurses Association.

RELATIONSHIPS

Koloroutis, M. (2004). *Relationship-based care: A model for transforming practice.* Minneapolis, MN: Creative Health Care Management.

Yager, J. (2004). *Who's that sitting at my desk?* Stamford, CT: Hannacroix Creek.

SUCCESSION PLANNING

Charan, R. (2005). Ending the CEO succession crisis. *Harvard Business Review, 83*(2), 72-82.

Ciampa, D. (2005). Almost ready: How leaders move up. *Harvard Business Review, 83*(1), 46-54.

Disser, A. (2002). Managing succession planning: The Inova Health System. *Seminars for Nurse Managers, 10*(4), 244-247.

Freeman, K. (2004). The CEO's real legacy. *Harvard Business Review, 82*(11), 51-58.

Griffin, N. (2003). Personalize your management development. *Harvard Business Review, 81*(3), 113-120.

Heller, B., Drenkard, K., Esposito-Herr, M., Romano, C., Tom, S., & Valentine, N. (2004). Educating nurses for leadership roles. *Journal of Continuing Education in Nursing, 35*(5), 203-210.

Kleinman, C. (2003). Leadership roles, competencies, and education: How prepared are our nurse managers? *Journal of Nursing Administration, 33*(9), 451-455.

Squires, A. (2001). Leadership development for the new manager in the small, acute care facility. *The Journal of Nursing Administration, 31*(12), 561-564.

TEAM BUILDING

Blanchard, K., & Bowles, S. (1998). *Gung Ho! Turn on the people in any organization.* New York: William Morrow, Harper Collins.

Blanchard, K., & Bowles, S. (2001). *High five! The magic of working together.* New York: William Morrow, Harper Collins.

Blanchard, K., Carew, D., & Parsi-Carew, E. (1990). *The one minute manager builds high performance teams.* New York: William Morrow, Harper Collins.

Kucera, K. (2002). Team building for case managers. *Inside Case Management, 9*(8), 9-12.

Labianca, J. (2004). The ties that blind. *Harvard Business Review, 82*(10), 19.

Majchrzak, A., Malhotra, A., Stamps, J., & Lipnack, J. (2004). Can absence make a team grow stronger? *Harvard Business Review, 82*(5), 131-138.

Roberts, L., Spreitzer, G., Dutton, J., Quinn, R., Heaphy, E., & Barker, B. (2005). How to play to your strengths. *Harvard Business Review, 83*(1), 74-82.

Triolo, P., Hanssen, P., Kazzaz, Y., Chung, H., & Dobbs, S. (2002). Improving patient satisfaction through multidisciplinary performance improvement teams. *Journal of Nursing Administration, 32*(9), 448-454.

TECHNOLOGY

American Academy of Nursing. (2003). Proceedings of the American Academy of Nursing Conference on Using Innovative Technology to Decrease Nursing Demand and Enhance Patient Care Delivery. *Nursing Outlook, 51*(3), S1-S49.

American Nurses Association. (2001). *Scope and standards of nursing informatics practice.* Washington, DC: The Author.

Androwich, I. M., Bickford, C. J., Button, P. S., Hunter, K. M., Murphy, J., & Sensmeier, J. (2003). *On clinical information systems: A framework for reaching the vision.* Washington, DC: American Medical Informatics Association/American Nurses Association.

Simpson, R. (2004). The softer side of technology: How IT helps nursing care. *Nursing Administration Quarterly, 28*(4), 302-305.

INDEX

Page numbers followed by f indicate figures, by b indicate boxes, and by t indicate tables.